PENGUIN REFERENCE

Medicines: A Guide for Everybody

Peter Parish is a Doctor of Medicine and a Professor Emeritus of the University of Wales. He has had a distinguished career and is recognized nationally and internationally for his valuable contributions to our knowledge and understanding of the prescribing and use of drugs. He is now retired.

Peter Weedle has revised and completely updated this new edition of *Medicines: A Guide for Everybody*. He is a previous research colleague of Professor Parish's, a community pharmacist and adjunct Professor of Clinical Pharmacy at University College Cork, Ireland.

D0230081

PETER PARISH & PETER WEEDLE

Medicines
A Guide for Everybody

NINTH EDITION

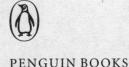

PENGUIN BOOKS

PENGUIN BOOKS

Published by the Penguin Group
Penguin Books Ltd, 80 Strand, London WC2R ORL, England
Penguin Putnam Inc., 375 Hudson Street, New York, New York 10014, USA
Penguin Books Australia Ltd, 250 Camberwell Road, Camberwell, Victoria 3124, Australia
Penguin Books Canada Ltd, 10 Alcorn Avenue, Toronto, Ontario, Canada M4V 3B2
Penguin Books India (P) Ltd, 11, Community Centre, Panchsheel Park, New Delhi – 110 017, India
Penguin Books (NZ) Ltd, Cnr Rosedale and Airborne Roads, Albany, Auckland, New Zealand
Penguin Books (South Africa) (Pty) Ltd, 24 Sturdee Avenue, Rosebank 2196, South Africa

Penguin Books Ltd, Registered Offices: 80 Strand, London WC2R ORL, England

www.penguin.com

First published 1976
Reprinted with revisions 1977
Second edition 1979
Third edition 1980
Fourth edition 1982
Fifth edition 1984
Reprinted with revisions 1987
Sixth edition 1987
Reprinted with revisions 1989
Seventh edition 1992
Eighth edition 1997
Ninth edition 2003
1

Copyright © Peter Parish, 1976, 1977, 1979, 1980, 1982, 1984, 1987, 1989, 1992, 1997
Copyright © Peter Parish & Peter Weedle, 2003

Typeset in Minion and TheSans
Typeset by Rowland Phototypesetting Ltd, Bury St Edmunds, Suffolk
Printed in England by Clays Ltd, St Ives plc

Contents

Drug Names

There has been an attempt to harmonize drug names internationally, so that we all use the same ones. It is now a requirement that the recommended 'International Non-proprietary' name be used. In general, the names used for medicines in the United Kingdom were the same as the international names, though a few differences did exist. Some were very minor variations in spelling, for example amphetamine is now spelt amfetamine, and we have used the new names in this edition. However, certain name changes might pose a major problem and cause confusion, such that there may be a danger to patients, for example adrenaline is now called epinephrine. In these instances, we have used both names, the new followed by the old in brackets; for example dosulepin(dothiepin). The old name is still listed in the A–Z, pointing to the new name, to help you in looking up particular medicines and to reduce any confusion.

Introduction

People are often confused by medicines being referred to as *drugs*, and this makes some patients anxious. But in fact all medicines *are* drugs, and coffee, tea, cola, cocoa, tobacco and alcohol are also drugs. The patient's anxiety is natural, because the word 'drugs' has become associated with the abuse of mind-active drugs by certain groups of people. This misconception has resulted in a belief that medicines are good and drugs are bad; as one headmaster said to another, 'If I were not on tranquillizers I think I would have finished up on drugs!' What then is a drug? A drug may be defined as any substance which can alter the structure or function of the living organism. Air pollutants, pesticides and vitamins, as well as virtually any chemical, may be regarded as drugs. Therefore, all medicines are drugs but not all drugs are medicines. Those drugs used as medicines have been selected because they possess or are thought to possess useful properties. They are used to relieve physical or mental symptoms, produce an altered state of mind, to treat, prevent or diagnose disease, and to prevent and end pregnancy.

The term drug does not indicate the way that it is used, whether medically or non-medically, legally or illegally, prescribed by a doctor or not. Similarly the term medicine does not refer specifically to a drug in liquid form; medicines can also be given as tablets, capsules, linctuses, inhalations, injections and so on.

The action of a drug is a complex physical and chemical process which affects living cells. In most cases we still know very little about how drugs actually act within the body; but we know a good deal about the effects of that action.

The effect of most drugs is to stimulate or to depress certain biochemical or physiological functions within the body. Some, such as the antibiotics, have little effect on the cells of the body; they have their effect instead on infecting organisms.

The effects of drugs can be used to attack disease in several different ways.

The most obvious example is the cure of disease by drugs such as antibiotics, which destroy the invading bacteria that were making the patient ill. Drugs whose effects are used in this way are known as antibacterial drugs. At the other end of the spectrum are the drugs whose effects can be used to prevent disease, such as the vaccines. In between these two extremes, there are drugs whose effects can be used to alter actual body processes, in order to change the course of a disease process. They include such drugs as anticoagulants (anti-blood clotting drugs), which are used, for example, in thrombosis, to lessen blood clotting. There are drugs which can be used to replace elements which the body cannot take in or absorb – such as vitamin B_{12} for the patient with pernicious anaemia – and there are drugs which can be used to give the body what it fails to manufacture for itself – such as thyroid hormone for the patient with an inactive thyroid gland. Finally, of course, there are all the drugs which are given because their effects relieve symptoms, and they include everything from pain-killers and tranquillizers to antacids and decongestants.

Any drug produces some undesired effects along with the desired effects for which it was administered. For a drug to be a useful medicine, it must produce more beneficial than harmful effects. If it does not make you better at least it should not make you worse. Unfortunately many people do not recognize adverse drug effects (sometimes called 'side-effects') in themselves. Drugs are described by their most important useful effect, and it does not occur to the patient that the morphine which he is considering only as a pain-reliever, an analgesic, is causing his constipation or his sleepiness or his tight chest. Sometimes doctors appear to be reluctant to consider the possibility that their treatment has made the patient worse; they may try to combat the new troubles with further drugs, thus starting up a new chain of adverse effects.

It must always be remembered that a drug's effects are like shotgun pellets – some land on target, others do not. We must therefore try to think of a drug in terms of its full spectrum of benefits and risks. This is discussed later in this Introduction.

Drug effects, both beneficial and harmful, are much affected by the way in which the drug is introduced into the body – the method of administration.

Methods of Administration

There are four main routes by which a drug may enter the body. Topical administration means applying the drug to the skin (e.g. ointments), to the eyes (e.g. eye drops), to ears (e.g. ear drops), or to the inner linings of the body – the mucous membranes, e.g. up the nose (intranasally), or up the vagina (pessaries). Inhalation means simply that the drug is breathed into the lungs (e.g. aerosols for asthma, or general anaesthetics). Enteral administration means that the drug is given by mouth. Parenteral administration means that the drug is given by any route other than by mouth but the term is often used to refer specifically to injections. An injection may be made directly into a nerve for local effect, as when the dentist deadens a painful tooth, or it may be made into the spinal cord fluid as in spinal anaesthesia. Otherwise, injections are either intravenous – made into a vein; intramuscular – made into a muscle; subcutaneous – made under the skin; or intradermal – into the skin.

Injections ensure that the drug reaches a high concentration in the blood very quickly. Intravenous injections may produce almost instantaneous effects, as mainlining drug abusers know. But no injection is without risk or difficulty. The drug has to be soluble; dosage must be very exact and the injection must take place under sterile conditions. Injections are therefore usually reserved for cases where a rapid effect is essential, or the drug is poorly absorbed from the intestine or the patient cannot take it by mouth.

Some intramuscular injections are given in prolonged-release forms. These are called 'depot' injections; the drug is slowly absorbed from the injection site over a period of hours, days or weeks – e.g. certain insulins, steroids and tranquillizers.

One way of administering a drug is to implant a special preparation deep in the tissues. The drug is released slowly over several months. Another way is to apply a drug to the skin in a skin patch (transdermal patch). The drug slowly passes through the skin and enters the bloodstream. Oestrogen skin patches are used in hormone replacement therapy (HRT).

The taking of drugs by mouth is the most convenient way. Some drugs may be absorbed from the mouth itself (e.g. glyceryl trinitrate tablets are allowed to dissolve under the tongue for the treatment of angina). Most are swallowed and absorbed from the stomach and intestine. There are some disadvantages to taking drugs by mouth – some drugs may irritate the stomach and produce vomiting; others may be destroyed by the acid in the stomach and may need a special coating (called enteric coating) to protect them until they reach the intestine.

All drugs that are taken by mouth pass through the liver first before being released into the general circulation. During their first-time passage through the liver, some drugs are broken down and therefore it is sometimes more effective to give such drugs by a parenteral route – e.g. inhaled, applied to the skin, via the rectum or by injection.

Absorption

The rate and extent to which a drug reaches the bloodstream (absorption) determines the time between taking the drug and the onset of its action. Injections ensure quick entry into the bloodstream, whereas absorption into the bloodstream from the intestine may be very variable. Rates of absorption can vary from person to person and from time to time in the same person. The best-known example is probably the absorption of alcohol. Hot food taken with alcohol delays its absorption. The presence of any food in the stomach also delays absorption to some extent, while alcohol taken when the stomach is empty will 'go to your head' almost immediately.

Rates of absorption are also dependent upon the solubility of the drug and of the other materials (excipients) used in making it into a tablet or capsule. Drugs given in solution are absorbed more quickly than tablets or capsules swallowed whole. Absorption from these depends upon many factors, including size and solubility of particles, chemical form, and various manufacturing processes such as the compression force used to make the tablet. These can all affect the rate at which a tablet breaks up and the particles separate in the intestine before dissolving, which is the important step in absorption.

Distribution

Once a drug has been absorbed into the bloodstream, its concentration in the tissue fluids around its target area will determine its effectiveness. This depends on the concentration of the drug in the blood. As we have seen, different routes of administration can give varying initial blood levels – with intravenous routes giving the highest levels quickly; and whatever the route of administration, different formulations of drugs can give different rates of absorption into the blood, with highly soluble drugs being absorbed most quickly. But even when a drug has been put into the body and absorbed into the bloodstream, different types of drug behave differently. Some can pass throughout the whole body, entering or passing through the plasma, the fluid inside as well as outside cells, the spinal fluid and across the placenta into an unborn baby. Other drugs are much more limited in their effects being, for example, 'filtered' by the placenta, or confined to action in the fluid outside cells.

When taken by mouth some drugs are fairly quickly absorbed, and well distributed around the body in the bloodstream, but are quickly broken down in the liver and excreted by the kidneys. Aspirin, for example, is normally excreted within a few hours, so that for a headache a once-only dose has time to be effective, but continuous treatment for the pain of arthritis requires regularly repeated doses.

Other drugs work quite differently, being very slowly excreted by the body because they accumulate in various tissues and form long-acting depots of the drug. At the beginning of treatment it takes several days for the depot of the drug to accumulate, so high starter doses are normally given. Once the drug has built up there is a balance between the concentration of the stored drug and the concentration of the free active drug in the bloodstream, and therefore smaller maintenance doses are needed to keep the level of the drug in the bloodstream adequate.

Some drugs bind themselves to proteins in the blood itself, which provides a means of transport for the drug and also acts as a depot from which the drug is released if the level of active-free drug in the blood falls.

Bones and teeth act as reservoirs for certain drugs. Lead, for example, accumulates in bones, while the antibiotic tetracycline is stored in both bones and teeth. Many unfortunate people have teeth yellowed by this drug, given to them when they were babies or young children, or to their mothers while they were in the womb.

Other tissues can act as reservoirs for some drugs. For example, the anti-malarial drug mepacrine reaches a concentration in the liver many times greater than the concentration in the blood after only a single dose. Even body fat can act as a storage depot of a fat-soluble drug, so that a fat person may store much more of such a drug than a thin person.

Drug Metabolism

Drug metabolism means the alteration of a drug from one chemical structure to another. This transformation within the body usually results in the inactivation of a drug so that it can be eliminated from the body. This may be called drug breakdown or biotransformation. Occasionally a drug is not active until it has been transformed in the body. For example, the drug pivampicillin is more readily absorbed from the intestine than ampicillin and converted (hydrolysed) in the liver to the active antibiotic ampicillin. A drug such as pivampicillin is described as a *pro-drug*. Drug metabolism involves complex chemical and physical processes which usually take place in the liver. Note how your body reacts to drugs; once a drug has been administered, the body's main concern is to try to get rid of it.

Elimination

The concentration of a drug in the tissues rises when the rate of absorption exceeds the rate of elimination. Eventually these rates become equal and thereafter elimination exceeds absorption. The kidneys are the important organ involved in the elimination or excretion of a drug: less important are the bile system, the lungs, sweat and other body secretions. Drugs excreted in the faeces are usually unabsorbed drugs which have been taken by mouth (note how dark your stools are when you take iron tablets) or breakdown products excreted in the bile. Drugs may also be excreted in breast milk and affect the baby. Ninety-five per cent of alcohol is metabolized and the small amount of unchanged alcohol is eliminated in the breath, urine and sweat.

Dosage

There is a relationship between dosage of a drug and its effectiveness. Unfortunately the relationship is a very complex one. Any drug will obviously be ineffective if the dose given is too small to produce effective levels in the bloodstream, or the formulation is such that the drug cannot be absorbed, or, with some drugs, the interval between doses is so great that the drug has been eliminated before the next dose starts to be absorbed. The effects of a drug can be increased by increasing the dosage. But by doing this you also increase whatever adverse effects the drug may have (see p. xvii). If we enjoy the relaxing effects of a glass of whisky, we cannot make ourselves more pleasurably relaxed by taking twice the quantity. We simply become unpleasantly drunk.

The dose of a drug required to produce a specified level of effect in 50 per cent of individuals is known as the median effective dose. The dose required to produce toxic effects in 50 per cent of individuals is known as the median toxic dose. The ratio of these two is called the therapeutic index and it gives an indication of a drug's safety and the relationship between benefits and risks.

Drug-Testing and the Placebo Effect

Therapeutic indices are initially worked out on animals but in the end they have to be applied to the effect of actual drugs given to real patients. Innumerable factors to do with the patient, such as the state of his or her digestion, his or her weight, age and so forth, may alter a drug's effects. To complicate drug-testing further the placebo effect operates in all sorts of unpredictable ways in different individuals. The word 'placebo' means 'I shall please'. It is used to describe any effect of a 'treatment' which is not due to the action or effects of the drug, but which occurs as a result of the patient's expectations of that treatment. Usually the effect of such a 'treatment' is good; if you think something will make you feel better it often will. But the placebo effect can operate the other way too: people given dummy tablets in drug trials may complain of side-effects such as headaches, nausea or giddiness.

Most of the medical practice of past centuries was based on placebos; there were very few effective drugs known, and treatment therefore rested on the faith the patient had in his doctor and his 'medicines'. Now many highly effective drugs have been discovered, and their very effectiveness has strengthened the faith which both patients and doctors have in drugs, so that the placebo effect is still as general as ever. It shows itself most clearly in the testing of pain-killers and sedatives. When such drugs are tried against dummy tablets, around four out of ten patients report improvement after taking the inactive tablets. And the effect does not only operate when you are given dummy tablets, it works when real medicine is given too. The more sure you are that the drug (or operation or other procedure) will do you good, the more likely it is to work well for you. *Your faith in the doctor who prescribes for you or the neighbour who suggests a pill or the advertisement which persuades you to buy one over the counter will all have some effect on how effective the drug will be for you.*

Scientific drug-testing has to allow for these faith-healing elements as well as all the other factors that influence a drug's effectiveness. In order to allow for them, it is necessary to know as much about them as possible. It is also essential to know as much as possible about the disorder which the drug is intended to cure or ameliorate. Perhaps the first essential is to understand the disorder's 'natural history'. For example, a cold (coryza) lasts for about three to four days if no treatment is given; an effective cold cure would have to shorten this duration of illness.

The selection of a proper sample of patients for the drug trial is important too. They must be representative of the population who are to be offered the new treatment, i.e. their age, sex, social group and many other factors should be considered as well as the disease being treated. The size of the sample of patients must be statistically representative, and the drug dosage must be carefully and realistically chosen.

Once a sample of patients and a drug regimen have been chosen, the drug-testers have to find a way of preventing placebo effects from distorting their results. This is usually done by using what is called a double-blind technique.

Identical tablets (or linctuses or injection ampoules) are made up, half containing the drug to be tested and the other half containing either an established drug (against which the new one is to show its worth) or some inert 'dummy' substance. Half the patients are given the true drug, half are given the dummy, and their responses are compared. Or half the patients may start with the real drug and then change to the dummy tablet after a suitable period, the other half of the sample starting with the dummy tablets and changing to the drug. The point, of course, is that neither the patient nor the prescribing doctor knows at any given time whether the 'drug' is real or fake, new or old. In this way the patient's expectations about treatment, and the extent to which he or she is influenced by his or her doctor, are kept out of the picture.

The results of the trials are subjected to highly complex statistical analyses. They may take several years from start to finish, and cost the drug companies a great deal of money, with no guarantee that at the end they will find that they have an effective, safe, marketable drug. So it is not surprising that many proprietary remedies in common use have never been subjected to such trials. Many of them would fail under scientific scrutiny, yet people swear by them. Because of the placebo effect many of us feel better, even before we swallow the first pill. Clearly our own opinions on effective 'cures' are often unreliable.

Unfortunately there are many disorders for which there is no cure. In the absence of a real cure and in the presence of patients, many of whom react favourably to *anything* which is done to help them, 'treatments' tend to proliferate. *It is a good rule of thumb that if many treatments are in use for the same disease it is because there is no real treatment known for that disease.* If one treatment had ever been scientifically shown to be effective, it would have displaced all other treatments for that disorder. But people find it very difficult to accept lack of treatment. Even the most unorthodox and expensive treatments will always be glowingly recommended by some patient who preferred any action to none. Private hair clinics and skin clinics, for example, perpetuate a range of expensive treatments largely on a basis of 'personal recommendation' from one patient to the next. Similarly, non-prescribed drugs, herbs and 'health' foods can be widely and profitably sold even where scientific testing would show them to be totally useless.

It should be obvious, then, that testimonials from people about a preparation are not worth the paper they were written on. Even less attention should be paid to preparations sponsored by actors and footballers and so on – they are paid to do it. Similarly, be careful about being taken in by television commercials and newspaper articles dealing with various preparations – the products advertised are nearly always expensive and gimmicky versions of drugs which are available much more cheaply.

Drug Regimens

Some drugs are taken occasionally as a single dose – for example, two aspirins for a headache. Others are taken daily as a single dose, such as a sleeping tablet taken each bedtime. A few drugs are prescribed to be taken when necessary, such as glyceryl trinitrate taken to relieve the pain of angina, or an antacid taken when indigestion is troublesome. But the majority of prescribed drugs are taken at intervals throughout the day for several days, or even for weeks or years at a time.

Decisions about dosage and the interval between doses are largely based on two considerations, both of which were discussed in detail earlier in this Introduction. First, the doctor must consider the length of time which this particular drug in this particular dosage takes to reach effective levels in the blood, and how quickly it starts to be eliminated from the body. Second, he or she must consider the therapeutic index for the drug. If the index is small, so that the effective level in the blood is rather close to the toxic level, then the dose will have to be very carefully controlled if adverse effects are to be prevented. If the index is large, then there is more leeway and more than adequate doses can be given without much risk of adverse effects which may reduce the number of doses to be taken daily.

Some drugs, for example antibiotics, can only do their work properly if the blood level is kept steady throughout the twenty-four hours. If the patient leaves a ten-hour gap between doses during the night, bacteria have a chance to reassert themselves so that the drug faces a two-steps-forward and one-back situation. In such cases the doctor will probably prescribe the drug to be taken six-hourly rather than four times daily.

Drugs which gradually build up and accumulate in the body are much more difficult to control than drugs which act rapidly and are readily excreted; for example, patients given a long-acting benzodiazepine for anxiety may not realize that even while their regular dosage is producing the desired effect, the drug is accumulating in their bodies, being put in faster than it can be excreted. When such a patient stops taking the pills he or she will still have the drug in his or her body for several days.

Obviously you should follow your doctor's instructions about taking any drug very carefully, and check with him or her before you alter either the dosage or the interval between doses. The way in which drugs are taken can be important too. Most drugs are absorbed better if they are taken when the stomach is empty. It makes sense therefore to take them before meals. But some drugs, for example aspirin and anti-rheumatic drugs, may irritate the stomach if it is empty. They are better taken with or after meals. Most drugs are better absorbed if they are taken in solution, so that soluble aspirin tablets taken in water will be more quickly effective than ordinary aspirin tablets which do not dissolve in water, but many pills and capsules are not soluble and must be swallowed whole with a good drink of water. A few drugs, such as tetracycline, are ineffective if taken with milk.

Many drugs are available in a wide variety of forms. For example, children can be given syrups and sweetened suspensions of drugs.* People who suffer irritation of the stomach from drugs can often take the same drugs in the form of suppositories or of specially coated tablets which protect the stomach from the drug until it reaches the intestines. Whatever the form of drug you are taking it is important to remember what it actually is. A suppository has just as much effect on the body as does a tablet. Some drugs should never be taken together, so that any doctor who is prescribing for you must be told of anything you are already taking – including alcohol – and so must the pharmacist from whom you buy medicines over the counter.

Often a drug will appear to have made you better before you have taken the full course prescribed by the doctor. To stop taking it without consulting him or her may be harmful. The most usual example is probably antibiotics given to children. The child has tonsillitis and a high temperature; the doctor prescribes an antibiotic to be given for five days, but in two days the temperature is down and the child feels better. The mother stops giving the drug and very probably puts it away in the medicine cupboard for use without consulting the

---

* Many medicines for children have a syrup base and may be harmful to teeth.

doctor, next time someone has a sore throat. The original patient may have got better because the disorder cured itself, but equally he or she may have got better because the antibiotic had started its work. In that case the bacteria have been decimated but not destroyed and the illness will reappear in a few days, but this time with the added complication that the bacteria may have become resistant to that antibiotic. At the same time the bottle of medicine which the mother stored away may have a short shelf-life, such that it becomes useless after ten days; it should not be stored or used on another occasion without the doctor's advice.

Anyone who is prescribed or buys over the counter a drug he or she does not intend to use immediately should tell the pharmacist. The form in which the drug is dispensed may well affect its shelf-life, and many formulations will only remain effective for a short period of time. An ancient bottle of antibiotic eye drops dredged from the back of a cupboard may well do more harm than good.

Interactions between Drugs

A drug interaction is the modification of the effects of one drug by another. Some drug interactions are used intentionally for therapeutic purposes, but most arise from unplanned combinations of drugs. Obviously the more drugs you take the more likely it is that some of them will react adversely with each other. The patient who takes over-the-counter drugs at the same time as prescribed ones, without telling the prescribing doctor what he or she buys from the pharmacist, may be at risk.

Most doctors are against the use of medicines containing several active drugs because it is impossible to vary the dosage or time schedule of each drug separately and because if adverse effects arise it is difficult to know which drug is responsible for them. For example, phenacetin was widely used for many years as one constituent in pain-killer preparations. A few patients who consumed such mixtures daily over a long period developed fatal kidney damage. Phenacetin is now considered to be the culprit, but it would have been identified sooner had its consumption not been confused with the use of aspirin and caffeine and other ingredients in such combined pain-relievers. Do not be impressed by advertisements which stress that products contain more than one active ingredient, and that they are approved by doctors. Several drugs are not necessarily more effective than one, and it would be surprising if such mixtures were not approved by doctors since the drug companies employ doctors to advise them!

If the combined effect of two drugs is greater than the effect of each alone they are said to act synergistically. If the combined effect is less than the sum of the two they are said to be antagonistic. The combined effects of drugs with similar actions are usually referred to as additive and these effects may be beneficial or harmful. The effects of a 'normal' dose of a drug may therefore be exaggerated if it is given with another drug which produces similar effects. Sleeping drugs, sedatives and tranquillizers, for example, have additive effects with alcohol. The patient who drinks moderately when taking one of these drugs may unexpectedly become very drunk indeed.

Drug interactions may cause adverse effects or simply make a drug ineffective. For example, the antibiotic tetracycline may interact with calcium salts (for instance, in milk) or magnesium salts (as in many indigestion remedies) to form an unabsorbable complex in the stomach. This interferes with the absorption of the antibiotic to a point where it cannot reach effective levels in the bloodstream.

Before taking more than one drug preparation, people should consider the possibility that their need for the second or third drug may in fact be caused by the harmful effects of the first drug. *All too often adverse drug effects arise because patients and doctors try to deal with the ill-effects of one drug by taking another, when it would be safer to stop the first drug.*

Adverse Effects of Drugs

Any unintended reaction from a 'normal' dose of a drug is an adverse effect. Most adverse effects of established drugs have been observed and recorded. However, with new drugs it is important to monitor every symptom that may be caused by the drugs in order to build up an information base on their benefits and risks.

If any of the processes involved in the body's breakdown or excretion of a drug are impaired (as, for example, in liver disease or kidney disease), the drug may have an excessive effect even when given in a 'normal' dose.

Some people may become allergic to certain drugs, and some suffer reactions which are idiosyncratic (i.e. peculiar to them). These become additional recognized adverse effects of that drug over time. The commonest allergic effects are skin rashes; there may also be fever, painful joints or a swollen face, or wheezing; occasionally sensitivity of the skin to sunlight may be produced by a drug. Very rarely a patient may drop dead from allergic shock following the injection of a drug to which he or she has become allergic during previous treatment (death from a second bee sting is an example of this). An idiosyncratic reaction may, for example, cause liver damage resulting in jaundice (e.g. to chlorpromazine).

Some rare adverse effects of drugs can be due to underlying genetic disorders which are not recognized until a drug touches them off. For example, barbiturates can trigger a first attack of a genetic disease called porphyria, which causes abdominal colic, polyneuritis (nerve damage), mental disturbances and sometimes death. Genetic factors may also influence the effect of a particular drug in a particular patient. The drug isoniazid, which is used in tuberculosis, is used up quickly in most patients. But in a few it is broken down and excreted very slowly, so that such patients run the risk of harmful effects from it.

Many people believe that once they have been on a drug for some time without obvious ill-effects, the appearance of adverse effects becomes unlikely. Unfortunately this is not true. The ill-effects of a drug taken for a long time may be cumulative – as they were with the long-term consumption of phenacetin, which was shown to cause kidney damage. Or ill-effects may arise spontaneously even when the patient has been on a drug for years. Furthermore certain drugs (e.g. prednisolone) can produce changes which may cause harmful effects long after the patient has stopped taking them (see Chapter 37).

The Use of Drugs in People who are Particularly Vulnerable to Adverse Drug Effects

The Use of Drugs in Elderly People

'Ageing' may be restricted to certain organs or tissues or may affect the whole body. Such changes may produce ageing before the person is old in years. Whenever its onset, the ageing process can alter the delicate physiochemical processes which are involved in drug action. Ageing does not mean disease, though the older you get the more chance you have of developing a disorder, particularly of the degenerative type (e.g. arthritis). In fact, older people are often found to have multiple disorders such as anaemia, arthritis and diseases of the arteries.

With advancing age, the body burns up energy more slowly, digestion may become affected, the acid in the stomach decreases, the gut wall may lose its muscular power and the emptying of the stomach and movement of the bowels may become less efficient. The circulation may be affected and the function of the liver, kidneys and brain may all be impaired.

Whether or not these actual deteriorations have taken place, the diet of an old person may lack the basic elements which are essential for normal body functioning and for the normal use of drugs by the body. So elderly people are at risk whenever they are given drugs. Aspirin may cause bleeding from the stomach in anyone: in an elderly person such bleeding may be serious because dietary deficiencies have already led to anaemia. Constipation caused by poor diet and weakened bowel action may become serious if the patient is given codeine. Sleeping pills, sedatives or tranquillizers in 'average' doses may make the elderly person confused and unsteady; a benzodiazepine sleeping drug which would be excreted by most patients within eight hours may 'hang over' the whole of the next day.

Clearly then, fixed 'average' doses and dosage schedules should not be applied to elderly people. They, even more than the rest of us, need careful tailoring of drug dosages to their particular needs, current health and social circumstances. Sometimes failure to provide this highly personal prescribing leads to tragic results. A patient who has become confused on tranquillizers may be considered senile and given more drugs to control the confusion – a vicious circle which may lead to the patient finishing his or her days confined to bed. The same kind of outcome may follow the prescribing of drugs to lower blood pressure in elderly people. The drugs may reduce the volume of blood reaching the brain, putting the patient at risk and mimicking symptoms of senility in someone who already has an insufficient blood supply to their brain. Another group of drugs called diuretics make the kidneys pass out more water and salt in the urine. This makes the patient empty his or her bladder more frequently, and, in the elderly, this often leads to incontinence. A drug-induced problem may be the final straw to a harassed family.

In order to avoid such tragedies, *the fewest possible drugs should be given to elderly people, in the minimum effective dosage and for the shortest duration of time possible.*

The Use of Drugs by Pregnant Women

In the early weeks of pregnancy the placenta (or afterbirth) is developing. Until it is fully formed, any drug circulating through the mother's body may enter the embryo. In later months the placenta acts as a barrier, protecting the developing baby from moderate doses of non-fat-soluble drugs. Fat-soluble drugs, and drugs given in high dosage, will continue to cross the barrier throughout pregnancy. Yet the baby's liver is not sufficiently developed to deal with the breakdown of drugs and its kidneys are not sufficiently developed to excrete them – but of course they return to the mother through the umbilical vein for her to break them down and excrete them from her body.

From the moment the female egg is fertilized, complex processes are set in motion. The egg embeds itself in the wall of the uterus (womb); the cells of the fertilized egg start to divide and redivide; under chemical control they start grouping and organizing themselves. Cells destined to be part of the brain, the liver, the eyes, the kidneys and so on position themselves, and the various organs start to develop. So the whole embryo baby is a group of cells, all dividing and being chemically organized.

At the beginning of the Introduction we stated that, while we know a good deal about the effects of drugs within the body, we know very little about how those effects are produced; how the drugs actually act on the cells. We know even less about how drugs act upon the cells that make up a developing baby. We really know little more than that some drugs may produce abnormalities (teratogenesis) and that these are more likely when the drug is taken within the twelve weeks after conception. You will not need to be reminded that thalidomide produced many abnormalities in newborn babies. It is particularly sad when it is realized that thalidomide was just another sedative with no particular advantage over other established drugs, and that it was taken for minor symptoms. However, this tragedy led, though at terrible cost to the children involved, to widespread publicity and recognition of the danger by the medical profession and by governments.

Governments and pharmaceutical companies have increased and improved the testing of *new* drugs for possible dangers during pregnancy. But there are still prescribed drugs and over-the-counter drugs on the market which have never been tested. Pregnant women take so many drugs, including tea, coffee, alcohol, cigarettes, aspirin and antacids, that it is often difficult to discover a relationship between any abnormality in the baby and drugs used by the mother in pregnancy. There is some evidence that mothers of abnormal babies tend to have taken more drugs than other mothers.

Only a few drugs are actually known to produce abnormalities. Smoking, for example, puts the unborn baby's life at risk and also leads to smaller babies; tetracycline can affect bone growth and stain teeth; anticonvulsant drugs have been associated with the risk of club foot and of cleft palate. Then there are a few drugs which can damage the baby by affecting its blood supply, which affects the placenta. Yet others may damage the baby after it is fully developed; hormones, for example, may affect sexual development; iodine and anti-thyroid drugs may lead to the baby being born with a thyroid goitre. Finally, of course, the baby may develop an overall reaction and even be born already addicted to narcotics.

What conclusions should we draw from this state of affairs? Without being alarmist *it is probably best to try to avoid regularly taking any non-essential drugs in pregnancy or if you are trying to become pregnant and this warning includes smoking, alcohol and caffeine-containing beverages.*

Drug Use During Breastfeeding

The taking of some drugs while breastfeeding may lead to toxic effects in the baby. Some drugs pass through the milk and work directly in the baby's body. Therefore, any drug should be taken with caution by breastfeeding mothers. Some drugs can become concentrated in the mother's milk, e.g. iodine, which can then produce goitre in the baby; some tranquillizers (e.g. diazepam, Valium) can produce lethargy and weight loss in the baby, oral anticoagulants can produce bleeding, and there are many other examples. *For many drugs there is insufficient information available, therefore any drugs should be taken with caution* by breastfeeding mothers. It is always best to consult your doctor or pharmacist.

The Use of Drugs in Babies and Children

As discussed earlier the way the body deals with drugs is very complex and relies on healthy, mature and functioning organs. You will remember that the liver has to bring about the breakdown of drugs, so that the kidneys can excrete them. In babies, the liver and kidneys are still immature. Some of the enzyme and other systems involved in drug breakdown and excretion are not fully developed. Ineffectively broken down or incompletely excreted, almost any drug may cause adverse effects.

Babies are also much more sensitive than older people to changes in the salt and water balance in their bodies. Drugs which alter this balance – such as drugs with a diuretic effect, or drugs which cause diarrhoea – may cause serious adverse effects. Equally any drug whose effect is made worse by a change in salt and water balance may have adverse effects in babies.

Infants are growing and developing. Drugs which have few adverse effects in an adult may interfere with growth or development in a baby, or may have adverse effects on the infant's mechanisms for controlling his body temperature or on his newly developing muscle control or coordination.

All these factors apply also to toddlers and, to a lesser extent, to children too. Dosage is therefore absolutely critical. Any liquid medicine should be administered via a 5 ml spoon given to you by the pharmacist. If the instructions say '1 teaspoonful' they mean 5 ml. A domestic teaspoon may hold 4 or 7 ml and such inaccuracy could be dangerous. Similarly if any dilution of the medicine is required, this should be carried out by the pharmacist when the drug is dispensed; it should never be left to the mother to estimate the right quantity of a drug with a label saying 'dilute in 5 parts of water'.

On the whole too many drugs are given to babies and children. Mothers have been led to expect a prescription every time they take their child to the doctor and many doctors seem unable to resist prescribing anti-diarrhoeal remedies, cough medicines and antibiotics. Antibiotics in particular are often used inappropriately. The mother says, 'Doctor always gives him an antibiotic when he gets these nasty colds.' The very statement is a command. Many of those 'nasty colds' are caused by viruses against which antibiotics are totally ineffective. In such a situation their only possible value is in protecting the child against the possibility that the cold may be followed by a bacterial invasion of the chest, throat or ears. With common colds and other virus infections of the nose and throat secondary infections are the exception rather than the rule. Doctors ought to stop thinking that patients expect drugs at every consultation and try giving reassurance, explanation and sound advice instead. Equally, mothers should not expect a prescription to relieve their child's every symptom.

Drug Use in Kidney Disease

Most drugs are excreted by the kidneys so that any impairment can lead to toxic levels of a drug or one of its breakdown products in the bloodstream. Drugs must therefore be used with *caution* in patients with impaired kidney function, particularly those that are excreted entirely by the kidneys. The dose of the drug must be decreased and/or the interval of time between doses should be increased. (*Note warning on drug use in the elderly.*) Drugs that are known to damage the kidneys should be avoided, but *always check with your doctor or pharmacist.*

Drug Use in Liver Disease

Many drugs are broken down in the liver so that severe liver disease may affect the metabolism of a drug and lead to toxic levels of the drug in the bloodstream. The liver is also involved in the manufacture of certain proteins in the blood to which drugs attach themselves. A serious liver disease will reduce the amounts of these proteins in the bloodstream (hypoalbuminaemia), thus allowing less protein for the drugs to attach themselves to and causing a toxic level of 'free' drugs in the bloodstream.

The clotting of blood depends on clotting factors made in the liver – any reduction in these by liver disease will lead to a greater sensitivity to oral anticoagulant drugs such as phenindione and warfarin.

All drugs should be given with caution to patients with liver disease, particularly drugs which depress brain function and drugs which affect fluid and salt balance in the body (e.g. carbenoxolone, corticosteroids).

Some drugs can actually damage the liver. These may be predictable effects and related to the dosage or they may be completely unpredictable and particular to the individual patient, i.e. they are idiosyncratic. You must be aware of the warnings with individual drugs and *always consult your doctor or pharmacist if you suffer from liver disease.*

The Use of Drugs by Drivers

To achieve the high degree of mental and physical skill, coordination and judgement required to drive any motor vehicle safely, a driver must be fully awake, alert, calm and concentrating. Yet every day thousands of motorists drive while under the influence of drugs which may affect their driving skills.

The drug most usually indicted after a motor accident is of course alcohol. Moderate amounts of alcohol can impair driving ability. Often this impairment is not noticed by drivers. Because the alcohol has relaxed them and made them less inhibited than usual they may even feel that they are driving particularly well. In high doses alcohol produces disorientation and confusion, blurred vision and poor muscle control. Such drivers are extremely lucky to get home without hurting themselves – or somebody else. Alcohol is not a suitable drug for drivers under any circumstances.

Unfortunately many of the other drugs which impair driving ability do this to an even greater extent if they are combined with even a very little alcohol. For example, many cough remedies and cold 'cures' contain drugs which affect the nervous system. Because they have been bought over the counter, individuals give no thought to the possible effects on their driving. On their own the drugs might not impair it seriously, but when individuals have also had a drink with their friends before driving home from work they may be quite unfit to drive.

Even more dangerous are some drugs which are prescribed by doctors. These include many of the most commonly prescribed groups of drugs such as antihistamines, stimulants, sleeping drugs, sedatives, tranquillizers, anti-depressants, slimming drugs, drugs used to treat blood pressure, anti-spasmodics, drugs used to treat nausea, vomiting or motion sickness, or to treat diabetes. Obviously it would be impossible to forbid any person taking any of these groups of drugs to drive a car. The effects depend on the person, the situation, the dose. What one can and must do is to point out the possible effects of these drugs on driving skill, and above all the danger of combining them with alcohol and then driving. *The rule is that any drug with an effect (whether intended or not) on the brain or the nervous system is likely to have some effect on driving ability.* If a drug prescribed for you makes you feel drowsy, nervous, tense, dizzy, faint, trembly, makes it difficult for you to concentrate or blurs your vision, then you can be sure that your driving skills are impaired. Other skills will also be impaired, particularly those calling for a combination of manual skills, experience and alertness. These may seriously affect those in charge of complex machinery, airline pilots, train drivers, etc.

The Use of Drugs in Patients with Stoma

Enteric-coated and **sustained-release** preparations of drugs should not be used, particularly by patients with ileostomies – they will not have time to release their active drug.

Laxatives, enemas and bowel wash-outs should not be used by ileostomy patients – they may produce severe dehydration. Bulk-forming laxatives (e.g. bran) are best. Codeine phosphate, loperamide and diphenoxylate may be used to treat diarrhoea.

Antacids containing magnesium salts may produce diarrhoea and those containing aluminium salts produce constipation.

Diuretics should be used with caution because they may easily produce dehydration and loss of potassium. If necessary, a potassium-sparing diuretic should be used (see p. 148).

Patients on **digoxin** should be given liquid preparations of potassium because of the dangers of low blood potassium levels in patients receiving digoxin (see p. 120).

Morphine and related pain-relievers (e.g. codeine, dextropropoxyphene) may produce troublesome constipation in colectomy patients.

Iron preparations may produce loose motions and may need to be given by intramuscular injections.

Warnings to Patients on Long-term Drug Treatment

Several groups of drugs, discussed in detail in the chapters that follow, may give rise to very serious adverse effects when other drugs are given to a person, or when an individual undergoes dental treatment, or requires emergency treatment even for a minor injury at an outpatient department. *The first rule for anyone undergoing long-term drug treatment should be to tell any medical personnel about their drugs.* In most cases warning cards are issued to such patients. If issued they should always be carried. In that way individuals can be sure that the hospital will have the information it needs should they be admitted unconscious after an accident.

1 Corticosteroids

These drugs, especially prednisolone, are frequently used to treat rheumatoid arthritis, allergic diseases, skin diseases, eye diseases and asthma.

During periods of anxiety, stress or injury, the body requires and produces more corticosteroids. This natural response by the adrenal glands is prevented by treatment with corticosteroids. The patient's body is already living with corticosteroids in the bloodstream, so the adrenal glands do not respond by producing extra in times of stress. Patients having such treatment are therefore liable to develop a state of acute adrenal insufficiency if they have an accident, a surgical operation or even an acute infection. Even the stress of an ordinary dental procedure can be enough, in such a patient, to produce faintness, weakness, nausea, vomiting and finally collapse.

If you are on these drugs or have had treatment with them even for only one month in the preceding two years, you should always carry your warning card with you.

2 Anticoagulants

These drugs lessen the blood's ability to clot. They are most often used to prevent the extension or recurrence of a thrombosis (clot) in a vein or in the chambers of the heart. Patients taking these drugs tend to bleed easily, and bleeding, even from a minor injury, can be difficult to stop.

You should always carry your warning card with you.

3 Anti-diabetic Drugs

Individuals on anti-diabetic treatment may experience a drastic fall in blood sugar (hypoglycaemia) with weakness, faintness or even collapse, if they miss out a meal in order to have an anaesthetic. Patients on anti-diabetic tablets must discuss any proposed dental anaesthetic with their dentist and with their doctor. Those who are taking insulin, especially if the total dose is high, should be admitted to hospital if they require dental anaesthesia.

4 Antidepressants

Those antidepressant drugs which belong to the group of monoamine oxidase inhibitors may produce adverse effects when taken with certain other drugs and with certain foods. *Patients on these drugs should be issued with warning cards, and should carry them.* Stimulant drugs, such as the amfetamines, and pain-relievers, such as pethidine and morphine, can be highly dangerous to patients on these drugs. Other antidepressant drugs may also cause problems; therefore dentists and casualty department doctors should be told if you are on an antidepressant.

5 Drugs Used to Treat Raised Blood Pressure

Many drugs used to treat raised blood pressure may react with a general anaesthetic to produce a severe drop in blood pressure which can be very dangerous. *If you are taking a drug of this type make sure you have a note on you.*

6 Sedatives and Tranquillizers

These may increase the depressant effects of general anaesthetics upon the brain, particularly the breathing centre. *Make sure you carry a warning card or note with you.*

Dependence on Prescribed Drugs

Everybody has their own picture of what they think a 'drug addict' is like. Yet many people would be hard put to define drug addiction in a way which covered all the possible types of person who might be addicted and all the possible types of drug they might be addicted to. Because of these problems of definition and because of the extent to which the term addiction has been misused in popular parlance, most authorities are now in favour of substituting the general term 'drug dependence' and then following it with a description of the type of dependence they mean.

In general, drug dependence can be defined as a psychological and/or physical state which results from the taking of a drug, associated with a compulsion to go on taking it either because of the 'desired' effects it produces, or because of the ill-effects if it is not taken, or both.

Defined in this general way it is clear that most of us are at least psychologically dependent on a great many substances we do not usually talk about as 'drugs'. Many of us feel we cannot start the day without coffee, cannot enjoy a rest without a cup of tea or are deprived if we do not have a much-more-than-adequate meal. And we are psychologically dependent on all kinds of other things in our daily lives too, from sex and sport to television and the newspapers. So psychological dependence is not *necessarily* a bad thing. What we have to decide is whether this dependence is producing problems – mentally, physically and/or socially – bearing in mind that different people will see different things as problems.

The person who is dependent on drugs may have such a craving for his or her drug, such a compulsion to go on taking it, that he or she goes on even when knowing full well that he or she is causing harm to him or herself (e.g. smoking).

Physical dependence is a condition in which repeated use of a drug leads to withdrawal symptoms when the drug is stopped. The 'withdrawal symptoms' that arise when a drug is taken away from someone physically dependent on it can be extremely severe. Among the commonest are vomiting, convulsions, trembling and confusion. Without the drug, the body goes to pieces. If no help is offered the patient may die. Physical withdrawal symptoms can always be instantly relieved by the administration of a dose of the drug which caused the dependence. In some cases one drug can replace another in this respect. Tranquillizers, for example, can relieve the symptoms of alcohol withdrawal. In instances like these, there is said to be cross-dependence between the two drugs.

Many of the drugs which can cause dependence also cause tolerance in the user. This simply means that the person's body becomes accustomed to a certain intake of the drug so that in order to derive a similar effect from it he or she has to increase the dose. The double scotch which makes a novice drinker feel pleasantly intoxicated will barely affect the seasoned drinker. Some drugs are capable of producing tremendous tolerance. Constant users of opium and morphine, for example, can take and tolerate doses which would be fatal to ordinary people.

Just as there can be cross-dependence between drugs, so too there can be cross-tolerance. A heavy drinker may need much more sleeping drug to 'knock him out' than a teetotaller.

A wide range of drugs which alter mood can cause drug dependence. But we are still very ignorant about who will become dependent on which drugs under what circumstances. Some drugs are highly likely to cause dependence and some individuals are highly likely to become dependent. On the whole dependence seems most likely to arise when three factors come together: a potential drug of dependence, a 'vulnerable' personality and some adverse aspect of the environment. Whether the risk becomes reality depends on many other complex socio-psychological factors which affect that individual.

Sleeping Drugs, Sedatives and Anti-anxiety Drugs

These drugs (e.g. barbiturates and benzodiazepines) depress brain function. They are all capable of producing drug dependence.

This dependence probably starts with the very first dose as the cells in the brain and nervous system begin to adapt to the presence of the drug. The degree of dependence will depend upon the dose and duration of use, which will determine the severity of withdrawal symptoms if the drug is stopped suddenly. The speed of onset and the intensity of withdrawal symptoms will also be influenced by the duration of action of the drug; for example, a short-acting drug will be cleared rapidly from its site of action and withdrawal symptoms will come on quickly and be intense. Withdrawal symptoms are opposite to the effects produced by the drug, e.g. anxiety and restlessness instead of calmness, and convulsions instead of sleep.

Sleeping drugs, sedatives and anti-anxiety drugs produce tolerance (see above) and cross-tolerance occurs between them and between any one of them and alcohol.

The symptoms of intoxication from sleeping drugs, sedatives and anti-anxiety drugs include difficulty in thinking coherently, slurred speech and lack of concentration. The individual becomes emotional, irritable, suspicious (paranoid), and sometimes depressed and suicidal. His or her gait may be unsteady and his or her vision blurred. In long-standing dependence there may also be a poor state of general health and nutrition associated with the dependence.

If an individual does become physically dependent on any of these drugs he or she may suffer from withdrawal symptoms (withdrawal symptoms of benzodiazepines are discussed in greater detail on p. 9) if they are suddenly stopped. These vary markedly in degree, depending upon which drug is responsible, how long the individual has been taking it and in what dosage. But they may include anxiety, restlessness, trembling, weakness, abdominal cramps, vomiting, hallucinations, delirium, fits and even death.

Amfetamines

The amfetamines are discussed in Chapter 6.

While different doses of amfetamines may produce different effects in different people, many individuals after a moderate dose taken by mouth feel alert, happy, full of energy. In the Second World War these drugs were widely used among the armed forces to combat fatigue. After the war their use spread. Students, nightshift workers and long-distance drivers found that they could stay awake and alert more easily with their help; athletes used them to increase their performance, while doctors prescribed them both to lift the mood of depressed patients and to help would-be slimmers.

Towards the end of the sixties many young multi-drug-users took to amfetamines and then discovered that their effects could be enormously increased (and distorted) if they were taken intravenously instead of orally. Such amfetamine use was known as a 'speed trip'.

But patients who took amfetamines in this way for 'kicks' sometimes experienced truly disastrous adverse effects. They became paranoid and extremely aggressive; they developed the symptoms of full-blown schizophrenia, together with physical ill-effects such as chest and abdominal pains, and fainting. Chronic users developed sores and ulcers, infections, liver damage, high blood pressure and sometimes bleeding into the brain. Users who developed bad effects ('bad trips') became known in their own drug-taking subculture as 'speed freaks', and the drug underworld itself turned against amfetamine use with such slogans as 'speed kills'. Over a period of a very few years there was a drastic reduction in the medical use of these drugs and their non-medical use. Unfortunately in recent years their non-medical use is beginning to rise again.

Tolerance develops to the amfetamines, to the adverse effects as well as the mood effects. Addicts may use hundreds of milligrams in a day – far above the dose that would kill an ordinary patient.

The type of physical dependence caused by these drugs is not fully understood. Withholding the drug from a chronic user does not produce the florid withdrawal symptoms of, say, alcohol or the barbiturates. Indeed it was claimed for years that the amfetamines produced no physical dependence and were therefore 'non-addictive'. But withdrawal does produce a marked 'let-down' effect, showing itself in extreme fatigue, lengthy sleep, increased appetite, depression and changes in electrical brain traces (electroencephalograph).

Narcotic (Opiate, Opioid) Pain-relievers (Opium, Morphine, Heroin, etc.)

Morphine and opiate pain-relievers are discussed in Chapter 30. The term 'narcotic' includes opiate drugs which are obtained from, or are pharmacologically related to, drugs obtained from the opium poppy plant, *Papaver somniferum*, but see p. 153.

The use of opium and opiate drugs goes back over thousands and thousands of years. The subjective effects produced by them vary considerably among individuals and in different situations. What may produce a warm feeling of peace in one person may produce nausea, drowsiness, lethargy, dizziness and mood changes in another. They reduce the desire for sex and food and reduce aggression. Some regular users may lead 'normal' lives, for example, doctors or other professionals with comparatively easy access to drugs; others may become social outcasts or steal to get the money to buy drugs on the black market.

Tolerance to the various effects of narcotics develops when the drugs are used frequently so that the addict who seeks a 'kick' or 'high' has continuously to increase the dose in order to achieve the same effects. In this way addicts may tolerate doses far in excess of those which would be tolerated by non-addicts. However, tolerance is not the same for the different effects produced by these drugs; for example, an addict who may tolerate very high doses of morphine may still show the small pupils and constipation which a non-addict would show with a 'normal' dose.

The development of physical dependence on narcotics is related to the size and frequency of dose taken, the length of time over which it is used, the particular drug and the personality of the user. In some individuals, regular use of small doses over even a few days (perhaps following a painful accident) can cause some degree of physical dependence. Others in similar circumstances would not notice when the drug was withdrawn provided that the pain it was given for had eased.

The severity of withdrawal symptoms is therefore closely related to all these factors. A patient who has been taking large doses of codeine for years is likely to have physical withdrawal symptoms if he or she stops. A baby born of a narcotic-dependent mother will be physically dependent and may die if his or her acute withdrawal symptoms are not recognized. The physically dependent person whose drugs are withdrawn will experience an overwhelming desire to obtain more. If he or she is unsuccessful his or her first withdrawal symptoms will include watery eyes, a running nose, yawning, sweating, restlessness and sleep. Later he or she will become irritable, develop tremors, sneeze and yawn continuously while nose and eyes run copiously. Later still there will be weakness, depression, nausea, vomiting, diarrhoea, chilliness, sweating, abdominal cramps, pain in the back and legs and kicking movements. At this stage the skin is cold and covered with gooseflesh, giving rise to the name 'cold turkey'. Without treatment these symptoms burn themselves out in seven to ten days. But at any point they can be dramatically reversed by giving a dose of any narcotic, since cross-dependence occurs between them all.

This cross-dependence is the basis for the commonly used methadone treatment of heroin and other opiate dependences. Methadone is long-lasting so that withdrawal effects are slow to develop and are less severe compared with heroin, etc.

1

Sleeping Drugs

Sleep

Sleep requirements vary from person to person and so 'normal' sleep is what suits you under ordinary everyday circumstances. The amount of sleep you need is as much a part of you as your appetite or your conscience. If your sleep is disturbed for only a night or two, this is usually of no consequence; but if the disturbance persists for two or more weeks then you have a sleep problem, and need to take action.

Insomnia really means sleeplessness, but nowadays it is used to describe most sleeping difficulties. These include difficulty in getting off to sleep, inability to stay asleep, frequent wakenings, restless sleep – often with nightmares, early morning wakening, and sleep which is not refreshing (you wake up and continue to feel as exhausted as you did when you went to bed).

There are many causes of sleep disturbance – these may be environmental, physical or mental. Among environmental causes are changes such as a strange bed or bedroom, changes in temperature, noise, motion, and changes of routine like going on night work. Pain from any cause, irritation of the skin, discomfort from indigestion and muscle cramps are some of the physical causes of disturbed sleep. Emotional disorders are a common cause of persistent insomnia. However, remember that environmental, physical and mental factors are all interrelated. Problems at work may produce anxiety which may produce insomnia. Persistent noise at night may interfere with sleep which may cause you to worry about lack of sleep, which may then produce tension and irritability resulting in further difficulty in sleeping. The death of a close friend or relative, the loss of a job, failure at work or in an examination may trigger off psychological symptoms, a prominent one of which may be disturbed sleep.

Insomnia must always be regarded as a symptom of some underlying environmental, physical or mental disorder. This is of particular importance in emotional disorders, especially in those patients who feel anxious, tense and/or miserable. In such patients insomnia may be only one of a group of mental and/or physical symptoms which they may experience. Therefore, it is inappropriate to take sleeping drugs as the only form of treatment.

Some drugs can cause insomnia. For example, caffeine in tea and coffee may keep you awake, particularly as you get older. Regular alcohol drinkers may find themselves waking early and people who take heroin or morphine may find their sleep impaired. Amfetamines, most slimming drugs, and some anti-depressant drugs may keep you awake. So may certain drugs used to treat nasal catarrh, colds and asthma.

We really know very little about sleep and its function. It is related to various anatomical structures in the brain and to certain chemical changes. It produces electrical changes in the brain, eyes and muscles. These can be measured by electrical tracings of muscles (electromyograph, EMG), eye movements (electro-oculograph, EOG) and brain waves (electroencephalograph, EEG). From these tests two main kinds of 'normal' sleep activity have been defined: a stage of non-rapid eye movements (NREM sleep) which is followed by a stage of rapid eye movements (REM sleep). NREM sleep is called orthodox sleep and is the stage when we 'think'; REM sleep is called paradoxical sleep and is the stage when we 'dream'. It seems that both stages of sleep are essential for health.

Sleeping Drugs

These drugs depress brain function; in small doses they are used as sedatives (to calm you down) and in larger doses as hypnotics (to send you to sleep).

Dependence (see p. xxv) Sleeping drugs are drugs of dependence and you can become psychologically and physically dependent upon them. The insomnia, nightmares, dreaming and restless sleep which results when you stop these drugs may strengthen your belief that you need to go on taking them, but you should realize that your disturbed sleep is caused by withdrawal symptoms due to physical dependence on the drugs. Other symptoms of withdrawal which indicate physical dependence include anxiety, trembling, weakness and dizziness.

Tolerance may develop to sleeping drugs within three–fourteen days of starting them. This means that you will get less effect from the same dose over time and therefore there is always the danger that you may increase the dose in order to obtain the same effects. With some of these drugs there may also be an increased breakdown in the liver, producing a decreased sleeping time and an increase in the average dose required to maintain sleep so that you start to wake earlier. Nevertheless, it is surprising how many patients stay on these drugs for years and years without increasing the dose. Even so, tolerance is a danger and if you find yourself having to increase the dose of your sleeping drug to get the same effect, then consult your doctor – you are in danger of becoming addicted.

If you drink alcohol regularly you ought not to take these drugs regularly. This is because alcohol is also a depressant of the brain and tolerance may develop to alcohol. It is quite easy to take an overdose of either and the combination may be fatal. Do not forget, therefore, that although you may be able to tolerate an increased dose of alcohol or sleeping drug the lethal dose of these drugs remains unaltered so that their combination can rapidly prove fatal. Another important point to remember is that sleeping drugs can actually make you anxious, irritable and depressed in the daytime. An increased dose will actually make you worse. This also applies to alcohol, so remember if you are getting anxious and miserable despite taking more alcohol and/or sleeping drugs, it is the drugs that are producing this effect. Many people have become trapped on this downward course which may end in suicide.

Like alcohol, sleeping drugs cause intoxication if taken in a dosage above that normally recommended. Further, elderly and debilitated patients and patients with impaired heart, kidney or liver function may develop intoxication at 'normal' dosage. Signs of intoxication are similar to those of alcohol – confusion, difficulty in speaking, unsteadiness on the feet, poor memory, faulty judgement, irritability, over-emotion, hostility, suspiciousness and suicidal tendencies.

The deliberate taking of an overdose with suicidal intent accounts for most cases of overdose, but accidentally self-administered overdose may occur. If you take a dose of sleeping drug and fail to fall asleep you may reach out and take another dose. The effects of this increased dose may make you confused and you may take further doses without knowing (or remembering sub-sequently). Therefore, never keep sleeping drugs by your bedside, keep them locked in a drug cupboard. Only take the recommended dose and leave the bottle in the locked cupboard. If you are responsible for, or live with, someone who is elderly, debilitated or depressed, and on sleeping drugs, then supervise their administration.

Do not forget that if you are tense or miserable, alcohol and sleeping drugs, although helping you at first, may eventually make you feel worse. You may sleep all right and awake feeling less tense, only to become tired, irritable and bad-tempered later in the day. One more important point to remember about these drugs (especially alcohol) is that they may reduce the effects of antidepressant drugs.

Sleeping drugs impair learned behaviour and interfere with your power to concentrate, therefore watch your driving. These drugs depress a wide range of functions in many vital organs, particularly nerves, muscles, respiration, and the heart and circulation. They may produce any state from mild sedation to confusion and unconsciousness. Like alcohol they may produce different effects according to the situation in which they are taken. At a discotheque they may produce excitement, while if taken on retiring to bed they may produce sleep. The combination of a strange environment (e.g. admission to a hospital ward) and a dose of sleeping drug may make elderly patients confused and disorientated. This is a warning against the habit of giving patients sleeping drugs as a routine just because they are in hospital; it is often not necessary and may lead to the development of a sleeping-drug habit when the patient returns home.

Do not forget that sleep produced by drugs is not natural. It may be appropriate to take sleeping drugs for a night or two during periods of stress (e.g. after a bereavement) or after periods of intense work when you just cannot relax, or intermittently through long periods of stress or when travelling overnight or working shifts. In such circumstances they should only be taken for a few nights in a row, because it is accepted that the sleeping-drug habit is a real risk after several nights of drug-induced sleep. If you have a persistent sleep problem, then you ought to consult your doctor. But, of course, it does little good if you get a quick consultation and a prescription for sleeping drugs with instructions to get further prescriptions from the receptionist when you need them. Do not forget that emotional problems are a common cause of sleep disturbance and these may produce many symptoms in addition to insomnia; for example, frequent headaches, feeling anxious or tense, sad, depressed or tearful, backaches, pains in the chest, indigestion, dizziness, no energy, feeling fed up, feeling irritable, fears about your health or about going out by yourself, loss of appetite, loss of interest in sex, loss of weight, palpitations, feelings of guilt, feeling not wanted or feeling that other people are talking about you. These are only some of the group of symptoms which should help your doctor diagnose a psychological disorder and organize appropriate treatment.

If you have a psychological disorder, the use of sleeping drugs may aggravate your condition, especially if you are feeling sad or miserable. It is important to recognize what are labelled as 'depressive symptoms'. These include characteristic sleep disturbances, and antidepressant drugs may be effective in relieving them. This again highlights the importance of the initial treatment of insomnia. You and your doctor need to consider together as many as possible of the factors which may be causing your insomnia.

What about those patients who have developed the habit of taking sleeping drugs every night? They are often elderly and many of them live alone or in residential homes. I think it would be wrong to give them guilt feelings about being on drugs but it may be advisable to wean them gradually off sleeping drugs, particularly if they are depressed, anxious or tense, drink alcohol regularly, show signs of intoxication or have impaired kidney, heart or liver function.

Breaking the Sleeping-drug Habit

If you have been taking sleeping drugs nightly for weeks, months or years and wish to stop them you must reduce the dose very slowly over many weeks and therefore it is better to consult your doctor, who will be able to advise you. A gradual reduction in dosage may enable you to break a long-lasting sleeping-drug habit. Even so, you are bound to have restless nights until your brain gets used to sleep without drugs – this may take several weeks or months.

In the treatment of insomnia there are many alternatives to sleeping drugs, such as a hot bath before retiring, reading a book, taking a walk, not having too large an evening meal, cutting down on coffee, tea or cocoa in the evening, reducing smoking, reducing alcohol intake, trying to get some regular exercise and fresh air during the day and probably most important of all – being taught how to relax. The ritual just before going to bed may condition you to go to sleep – undressing, washing, etc. A milk-cereal drink may help you sleep more peacefully. A warm drink and a biscuit often helps the older patient to get off to sleep and, of course, patients with pain, discomfort and irritation of the skin need more specific treatment, as do those with other physical or psychological symptoms.

Sleeping Drugs

- *Benzodiazepines*

*Long-acting (six–ten hours):
  flunitrazepam (Rohypnol)
  flurazepam (Dalmane)
  nitrazepam (Mogadon, Remnos, Somnite)
Short-acting (up to six hours):
  loprazolam (Dormonoct)
  lormetazepam
  temazepam

- *Other Sleeping Drugs*
  chloral hydrate (Welldorm elixir)
  clomethiazole (Heminevrin)
  cloral betaine (Welldorm tablets)
  triclofos
  zaleplon (Sonata)
  zolpidem (Stilnoct)
  zopiclone (Zimovane)

* Note: Long-acting preparations in normal doses may produce hangover effects the next day, especially in the elderly. These long-acting drugs can accumulate in the body and cause elderly patients to become confused and unsteady, particularly on their feet. This may cause them to fall and injure themselves.

● *Sedative Antihistamines*
  diphenhydramine (**Medinex, Nytol**)
  promethazine (**Phenergan, Sominex**)

● *Barbiturates*
  amobarbital (**Amytal**)
  amobarbital (**Sodium Amytal**)
     with secobarbital (**Tuinal**)
  butobarbital (**Soneryl**)
  secobarbital sodium (**Seconal Sodium**)

Benzodiazepines are discussed in Chapter 2. They are the most commonly used sleeping drugs. Because of the risk of dependency they should only be used to treat insomnia that is causing distress and should only be taken nightly for no more than two to three weeks. It is best to take them intermittently.

Chloral hydrate (**Welldorm elixir**) is the oldest sleeping drug. It tastes horrible, irritates the stomach, causes hangover effects and is dangerous in overdose.

Trichlorethanol is the active breakdown product of chloral hydrate and a stable form of this is available as **triclofos elixir**. It irritates the stomach less than chloral hydrate. Another preparation with effects similar to chloral hydrate is **cloral betaine** (**Welldorm tablets**) which is broken down in the body to chloral hydrate. Contrary to what is often claimed, chloral hydrate is not of especial use in elderly people. Very occasionally it may be used in children.

Clomethiazole (**Heminevrin**) has a short duration of action and may occasionally be useful in elderly patients who easily suffer from hangover effects with longer-lasting drugs, but there is a risk of dependence and dangerous effects with alcohol.

Zaleplon (**Sonata**), **zolpidem** (**Stilnoct**) and **zopiclone** (**Zimovane**) act like the benzodiazepines, but are more sedative in their actions on sleep mechanisms. They are short-acting and act very rapidly with little or no hangover effect. They may be used to help patients who have difficulty getting to sleep, or who wake in the night and cannot get back to sleep. They should be taken nightly for no more than two to three weeks. Preferably, they should only be taken intermittently.

Sedative antihistamine drugs (see above) in addition to their antihistamine effects produce drowsiness as a side-effect and this is sometimes used to promote sleep. They may be useful for promoting sleep in patients with skin irritations or allergic symptoms.

There are dangers in using them to treat insomnia because sleep cannot be improved just by increasing the dose. Rather, the reverse happens and after a large dose, excitation occurs which may result in restlessness and agitation. Sedative antihistamines have a long duration of action and may produce hangover effects the next day. Some experts consider that it is not appropriate to use them as sleeping drugs.

Barbiturates produce tolerance, psychological dependence, physical dependence and withdrawal symptoms (see p. xxvii); they increase the action of alcohol and they were a common agent in accidental or intentional overdose. The signs of intoxication are similar to those produced by alcohol. They are involved in complex chemical processes in the liver which may affect the effectiveness of other drugs. In patients suffering from a disease called porphyria (a rare congenital metabolic disease) they can trigger off an acute attack resulting in abdominal colic, paralysis, confusion and even death.

Barbiturates and their salts should only be used very occasionally to induce sleep.

Remember: All sleeping drugs and sedatives depress brain function and they may produce tolerance and dependence, increase the effects of alcohol, interfere with ability to drive motor vehicles and operate moving machinery, and produce intoxication like alcohol. They may produce hangover effects the next day especially in elderly patients who may become confused and unsteady on their feet and may fall and injure themselves.

Sleeping drugs should only be used occasionally. They should not be taken every night for more than two to three weeks because of the risk of withdrawal effects and dependence.

2

Drugs Used to Treat Anxiety

Drugs used to treat anxiety are referred to as *anti-anxiety drugs or anxiolytics*. Sometimes they are referred to as anxiolytic-sedatives, sedatives, tranquillizers or minor tranquillizers. The most frequently used group of anti-anxiety drugs is the benzodiazepines. They are also the most frequently used type of sleeping drug (*see previous chapter*).

Benzodiazepines

The benzodiazepines have four main uses – to induce sleep, to relieve anxiety, to relax skeletal muscles and to treat epilepsy.

Benzodiazepines Used to Treat Anxiety

Intermediate-acting:
    bromazepam (Lexotan)
    chlordiazepoxide (Librium, Tropium)
    lorazepam (Ativan)
    oxazepam
Long-acting:
    alprazolam (Xanax)
    clobazam (Frisium)
    clorazepate dipotassium (Tranxene)
    diazepam (Dialar, Diazemuls, Rimapam, Stesolid,Tensium, Valclair, Valium)

Common adverse effects produced by benzodiazepines include drowsiness, light-headedness, and loss of control over voluntary movements (ataxia). (See A–Z of Medicines.) They should be used in the smallest possible effective dose for the shortest possible duration of time.

Warnings

Benzodiazepines should be used with the utmost caution in *pregnancy*. The use of high doses during labour or prolonged use of daily doses in the last three months of pregnancy may depress breathing and cause floppy limbs and poor sucking in newborn babies for a few days, and occasionally withdrawal symptoms.

They should not be taken regularly by breastfeeding mothers because they may produce lethargy and weight loss in the baby, and they should not be used in patients with severe phobias or obsessional illness or to treat depression or serious mental illness (e.g. schizophrenia).

The dose of benzodiazepines should be reduced in patients with long-standing kidney or liver disease and in patients with severe, long-standing chest diseases such as chronic bronchitis and emphysema.

They can reduce ability to carry out skilled tasks so that they can affect the ability to drive motor vehicles and operate moving machinery. They can increase the effects of alcohol.

Benzodiazepines should be used with great caution in elderly patients because of the risks, particularly of confusion and unsteadiness on their feet (ataxia) which may lead to falls. Elderly patients should be given no more than half the normal recommended daily dose for adults.

These drugs can produce opposite effects (paradoxical effects) in some people. Instead of acting as 'downers', they act as 'uppers', and the patients become excited, aggressive and confused. Underlying depression may be triggered and the patient might become suicidal.

They can increase the effects of other drugs which depress brain function (e.g. sleeping drugs, antidepressants, pain-relievers and anaesthetics). These effects when given with other drugs can be dangerous in elderly patients. They can increase the adverse effects associated with some anticonvulsant drugs, e.g. hydantoins and barbiturates.

Addiction to Benzodiazepines

The benzodiazepines are 'downers', they calm you down and send you to sleep. But you may develop tolerance to them, cross-dependence with other depressants of the brain (e.g. sleeping drugs, alcohol) or addiction (see p. xxvii).

Benzodiazepine Withdrawal Symptoms

A substantial number of individuals who have taken a benzodiazepine regularly every day for more than two to three weeks will experience some withdrawal effects if they stop the drug abruptly, particularly if they have been using higher than average doses. They may experience a few or many of the following symptoms: increased anxiety, tension and panic, depression and feelings of suicide, irritability and outbursts of rage, overactivity and poor concentration, poor sleep and unpleasant and sometimes terrifying dreams, headaches, nausea and loss of appetite, a metallic taste in the mouth, palpitations, trembling, faintness, dizziness and sweating, flu-like symptoms, tight chest and pains in the stomach, pain and stiffness in the jaw, face, head, neck and shoulders. They may become aware of sensations in their body, for example, creeping sensations in the skin, and they may become very sensitive to light, noise, touch and smell. They may get strange feelings of movement, feel depersonalized as if they are not themselves, feel unreal as if they are in a dream and develop a fear of going out. Their arms and legs may feel heavy and wobbly and they may develop pins and needles in them.

These symptoms may occur within a few hours of stopping a short-acting benzodiazepine, two–three days after stopping an intermediate-acting, and about seven–twenty-one days after stopping a long-acting one. Symptoms usually last from one–three weeks, but may go on for months.

Rebound Anxiety on Stopping Benzodiazepines

Rebound anxiety may be a serious problem after stopping benzodiazepines. The individual may develop panic attacks which are so severe that he or she may become housebound and never want to go out for fear of developing an attack. During an attack, breathing may become rapid, the heart may beat quickly, and there may be light-headedness and dizziness. Sweating and trembling may occur and the legs may go like jelly. A feeling of complete panic may develop, as if something totally catastrophic is going to happen. These attacks only last for a few seconds and nothing *does* happen, but the individual is left feeling totally exhausted. Many of these symptoms may be caused by rapid breathing and there is no doubt that controlled breathing (from the abdomen) may stop most of them from developing.

How to Withdraw Benzodiazepines

If you have been taking benzodiazepines regularly every day for weeks, months or years and wish to stop the drug with a minimum of withdrawal symptoms, it is important to reduce the daily dose of your drug slowly (e.g. every two weeks) and to be prepared to experience a few or many symptoms in varying degrees of intensity. It may take you weeks, months or even a year to be able to stop your drug completely without developing unpleasant symptoms. If you are on an intermediate-acting benzodiazepine it is important that you switch to a long-acting one such as diazepam and take the full dose at bedtime.

In addition to switching to diazepam and then reducing the daily dose by

2.0 to 2.5 mg every two weeks, you will need advice and counselling from your doctor or other health-care worker, particularly a clinical psychologist. You may also find it useful to attend a self-help group.

If withdrawal symptoms occur, maintain the dose until symptoms improve and then start to reduce again but more slowly. Remember the time needed to withdraw from benzodiazepines may take anything from four weeks to over a year. Beta-blockers should only be tried if other measures fail. Avoid antipsychotic drugs because these may worsen benzodiazepine withdrawal symptoms. Antidepressants should only be used if clinically depressed. Equivalent doses of benzodiazepines are diazepam (5 mg), chlordiazepoxide (15 mg), loprazolam (0.5–1 mg), lorazepam (0.5 mg), lormetazepam (0.5–1 mg), nitrazepam (5 mg), oxazepam (15 mg) and temazepam (10 mg).

Benzodiazepines should be used only for the short-term (two–four weeks) relief of anxiety that is interfering with an individual's ability to cope with the everyday stresses and strains of living. Do not use to relieve mild anxiety.

Miscellaneous Drugs Used to Treat Anxiety

Barbiturates (**Amytal**, **Sodium Amytal**, **Soneryl**, **Seconal Sodium**, **Tuinal**) are much more dangerous than benzodiazepines in overdosage and have produced many deaths, particularly when taken with alcohol. *They should not be used to treat anxiety.*

Meprobamate (in **Equagesic**) is less effective than the benzodiazepines. It carries a higher risk of drug dependence and is more dangerous in overdose. It produces more adverse effects and has no benefit over the benzodiazepines.

Antipsychotic drugs are occasionally used to treat severe, acute anxiety. **Oxypertine**, **fluphenazine** (**Moditen**, in **Motipress**, in **Motival**), and **trifluoperazine** (**Stelazine**) may occasionally be used to treat anxiety/depression.

Beta-adrenoceptor blocking drugs (**Beta-blockers**) are discussed in detail on p. 114. They are useful for relieving physical symptoms of anxiety such as palpitations, sweating, nervous stomach symptoms and tremor. Betareceptor blockers used to treat anxiety include **oxprenolol** (e.g. **Trasicor**) and **propranolol** (e.g. **Inderal**).

Buspirone (**Buspar**) is an anti-anxiety drug not related to the benzodiazepines. It produces less sedation than the benzodiazepines and there is no cross-tolerance with them. It takes up to two weeks to produce beneficial effects.

Hydroxyzine (**Atarax**, **Ucerax**) is an antihistamine used very occasionally, but inappropriately, to relieve anxiety.

3

Drugs Used to Treat Psychoses and Related Disorders

Antipsychotic Drugs

These drugs are used to control acute symptoms and to prevent relapse in patients suffering from schizophrenia and mania. They are also used to treat acute confusional states and to treat certain symptoms produced by dementia and brain damage. In addition they may be prescribed (in small doses) for the treatment of anxiety, tension and agitation and some of them are used to treat dizziness, nausea and vomiting (see Chapter 18).

They are called **antipsychotic drugs** but were previously referred to as major tranquillizers. They may also produce a state of emotional quietness and indifference called neurolepsy and hence they are sometimes called **neuroleptics**.

Antipsychotic Drugs

amisulpride (**Solian**)
benperidol (**Anquil**)
chlorpromazine (**Chloractil, Largactil**)
clozapine (**Clozaril**)
flupentixol (**Depixol**)
fluphenazine (**Moditen**)
haloperidol (**Dozic, Haldol, Serenace**)
levomepromazine (**Nozinan**)
loxapine (**Loxapac**)
olanzapine (**Zyprexa**)
periciazine (**Neulactil**)
perphenazine (**Fentazin**, in **Triptafen**)
pimozide (**Orap**)

prochlorperazine (**Stemetil**)
promazine, sulpiride (**Dolmatil, Sulparex, Sulpitil**)
quetiapine (**Seroquel**)
risperidone (**Risperdal**)
thioridazine (**Melleril**)
trifluoperazine (**Stelazine**)
zotepine (**Zoleptil**)
zuclopenthixol (**Clopixol**)

● *Depot Injections*
flupentixol decanoate* (**Depixol**)
fluphenazine decanoate* (**Modecate**)
haloperidol decanoate* (**Haldol Decanoate**)
pipotiazine palmitate* (**Piportil Depot**)
zuclopenthixol decanoate* (**Clopixol**)

* Indicates that the long-acting form of the drug is used.

These compounds are similar in their effects and uses. They calm a person down without affecting consciousness and without producing paradoxical excitement. By blocking dopamine activity (see p. 40) they produce changes in all parts of the nervous system. They may cause involuntary movements such as tremor, dystonias (abnormal face and body movements), akathisia (restlessness), tardive dyskinesia (involuntary movements of jaws, tongue, face, lips and limbs) and parkinsonism. The blocking of dopamine activity also affects the pituitary gland leading to an increased production of the milk-producing hormone (prolactin) which results in enlargement of the breasts (gynaecomastia) and milk production (galactorrhoea) in males and females. By causing dilatation of the blood vessels in the skin and by acting on control centres in the brain they may cause the body to cool (hypothermia), affect the heart and lower blood pressure. These effects can be dangerous in the elderly. They may increase the effects of all depressant drugs – alcohol, hypnotics, sedatives and anaesthetics.

They control over-active and manic patients without impairing consciousness. They relieve many symptoms of schizophrenia and modify behaviour. They calm agitation and are useful in the treatment of drug- or disease-induced vomiting but they are of no value in treating motion sickness.

Antipsychotic drugs differ in the amount of sedation they produce, in their effects upon blood pressure, and in the production of adverse effects such as parkinsonism and movement disorders. The use of these drugs depends upon balancing the benefits with the risks. The choice of drug depends upon the degree of sedation required and consideration of the wide variation in response which may be expected between patients, particularly to adverse effects. The antipsychotic drugs therefore differ in the predominance of the effects they produce and in their adverse effects. Parkinsonism adverse effects may be suppressed by anticholinergic drugs (see p. 78), but they make tardive dyskinesia worse and should not be used routinely.

Antipsychotic drugs are valuable in the treatment of schizophrenia and have enabled patients to be treated in the community rather than being locked away in psychiatric hospitals. They are not curative but they do relieve distressing symptoms such as thought disturbances, paranoid symptoms, hallucinations, delusions, loss of self-care, social withdrawal, anxiety and agitation. Patients may need to take a daily maintenance dose for many years because it has been observed that failure to take a regular dose may lead to relapse, necessitating referral to hospital.

Clozapine (**Clozaril**) and **olanzapine** (**Zyprexa**) relieve both the positive symptoms of schizophrenia (e.g. paranoia and hallucinations) and the negative symptoms (poverty of speech, thought disorder and depression). The other antipsychotic drugs are generally more successful against the positive symptoms of the disease.

The effects of withdrawing antipsychotic drugs should be carefully monitored because of the serious risk of relapse. Therefore it is important that patients are seen regularly by a psychiatrist, particularly when it is realized that relapse may take from two to eight weeks after stopping the drugs.

● Depot Injections

Long-lasting injections of antipsychotic drugs are used as maintenance treatment because it is one way of ensuring that the patient takes the required dose. However, the risk of adverse effects such as parkinsonism are greater than with oral treatment and patients must be seen regularly by a psychiatrist. Also, adverse effects may take up to a month to clear up after depot injections have been stopped.

● Antipsychotic Drugs and Depression

Some antipsychotic drugs also have antidepressant effects, e.g. chlorpromazine, thioridazine and flupentixol, whereas others can make depression worse, e.g. fluphenazine, pimozide and pipothiazine.

4

Antidepressant Drugs

Depression

Antidepressant drugs are prescribed to patients who are 'labelled' by their doctors as suffering from 'depression'. But what is depression? We can all feel sad or happy and some of us at times may feel very happy or very sad. These feelings are part of everyday life, so why do doctors talk about depression and why do some patients need drugs? Why can't they 'just pull themselves together'? The fact is that many patients who go to their doctors for help have got sick of trying to pull themselves together. They may complain of various mental and/or physical symptoms and not feel or recognize they are suffering from a psychological disorder.

Of course it is impossible to separate social, physical and mental factors, but it is possible to recognize a group of symptoms which, for want of a better label, doctors call 'depression'. Admittedly there is a continuum from feeling blue to feeling severely depressed and suicidal, and from feeling tired and fed up to possessing symptoms which totally interfere with your capacity to cope with your everyday life. If you feel sad and miserable for long periods, then this is not just 'feeling blue'. There can be many reasons for depression: social factors – for example, unemployment or bereavement; physical factors – after virus infections such as influenza, because of continuous pain, irritation or discomfort and after surgery or a heart attack. Women may feel severely depressed after childbirth, during the menopause or just before a period; vitamin deficiencies can also make you feel depressed; but you may also be severely depressed for no obvious reason.

Along with feelings of depression (sad, miserable, weepy, suicidal) patients may develop changes in behaviour. They may stop wanting to mix socially and start staying at home in the evenings. They may develop physiological changes such as alterations in sleep rhythm (particularly difficulty in getting off to sleep or early morning wakening), alteration in appetite, weight or sex drive, and loss of energy. They may develop physical symptoms; for example, headaches, dizziness, chest pains, palpitations, dyspepsia, diarrhoea and backache. These symptoms may make them worry about physical disease so that they become hypochondriacal and think they have a cancer, or heart disease. They may develop mental symptoms and feel unreal, divorced from themselves, as if they are looking from outside at themselves; they may have difficulty in concentrating; in thinking; their memory may be affected and they may keep thinking morbid thoughts about death, dying and suicide. They may become very tense and anxious (as if something dreadful is going to happen all the time). Some develop fears (e.g. fear of seeing people; fear of going out). They may become very agitated and irritable or very withdrawn and quiet. Some become obsessive, having to do things over and over again, and some feel guilty. They may recall all sorts of things from their past lives.

This has been a very sketchy description of what doctors label as depression. Patients may experience a few or many of these symptoms. Some symptoms may be mild and some intense, and according to all sorts of factors in upbringing, culture, personality and environment, the person will react in different ways. Certainly in Western society the puritan ethic of 'being firm and standing on one's own two feet' may produce awful feelings of guilt and unworthiness in which suicide appears to be the only way out. The whole problem is far too complex to be simply labelled 'depression'.

The Use of Drugs to Treat Depression

The antidepressant drugs introduced since 1958 have greatly improved the treatment of depression. This has resulted in an impressive relief from suffering in many patients and their relatives, a reduction in hospitalization and in electroconvulsive treatments, and an increasing involvement of family doctors in the treatment of disorders of this kind. We must remember that they do not 'cure', but they provide relief from distressing symptoms until such time as the underlying 'disorder' resolves itself – which happens in the vast majority of patients. Doctors prescribe these drugs because within a few weeks of treatment, crippling symptoms may be relieved and the patient is able to cope – sleep improves, energy and appetite return, interests return, the mood lifts and the person may begin to see how dreadful life has felt for months or years. The process of rebuilding one's life can begin. Here is the crunch for doctors; having relieved the patient's symptoms they must not forget to treat the patient. The duration of treatment may be short or long and may need the help of a clinical psychologist or psychotherapist or psychiatrist; however, because the patient's symptoms are relieved there may be a much better response to such therapy. This does not mean that all depressed patients need drugs – the decision to use antidepressants should only be taken after careful consideration of all the facts by the doctor and a detailed discussion with the patient.

Some of us can tolerate physical pain better than others and some of us can tolerate mental pain better than others – but at some stage we all may need help. Some of us may respond better to one drug and not to another or to one doctor and not another. Some will respond to individual therapy and others to group therapy. We all vary and it is, therefore, wrong to say that all depressed patients should receive drug therapy and it is equally wrong to say they should all have psychotherapy. What is certain, however, is that doctors within the limits of their present knowledge must aim at giving maximum benefit with minimum risks to the maximum number of patients. At present, the responsible and rational use of drugs appears to offer the most hope in this direction.

Antidepressant Drugs

There are several groups of antidepressant drugs:

Tricyclic Antidepressants (TCADs)

These antidepressants share a basic structure which consists of three chemical rings. They include:
    amitriptyline (Elavil, Lentizol, in **Triptafen**, in **Triptafen-M)**
    amoxapine (Asendis)
    clomipramine (Anafranil)
    dosulepin/dothiepin (Dothapax, Prepadine, Prothiaden)
    doxepin (Sinequan)
    imipramine (Tofranil)
    lofepramine (Gamanil, Lomont)
    nortriptyline (Allegron, in **Motipress**, in **Motival)**
    trimipramine (Surmontil)

The manner in which tricyclic antidepressants relieve the symptoms of depression is not yet fully understood. However they may produce an increased quantity of stimulating nerve transmitters (i.e. noradrenaline(norepinephrine) and serotonin) at nerve endings by blocking their re-uptake into nerve cells, and they may produce a reduction in neurotransmitter receptors. They lift the mood but they do not produce a 'high'. They may cause anticholinergic effects (see Chapter 9) such as dryness of the mouth, constipation, difficulty in passing urine, blurred vision, palpitations and rapid heart beat. Because tricyclic antidepressants may affect the eyes they should be given with utmost caution to patients with glaucoma. Similarly, their effect upon the bladder makes caution necessary when using them in patients who have an enlarged prostate gland.

For adverse effects and precautions see A–Z of Medicines.

Tolerance develops to anticholinergic adverse effects such as dry mouth, blurred vision, etc. and within one or two weeks patients notice these symptoms less and less. At the same time their mental and physical symptoms start to disappear and they begin to feel better as each day goes by. This knowledge is important to anyone prescribing or taking antidepressant drugs because with some of them their beneficial effects are slow to develop (up to two or five weeks from starting), whereas anticholinergic effects come on straight away. Therefore, it helps if initial daily doses are low and are then increased gradually as adverse effects lessen.

The tricyclics are useful because they offer a choice of drug to treat different depressive symptoms. For example, clomipramine, imipramine, lofepramine and nortriptyline produce only mild sedation and are therefore used to treat depressed patients who are slow and withdrawn (melancholic). Amitriptyline, dosulepin(dothiepin), doxepin and trimipramine have a more pronounced sedative effect and are therefore useful for treating depressed patients who are tense, anxious or irritable. Protriptyline stimulates and is useful for severely withdrawn patients. Amitriptyline and trimipramine are particularly useful for patients with sleep disorders if the whole daily dose is given at night, as this helps to improve sleep.

Tetracyclic Antidepressants

These antidepressants have four rings (tetracyclic) and appear to act differently from the tricyclics.

Maprotiline (**Ludiomil**) mainly blocks the re-uptake of noradrenaline(norepinephrine). It produces fewer antimuscarinic effects, and effects on the heart, than the tricyclics. However, it may cause skin rashes and occasionally convulsions in high doses.

Mianserin increases the amount of the stimulant neuro-transmitters noradrenaline(norepinephrine) and serotonin in the brain. It produces fewer anticholinergic effects than the tricyclics (e.g. dry mouth, blurred vision, constipation) and fewer effects on the heart, but it may cause sedation and occasionally serious blood disorders. Rarely it may cause jaundice.

Selective Serotonin Re-uptake Inhibitors (SSRIs)

These antidepressant drugs block the mopping-up of the nerve transmitter serotonin. This results in an increase in the amount of serotonin at nerve junctions in the brain and nervous system. They are less sedative than the tricyclics and produce fewer adverse effects on the heart and fewer antimuscarinic effects. They include **citalopram** (**Cipramil**), **fluoxetine** (**Felicium**, **Prozac**), **fluvoxamine** (**Faverin**), **paroxetine** (**Seroxat**) and **sertraline** (**Lustral**).

Serotonin/Noradrenaline(Norepinephrine) Re-uptake Inhibitors (SNRIs)

Venlafaxine (**Efexor**) produces fewer adverse effects than the tricyclics. It has a rapid onset of action (within two–four weeks).

Selective Noradrenaline(Norepinephrine) Re-uptake Inhibitors (NARIs)

Reboxetine (**Edronax**) is a selective inhibitor of noradrenaline(norepinephrine) which produces fewer adverse effects because it has a selective action on inhibiting serotonin and noradrenaline(norepinephrine) re-uptake.

Noradrenaline(Norepinephrine) and Selective Serotonin Antagonists (NASSAs)

Mirtazapine (**Zispin**) increases central noradrenergic and serotonergic neurotransmission, it causes less sedation during initial treatment and produces fewer adverse effects such as anxiety, agitation and sexual dysfunction.

5HT$_2$ Antagonists

Nefazodone (**Dutonin**) inhibits re-uptake of serotonin and also blocks serotonin receptors. It helps sleep and has less effect on sexual function than the SSRIs.

Monoamine Oxidase Inhibitor Antidepressant Drugs (MAOIs)

Monoamine oxidases (MAO-A and MAO-B) are enzymes present in the intestine, liver and brain that break down a group of stimulant neurotransmitters known as catecholamines, e.g. adrenaline(epinephrine) and noradrenaline(norepinephrine). Monoamine oxidase inhibitors (MAOIs) irreversibly block these enzymes and, therefore, prolong the action of stimulant neurotransmitters. This action has a beneficial effect on the symptoms of depression in some people. However, their use has two major drawbacks – they also block the breakdown of other stimulant drugs and they can block the breakdown of stimulant chemicals in certain foods to produce serious harmful effects. (See A–Z of Medicines.)

Monoamine oxidase inhibitor drugs (MAOIs) include:
Isocarboxazid
phenelzine (**Nardil**)
tranylcypromine (**Parnate**)

● *The Dangers of MAOIs Blocking the Breakdown of Stimulant Drugs*

When monoamine oxidase is blocked, the body cannot break down naturally occurring stimulants such as adrenaline(epinephrine) and noradrenaline (norepinephrine); neither can it break down stimulant chemicals in medicines. MAOIs therefore increase the effects and dangers of stimulants such as sympathomimetic bronchodilator drugs used to treat asthma (e.g. isoprenaline, ephedrine); sympathomimetic drugs used as decongestants in cough and cold remedies (e.g. ephedrine, pseudoephedrine, phenylpropanolamine); amfetamine drugs used as stimulants and amfetamine-related drugs used to suppress the appetite and as stimulants (e.g. methylphenidate).

MAOIs also block the breakdown of dopamine, another stimulant nerve messenger, and if they are given with levodopa (a drug that is converted into dopamine by nerve cells and is used to treat parkinsonism) an excess level of dopamine may occur in the brain.

If an individual who is on MAOI treatment takes one of the above drugs a *hypertensive crisis* may occur. The blood pressure shoots up and the individual develops a severe headache, sweating, flushing, nausea, vomiting and palpitations. The rise in blood pressure may cause an artery in the brain to burst and bleed into the brain, which may cause death.

Severe reactions may also occur if an MAOI is taken with a tricyclic antidepressant, especially amitriptyline or imipramine. A combination of the MAOI tranylcypromine and the tricyclic clomipramine is particularly dangerous. Morphine and narcotic pain-relievers may interact with MAOIs to produce a serious reaction, especially pethidine, which may produce alarming effects that include flushing, sweating, restlessness, muscle rigidity, depression of breathing, a fall in blood pressure and coma.

MAOIs may also prolong and intensify the effects of general anaesthetics, antihistamines, antimuscarinic drugs, barbiturates and possibly other sleeping drugs, insulin and oral anti-diabetic drugs, and blood pressure lowering drugs such as methyldopa, reserpine and guanethidine.

● *The Dangers of MAOIs Blocking the Breakdown of Stimulant Chemicals in Food*

A most serious risk of MAOIs is that they can block the breakdown of stimulant chemicals in food and drink, for instance tyramine in cheese and Chianti and other stimulants in food (e.g. caffeine in chocolate and beverages and levodopa in broad bean pods). In someone who is receiving treatment with MAOIs these stimulants are not broken down in the intestine and liver and excessive amounts enter the main bloodstream and cause stimulation of the nervous system. This can produce a *hypertensive crisis* (see above).

The amount of tyramine in foods varies depending on their manufacture and storage, and the amount of tyramine taken into the body will depend on the amount of tyramine-containing foods that are eaten. Protein foods that have been fermented, pickled, smoked or have gone off contain an increased amount of tyramine.

Warning: *Stimulant drugs (see above) and foods and drinks containing stimulant chemicals should not be taken while on treatment with an MAOI and for two weeks after stopping such treatment.*

● MAOIs Should Be Used with Caution

MAOIs are potentially dangerous drugs because of the harmful effects they may produce when taken with certain other drugs and foods. However, they may produce improvement in some people who are severely incapacitated by their depressive symptoms and in whom no other drug treatment seems to work. In particular, individuals with atypical depression in which anxiety and physical symptoms may be dominant and people who have severe phobias (e.g. agoraphobia) may be greatly helped by these drugs.

Foods and drinks high in stimulants include:
- Pickled herring, liver, dry sausages (salami, pepperoni), game, broad bean pods (fava bean pods), flavoured textured vegetable proteins, cheese (cottage cheese and cream cheese are allowed), yoghurt, banana skins.
- Beers, lagers and wines – it is best to avoid all alcoholic drinks, including low-alcohol ones.
- Yeast extracts (e.g. Marmite), meat extracts (e.g. Bovril, Oxo).
- Large amounts of chocolate and drinks containing caffeine (tea, coffee, cola).
- Any foods that have undergone protein changes due to ageing, pickling, fermentation or smoking to improve flavour, particularly fish, meat, poultry and offal.

Medicines that contain stimulants include:
- *Over-the-counter medicines*: Cough and cold medicines; nasal decongestants; hayfever remedies; sinus remedies; asthma inhalant remedies; slimming remedies; 'pep' pills.
- *Prescription medicines*: Amfetamines; cocaine; methylphenidate and pemoline used as stimulants; dopamine and dopamine precursors (e.g. levodopa, used to treat parkinsonism); adrenaline(epinephrine), ephedrine and related bronchodilator sympathomimetic drugs used to treat asthma; phenylpropanolamine and other sympathomimetic drugs used in nasal decongestants, cold and cough remedies and hayfever preparations; methyldopa used to treat raised blood pressure; phenylalanine, an amino acid which is an essential constituent of the diet

and is used as a dietary supplement; tyrosine, an amino acid used as a dietary supplement.

Reversible, Selective MAOIs

Reversible, selective MAOIs such as **moclobemide** (**Manerix**) produce selective reversible effects on MAO-A. It produces fewer adverse effects, and a reduced risk of interaction with foods and drugs.

Other Antidepressant Drugs

Trazodone (**Molipaxin**) is an antidepressant that is not related to the tricyclic antidepressants. Its mode of action in relieving depression is not fully understood. It produces sedation and fewer antimuscarinic effects than the tricyclics. It is safer in overdose.

Flupenthixol (**Fluanxol**) is an antipsychotic drug which has antidepressant properties (see p. 12). It is useful in patients who are withdrawn and apathetic.

Tryptophan (**Optimax**) is an essential amino acid in the diet. It is a precursor of the stimulant nerve transmitter 5HT (or serotonin). On its own, combined with pyridoxine (vitamin B$_6$) or with another antidepressant, it was previously used to treat depression. However, tryptophan is now restricted to hospital use because of reports that products containing tryptophan may cause a serious disorder called oesinophilia-myalgia which results in fever, skin rashes, painful muscles, fluid retention and lung and nerve disorders.

Lithium salts (**Camcolit**, **Li-Liquid**, **Liskonum**, **Lithonate**, **Priadel**) are used to prevent and treat mania and manic-depression and to prevent recurrent depressive episodes in some people. Lithium competes with sodium salts in the body and changes the composition of the body fluids. It has a wide range of actions on nerve transmitters and nerves but it is not fully understood how it works. It is accumulative and adverse effects are related to dosage. When these appear the drug must be *stopped* immediately. Lithium should only be given under hospital supervision and weekly blood tests to estimate the plasma level should be carried out. When the dosage is stabilized these can be reduced to once every two to four weeks. Duration of treatment should preferably be for not more than three–five years because of a possible risk of kidney damage. Read the entry on lithium in A–Z of Medicines.

Carbamazepine (**Tegretol**) is used to treat epilepsy. It is also useful for preventing manic-depressive episodes in patients who do not respond to lithium.

Warning on the Use of Antidepressants: After about eight weeks of daily treatment with an antidepressant, suddenly stopping the drug may produce withdrawal effects that include nausea, vomiting and diarrhoea, chills, poor sleep, restlessness, panic attacks and over-excitability. Therefore, the daily dose of an antidepressant should be tapered off slowly over a period of at least two weeks. All types of antidepressant drugs may cause the blood potassium level to fall, particularly in elderly people. This may cause drowsiness, confusion and rarely convulsions.

Hypericum (**St John's Wort**) is widely used as a herbal antidepressant. How Hypericum works in the treatment of depression is unclear. Hypericum has been shown to have monoamine oxidase inhibiting activity; however, whether this is relevant in practice is currently unclear. Recently concern has been expressed about its unrestricted use, due to the number of interactions which are associated with it.

These include interactions with:

- *other antidepressants*: amitriptyline, citalopram, fluoxetine, fluvoxamine, nefazodone, paroxetine, sertraline, venlafaxine;
- *anticonvulsants:* carbamazepine, phenobarbitone, phenytoin;
- *antivirals:* delavirdine, efavirenz, indinavir, nelfinavir, nevirapine, ritonavir, saquinavir, zidovudine;
- also cyclosporin, digoxin, rizatriptan, theophylline, warfarin and oral contraceptives.

Care should be taken if you intend to take Hypericum. If you are in doubt, consult your doctor or pharmacist to see if it is safe for you to take Hypericum.

5

Stimulant Drugs – Tea, Coffee and Cola

Coffee contains the drug caffeine, plus certain oils; tea contains caffeine, theobromine and tannin; cola contains caffeine, and cocoa contains caffeine, theobromine and tannin. Caffeine is also present in numerous over-the-counter tonics, 'pick-me-ups', and pain-relievers. The drugs caffeine, theophylline and theobromine are usually referred to as xanthines because of their chemical structure. They produce stimulation of the nervous system, make the kidneys produce more urine, stimulate heart muscle, relax the muscles of the bronchial tubes and affect the blood pressure and circulation. Caffeine is used as a stimulant and theophylline in the treatment of bronchial spasm (e.g. asthma). The xanthines also possess other properties which affect the heart and circulation; they increase the blood supply to the heart, dilate blood vessels in the skin, and constrict blood vessels which supply the brain. Theobromine produces fewer of these effects than caffeine or theophylline.

Caffeine

The use of caffeine (e.g. a strong cup of tea or coffee) to wake you up or to help you after a hangover is well founded. Caffeine stimulates the brain and all parts of the central nervous system. It stops you feeling tired and makes you think clearly. It lessens fatigue and increases muscular power to do physical work. After a dose of caffeine typists are said to type faster and with fewer mistakes. The dose of caffeine to produce stimulation varies from 100–300 mg. The final caffeine content of a cup of tea or coffee varies according to how strong a person likes the drink. The average caffeine content in a cup of tea is 40–100 mg, in coffee 80–100 mg and in cocoa 5 mg per cup. An average cola drink contains 35–55 mg of caffeine.

The effects of caffeine vary from person to person but a dose of 1,000 mg or over will produce adverse effects such as difficulty in sleeping, restlessness, excitement, trembling, rapid beating of the heart with extra beats, increased breathing, desire to pass water, ringing in the ears and flashes of light in front of the eyes. Caffeine increases the production of acid in the stomach and therefore patients with indigestion or stomach ulcers should restrict the amount of tea, coffee, cola or cocoa that they drink. They should preferably drink their tea or coffee with meals and add milk to the drinks. The oils in coffee may cause irritation of the intestine and the tannin in tea may produce constipation.

Psychological dependence and tolerance to caffeine obviously develop and it must be accepted that the majority of us are dependent upon our daily supply of tea and/or coffee, cocoa or cola.

Warning: Abrupt withdrawal of caffeine may be associated with headaches and other nervous symptoms which are relieved by taking caffeine. High caffeine intake should be reduced significantly during pregnancy, in patients with raised blood pressure or heart disease, and in those who are anxious, stressed or suffer from palpitations.

6

Stimulant Drugs – Amfetamines

Amfetamines

The **amfetamines** are synthetic compounds which cause an increased concentration of stimulant nerve transmitters (noradrenaline(norepinephrine) and dopamine) in the brain and nervous system. They lift mood and are drugs of abuse (see p. xxvii). They include **amfetamine** and **dexamfetamine** (**Dexedrine**).

The effects produced by amfetamines vary with dose and the rate of administration. Children respond differently to adults; in fact, amfetamines are occasionally used to calm hyperactive children (now usually known as attention deficit hyperactivity disorder (ADHD)). In moderate dosage they increase heart rate, blood pressure and blood sugar. The pupils dilate, respiration increases and the appetite decreases.

The effects on mood vary tremendously between individuals and are influenced by many factors in the environment and in the personality. In some individuals there is increased wakefulness and alertness. They become more active physically and mentally, and fatigue is delayed; thinking gets clearer and they become more responsive and aware of their surroundings – in effect more sociable. However, other individuals may become restless, irritable and anxious.

Amfetamines may cause nausea, headache, dry mouth, trembling, difficulty in passing water, rapid beating of the heart and chest pains, diarrhoea, constipation and inability to concentrate. Higher doses may produce panic, confusion, aggression, hallucinations, mental breakdown and heart irregularities.

On stopping the use of moderate doses patients become fatigued, drowsy and depressed. They feel 'let down' and have a strong desire to take another dose to lift themselves again. Dependence on amfetamines is discussed on p. xxviii. Amfetamines should not be used as slimming drugs, and in depression they will do more harm than good.

Other Stimulants

Methylphenidate (**Equasym**, **Ritalin**) is a mild stimulant that produces effects similar to those of the amfetamines, but causes fewer adverse effects.

Modafinil (**Provigil**) is a stimulant used for the treatment of narcolepsy, a rare disorder that causes the individual to keep falling asleep during the daytime. However, it may cause dependence and therefore should be used with great care.

Dexamfetamine (**Dexedrine**) and **methylphenidate** (**Equasym**, **Ritalin**) are used to treat children with hyperkinesia (over-activity) or attention deficit hyperactivity disorder (ADHD) where psychotherapy has failed to help. They are used in low daily doses. If there is an improvement after four to eight weeks, they may be continued up to the age of ten years. The daily dose should be reduced and the drugs stopped once a year to check whether their continued use is necessary. Dexamfetamine (Dexedrine) is also used to treat narcolepsy.

7

Tonics

Millions of pounds are spent every year on tonics and yet most doctors accept that there is no single substance which may be called a tonic. Many medical experts are highly critical of the whole concept of tonics and their criticism has influenced prescribing doctors. However, although medical fashions can change quickly, patients' expectations often do not. Doctors' prescribing habits influence patients' demands so that patients often expect what they have been led to expect. For decades doctors prescribed tonics for everybody and everything and the idea of a tonic is still appealing to many patients.

If you think something will do you good, then it most probably will – the least it should do is cause you no harm. A tonic is something that we hope will help us to feel better. However, drug tonics are usually taken because the individual is feeling persistently run-down, physically or mentally. They are often, and quite wrongly, taken for a multiplicity of mental and/or physical symptoms, the cause of which may be fairly straightforward – such as convalescence from an attack of influenza – or quite complex and due to a serious underlying physical or psychological disorder. The reasons which make people feel that they need a tonic are complex and include social, physical and mental factors. Therefore, there is no such thing as a universal tonic – someone who is anaemic will require a blood test and specific treatment; someone who is depressed needs specific treatment, as does someone with an underlying physical disease. The idea that a tonic can help anybody just is not true.

If you feel persistently run-down and/or fed-up, then see your doctor. Your medical history can be checked, your physical, mental and social state can be assessed and you can be advised and treated accordingly.

Many over-the-counter tonics are based on the principle that if you belch and have your bowels opened, then you are living life to the full. Some tonics are just very expensive foods. A popular 'tonic' these days contains about 2 per cent liquid glucose which is no substitute for a well-balanced nutritious diet.

Iron salts are often included in tonics because many individuals have been led to believe that anaemia is a common cause of feeling run-down. You may develop iron-deficiency anaemia because you are losing blood regularly through, for example, heavy periods or a bleeding peptic ulcer. However, iron deficiency is only one cause of anaemia and doctors cannot recognize the type of anaemia from which you may be suffering without carrying out blood tests. Incredible variations have been reported when groups of doctors have been asked to estimate the degree of anaemia in a particular patient. Yet patients still believe that a doctor has some magical power to diagnose anaemia without blood tests. The same applies to vitamins; there is an optimum daily intake to prevent vitamin-deficiency disorders and there is a recommended dose for treating these disorders. The principle that if 100 units will make you feel good, then 1,000 units will make you feel even better just is not true.

Many decades ago it was found that nerve cells contain glycerophosphates; because of this the manufacture and sale of nerve tonics containing glycero-phosphates and hypophosphates has proved an extremely lucrative business. This has happened despite the fact that the use of these drugs has never been shown to produce any benefit over and above that which would be produced by an inert substance. However, they are harmless and therefore useful as a placebo. Unfortunately, they are mixed with all sorts of bitters (appetite stimulants), laxatives and stimulants. Some of these may produce adverse effects if taken regularly over time. Tonic wines contain hypophosphates and vitamins but people who take them must realize that it is probably the wine that makes them feel better.

Bitters, which appear in many tonics, stimulate salivation and the pro-duction of gastric juice by taste and smell. Certain alcoholic drinks are used for this purpose (aperitifs); but persistent loss of appetite is not the sort of symptom you should treat yourself.

Yeast is the basis of many tonics; again it can do you no harm on its own and it supplies you with a few vitamins. It may be combined with other drugs such as caffeine (you would get the same degree of stimulation from the caffeine in a cup of tea), or a pain-reliever.

Over-the-counter remedies containing digestive enzymes such as pepsin and pancreatin, liver salts and bile salts are valueless. Some contain small quantities of obsolete laxatives. Health salts have nothing to do with health, and honey may make you feel beautiful if you believe that it will. There is also no evidence that if you stuff yourself full of vitamin E, you will look younger and feel more sexy.

Finally, there is no substitute for a good healthy diet and reasonable exercise and sleep. If you feel you really need a tonic then you ought to see your doctor. Remember, the only part of a tonic that is really guaranteed to make you feel better is your belief that it is going to work.

8

Slimming Drugs

Being overweight is considered to be the commonest nutritional disorder in Western countries. However, this implies that there is a range of normal weights to which we should conform. In order to persuade us that this is true and in order to help us conform to these 'normal weights' a multi-million-pound slimming industry has developed since the Second World War.

Being overweight may be due to having a big frame but is usually due to fat. Stand naked in front of a mirror – if you have got rolls which shake when you jump up and down then you are fat! Being fat is mainly due to eating more food, particularly foods containing a large number of calories, than we require for our everyday needs. This results in the storage of fat in some of us, but others appear to be able to use up the extra calories. Lack of physical exercise also predisposes to the laying down of fat. Women have more fat cells than men and there is a relationship between the number of fat cells, their size and being overweight. Hereditary factors may influence the number of fat cells we have (fat parents may have fat children – but children may also 'inherit' their parents' eating habits). The number of our fat cells may also increase up to about the age of twenty and they may increase as a result of overeating in childhood so that fat children may become fat adults. We may also become fat if our fat cells store a lot of fat and increase in size. This is due to the way we use up fats and sugars, and is related to diet and exercise. There are also glandular influences which make us put on weight and which must be regarded as normal; for example, women may put on weight in their early teens, after pregnancy and during the menopause. These may be short-term increases in weight but we must not forget that we all put on weight as we get older; women more than men. Women tend to put fat on round their bottoms and breasts and men around their abdomens.

Our appetites and the foods that we eat often have little to do with our requirements and are more determined by the eating habits we have acquired from childhood. These are related to family and environmental factors, our economic status, various customs and social requirements. Further, over-eating may be as much a problem of habit as alcoholism, drug-taking or smoking, and as such is as much related to our personality as it is to social and hereditary factors.

The Use of Slimming Drugs

Doctors consider that obesity requires treatment when fat deposits have raised the body weight by 20 per cent or more above the standards for people of the same age, sex and race. They point out what they think are the hazards of being fat. These include flat feet, varicose veins, osteo-arthritis, gall-bladder disorders, high blood pressure, bronchitis, diabetes, complications after surgical operations, degenerative changes in heart muscle and a shortening of our lives. Doctors have certainly been successful in giving some of us the motivation to lose weight.

Since the commonest cause of being fat is taking in more calories than is required, the only sensible way to reduce weight is to reduce the amount of food you eat and alter your eating habits so that you eat a balanced diet and take in fewer calories. You should also take more physical exercise.

Drugs Used to Aid Slimming

Drugs which Block the Absorption of Fat

Orlistat (**Xenical**) blocks the action of an enzyme (pancreatic lipase) that is reponsible for digesting fats in the gut. This reduces the amount of fat absorbed from food. Orlistat treatment should only be started if diet alone has reduced weight loss, over a four-week period, by at least 2.5 kg. Orlistat can cause very liquid, oily stools and an urgency to go to the toilet as well as flatulence. However, these effects can be reduced by significantly reducing the amount of fat in the diet, which in turn will contribute to weight loss.

Drugs which Cause Loss of Fluids

Laxatives such as **cascara** or rhubarb are contained in some slimming remedies. These cause a loss of water from the bowel and therefore from the tissues, resulting in weight reduction. The body immediately puts to rights this water loss the next time you drink and so such medicines are useless. They could be harmful if taken regularly.

Diuretics (water tablets, see p. 146) act on the kidneys to make them excrete more salt and this takes water with it. The loss of water and salt results in a fall in the volume of body fluids and a subsequent temporary reduction in body weight. Diuretics also alter the body's excretion of other salts. They may be harmful and should not be taken to lose weight.

Drugs which Increase the Bulk of Food

These slimming remedies contain **methylcellulose** (**Celevac**) or a similar substance in tablet form. They absorb water from the stomach, swell and are supposed to make you feel less hungry if taken before meals. They are not absorbed and increase the bulk of the motions, taking some water with them. As slimming aids these preparations have not been proved to be of value.

Thyroid Drugs

Thyroid drugs affect the rate at which you burn up energy. They may produce loss of weight because fat is burned up as a source of energy. However, for slimming they are ineffective in small doses and dangerous in high doses (see A–Z of Medicines). They should not be used.

Drugs which Suppress the Appetite

Amfetamines have been widely used in the past because they stop you feeling hungry but they lose this effect after a few weeks. They do, however, give you more energy, but only for a short period of time. These effects cause some people to increase the dosage which may eventually lead to drug dependence and mental breakdown. Any possible benefit is outweighed by the dangers.

Starch Blockers

These comprise a protein component (phaseolansin) from red kidney beans which is claimed to prevent the digestion of dietary starch – the protein is said to 'lock' into amylase (an enzyme in the intestine which converts starch to sugar) without changing it chemically or being absorbed. For many years several preparations on the market in the USA just contained ground-up kidney beans and there were many reported adverse effects which led to the drugs being withdrawn from the market.

Herbal Remedies

Herbal remedies usually contain drugs that are supposed to make you feel full and eat less, or drugs that make your kidneys pass more water and/or 'laxatives' that make you lose water in your motions. With many herbal preparations you will lose weight because you are losing water from your body. This dehydration may be harmful. As soon as you stop these drugs the body adjusts its water level back to normal by reducing the amount of urine you pass and your weight will go back to what it was before you started such treatment. They do not produce any loss of fat. Herbal remedies should not be used to aid slimming.

Chitosan (Fat Attract, Fat Binder, Fat Magnet)

Chitosan is obtained from chitin, which is a complex sugar (polysaccharide) that forms the shells of crustacea (e.g. shells of crabs and shrimps). It is insoluble and indigestible and corresponds to cellulose in plants. Because it is insoluble it has been used in the food industry as a bulking agent and as a bulk laxative. However, recent interest centres on claims that if taken before a fatty meal, chitosan combined with vitamin C is capable of binding to fats in the food and reducing their absorption from the intestine – which is of obvious interest to slimmers. It also helps to reduce the blood cholesterol level. Chitosan can bind up to six times its weight in fats and the risk is that it will interfere with the absorption of essential fatty acids and fat-soluble vitamins (A, D, E, K). It should be taken with plenty of fluids. The overall benefits to risks of taking chitosan over the medium to long term are not known. It is only a short-term aid to slimming and should not replace lifestyle changes such as a sensible, well-balanced diet and fat-burning exercises.

Comment: *Being overweight is a lifelong problem and you must re-educate yourself to accept a change in eating and exercise habits for life. Crash diets and slimming pills have only a transient effect and are best avoided.*

9

Drugs which Act upon the Autonomic Nervous System

The autonomic nervous system, as the name implies, is not under voluntary control. It supplies internal organs, e.g. the stomach, intestine, bronchi (the lungs), heart, blood vessels, sweat glands, bladder and the eyes. Therefore, it controls all sorts of functions – from breathing to sexual activity and from sweating to digestion. It consists of two divisions – **sympathetic** and **parasympathetic**. These divisions oppose each other but a careful balance is maintained by special centres in the brain.

Impulses from the brain and spinal cord join the autonomic network of nerves along nerve fibres which run into ganglia (rather like electrical switch-boxes). The impulses are transmitted at these junctions by chemical transmitters (nerve transmitters). The nerve fibres running to the junctions are called *pre*-ganglionic nerve fibres and they all use the same chemical transmitter – **acetylcholine**. This only works for a very short time because once it is liberated at nerve junctions to act as a nerve transmitter another chemical starts to break it down. This chemical is an enzyme called **cholinesterase**. Nerve fibres running *from* the nerve junctions (ganglia) are called *post*-ganglionic nerves.

Parasympathetic post-ganglionic nerves also use acetylcholine as a nerve transmitter – they are therefore known as cholinergic nerves, but the sympathetic post-ganglionic nerve fibres use **adrenaline**(epinephrine) and **noradrenaline**(norepinephrine) as chemical transmitters and therefore these are known as adrenergic nerves. The central part (medulla) of the adrenal glands also produces adrenaline(epinephrine) and noradrenaline(norepinephrine).

Drugs which Act on the Parasympathetic Nervous System

Drugs which act like acetylcholine were called **cholinergic drugs** – they are now called **parasympathomimetic** because they mimic the actions of the parasympathetic nervous system.

Stimulation of the parasympathetic division produces stimulation of secretory glands – salivary, tear, bronchial and sweat. It slows the heart rate, constricts the bronchi, produces increased movement of the intestine, contracts the bladder and constricts the pupil. Parasympathomimetic drugs also stimulate nerve endings in voluntary muscles, stimulate and then depress the brain, and dilate blood vessels.

Parasympathomimetic Drugs

Parasympathomimetic drugs mimic the actions of **acetylcholine**. There are three groups:

1. Choline esters (e.g. **carbachol**, **bethanechol**) – these are related to acetylcholine and act at all sites like acetylcholine.
2. Alkaloids (e.g. **pilocarpine**) – these are obtained from plants and act selectively on those nerve endings which respond to acetylcholine.
3. Cholinesterase inhibitors or anticholinesterase drugs (e.g. **pyridostigmine, neostigmine**) – these inactivate the enzyme (cholinesterase) which is responsible for breaking down acetylcholine into acetic acid and choline, and thereby inactivating it. This allows acetylcholine to go on working. Cholinesterase inhibitors are also used in the treatment of Alzheimer's disease due to evidence which shows that they can enhance cognitive function. They include **donepezil (Aricept)**, **galantamine (Reminyl)** and **rivastigmine (Exelon)**.

Parasympathomimetic drugs produce similar effects to stimulating the parasympathetic division. But not all effects occur with each drug and also the intensity of effects varies. Acetylcholine is not usually used in drug treatments. **Carbachol (Isopto Carbachol)** and **Pilocarpine (Isopto Carpine, Pilogel, Salagen)** are used to constrict the pupil and decrease the pressure inside the eye in patients with glaucoma. **Carbachol** may also be used to stimulate bowel and bladder function after surgical operations. It may be given by injection under the skin or by mouth. **Bethanechol (Myotonine)** is related and may be given by mouth to treat acid reflux (reflux oesophagitis) and retention of urine.

The anti-cholinesterase drug **neostigmine (Robinul)** may be used to stimulate the bowel and bladder after surgery. **Edrophonium** is used to diagnose, and **neostigmine (Robinul)** and **pyridostigmine (Mestinon)** are used in the treatment of myaesthenia gravis (a disease caused by defective transmission of impulses by acetylcholine and characterized by severe muscle weakness and fatigue). They are used as antidotes to neuromuscular blocking drugs (see

p. 41). **Pyridostigmine** (**Mestinon**) is also used to treat paralysis of the bowel (paralytic ileus). **Distigmine** (**Ubretid**) is longer-acting than pyridostigmine and is used to stimulate the bowels after surgery, to treat myasthenia gravis and to treat incontinence of the bladder. Many related drugs are also 'used' as nerve gases and some are pesticides.

Drugs which Oppose Acetylcholine Activity

These may be called **acetylcholine antagonists** or **parasympatholytics**. They prevent acetylcholine from acting as a transmitter.

One of the main classes of *anticholinergics* is referred to as *antimuscarinics* because they block the actions of acetylcholine at muscarinic receptors. This is a more accurate term for the anticholinergics used as medicines. The other main group of anticholinergics work on nicotine receptors. In medicine they are used as ganglion blockers and skeletal muscle relaxants.

There are three groups:
1 **Antimuscarinic drugs** which act principally at parasympathetic nerve endings.
2 **Ganglion blocking drugs** which act on ganglia (and don't forget that acetylcholine is the chemical transmitter in all ganglia – both in the parasympathetic and sympathetic divisions).
3 **Neuromuscular blocking drugs** – these act on nerve endings in voluntary muscles.

1 *Antimuscarinic drugs.* Antimuscarinic drugs block the action of acetylcholine on acetylcholine receptors in the tissues and organs of the body. In addition, some of them have a weak effect in blocking acetylcholine in the main switchboxes (ganglia) of the autonomic nervous system (affecting both sympathetic and parasympathetic divisions). No antimuscarinic drug blocks the action of acetylcholine at nerve endings in voluntary muscles, except propantheline in very high doses.

There are several groups of antimuscarinic drugs which produce differing degrees of effects in the body. For example, some produce more effects on the brain and/or the eyes than the others, some produce more effects on the stomach or intestine, and some are much more selective in their actions than others.

Antimuscarinic drugs obtained from plants include **atropine, belladonna** and **hyoscine**. They produce similar effects and their uses are listed later.

Synthetic antimuscarinic drugs may be divided into three groups according to whether their principal actions are in drying up secretions and reducing movements of the intestines (anti-secretory and anti-spasmodic); whether they reduce the shaking and excessive salivation in patients with parkinsonism (anti-parkinsonism effects); or whether their main effects are upon the eyes (mydriatic and cyclopegic effects).

Those used mainly for their anti-secretory/anti-spasmodic effects include **dicycloverine**(dicyclomine) (**Merbentyl**, in **Kolanticon**), **glycopyrronium** (**Robinul**) and **propantheline** (**Pro-Banthine**).

Those used mainly to treat parkinsonism include **trihexyphenidyl**(benzhexol) (**Broflex**), **benzatropine** (**Cogentin**), **biperiden** (**Akineton**), **orphenadrine** (**Biorphen, Disipal**) and **procyclidine** (**Arpicolin, Kemadrin**).

Those used mainly to treat eye disorders include **cyclopentolate** (**Mydrilate**) and **tropicamide** (**Mydriacyl**).

The principal uses of antimuscarinic drugs therefore include the treatment of parkinsonism and motion sickness, as sedatives, to dilate the pupils, to dilate the bronchi and reduce bronchial secretions, to reduce acid production by the stomach in the treatment of peptic ulcers, to treat colic, to reduce sweating and occasionally to treat heart block and slow pulse rates.

2 *Ganglion blocking drugs.* These have been used in the past to treat raised blood pressure. They lower blood pressure by producing dilatation of blood vessels and therefore a fall in peripheral resistance. They included **hexamethonium, mecamylamine, pempidine** and **pentolinium**. Because they are not selective and block ganglia in both parasympathetic and sympathetic divisions, they produce numerous adverse effects. **Trimetaphan** is used to keep the blood pressure low during surgery.

3 *Neuromuscular blocking drugs (myoneural blocking drugs).* When an impulse passes down a nerve to a voluntary muscle it causes the release of acetylcholine at the nerve ending which acts as a chemical transmitter stimulating the muscle to contract. Neuromuscular blocking drugs interfere with this chemical transmission. **Curare**, used on poisoned arrows by the natives of South America, is the most famous example of this group of drugs. There are two main ways in which neuromuscular blocking drugs work. **Atracurium** (**Tracrium**), **cisatracurium** (**Nimbex**), **gallamine** (**Flaxedil**), **mivacurium** (**Mivacron**), **pancuronium** (**Pavulon**), **rocuronium** (**Esmeron**) and **vecuronium** (**Norcuron**) compete with acetylcholine and block the impulse being transmitted to the receptor organ in the muscles. They cause a prolonged paralysis of voluntary muscles. They are referred to as *competitive neuromuscular blocking drugs* (or non-depolarizing muscle relaxants) and are used to relax muscles during surgery and in long-term mechanical ventilation. Drugs such as **suxamethonium** (**Anectine**) mimic the action of acetylcholine – at first they cause the muscles to contract but this effect wears off quickly and they leave the muscle no longer receptive to stimulation by acetylcholine. They are referred to as *depolarizing neuromuscular blocking drugs* because they block the complex physicochemical process called polarization. Suxamethonium produces its effects for only a few minutes and it is used to provide muscle relaxation for procedures such as passing a tube into the lungs.

Drugs which Act on the Sympathetic Nervous System

Those drugs that imitate the effects of stimulation of the sympathetic division are called **sympathomimetic** drugs. Those that oppose its effects are called **sympatholytic**.

Sympathomimetic Drugs

This group of drugs includes **adrenaline**(epinephrine) and **noradrenaline** (norepinephrine), which are secreted by the medulla of the adrenal glands. **Noradrenaline**(norepinephrine) is also the main chemical transmitter at post-ganglionic sympathetic nerve endings. These nerves are therefore called adrenergic nerves and drugs which stimulate them are called **adrenergic drugs** – those that oppose their action are called **adrenolytic**.

Noradrenaline(norepinephrine) is produced and stored at adrenergic nerve endings and can be liberated from these stores by stimulating the nerve, or by drugs such as amphetamines, ephedrine, reserpine and guanethidine. Sympathomimetic drugs (or adrenergic drugs) may act directly on the receptors at the nerve endings of the sympathetic nervous system (e.g. **adrenaline** (epinephrine), **noradrenaline**(norepinephrine), **isoprenaline** (**Saventrine**)); indirectly by stimulating the liberation of noradrenaline(norepinephrine) from the stores at the nerve endings (e.g. **amphetamines**); or by both indirect and direct actions (e.g. **ephedrine**, **metaraminol** (**Aramine**)).

Sympathomimetic drugs act on adrenergic receptor sites which are found widely distributed throughout the body. These receptors are classified simply into alpha (α) and beta (β_1 and β_2) receptors. Stimulation of alpha receptors produces what are called alpha effects – constriction of arteries in the skin and intestine, sweating and dilatation of the pupils. β_1 receptors are principally located in the heart; stimulation produces an increase of heart rate and increased output of blood from the heart. Stimulation of β_2 receptors produces relaxation of bronchial muscles, relaxation of the uterus, dilatation of arteries (chiefly in muscles), and tremor of skeletal muscles.

Adrenaline(epinephrine) produces both alpha and beta effects, **noradrenaline**(norepinephrine) produces chiefly alpha effects and **isoprenaline** produces beta effects.

Sympathomimetic drugs are principally used:

- *as nasal decongestants:* read Chapter 10 on drugs used to treat the common cold.
- *to treat bronchospasm:* read Chapter 14 on drugs used to treat bronchial asthma.
- *to treat low blood pressure:* those sympathomimetics that constrict arteries are occasionally used to raise the blood pressure in severe states of low blood pressure caused by coronary thrombosis, anaesthetics or drug

overdose. They include **ephedrine**, **metaraminol**, **methoxamine**, **noradrenaline**(norepinephrine) and **phenylephrine**.

● *to treat premature labour:* **ritodrine** (**Yutopar**), **salbutamol** and **terbutaline** cause relaxation of the womb and are used to stop premature labour.
● *to treat heart failure* (see p. 123).

Drugs which Oppose Sympathetic Activity

These drugs oppose sympathetic activity:

1 *Adrenergic neurone blocking drugs.* These block transmission of nerve impulses along post-ganglionic sympathetic nerves (adrenergic nerves) or their nerve endings. They include **debrisoquine** and **guanethidine** (**Ismelin**). These drugs are discussed in Chapter 25 – drugs used to treat raised blood pressure.

2 *Alpha-adrenoceptor blocking drugs.* These include **alfuzosin** (**Xatral**), **doxazosin** (**Cardura**), **indoramin** (**Doralese, Baratol**), **phentolamine** (**Rogitine**), **phenoxybenzamine** (**Dibenyline**), **prazosin** (**Hypovase**) and **terazosin** (**Hytrin**). The principal effect of these drugs is to produce dilation of arteries. They are also discussed in Chapter 25. They are also used (except for phentolamine and phenoxybenzamine) to improve the flow of urine in men with enlarged prostate glands (see page 284).

3 *Beta-receptor blocking drugs.* These are used to treat angina, disorders of heart rhythm, raised blood pressure, over-active thyroids, anxiety and migraine. They are discussed on p. 114.

Summary: Drugs which Act on the Autonomic Nervous System

Parasympathetic Division

Parasympathomimetic drugs
choline esters (e.g. **carbachol**)
alkaloids (e.g. **pilocarpine**)
cholinersterase inhibitors (e.g. **neostigmine**)

Parasympatholytic drugs
Antimuscarinic drugs, e.g. **atropine**
Ganglion blocking drugs (block ganglia in both parasympathetic and sympathetic divisions)

Sympathetic Division

Sympathomimetic drugs
alpha-receptor stimulants (e.g. **noradrenaline**(norepinephrine))
alpha-and beta-receptor stimulants (e.g. **adrenaline**(epinephrine))
beta-receptor stimulants (e.g. **isoprenaline**)

Sympatholytic drugs
Adrenergic neurone blocking drugs, e.g. **guanethidine**
Alpha-adrenoceptor blocking drugs, e.g. **phentolamine**
Beta-receptor blocking drugs, e.g. **propranolol**
Alpha and beta blocking drugs, e.g. **labetolol**

Other Nerve Transmitters

Dopamine

Dopamine stimulates dopamine receptors in the brain and nervous system and also alpha and beta adrenoreceptors. It can also stimulate the release of noradrenaline(norepinephrine) from nerve endings. It is used to stimulate the heart in acute heart failure and in heart surgery.

● *Dopamine-stimulants*
Amantadine (**Symmetrel**) is used to treat parkinsonism (see Chapter 16). It stimulates an increase in concentration of dopamine in the brain.

Bromocriptine (**Parlodel**) is a selective dopamine receptor stimulant. It is used to suppress milk production after childbirth because it blocks the release of the milk-producing hormone prolactin by the pituitary gland, and to treat tumours which produce excessive amounts of prolactin. It also blocks the release of growth hormone by the pituitary gland and may be used to treat overproduction of this hormone (e.g. acromegaly). Another main use of bromocriptine is to treat parkinsonism (see Chapter 16).

Levodopa is a precursor of dopamine and is used to treat parkinsonism (see Chapter 16).

Lisuride and **Pergolide** (**Celance**) are selective dopamine receptor stimulants used to treat parkinsonism (see Chapter 16).

Selegiline (**Eldepryl**, **Zelapar**) is a selective blocker of the enzyme that breaks down dopamine and is used to treat parkinsonism (see Chapter 16).

● *Dopamine-blockers*
Certain antipsychotic drugs (e.g. **phenothiazines**) used to treat serious mental disorders block dopamine receptors. They may produce adverse effects similar to parkinsonism which is caused by a deficiency of dopamine in the brain (see

Chapter 16). They are also used to treat nausea and vomiting (see Chapter 18).

Other dopamine blockers (e.g. **domperidone** (**Motilium**) and **metoclopramide** (**Maxolon, Gastrobid, Continus, Gastroflux, Primperan**)) are also used to treat nausea and vomiting (see Chapter 18).

Tetrabenazine reduces the concentration of dopamine in the brain and nervous system and is used to treat disorders of movement such as Huntington's chorea.

5-Hydroxytryptamine (5HT, serotonin)

This chemical is present in many cells in both plants and animals. It has a wide spectrum of activity by stimulating and blocking nerves in smooth muscles (particularly in the breathing tubes, producing wheezing), and in blood vessels; it also produces constriction in some muscles. It produces a slowing of the heart rate, a fall in blood pressure and affects the movements of the stomach and intestine. It also acts as a nerve transmitter in the brain and affects mood and behaviour.

Most of the 5HT in food is destroyed in the walls of the intestine and, if it is absorbed, in the liver and the lungs. Therefore, it is manufactured in the body from tryptophan (an essential amino acid in the diet).

● *5HT stimulants*

Drugs that increase the amount of 5HT (serotonin) available in the brain are used to treat depression. They are discussed in Chapter 4 (see p. 18).

● *5HT Blockers*

Methysergide (**Deseril**) blocks 5HT at its receptor sites and is used to prevent migraine (see Chapter 34). **Pizotifen** (**Sanomigran**) is a 5HT blocker that is also used to prevent migraine.

Antipsychotic drugs block the activity of dopamine in the brain and they may also block the activity of 5HT.

Cyproheptadine (**Periactin**) is an antihistamine that also blocks the effects of 5HT. It is used to treat migraine.

Granisetron (**Kytril**), **ondansetron** (**Zofran**) and **tropisetron** (**Navoban**) are selective 5HT blockers used to treat nausea and vomiting caused by anti-cancer drugs and radiation treatment. See Chapter 18.

Drugs which Enhance Neuromuscular Transmission

In conditions such as myasthenia gravis, anticholinesterase drugs are used. They prolong the action of acetylcholine by inhibiting the action of the enzyme acetylcholinesterase which breaks down acetylcholine. They may produce adverse effects such as increased sweating, salivation, and gastric secretion, increased contractions in the gut and uterus, and slowing of the heart rate. These drugs include **distigmine** (**Ubretid**), **edrophonium**, **neostigmine** and **pyridostigmine** (**Mestinon**). They vary according to their duration of action. Their effects can be stopped by giving atropine.

Muscle Relaxants Used in Anaesthesia

Drugs which block the transmission of nervous impulses at neuromuscular junctions are used in anaesthesia. They are usually referred to as *neuromuscular blocking drugs* or *myoneural blocking drugs*. They make muscles relax during surgery (e.g. abdominal muscles) and they make the vocal cords relax so that a tube can be passed down into the lungs in order to give anaesthetic gases. As stated earlier, there are two groups of neuromuscular blocking drugs. The first are those that compete with acetylcholine and block its effects (*non-depolarizing muscle relaxants*). They include **atracurium** (**Tracrium**), **cisatracurium** (**Nimbex**), **gallamine** (**Flaxedil**), **mivacurium** (**Mivacron**), **pancuronium** (**Pavulon**), **rocuronium** (**Esmeron**), **vecuronium bromide** (**Norcuron**). The second group are *depolarizing muscle relaxants* which mimic the action of acetylcholine and cause blockage of impulses at neuromuscular junctions. **Suxamethonium** (**Anectine**) is the most commonly used.

Skeletal Muscle Relaxants

Muscle relaxants used to relieve pain and spasm in skeletal muscles act principally on the brain and spinal cord. Drugs used include benzodiazepines, e.g. **diazepam** (see p. 8) and **baclofen** (**Baclospas, Balgifen, Lioresal**). **Dantrolene** (**Dantrium**) acts directly on skeletal muscles to produce relaxation but produces adverse effects on the brain. **Quinine** is useful for relieving leg cramps in bed at night. Other muscle relaxants include **carisoprodol** (**Carisoma**) and **methocarbamol** (**Robaxin**). **Tizanidine** (**Zanaflex**) is an alpha$_2$-adrenoceptor agonist indicated for spasticity associated with multiple sclerosis or spinal cord injury.

10

Drugs Used to Treat the Common Cold

There is no such drug as a cold cure. There is no drug on the market which prevents colds or reduces their duration. But, because there is no cure, there are numerous remedies.

The common cold produces swelling and inflammation of the lining membrane of the nose which produces blockage and a runny nose. This may be accompanied by a sore throat, cough, headache, aching back or limbs and a mild fever. In an attempt to relieve these symptoms drug companies produce nose drops, inhalants, sprays, aerosols, ointments, tablets, powders, capsules, linctuses and mixtures in all shapes, colours and sizes. Treatment is aimed at two target groups of symptoms – aches, pains and fever; blocked and runny nose.

Relief of Aches, Pains and Fever

Mild pain-relievers will relieve your aches and pains and will bring down your temperature. They must be taken according to the instructions on the package and with plenty of fluids. They will have no effect upon the duration or outcome of the cold. There are many pain-relieving preparations on the market and yet the choice boils down to **paracetamol** or **ibuprofen** with soluble **aspirin** as an alternative.

Aspirin should not be used for children under twelve years of age or by breastfeeding mothers because of the risk of Reye's Syndrome (see p. 159).

Products which Contain **Aspirin** and **Paracetamol** only

Disprin Extra

Products which Contain **Aspirin** and **Paracetamol** and Other Ingredients

- *Caffeine:*
  Anadin Extra Soluble
  Nurse Sykes' Powders

- *Codeine*
  Veganin

Products which Contain **Aspirin** only

Aspro Clear	**Disprin**
Beechams Lemon Tablets	**Disprin CV**
Mrs Cullen's Powders	**Disprin Direct**

Products which Contain **Aspirin** and Other Ingredients

- *Caffeine*
  Anadin
  Anadin Maximum Strength
  Beechams Powders
  Phensic

- *Codeine*
  Codis

- *Caffeine & Chlorphenamine & Phenylephrine*
  Dristan Tablets

Products which Contain **Paracetamol** only

Anadin Paracetamol	**Hedex**
Boots Children's 3 Months Plus Pain Relief	**Infadrops**
	Mandanol
Boots Cold Relief Hot Blackcurrant	**Medinol**
Boots Cold Relief Hot Lemon	**Panadol**
Calpol	**Panaleve Junior**
Calpol 6 Plus	**Panaleve 6+**

Disprol
Fennings Children's Cooling
  Powders
Galpamol

Paracets
Paraclear
Placidex
Tixymol

Products which Contain **Paracetamol** and Other Ingredients

- *Caffeine*
  De Witt's Analgesic Pills
  Hedex Extra
  Panadol Extra

- *Codeine*
  Panadol Ultra
  Paracodol
  Solpadeine Max

- *Dihydrocodeine*
  Paramol

- *Diphenhydramine*
  Benylin Day and Night – night tablets
  Dozol
  Panadol Night

- *Phenylephrine*

  Beechams Cold And Flu
  Beechams Flu-Plus Berry Fruits
  Beechams Flu-Plus Powder
  Beechams Hot Blackcurrant
  Beechams Hot Lemon
  Beechams Hot Lemon And Honey

  Lemsip Blackcurrant
  Lemsip Cold + Flu Breathe Easy
  Lemsip Cold + Flu Max Strength
  Lemsip Lemon
  Lemsip Max Strength

- *Phenylpropanolamine*
  Benylin Day and Night – day tablets
  Mu-Cron Tablets
  Sinutab

- *Promethazine*
  Medised

- *Pseudoephedrine*
  Lemsip Power & Paracetamol
  Sudafed-Co

- *Caffeine & Codeine*
  Solpadeine

- *Caffeine & Phenylephrine*
  Anadin Cold Control   **Catarrh-Ex**
  Beechams Flu-Plus Caplets   **Lemsip Cold+Flu Combined Relief**
  Beechams Powders Capsules   **Paracets Plus**
  Boots Cold And Flu Relief Tablets

- *Dextromethorphan & Phenylpropanolamine*
  Day Nurse

- *Dextromethorphan & Promethazine*
  Night Nurse

- *Diphenhydramine & Pseudoephedrine*
  Benylin 4 Flu

- *Guaifenesin & Phenylephrine*
  Beechams-All-In-One

- *Phenylpropanolamine & Phenyltoloxamine*
  Sinutab Nightime

- *Pholcodine & Pseudoephedrine*
  Nirolex Day Cold Comfort

- *Caffeine & Codeine & Diphenhydramine*
  Propain

- *Dextromethorphan & Doxylamine & Ephedrine*
  Vicks Medinite

- *Diphenhydramine & Ephedrine & Caffeine*
  Dolvan

- *Pseudoephedrine & Diphenhydrate & Pholcodeine*
  Nirolex Night Cold Comfort

- *Caffeine & Codeine & Diphenhydramine & Phenylephrine*
  Uniflu with Gregovite C.

Products which Contain **Ibuprofen** only

Advil	Inoven
Anadin Ibuprofen	Novaprin
Anadin Ultra	Nurofen
Boots Children's 6 Years Plus Fever	Obifen
and Pain Relief	Pacifene
Cuprofen	PhorPain
Galprofen	Proflex
Hedex Ibuprofen	Relcofen
Ibrufhalal	

Products which Contain **Ibuprofen** and Other Ingredients

- *Codeine*
  Nurofen Plus
  Solpaflex

- *Pseudoephedrine*
  Advil Cold and Sinus
  Lemsip Power Plus
  Nurofen Cold and Flu

Nasal Sprays

The majority of decongestant drugs belong to a group known as sympathomimetic drugs (see p. 38).

When applied locally to the surface of the nose they reduce swelling and secretions by constricting blood vessels. They are used to relieve runny nose and nasal congestion. They all share the disadvantage that their use may be followed by an increase of nasal congestion ('rebound' or 'after congestion'). Some irritate the lining of the nose and sting when applied. They may produce headache and rapid beating of the heart (see warnings with oral preparations, p. 48) and they may cause children to become hyperactive. Their repeated use may damage the lining membrane of the nose and produce permanent blockage.

The commonly used sympathomimetic drugs in nasal decongestant preparations include **ephedrine**, **oxymetazoline** (**Afrazine Nasal Spray**, **Dristan**, **Sudafed Nasal Spray**, **Vicks Sinex**), **phenylephrine** (**Fenox**), and **xylometazoline** (**Otradrops**, **Otrivine**, **Tixycolds**). The sympathomimetic drugs in nasal decongestant sprays may be absorbed into the bloodstream through the lining of the nose and produce adverse effects. They should be used with the utmost caution in pregnancy. Do not use daily for more than seven days and only use occasionally.

Overdose of naphazoline and xylometazoline may cause coma and a fall in body temperature, especially in infants.

Nasal Decongestants by Mouth

Nasal decongestants are usually applied locally in the nose by nasal spray or drops (see p. 47), but they may also be taken by mouth. However, the arteries supplying the lining membranes of the nose have not been shown to be more sensitive to these drugs than any other vessels in the body. Nasal decongestants taken by mouth will therefore produce constriction of other arteries in the body and increase the blood pressure. This may be dangerous in patients at risk of developing a stroke, who suffer from angina, coronary thrombosis, high blood pressure, diabetes or overworking of their thyroid glands, and in patients who are receiving monoamine oxidase inhibitor antidepressant drugs. Their adverse effects include giddiness, headache, nausea, vomiting, sweating, thirst, palpitations, difficulty in passing urine, weakness, trembling, anxiety, restlessness and insomnia. Some individuals may be very sensitive to them while others may be able to tolerate high doses. They do not cause rebound congestion of the nose when their effects have worn off but they are of doubtful value.

The main decongestants included in oral preparations are **phenylephrine**, **phenylpropanolamine** and **ephedrine** (see lists above for products which contain these drugs).

Other Cold Remedies

Antimuscarinic drugs (see p. 36) reduce secretions in the upper and lower respiratory tract. They are a constituent of some cold remedies, usually in such small doses as to be ineffective. But, of course, if they were given in effective doses by mouth they would produce unpleasant adverse effects.

Antihistamines (see p. 84) are present in some common cold remedies but there is disagreement about their benefits. Some of them may cause drowsiness and interfere with your ability to drive a motor vehicle, and their effects are increased by alcohol.

Vapour rubs and inhalations may provide very transient relief of cold symptoms in some people but they should be used with caution, and not in infants under three months of age in whom strong applications may interfere with breathing.

Vitamin C. There is no convincing evidence that taking vitamin C helps to prevent colds, reduce the severity of cold symptoms or shorten the duration of a cold.

Soothing throat lozenges and pastilles may provide transient relief of symptoms in some people but there is a large 'psychological' element to their effectiveness. Many are high in sugar and sucking between meals may be harmful to teeth. They should not be used by diabetics unless they are sugar-free.

Antibacterial throat lozenges are of no use in treating a virus infection (the commonest cause of sore throats) and **antiseptic preparations** are usually so weak as to have no beneficial effect and the same criticism applies to **gargles**.

Catarrh

Catarrh is an inflammation of the lining membranes of the air passages. It may affect the nose (nasal catarrh), the space at the back of the nose (post-nasal catarrh), or any part of the air passages. It may be acute and caused by a cold or it may be chronic and aggravated by smoking and a dry atmosphere. It may also be caused by many other factors: for example, allergy (e.g. hayfever), a dusty dry atmosphere, or fungal spores in the air. Acute catarrh may produce a soreness of the affected area, or it may produce a mucous discharge: for example, runny nose, mucus at the back of the throat, phlegm on the chest, or snuffles in a baby. The mucus may become sticky and hard to clear and it may become yellowish-green due to secondary bacterial infection.

Treatment of Catarrh

In treating acute catarrh it is important to treat the cause, for example, hayfever, to stop smoking if you smoke, and avoid dry, dusty and/or smoky atmospheres if possible. Parents of snuffly babies should not smoke in the home. This general advice also applies to the treatment of chronic catarrh.

Steam inhalation may help to clear catarrh; so may nasal decongestants but note the dangers of regular daily use and dangers in infants (see p. 48). Vapours and inhalations may help some people but they should be used with caution, and preferably not in infants under three months of age in whom strong applications may interfere with breathing.

There is no convincing evidence from adequate and well-controlled studies that mucolytics (drugs that dissolve phlegm) are beneficial in treating chronic catarrh despite their being heavily advertised. Preparations containing more than one drug are best avoided because the dose of one drug cannot be changed without changing the dose of the other drug or drugs. Furthermore, such preparations expose you to the risk of harmful effects from more than one drug.

11

Drugs Used to Treat Coughs

Coughs frequently serve a useful purpose, for example, to get rid of an inhaled foreign body or to cough up sputum. These coughs are said to be productive. A cough which is just dry and irritating is said to be unproductive and serves no purpose. As with cold remedies the marketing of cough medicines is a lucrative business and so the market is flooded with preparations. Many of these are mixtures containing such small doses of individual drugs as to render them pharmacologically ineffective. But, of course, a large proportion of us respond to inert mixtures – some of us responding better to one colour or taste than to others.

The aim of using cough medicines is to give comfort to those people with a productive cough and to help them cough up their sputum. For those people with a dry, irritating, unproductive cough, the aim is to suppress it. We therefore have two main groups of drugs which are used to treat coughs – expectorants and cough suppressants. Expectorants are given with the aim of liquefying the sputum, so that it is easier to cough up. Cough suppressants either work locally at the site of the irritation in the throat or they act on the cough centre in the brain, reducing the desire to cough. Some cough mixtures contain drugs which act on the conscious part of the brain producing drowsiness and therefore making you less aware of the irritation in your throat.

Expectorants

These act by irritating the lining of the stomach which by reflex stimulates the nerves supplying the glands in the bronchi. This is said to result in an increased production of secretions thus making the sputum more watery and easier to cough up. However, the dose required to do this would, with most of these drugs, produce stomach pains and vomiting. They include ammonium chloride, acetates, acetic acid, benzoin compounds, bicarbonates, creosote, eucalyptus, ipecacuanha, menthol, peppermint, potassium iodide, sodium benzoate, sodium citrate, tolu and guaiacols (e.g. guaifenesin). They are present in many cough medicines, and from the point of view of effectiveness you may as well choose them by taste or colour.

The stickiness of sputum depends on its degree of water content, which in turn depends upon the general degree of hydration of the body. Patients with chronic bronchitis and other chest disorders which produce dry sticky sputum may well benefit from increasing their fluid intake. **Inhalation of water or steam** may also be very useful and it does not really matter whether these are made to smell pleasant by the addition of **menthol**, **eucalyptus** or **benzoin**.

Drugs that Dissolve Sputum (Mucolytic Drugs)

Some drugs have been shown to 'digest' sputum in the laboratory, but their effect upon sputum in the bronchial tubes has been variable. Cysteine compounds, e.g. **carbocisteine** (**Mucodyne**) and **mecysteine** (**Visclair**) by mouth may liquefy sputum and help patients with cystic fibrosis to cough up phlegm. **Dornase alfa** (**Pulmozyme**) is a bioengineered human enzyme that dissolves sputum. It is given by inhalation using a jet nebulizer in patients with cystic fibrosis.

Cough Suppressants (Antitussives)

The most important cough suppressant in people who smoke is to stop smoking. For coughs which are caused by irritation or inflammation in the throat above the larynx (voice-box) there are many different makes of soothing cough preparation; they include sweets, pastilles, lozenges, cough drops and linctuses. A few contain **antiseptics** (such as benzoin, cetylpridinium, chloroxylenol, creosote, domiphen, thymol) in doses which are totally useless but which, if given in effective antiseptic doses, could be harmful.

Most cough sweets contain **demulcents**, which are soothing substances which act on the surface of the throat, e.g. honey, liquorice, glycerin. Such preparations also contain pleasant-smelling and tasting substances, like peppermint, eucalyptus, cinnamon, lemon, clove, aniseed. Others contain menthol, camphor, chloroform. The main effect of these preparations is that their smell or taste may help you feel better. They may increase the production of saliva, which is soothing and helps to wash the inflamed surfaces of the throat. Some preparations contain a topical anaesthetic (e.g. **benzocaine**), which may reduce the pain of inflammation. Cough medicines which contain the same ingredients in liquid form are even more irrational since they are swallowed directly into the stomach and only have a fraction of a second to work locally on the throat. There is no evidence that any of these cough preparations are any more effective than sucking ordinary sweets or chewing gum.

For non-productive irritating coughs caused by inflammation below the larynx, **steam inhalations** may be very useful and can be made to smell nice by adding substances such as **menthol**.

Opiate Cough Suppressants

Powerful opiate drugs reduce the sensitivity of the cough centre in the brain. They are used to suppress severe coughs (e.g. in cancer of the lung). They include **diamorphine** (**heroin**), **methadone** (**Physeptone**) and **morphine**. These are discussed in Chapter 30. They also tend to dry up and thicken bronchial secretions. These drugs can cause addiction.

Codeine is a much less powerful opiate than morphine. In appropriate dosage it may help to suppress a dry or painful cough but not a severe cough. It may cause constipation and regular daily use may produce addiction.

Milder opiate cough suppressants include **pholcodine** and **dextromethorphan** (present in many cough mixtures). They are less constipating and less effective but they are not addictive.

> *Cough medicines containing codeine or some other opiate should be used with utmost caution in children and not in infants under one year of age.*

Cough Mixtures

In addition to containing small doses of a cough suppressant and/or an expectorant many of these mixtures contain soothing substances (*demulcents*) such as sorbitol, glycerol, syrup and flavourings, for example, peppermint, eucalyptus, lemon, clove, aniseed and menthol.

Some compound cough medicines contain **antihistamines**. Yet there is doubt about their benefits. They may dry the surface of the upper respiratory tract. Cough medicines that contain a sedative antihistamine, e.g. promethazine and diphenhydramine, are used at night because they cause drowsiness; but see warnings on antihistamines in A–Z of Medicine.

Selecting a Cough Medicine

For a dry or painful throaty cough (i.e. caused by inflammation or irritation above the larynx) anything that may be sucked will help. If the cough is very irritating it may help to take a dose of codeine linctus along with something to suck or chew.

For a cough which is on the chest (below the larynx) which is dry and irritating, a single cough suppressant may help, e.g. linctus **codeine** or **phol-**

codine. For the ordinary dry cough associated with a common cold only three or four doses at appropriate intervals will be required.

Products containing codeine and pholcodine include:

Codeine:	*Pholcodine:*
Benylin with Codeine	**Benylin Children's Dry Cough**
Boots Catarrh Cough Syrup	**Boots Children's 1 Year Plus Night Time Cough Syrup**
Dimotane Co	**Expulin**
Dimotane Co Paediatric	**Expulin Dry**
Famel Original	**Expulin Paediatric**
Galcodine	**Galenphol**
Galcodine Paediatric	**Galenphol Strong**
Pulmo Bailly	**Hill's Balsam Adult Expectorant**
Robitussin Night-Time	**Hill's Balsam Cough Suppressant**
	Nirolex Day Cold Comfort
	Nirolex for Night Time Coughs
	Pavacol D
	Tixylix Cough and Cold
	Tixylix Daytime
	Tixylix Night-time

Steam inhalations are of benefit to both dry throaty coughs and to nonproductive chesty coughs. If you find yourself having to take a cough suppressant for more than a few days then see your doctor. Also see your doctor if the cough does not clear up after one or two weeks, if your sputum turns yellow or green (you may need an **antibiotic**), if there is blood in your sputum, if your cough is associated with chest pain and/or fever or if it is associated with breathlessness.

A chesty productive cough (i.e. when you cough up sputum) may be helped by **warm drinks** and/or **steam inhalations**, stopping smoking and avoiding dry, dusty atmospheres. Cough medicines are of little use.

Diamorphine (**heroin**), **methadone** and **morphine** are effective cough suppressants used to control coughs in patients suffering from lung cancer or other severe disorders.

> *Patients with kidney or heart disorders, or with raised blood pressure, or on a reduced sodium intake, should check the sodium content of any cough medicine that they purchase from their pharmacist.*

12

Drugs Used to Treat Disorders of the Mouth and Throat

Thrush, Cold Sores and Mouth Ulcers

Thrush of the mouth is caused by a fungus, *candida albicans*. It is treated with an antifungal drug such as **nystatin** suspension (**Nystamont, Nystan**) or with **amphotericin** lozenges (**Fungilin**). **Miconazole** oral gel (**Daktarin**) or **fluconazole** (**Diflucan**) are useful for severe fungal infections.

Herpes infection (cold sores) of the mouth is very difficult to treat. The antiviral drug **aciclovir** (in **Boots Avert, Herpetad, Soothelip, Viralief, Virasorb, Zovirax** cream) should be used at the first sign of a sore. A protective such as petroleum jelly (**Vaseline**) may help. Corticosteroid applications should *not* be used and drying agents may trigger secondary infection. A **tetracycline** rinse may help. A **chlorhexidine** mouthwash (**Chlorohex, Corsodyl**) should be used to prevent dental plaque if the mouth is too painful to use a toothbrush.

Recurrent mouth ulcers (aphthous ulcers) can be very painful and treatment very disappointing. Local treatment aimed at soothing the pain and helping healing is not usually very effective. Preparations available include:

- *mechanical protectives* e.g. **Orabase** ointment (**carmellose sodium**, pectin and **gelatin**); *corticosteroids* in lozenges or pastes e.g. **Adcortyl** (**triamcinolone**) in **Orabase** paste; **Corlan** pellets (**hydrocortisone**);
- *local anaesthetic gels and lozenges* e.g. **benzocaine** lozenges, **benzocaine** compound lozenges (contain **menthol** as well);
- *local pain-relievers* such as **Bonjela** and **Teejel** (**choline salicylate** paste), **Pyralvex** (**anthraquinone** and **salicylic acid**) and **Difflam** (**benzydamine**);
- *antibiotic mouthwashes* (e.g. **tetracycline** mouthwash).

Other preparations include:
   Anbesol (**cetylpyridinium, chlorocresol, lidocaine**(lignocaine))
   Bansor (**cetrimide**), **Bioral Gel** (**carbenoxolone sodium**)
   Bonjela Pastilles (**aminoacridine**(aminacrine), **lidocaine**(lignocaine))

Frador (**chlorbutanol, menthol**)
Medijel (**aminoacridlne**(aminacrine), **lidocaine**(lignocaine))
Oragard (**cetylpyridinium, lidocaine**(lignocaine))
Rinstead Gel (**benzocaine, chloroxylenol**)
Rinstead Pastilles (**chloroxylenol, menthol**)

Acute ulceration of the gums (Vincent's infection) requires treatment with
the antimicrobial drug **metronidazole** (**Flagyl**).

Mouth Washes and Gargles

Mouth washes and gargles clean and freshen the mouth and are helpful in the
care of the mouth in debilitated patients. The mouth washes include compound **sodium chloride** (salt), compound **thymol glycerine**, **hydrogen peroxide**
(**Peroxyl**) and **phenol** mouth washes. Brand preparations include **cetylpyridinium** (**Merocet**), **chlorhexidine** (**Chlorohex, Corsodyl,** in **Eludril**) which is useful
for preventing plaque formation on teeth which may lead to the development
of caries, **hexetidine** (**Oraldene**), **povidone-iodine** (**Betadine**) and **sodium perborate** (**Bocasan**).

Drugs Used to Treat Sore Throat

The commonest cause of a sore throat is a virus infection, for which there is
no specific treatment apart from sucking a sweet or a throat lozenge and
taking a pain-reliever such as paracetamol or ibuprofen.

Antiseptic throat sprays and lozenges, while very popular, have very little
evidence to support their use. They can cause irritation and sore tongue and
lips. Some of these medicines contain local anaesthetics which relieve pain
but may cause sensitization.

A list of these preparations include:

AAA (**benzocaine**)
Beechams Throat Plus
  (**benzalkonium,**
  hexylresorcinol)
Bradosol (**benzalkonium**)
Bradosol Plus (**domiphen,**
  lidocaine(lignocaine))
Dequacaine (**benzocaine,**
  dequalinium)
Dequadin (**dequalinium**)
Eludril spray
  (**tetracaine**(amethocaine),
  chlorhexidine)

Merocets (**cetylpyridinium**)
Merothol (**cetylpyridinium,**
  menthol)
Strepsils (**amylmetacresol,**
  dichlorobenzyl alcohol)
Strepsils Extra (**hexylresorcinol,**
  menthol)
Strepsils Pain Relief Plus
  (**amylmetacresol,**
  dichlorobenzyl alcohol,
  (**lidocaine**(lignocaine))
Strepsils Pain Relief Spray
  (**lidocaine**(lignocaine))

Labosept (dequalinium)
Meggezones (menthol)
Mentholatum (amylmetacresol,
   menthol)
Merocaine (benzocaine,
   cetylpyridinium)

TCP pastilles (phenols)
Tyrozets (benzocaine, tyrothricin)
Valda (menthol, thymol)
Vicks Ultra Chloraseptic
   (benzocaine)

The commonest bacterial infection of the throat is caused by a streptococcal infection (a strep sore throat). This infection can cause tonsillitis and complications such as rheumatic fever and kidney disease. It needs treating quickly and effectively with **phenoxymethylpenicillin**(penicillin V) (**Tenkicin**) by mouth for ten days. If the infection is severe an initial injection of **benzylpenicillin**(penicillin G) (**Crystapen**) should be given into a muscle. Amoxicillin by mouth is an alternative to phenoxymethylpenicillin. If the patient is allergic to penicillin, **erythromycin** (**Erymax, Erythrocin, Erythroped, Rommix, Tiloryth**) should be used.

Treatment of Laryngitis

Laryngitis is an inflammation of the voice-box which affects the vocal cords, producing a hoarse voice. Acute laryngitis is often due to a virus infection (e.g. a cold virus). It may also occur from shouting, over-singing, allergy and inhaling irritant fumes. Chronic laryngitis is often due to shouting or over-singing, what the specialists politely call 'vocal abuse'. It occurs particularly by straining the voice during an acute attack of laryngitis. It is made worse by coughing and smoking.

The best treatment for acute laryngitis is to rest the voice, inhale steam and avoid irritants (e.g. smoking). If hoarseness persists for more than a week or so you should ask your doctor to send you to see an ear, nose and throat specialist for a check-up.

13

Drugs Used to Treat Disorders of the Ears and Eyes

1 Disorders of the Ear

Removal of Ear Wax

Wax (cerumen) in the ear is normal and it helps to protect the lining of the outer ear. It only needs removing if there is so much that it is causing deafness or if the doctor cannot examine the ear drum properly in a patient with some other ear complaint. To clean the wax out, the ear should be syringed with warm water by a doctor or nurse. If the wax is very hard, it can be softened before syringing by applying sodium bicarbonate ear drops, warm olive oil or almond oil. Preparations that contain a wetting agent (e.g. **docusate sodium**) or **urea hydrogen peroxide** may be equally effective.

Ear drops used to remove wax from the ears include:
Cerumol (**chlorbutanol**, paradichlorobenzene, **arachis oil**)
Exterol (**urea hydrogen peroxide, hydroxyquinoline and glycerol**)
Molcer (**docusate sodium**)
Otex (**urea hydrogen peroxide, hydroxyquinoline and glycerol**)
sodium bicarbonate (**sodium bicarbonate in glycerol**)
Waxsol (**docusate sodium**)

Inflammation of the Outer Ear (Otitis Externa)

Otitis externa is inflammation of the skin lining the outer ear canal, caused by eczema and/or infection. Acute attacks are treated by drying and cleaning the ear and the application of a ribbon gauze (gauze wick) soaked in **aluminium acetate solution** to dry the surface, or a weak solution of a **corticosteroid** to relieve any inflammation. Chronic otitis externa is often accompanied by a discharge, itching and irritation. Cleaning, drying and drying drops (aluminium acetate solution) may help. Corticosteroid drops (**betamethasone**

(**Betnesol**, **Vista-methasone**), **prednisolone** (**Predsol**)) are very helpful and if infection and inflammation are present a combined **corticosteroid/antibacterial** preparation should be used. Combined corticosteroid/antibacterial preparations include:

betamethasone/neomycin (**Betnesol-N, Vista-Methasone-N**)
dexamethasone/neomycin (**Otomize**)
dexamethasone/framycetin/gramicidin (**Sofradex**)
flumetasone/clioquinol (**Locorten-Vioform**)
hydrocortisone/gentamicin (**Gentisone HC**)
hydrocortisone/neomycin (**Neo-Cortef**)
hydrocortisone/neomycin/polymyxin B (**Otosporin**)
prednisolone/neomycin (**Predsol-N**)
triamcinolone/neomycin (**Audicort**)
triamcinolone/gramicidin/neomycin/nystatin (**Tri-Adcortyl Otic**)

Infection should be treated with a topical non-systemic broad spectrum **antibacterial** drug (**chloramphenicol**, **gentamicin** (**Cidomycin**, **Garamycin**, **Genticin**)). Treatment for more than one week may trigger a fungus infection which can be very difficult to treat. Allergy to the antibiotic or solvent may occur and resistance to the antibiotic may develop. If a fungal infection is suspected, an antifungal drug, e.g. **clotrimazole** (**Canesten** solution) should be added to the treatment.

Corticosteroids rapidly reduce swelling when applied to an inflamed non-infective otitis externa. They should be used with caution for long-term treatment and prolonged treatment in pregnancy should be avoided. Prolonged use of topical corticosteroid and antibacterials should be avoided because of the risk of the antibacterial producing damage to the ear (e.g. hearing loss) and bacterial resistance to the antibiotic (see p. 264). If a fungal infection is suspected, an antifungal drug (e.g. clotrimazole (Canestan Ear)) should be used, alone or in combination with an antibacterial drug.

Patients suffering from otitis externa should have their ear drums examined carefully to see if there is a perforation, because sometimes a discharge may come from the *middle ear* through a perforation in the ear drum. In these patients, it is important to be careful and not to apply antibacterial drugs to the outer ear which, if they were to enter the middle ear, could cause deafness; for example, the antibiotics **framycetin**, **gentamicin**, **neomycin**, or **polymyxin B**, or the antiseptic **chlorhexidine**.

Choline salicylate (**Audax**) is a mild analgesic which is of doubtful benefit when applied locally.

Inflammation of the Middle Ear (Otitis Media)

Infection in the middle ear causes pain, often with fever and deafness. Pain should be treated with paracetamol. If it is caused by a virus no antibiotic treatment is necessary; if it is bacterial, then antibiotics should be given immediately. An injection of **benzylpenicillin**(penicillin G) (**Crystapen**) should be given to start treatment and then **phenoxymethylpenicillin**(penicillin V), (**Tenkicin**) by mouth. Treatment should continue for five–ten days. Recurrent otitis media should be prevented by giving an antibacterial drug daily during the winter months, e.g. trimethoprim or erythromycin.

2 Disorders of the Eyes

Antibacterial Drugs Applied to the Eyes

As with antibacterial drugs used to treat skin and ear disorders, those antibiotics which are never, or seldom, used internally, should be used. This is to reduce the risk of the patient becoming allergic to an antibiotic applied topically to the eyes and then subsequently running the risk of a serious allergic reaction if that drug is then taken by mouth or injection at some future date.

Antibiotics with a wide spectrum of activity against bacteria are used locally. They include **chloramphenicol** (**Chloromycetin**, **Sno Phenicol**), **ciprofloxacin** (**Ciloxan**), **framycetin** (**Soframycin**), **gentamicin** (**Cidomycin**, **Garamycin**, **Genticin**), **lomefloxacin** (**Okacyn**), **neomycin** (**Neosporin**), **ofloxacin** (**Fxocin**). Gentamicin is effective against a particularly nasty infection caused by *Pseudomonas aeruginosa* and **fusidic acid** (**Fucithalmic**) is effective against bacteria that also cause boils (staphylococcus). **Chlortetracycline** (**Aureomycin**) and **tetracycline** are used to treat chlamydial infections of the eyes, including trachoma.

Antiviral Drugs Applied to the Eyes

The herpes simplex virus that produces cold sores can infect the eyes, producing ulcers of the cornea; so too can the herpes zoster virus that produces shingles. They are treated with **aciclovir** (**Zovirax**) applications.

Retinitis caused by the cytomegalovirus in patients with AIDS can be treated with **fomivirsen** (**Vitravene**) which is administered by injection into the eye.

Corticosteroid Drugs Applied to the Eyes

The most effective anti-inflammatory drugs used to treat inflammatory conditions of the eyes are the corticosteroids. They are used to reduce inflammation in inflamed and allergic eye diseases and to reduce inflammation following eye surgery. They may be used as local applications, local injections under the conjunctivae or by mouth. They include **betamethasone** (**Betnesol**, **Vista-Methasone**), **clobetasone** (**Cloburate**), **dexamethasone** (**Maxidex**), **fluorometholone** (**FML**), **hydrocortisone** (**Neo-Cortef**), **prednisolone** (**Pred Forte**, **Predsol**), **rimexolone** (**Vexol**).

It is very important to restrict the use of corticosteroid eye preparations and not to use them to treat acute red eye (e.g. allergic or bacterial conjunctivitis) or to treat inflammation of the eyelids. A corticosteroid *should only be used* after a full eye examination has been carried out (including sight test) and fluorescein eye drops have been inserted in the eye to check for any ulcers or scarring of the cornea. If these are present the patient should be referred to an eye specialist. The patient should also see an eye specialist if there is no improvement after one–two weeks of treatment.

Corticosteroids applied to the eye can lower defence mechanisms and make an eye infection worse, particularly if it is due to a viral or fungal infection. They may lower resistance to an infection, especially to bacteria. If corticosteroid applications are used over the long term they may cause thinning of the cornea, perforation, raised pressure in the eye (glaucoma) and cataracts. Long-term use in young people may produce generalized toxic effects (see Chapter 37). Therefore, the use of a corticosteroid and an anti-infective combined is rarely justified. Those commonly prescribed are **betamethasone/ neomycin** (**Betnesol-N**, **Vista-Methasone N**), **dexamethasone/neomycin/poly- myxin B** (**Maxitrol**), **dexamethasone/framycetin/gramicidin** (**Sofradex**), **pred- nisolone/neomycin** (**Predsol-N**).

Anti-inflammatory Drugs Applied to the Eyes

Ketorolac trometamol (**Acular** eye drops) are used to prevent and reduce inflammation of the eye following surgery.

Anti-allergy Drugs Applied to the Eyes

Eye drops containing an antihistamine may help to relieve the redness and itching of allergic conjunctivitis, for example, **antazoline** (**Optilast**) combined with a decongestant **xylometazoline** (**Otrivine-Antistin**), but they should only be used for a few days at a time. **Levocabastine** (**Livostin** eye drops) is an antihistamine applied topically that is quick to act and produces prolonged effects. **Emedastine** (**Emadine**), **Iodoxamide** (**Alomide**), **nedocromil sodium** (**Rapitil**) and **sodium cromoglycate** (**Clariteyes**, **Hay-crom**, **Opticrom**, **Optrex Allergy**, **Viz-on**, **Vividrin**) are effective anti-inflammatory/anti-allergy drugs.

Soothing Eye Applications

Soothing preparations are included in eye drops to soothe and relieve irri- tation. The safest ones to use are polymers which are soluble in water (e.g. **hypromellose**).

Drugs Used to Treat Dry Eyes

Eye lubricants include **carmellose sodium** (**Celluvisc**), **hypromellose** (**Artelac, Isopto** preparations, **Tears Naturale**), **polyacrylic acid** (**GelTears, Viscotears**), **hydroxymethylcellulose** (**Minims Artificial Tears**), **liquid paraffin** (**Lacri-Lube, Lubri-Tears**), **polyvinyl alcohol** (**Hypotears, Liquifilm Tears, Sno Tears**) and **povidone** (**Oculotect**). **Acetylcysteine** (**Ilube**) helps to lubricate and also break down mucus.

Other Preparations

Sodium chloride solution (sterile) is useful for washing out the eyes and **zinc sulphate** eye drops have been used to dry the eyes. Decongestant cye drops (**ephedrine** and **phenylephrine**) relieve congestion but repeated use can cause redness of the eyes.

Drugs which Work on the Pupils

● *Drugs which Dilate the Pupils*

Drugs which dilate the pupils are called mydriatics. They cause the pupil to dilate by paralysing the circular muscles of the iris, by stimulating it to contract or by a mixture of both actions. Those that paralyse the circular muscles may be referred to as cycloplegics and they may produce prolonged effects.

Anticholinergic drugs (see Chapter 9) produce these effects and they are used in eye drops to dilate the pupils. Short-acting anticholinergic drugs such as **tropicamide** (**Mydriacyl**) are used by eye specialists to dilate the pupils so that they can examine the inside of the eyes more easily. Longer-acting anticholinergic drugs are used to rest the pupil in patients who have an infection of the pupil. The effects of **tropicamide** last about three hours; **cyclopentolate** and **homatropine** about twenty-four hours, and the effects of **atropine** may last for over a week.

● *Drugs that Constrict the Pupils*

Drugs that cause the pupils to constrict (become small) are called *miotics*. They act in an opposite way to the anticholinergic drugs. They constrict the muscle that works the iris, so that the pupil becomes small and opens up the drainage canal in the front chamber of the eye. They are used to constrict the pupil after a patient has had a mydriatic applied to dilate the pupil for an eye examination, particularly in patients over the age of forty, in order to avoid the risk of triggering off an attack of glaucoma. They are also used to treat open-angle glaucoma in order to reduce the pressure in the front of the eye (see below).

Drugs that constrict the pupils (*miotics*) include drugs which act like acetylcholine, for example **carbachol** and **pilocarpine** (**Pilogel**). For a discussion of the actions and effects produced by these drugs, read Chapter 9.

> **Warning:** *Drugs which constrict the pupils and are applied to the eyes may be absorbed directly into the bloodstream. Also, eye drops may run down the nose and down the cheek into the mouth and be absorbed from the nose or mouth into the bloodstream. Therefore, they may produce generalized harmful effects which include increased salivation, sweating, slow heart rate, stomach pains and wheezing.*

Glaucoma

Glaucoma is a term used to describe an increase in pressure inside the eye and the damage that it produces. About 1 person in 100 over forty years of age develops glaucoma, and about 5 in 100 of those over sixty-five years.

In *glaucoma* the pressure of the fluid in the front chamber of the eyes (between the lens and the cornea) is raised due to a defective draining away of the fluid while the inflow remains steady. The increase in pressure affects the transparency of the cornea (the window of the eye) and compresses the blood vessels that supply the main optic nerve that links the eye to the brain. The latter may produce irreversible damage to the optic nerve resulting in a permanent loss of vision. This loss of vision may come on suddenly over a few days or may develop slowly over years.

There are two principal types of glaucoma – *open-angle* and *closed-angle* glaucoma.

● Open-angle Glaucoma (Chronic Simple Glaucoma)

This is the commonest type of glaucoma. It comes on slowly and is commonest in elderly people. The increase in pressure is caused by a decreased outflow from the front chamber of the eye which probably results from a degeneration of the outlet mechanisms. It causes no early symptoms but may lead to a slow and progressive reduction in the outer fields of vision (the peripheral vision) and eventually to blindness. Both eyes are nearly always affected, although one eye may be more severely affected than the other and the loss of vision may not be noticed for months or years. *There is no pain with open-angle glaucoma and no sudden onset of symptoms.*

● Closed-angle Glaucoma (Narrow-angle Glaucoma; Acute Glaucoma; Congestive Glaucoma)

This develops when the drainage of fluid from the front chamber of the eye is *suddenly* blocked. This may occur in patients who are *predisposed to develop closed-angle glaucoma* because they have a small eyeball in which the drainage angle for fluid in the front chamber of the eye between the iris and the lens is very narrow and it may easily become *closed off* by a swelling of the iris or lens (i.e. 'closed-angle'). When the pupil dilates, the circular muscles of the iris are more bulky than when the pupil is constricted. This bulkiness may block off the narrow angle between the iris and the lens and interfere with the drainage of fluid. *A number of drugs may close this angle by causing dilation of the pupil and may trigger off an acute attack in someone prone to develop glaucoma.*

When the angle is blocked the pressure builds up rapidly and the patient complains of a sudden onset of blurred vision, perhaps preceded by seeing haloes around objects, severe pain in the affected eye and usually some headache, nausea and vomiting. On examination the pressure in the affected eye is found to be increased and there is a loss of vision, the eye is red and painful, and the pupil looks cloudy. It may be very serious and requires *immediate treatment* from an eye specialist.

● *Drugs which may Trigger off an Attack of Glaucoma in Patients Prone to Develop Closed-angle Glaucoma*

antimuscarinic drugs (e.g. **atropine** and **hyoscine**)
antihistamines
chlorpropamide used to treat diabetes
corticosteroids
cough and cold remedies containing **antimuscarinic drugs** or **antihistamines**
indomethacin used to treat rheumatoid arthritis
monoamine oxidase inhibitor antidepressants
oral contraceptives
tricyclic antidepressant drugs

Treatment of Glaucoma

● *Drugs Used to Treat Glaucoma and How They Work*

Miotic eye drops (e.g. **carbachol**, **pilocarpine** (**Pilogel**)) decrease the pressure in the front chamber of the eye by improving the drainage of the fluid. Unfortunately, they constrict the pupil and may produce blurring of vision and an aching in the brow.

Adrenaline(epinephrine) (**Eppy, Simplene**) eye drops help to improve the drainage of fluid in the front chamber of the eye and may decrease its rate of production. The net result is a reduction in the pressure in the eye. Adrenaline(epinephrine) may produce severe smarting and redness of the eye and it should not be used in closed-angle glaucoma (see earlier) because adrenaline(epinephrine) dilates the pupil and this may interfere with drainage. **Dipivefrine** (**Propine**) eye drops are formulated to pass quickly through the cornea and enter the fluid in the front chamber of the eye where the dipivefrine is converted into adrenaline(epinephrine). Adrenaline(epinephrine) and related preparations applied to the eye reduce the production of fluid in the anterior chamber and increase its drainage. They have minimal effects on the heart and circulation and do not affect breathing.

Brimonidine (**Alphagan**) and **apraclonidine** (**Iopidine**) are **Alpha$_2$-Adrenoceptor Stimulants**. Brimonidine is more selective in its actions than apraclonidine and does not cause blanching of the conjunctivae or mydriasis. They are used in the treatment of open-angle glaucoma or hypertension in the eye.

Guanethidine (**Ganda**) is used to treat raised blood pressure (see Chapter 25). It is applied as eye drops to treat glaucoma because it helps to reduce the pressure inside the eye by slowing the rate of production of the fluid in the front chamber of the eye and increasing its drainage outflow. It has a slow constricting effect on the pupil, although at first it may cause the pupil to dilate. It increases and prolongs the effects of adrenaline(epinephrine).

Beta-blockers are discussed in detail in Chapter 22. Several are used as eye drops for treating glaucoma. They are thought to reduce the pressure inside the eye by reducing the rate of production of the fluid in the front chamber of the eye.

Beta-blockers used as eye drops include the selective blocker **betaxolol** (**Betoptic**), and the non-selective blockers **carteolol** (**Teoptic**), **levobunolol** (**Betagan**), **metipranolol** and **timolol** (**Timoptol**).

Like any drug applied to the eyes, beta-blockers may be absorbed directly into the bloodstream and also from the nose and mouth if the drops run into them. This absorption may produce harmful effects, particularly in patients who suffer from asthma; in patients with a slow heart rate; and in patients with heart failure because they may make the condition worse. A sufficient amount of drug may also be absorbed to interact with other drugs: for example, with the drug **verapamil**, used to treat angina and disorders of heart rhythm. The absorbed beta-blocker may interact with the verapamil to cause a fall in blood pressure, heart failure and may, very rarely, stop the heart from beating. Beta-blocker eye drops may produce dry eyes, conjunctivitis and allergic inflammation of the eyelids.

Diuretics (water tablets) are discussed in detail in Chapter 29. One of these drugs, **acetazolamide** (**Diamox**), is used to reduce the pressure in the eye. It reduces the volume of fluid in the front chamber of the eye by blocking the production of bicarbonate which causes a reduction in the production of water into the fluid.

Dorzolamide (**Trusopt**, in **Cosopt**) and **brinzolamide** (**Azopt**) are diuretics similar to acetazolamide that can be applied directly to the eye instead of being taken by mouth.

The prostaglandin analogue **latanoprost** (**Xalatan**) increases the outflow of fluid from the eye. It is used for open-angle glaucoma and hypertension in the eye when other drugs are inappropriate. Latanoprost can affect the colour of the eyes increasing the brown colour. Therefore, particular care is required in patients with mixed coloured eyes or when only one eye is being treated.

● *Drug Treatment of Open-angle Glaucoma (Chronic Simple Glaucoma)*

In this condition drug treatment is used to reduce the pressure inside the eye and to maintain this pressure at a normal level, usually for the rest of the patient's life. Effective drug treatment (if taken as directed) prevents further deterioration in vision, but of course it cannot restore any damage that has already occurred and this is why early diagnosis is important.

Treatment usually starts with **beta-blocker** eye drops (see above) to reduce the rate of production of fluid in the eye and then a drug which constricts the pupil and improves drainage of fluid from the eye may be added. **Pilocarpine** (**Pilogel**) is one of the most commonly used drugs for this purpose and it is often preferred in older patients. However, younger people and short-sighted people may find that the constriction of the pupil produced by pilocarpine affects their vision, while other people may find that the drops actually help them to focus. Over time it may be necessary to add **adrenaline**(epinephrine) (**Eppy, Simplene**) to the beta-blocker and pilocarpine.

Because pilocarpine constricts the pupils, anyone who has a disorder of the lens (e.g. early cataract) may find that their vision is further impaired. In these patients it is best to try a beta-blocker first and then add adrenaline (epinephrine) eye drops if necessary.

If these treatments are not beneficial the addition of **acetazolamide** (**Diamox**) by mouth may help. An alternative is **dorzolamide** (**Trusopt**) eye drops which may be given on its own if beta-blockers are contra-indicated or are ineffective, or as additional treatment to beta-blockers. A combination product of **dorzolamide** with **timolol** (**Cosopt**), a beta-blocker, is available.

● *Drug Treatment of Acute (Closed-angle) Glaucoma*

A person who has developed acute glaucoma needs urgent medical treatment in order to prevent loss of vision. Drugs are used to bring down the pressure in the eyes and then laser treatment or surgery may be carried out to provide drainage of the fluid and to prevent a recurrence of the problem. It is not usual for drug treatment to be continued for very long.

Acetazolamide (**Diamox**) is normally the first drug to be given, at first by injection and then by mouth. Eye drops to constrict the pupil are then applied at frequent intervals and occasionally a thiazide or other osmotic diuretic is given by mouth (see Chapter 29) to draw fluid out of the tissues.

Other Eye Preparations

For diagnostic purposes **fluorescein sodium** and **rose bengal** are both used. They stain the eye and are used for locating any damaged areas of the cornea.

Diclofenac sodium (**Voltarol Ophtha**) and **flurbiprofen** (**Ocufen**) are anti-inflammatory drugs used to reduce inflammation in the eye following surgery.

14

Drugs Used to Treat Bronchial Asthma

1 Drugs Used to Relieve the Symptoms of Asthma

Bronchodilators

Drugs which open up the airways are called bronchodilators because they act by dilating (opening up) the bronchial tubes. They are used to reverse or decrease obstruction to the flow of air to the lungs caused by narrowing of these tubes. This occurs in bronchial asthma which is a chronic inflammation, causing spasm of the muscles in the bronchial tubes (bronchospasm), swelling of the lining surfaces and an increased production of secretions. Narrowing of the airways may also occur in chronic chest disorders such as emphysema and bronchitis. In these disorders the small bronchial tubes are scarred, distorted and narrowed by repeated infections (e.g. bronchitis). In addition, repeated infections affect the secretory glands in the walls of the bronchial tubes and in the lining membranes. These increase in size and produce more secretions (sputum or phlegm), resulting in a productive cough. Also in such disorders as emphysema the lung tissues lose their normal 'elastic' action and this causes many small bronchial tubes to close up on breathing out. Thus the two types of obstruction to the airways produced by asthma and chronic bronchitis differ; the extent to which they can be treated by drugs also differs. Much more benefit from bronchodilator drugs may obviously be obtained when the airways are obstructed due to spasm, as in asthma, than when it is due to scarring as in chronic bronchitis. Breathing tests show that bronchodilator drugs are highly effective in improving the airways in patients suffering from bronchial asthma and may be effective in patients with chronic obstructive airways disease (e.g. chronic bronchitis and emphysema).

There are three main groups of bronchodilator drugs – sympathomimetic drugs, theophylline derivatives and antimuscarinics.

Sympathomimetic Drugs

These drugs, as their name implies, mimic the effects of stimulating the sympathetic division of the autonomic nervous system (see p. 38). They include chemicals which are produced in the body, e.g. **adrenaline**(epinephrine) and **noradrenaline**(norepinephrine) (which is the main chemical messenger at nerve endings of the sympathetic nervous system). Numerous drugs also mimic stimulation of the sympathetic nervous system, e.g. **isoprenaline** and **ephedrine** (see Chapter 9).

Drugs which stimulate beta adrenoreceptors (beta-stimulants, beta agonists) (see p. 38) are used to treat acute bronchospasm (wheezing) because they relax bronchial muscles. Original sympathomimetic bronchodilator drugs act on both β_1 and β_2 receptors, so that in addition to relieving bronchospasm (a β_2 effect) they also produce unwanted effects upon the heart and circulation (a β_1 effect) and may produce disorders of heart rate and rhythm. They are called **non-selective adrenoreceptor stimulants**. Drugs which stimulate mainly β_2 receptors to dilate bronchial muscles but produce less effect upon the heart are called **selective adrenoreceptor stimulants**.

The **adrenoreceptor stimulants drugs** used to treat asthma include:

- *Selective Stimulants*
  bambuterol (**Bambec**)
  formoterol(eformoterol) (**Foradil, Oxis**)
  fenoterol* (in **Duovent**)
  reproterol* (**Bronchodil**)
  salbutamol* (in **Aerocrom, Aerolin, Airomir, Asmasal, Asmaven**, in **Combivent, Maxivent, Salamol, Salbulin, Ventmax**, in **Ventide, Ventodisks, Ventolin, Volmax**)
  salmeterol (**Serevent**)
  terbutaline* (**Bricanyl, Monovent**)
  tulobuterol* (**Respacal**)
  orciprenaline (**Alupent**): partially selective

* Short-acting bronchodilators.

Inhalation devices (e.g. aerosols) are the most effective and convenient way of taking these drugs. Inhalations of short-acting bronchodilators provide relief for three–six hours. They act rapidly and should be used *when needed* to treat acute attacks of asthma in patients with normal lung function who suffer infrequent attacks, and to prevent an asthma attack during exercise. *They should not be used on a regular basis*. Reduction in the duration of their effects or an increase in their use indicates that the asthma is getting worse, and that further treatment is needed. In general children do better on inhalers than on preparations by mouth. Long-acting bronchodilators (**bambuterol**,

formoterol(eformoterol) and **salmeterol**) may be used on a long-term basis to prevent, for example, asthma attacks during the night and exercise-induced symptoms. Salmeterol by inhalation is slow to act and works for about twelve hours. Formoterol(eformoterol) by inhalation acts rapidly and works for about twelve hours. Bambuterol is a pro-drug of terbutaline which is taken by mouth and works for up to twenty-four hours. They should not be used to treat an acute attack or to replace other preventative drug treatments (see below).

Special devices to help inhalation are available and the inhalation of aqueous solutions using a **nebulizer** (a powered machine that produces a fine spray) may be very useful in some patients, but be warned, the doses are higher than in aerosols.

Preparations by mouth are available for people who cannot manage inhalers. They are slower to work than inhalers but their effects last longer. Sustained-released preparations may be useful for preventing night attacks of asthma.

For adverse effects and precautions in using adrenoreceptor stimulants, see A–Z of Medicines.

Warning: *If over-used, all these bronchodilators (beta stimulants) may cause dose-related increases in heart-rate, tremor of the hands, a rise in blood glucose levels and a potentially serious fall in the concentration of potassium in the blood.*

Theophylline and Related Drugs (Xanthines)

Theophylline and related drugs relax bronchial muscles and relieve wheezing. They may be given by injection, by mouth and as suppositories. Their effectiveness depends upon the amount of theophylline which enters the bloodstream. **Aminophylline** is a mixture of theophylline and ethylinediamine which makes a more soluble preparation for injection.

Modified release preparations of theophylline by mouth may be used as additional treatment when a patient is not responding to anti-inflammatory drugs (e.g. corticosteroids) plus the use of a bronchodilator when necessary. They are useful when given at night for controlling night attacks of asthma and for preventing early morning attacks of wheezing. Treatment should start with small doses and be gradually built up. Treatment needs to be individualized and regular measurements of the blood level of theophylline should be carried out because there is a narrow gap between the level that relieves and prevents wheezing and the level that produces adverse effects. There is also a marked variation in response between individuals.

Theophylline preparations include:

aminophylline (Amnivent*, Min-I-Jet, Norphyllin SR*, Phyllocontin Continus*)

theophylline (Nuelin, Nuelin SA*, Slo-Phyllin*, Theo-Dur*, Uniphyllin Continus*)

* Modified-release preparations.

> *Note: the duration of the action of **theophylline** is reduced by smoking and alcohol. It is increased by virus infections and in patients suffering from liver disease and heart failure. This may result in high blood levels, producing nausea and vomiting in these patients on what appears to be a 'normal' dose. Blood level monitoring should be carried out on patients receiving a theophylline preparation. Several drugs can affect the blood level of theophylline; see A–Z of Medicines.*

Antimuscarinic Drugs

Ipratropium (Atrovent, in Duovent, Respontin) and **oxitropium (Oxivent)** are *selective* acting antimuscarinic drugs. They are given by inhalation and relax the bronchial muscles and dry up secretions for eight–twelve hours. They are used to relieve wheezing especially in chronic bronchitis. They are a useful addition to treatment when anti-inflammatory drugs (e.g. corticosteroids) and a selective adrenoreceptor stimulant (used when necessary) are not providing adequate relief.

> *Warning: Combined preparations of bronchodilators and/or other anti-asthma drugs should not be used because the dose of each cannot be changed without changing the dose of the other drug.*

2 Drugs Used to Prevent Asthma

Non-steroidal Anti-inflammatory Drugs

Sodium cromoglycate (in Aerocrom, Cromogen, Intal) and **nedocromil sodium (Tilade)** act on the surface of special cells (mast cells) to prevent the release of chemicals (in response, for example, to an allergen) which cause bronchospasm (wheezing) and inflammation of the lining of the bronchial tubes. They are used to *prevent* attacks of asthma but are not effective if taken after the reaction has started. They should be tried on adults who need to use a bronchodilator more than once a day and who get night symptoms and/or who should not take corticosteroids. Sodium cromoglycate should be tried for at least six weeks in children before using corticosteroids. They are also effective for preventing wheezing triggered by exercise, aspirin, industrial dusts, chemicals and cold air. Nedocromil should not be used in children.

Steroidal Anti-inflammatory Drugs

Corticosteroids

These are discussed in Chapter 37. They relieve inflammation in the bronchial tubes and are usually taken by inhalation or by mouth.

Corticosteroids by inhalation are the treatment of choice to prevent asthma attacks in children and adults who need to use an adrenoreceptor stimulant bronchodilator more than once a day or who get night symptoms. They are of doubtful value in chronic bronchitis and emphysema. They take three–seven days to produce maximum benefit and they are best used with a spacer device to prevent deposits in the mouth and throat causing thrush. Preparations of corticosteroids for inhalation include **beclometasone** (**AeroBec**, **Asmabec**, **Beclazone**, **Becloforte**, **Becodisks**, **Becotide**, **Filair**, **Qvar**, in **Ventide**), **budesonide** (**Pulmicort**) and **fluticasone** (**Flixotide**, in **Seretide**). *Note that only a small proportion reaches the lungs; the rest is swallowed and absorbed into the blood-stream. Over time, this may produce corticosteroid adverse effects (see p. 184). Absorption can be minimized by rinsing the mouth out after inhalation.*

Severe acute attacks of asthma will be helped by a short course of oral corticosteroids (e.g. **prednisolone**), Some patients will benefit from intermittent courses when necessary, but a few will need a maintenance daily dose of prednisolone with increased dosage during an acute attack. In order to minimize adverse effects from maintenance treatment oral corticosteroids should, whenever possible, be given as one dose in the morning in the smallest effective dose, along with high doses by inhalation, divided throughout the day.

Anti-allergic Drugs

Ketotifen (**Zaditen**) is an antihistamine which produces anti-allergic effects. It is taken by mouth and may produce drowsiness. It may be of greater use in infancy than in older children.

Montelukast (**Singulair**) and **zafirlukast** (**Accolate**) belong to a group of drugs called **leukotriene receptor antagonists.** These work by blocking the effects of cysteinyl leukotrienes in the airways. Leukotrienes are the main chemicals which tighten the bronchial tubes (i.e. bronchoconstrictors). Therefore, leukotriene receptor antagonists are used in the treatment of mild to moderate asthma in patients where the asthma is not controlled with an inhaled corticosteroid and a short-acting beta₂-stimulant. They may be of benefit in exercise-induced asthma and in those who also suffer from rhinitis (nasal allergy).

Emergency Treatment of Asthma

Emergency treatment of asthma involves the use of oxygen and **salbutamol** or **terbutaline** by nebulizer and an intravenous injection of **hydrocortisone** or **prednisolone** by mouth. If there is no improvement, **ipratropium** by nebulizer may be added to the treatment and **aminophylline** given by slow injection into a vein, provided that the individual is not already taking theophylline by mouth (in high dosages), otherwise **salbutamol** or **terbutaline** should be given by subcutaneous injection.

15

Drugs Used to Treat Epilepsy

Epilepsy is a general term for a group of disorders of the brain which produce sudden and transitory attacks or seizures which may affect various parts of the brain. The attacks are caused by an excessive or disordered 'electrical' discharge from nerve cells in the affected part of the brain. Electrical tracings of the brain show that epileptic attacks are due to electrical discharges spreading outwards from a focus. If such a focus affects the part of the brain that controls movements, then it produces a convulsion; if it affects the part that controls behaviour, then it produces abnormal behaviour, and if it affects a sensory area, then it may produce increased sensations, e.g. an abnormal sense of smell.

In most cases of epilepsy the cause is unknown and we refer to them as primary or idiopathic epilepsies. Where there is a cause such as a tumour, infection or injury we call them secondary or symptomatic epilepsies.

When discussing epilepsy, the term *seizure* (or fit) refers to an 'episode' or an 'attack' of epilepsy caused by an excessive amount of electrical activity in parts of the brain. Such an episode may or may not produce a convulsion.

A *convulsion* is a violent involuntary contraction of the muscles which may be prolonged or occur in spasms. Depending upon the type of seizure, it may affect a few muscles (e.g. just in the thumb) or many (e.g. the whole body).

Drug Treatment of Epilepsy

Normally there is a relatively low level of electrical activity in the brain but in a seizure there is a build-up of excessive electrical activity starting in one place (or focus) and spreading outwards to cause uncontrolled stimulation of other parts of the brain – for example, stimulation of the brain cells that bring about movement will cause increased activity of those muscles under the nervous control of those brain cells – this will cause the muscles to twitch and go rigid (a convulsion). Most anti-epileptic drugs (or anticonvulsant drugs) damp down the electrical activity of brain cells and prevent any excess build-up of electrical activity which could result in a seizure.

An epileptic attack may be stopped by any drug that depresses the brain function, for example, a sleeping drug or an anaesthetic. Drugs selected to treat epilepsies should block the electrical discharges but produce as little depression of the brain as possible – you don't want a drug that controls seizures but sends the patient fast asleep or changes the behaviour. Patients have got to have their seizures controlled and yet be able to go to work or school as normal. This is a particularly important point because the first aim of treatment is to prevent attacks developing.

Risks in Pregnancy

There is a rare risk of damage to the baby when anti-epileptic drugs are taken during pregnancy but this risk must be balanced against risks to the baby of inadequately controlled seizures in the mother.

Requirements for anti-epileptic drugs during pregnancy may change because blood levels may fall and cause an increase in frequency of seizures. Therefore, it is important to carry out regular estimations of the blood levels of the drug during pregnancy and to adjust the dose accordingly, in order to keep it within effective and safe limits.

Babies born from mothers who have taken anti-epileptic drugs during pregnancy may have an increased risk of developing spinal cord defects.

Risks in Breastfeeding

Anti-epileptic drugs should be used with caution in breastfeeding mothers, particularly barbiturates (e.g. **phenobarbital**, **methylphenobarbital**) and **primidone** (which is converted to phenobarbital in the body) and **ethosuximide**. If possible, these should not be used.

Epileptic Emergencies

Repeated and prolonged epileptic seizures without recovery of consciousness between attacks is called *status epilepticus*. It is an emergency because if it is not treated the patient may die. The immediate treatment is to give a dose of **diazepam**, **clonazepam** or **lorazepam** directly into a vein (intravenous). If it is not possible to get a needle into a vein, then diazepam may be given as a solution into the rectum. These drugs should work effectively in about nine out of ten patients. To prevent recurrence **phenytoin sodium** or **phenobarbital sodium** should be given by slow intravenous injection. **Fosphenytoin** is converted in the body to **phenytoin** which is used in *status epilepticus* and has the advantage of causing fewer injection site reactions. **Paraldehyde** by injection into a muscle or by rectum was popular in the past and is still used occasionally; so is **chlormethiazole** by intravenous infusion.

All these drugs may depress breathing and facilities for keeping the airways open and for mechanical respiration should be on hand.

Driving

Patients suffering from epilepsy may drive a motor vehicle (but not a heavy goods or public transport vehicle) if they have not had a seizure for one year or if they have suffered only attacks in the night and not when awake for the last three years. If treatment makes you feel drowsy, then do not drive or operate moving machinery.

Drugs Used to Treat Epilepsy

The following drugs are used to treat epilepsy:

● *Benzodiazepines*
 clobazam (**Frisium**)
 clonazepam (**Rivotril**)
 diazepam (**Diazemuls, Stesolid, Valium**)
 lorazepam (**Ativan**)

● *Barbiturates*
 methylphenobarbital (**Prominal**)
 phenobarbital (**Gardenal Sodium**)

● *Others*
 acetazolamide (**Diamox**)
 carbamazepine (**Epimaz, Tegretol, Teril CR, Timonil Retard**)
 chlormethiazole (**Heminevrin**)
 ethosuximide (**Emeside, Zarontin**)
 fosphenytoin (**Pro-Epanutin**)
 gabapentin (**Neurontin**)
 lamotrigine (**Lamictal**)
 levetiracetam (**Keppra**)
 oxcarbazepine (**Trileptal**)
 paraldehyde
 phenytoin (**Epanutin**)
 piracetam (**Nootropil**)
 primidone (**Mysoline**)
 sodium valproate (**Convulex, Epilim**)
 tiagabine (**Gabitril**)

topiramate (**Topamax**)
vigabatrin (**Sabril**)

Commonly Used Drugs to Treat Different Types of Epilepsy

● *Generalized Tonic/Clonic Seizures (grand-mal)*

carbamazepine (**Epimaz, Tegretol, Teril CR, Timonil Retard**)
oxcarbazepine (**Trileptal**)
phenytoin (**Epanutln**)
sodium valproate (**Epilim**)
phenobarbital sodium (**Gardenal Sodium**)
primidone (**Mysoline**)
clonazepam (**Rivotril**)
vigabatrin (**Sabril**)
lamotrigine (**Lamictal**)

● *Partial Seizures (focal, local seizures)*

carbamazepine (**Epimaz, Tegretol, Teril CR, Timonil Retard**)
oxcarbazepine (**Trileptal**)
phenytoin (**Epanutin**)
phenobarbital sodium (**Gardenal Sodium**)
primidone (**Mysoline**)
sodium valproate (**Epillm**)
clonazepam (**Rivotril**)
clobazam (**Frisium**)
acetazolamide (**Diamox**)
vigabatrin (**Sabril**)
gabapentin (**Neurontin**)
lamotrigine (**Lamictal**)
tiagabine (**Gabitril**)
topiramate (**Topamax**)
levetiracetam (**Keppra**)

● *Absent Seizures (petit-mal)*

ethosuximide (**Emeside, Zarontin**)
sodium valproate (**Convulex, Epilim**)

● *Myoclonic Seizures (myoclonic jerks)*

sodium valproate (**Convulex, Epilim**)
clonazepam (**Rivotril**)
ethosuximide (**Emeslde, Zarontin**)

● *Atypical Absence, Atonic and Clonic Seizures*
   phenytoin (**Epanutin**)
   sodium valproate (**Convulex, Epilim**)
   clonazepam (**Rivotril**)
   ethosuximide (**Emeside, Zarontin**)
   phenobarbital sodium (**Gardenal Sodium**)
   lamotrigine (**Lamictal**)

Balancing the Benefits to Risks

The aim of anti-epilepsy drug treatment is to prevent seizures and keep adverse effects to a minimum. This is best achieved by a stepwise approach, starting with a small daily dose and gradually increasing the dose. Estimations of the concentration of an anti-epileptic drug in the bloodstream enable the dose to be adjusted in order to achieve maximum benefits from the smallest dose, ensuring that the risk of harmful effects is kept to a minimum.

Anti-epileptic drugs should not be stopped suddenly because of the risk of triggering a seizure (particularly barbiturates and benzodiazepines). They should be withdrawn gradually, reducing the daily dosage by a small amount every few weeks over a period of several months. Likewise, any changeover of drug treatment should be carried out gradually and with great caution.

Combination Treatment

It is usually more effective and safe to use a single drug (monotherapy) in appropriate daily dosages than to use a combination of drugs. A second drug should be added if adverse effects appear and yet seizures continue. The use of more than two drugs is seldom necessary.

If the maximum daily dose of a single drug fails to provide control of the seizures, its daily dose should be slowly decreased and another drug slowly introduced. Patients should have regular checks of their kidneys and liver function because any decrease in function can affect the blood level of an anti-epileptic drug, leading to a change in seizure control and/or the appearance of adverse effects. Many anti-epileptic drugs affect how the liver deals with other drugs and this can affect their rate of breakdown – see drug interactions, p. xvi.

Risk of Drug Interactions

There is always a risk of one anti-epileptic drug interacting with another, causing a decrease or increase in the blood level of one of the drugs. The result may be an increase in toxicity without improved seizure control. Because these interactions vary considerably and are, in general, unpredictable, patients on two drugs should have the blood level of each drug monitored.

16

Drugs Used to Treat Parkinsonism

Parkinsonism is a disorder of the nervous system in which voluntary movement is disturbed, involuntary movements occur and the tone of muscles is altered. Voluntary movements become slow and shaky (tremor) and muscles become stiff (rigidity). The group of signs and symptoms produced are usually referred to as the 'Parkinson's syndrome' or simply as 'parkinsonism'. There are several causes and the severity of the disorders varies between patients. A common cause these days is the long-term use of antipsychotic drugs (see Chapter 3).

To function properly, centres in the brain responsible for controlling movement are kept in balance by two nerve transmitter systems, **acetylcholine** and **dopamine**. These two systems in the brain are often referred to as the cholinergic system and the dopaminergic system respectively. In parkinsonism the dopaminergic system appears to be defective so that the control mechanisms of movement become unbalanced and the cholinergic system dominates, producing the abnormal movements and rigidity seen in parkinsonism. Chemical suppression of this dominance may, therefore, be applied by the use of drugs which block or interfere with the action of acetylcholine (e.g. by the use of antimuscarinic drugs). Alternatively, drugs which increase the effect of the dopaminergic system will have beneficial effects (e.g. the use of **levodopa**).

The main aim of treatment in parkinsonism is to try to improve both the difficulty in starting movements and the slowness of movement (bradykinesia), and to reduce tremor and muscle rigidity.

For over a century parkinsonism has been treated with antimuscarinic drugs. Atropine was the first to be used and since then many atropine-like drugs have been used. Antihistamines have also been used (such as promethazine and diphenhydramine) but these may have helped because they produce mild antimuscarinic effects (see Chapter 17). Many other drugs have been claimed to be of benefit in treating patients suffering from parkinsonism but the real advance was the discovery of levodopa and other drugs that improve the dopaminergic system.

Antimuscarinic Drugs

There is a choice of antimuscarinic drugs available for the treatment of parkinsonism. These include **benzatropine** (**Cogentin**), **biperiden** (**Akineton**), **orphenadrine** (**Biorphen, Disipal**), **procyclidine** (**Arpicolin, Kemadrin**) and **trihexyphenidyl**(benzhexol) (**Broflex**).

The antimuscarinic drugs are discussed on p. 36. Their beneficial effects in parkinsonism are limited. Muscle rigidity and tremors may be helped but bradykinesia (slowness of movement), one of the most disturbing effects of parkinsonism, is unaffected by them. They dry up the mouth and may help reduce dribbling.

Antimuscarinic drugs are useful in patients with mild early symptoms of parkinsonism who may improve on these drugs *before* they need to take levodopa. Patients with post-encephalitic parkinsonism (principally affects those less than forty years of age and with a history of varying degrees of lethargy) appear to respond better to antimuscarinic drugs than patients with idiopathic (no apparent cause) parkinsonism. They are also useful for reducing drug-induced parkinsonism in patients receiving antipsychotic drugs. Tardive dyskinesia (see Chapter 3) is not improved by anticholinergic drugs and may be made worse. The choice of drug is not critical and they may be taken before food if dry mouth is a problem or after food if they produce stomach upsets.

Different people respond differently to any one of the antimuscarinic drugs; therefore if one drug does not work it is worth trying another.

Dopaminergic Drugs

Levodopa (in **Madopar**, in **Sinemet**) is the chemical precursor (forerunner) of **dopamine**. It improves some of the worst features of parkinsonism – difficulty in starting movement and slowness of movement. This is often impressive, resulting in improvement in walking, eating and talking. The rigidity is also helped and other effects of parkinsonism such as difficulty in balancing, drooling of saliva from the mouth and involuntary eye movements may also improve slowly. Shaking is less frequently improved.

Levodopa may produce many adverse effects which are related to dosage (see under levodopa, A–Z of Medicines).

A major problem with levodopa is that it is rapidly metabolized in the body into dopamine which cannot cross the blood-brain barrier, whereas levodopa can. When given in high dosage sufficient levodopa enters the brain, where it is converted into dopamine. However, adverse effects of levodopa are dose-related. **Carbidopa** and **benserazide** block levodopa metabolism in the body by inhibiting the enzyme dopa-decarboxylase but do not enter the brain. Therefore, they cannot interfere with the conversion of levodopa to dopamine in the brain. When these are given along with levodopa, the metabolism of levodopa outside the brain is blocked and the blood level of levodopa increases. An effective treatment, therefore, is to give a dose of levodopa and carbidopa or benserazide together. This enables the dose of levodopa to be reduced. When giving carbidopa or benserazide and levodopa separately there is a risk that too high a dose of levodopa may be given. Therefore a fixed-dose preparation is used, e.g. **carbidopa** and **levodopa** (**co-careldopa**, **Sinemet**) or **benserazide** and **levodopa** (**co-beneldopa**, **Madopar**). This ensures that the appropriate dose of each is given.

During the first six–eighteen months of treatment with levodopa there may be a slow improvement which is then maintained. Unfortunately, after several years of treatment there may be variations in response, with attacks of weakness lasting for a few hours. These 'on/off' effects are a problem but can be treated by decreasing the interval between doses or by adding other drugs to the treatment. The duration of benefit after each dose of levodopa may decrease over time ('end-of-dose' effect) and this may be helped by giving modified release preparations.

Amantadine (**Symmetrel**) is an antiviral drug used to treat influenza. In parkinsonism it is thought to work by increasing the concentration of dopamine in the brain. It produces mild improvement of slowness of movement, tremor and rigidity. Only a few patients benefit and its effects are short-lived. It may increase the effects of antimuscarinic drugs. It is sometimes used in combination with levodopa, particularly in patients who are unable to tolerate full doses of levodopa.

Bromocriptine (**Parlodel**) stimulates dopamine receptors. It produces similar effects to levodopa but has a long duration of action which may be useful if taken at bedtime by patients who have severe early-morning disability. It is reserved for patients in whom levodopa no longer works and for those who cannot tolerate levodopa. When taken with levodopa it may cause movement disorders and confusion.

Selegiline (**Centrapryl**, **Eldepryl**, **Zelapar**) is a monoamine oxidase (B) inhibitor which blocks the enzyme that breaks down dopamine. It is generally used when the effects of levodopa begin to wear off. It does not produce the adverse effects of other MAOIs: see Chapter 4. It may help to slow down the disease in previously untreated patients and when given with levodopa it may help to reduce the wearing-off effects (end-of-dose effects) that may occur between doses with levodopa. It enables the dose of levodopa to be reduced.

Cabergoline (**Cabaser**), **lisuride**, **pergolide** (**Celance**), **pramipexole** (**Mirapexin**) and **ropinirole** (**Requip**) are selective dopamine stimulants. They can be used with levodopa to reduce the fluctuations in response and end-of-dose effects which may occur with levodopa. They enable the dose of levodopa to be reduced.

Entacapone (**Comtess**) helps to stop the breakdown of levodopa in the body and is used as an add-on treatment to co-beneldopa or co-careldopa for patients who experience end-of-dose deterioration and cannot be stabilized on the combinations.

Apomorphine (**APO-go**, **Britaject**) is a power stimulator of dopamine receptors and may be beneficial in patients who experience 'on/off' effects with levodopa. The anti-vomiting drug domperidone should be given to prevent vomiting during treatment and for three days before treatment starts.

17

Antihistamine Drugs and Immunosuppressants

Allergy

In defence against infecting organisms, the body produces antibodies which combine with protein in the organisms to neutralize any effects which they may have upon the body. By means of this defence mechanism the body develops resistance or immunity. This often gives protection against reinfection by the same organism (e.g. you never get chickenpox twice). An antibody is a protein (globulin) which reacts only with the protein of the infecting organism (usually called an antigen) responsible for its formation. There is no cross-antibody formation to other organisms (cross-immunity), for example, between measles and polio. Sometimes renewed exposure to an infection produces a different or altered response – this is called allergy, which is the result of the body having been sensitized to that organism. Allergy to organisms is rare and most allergy is to a foreign protein (i.e. a protein not made by your body and not known to your own defence systems).

Foreign proteins (allergens) include drugs, house dust, pollens, certain foods and all sorts of things. These are usually grouped under the general term allergens. The reason why some people become sensitized and not others is not understood – we are all, for example, exposed to pollen grains and yet some of us will develop hayfever and others will not. Nor is the nature of allergic reactions fully understood; it may be a fault in the immunity mechanisms resulting in faulty antibody production or it may be due to an inherited defect in the tissues concerned.

The features of the allergic reaction are largely due to the release locally or into the bloodstream of a chemical called histamine and several other chemicals. A single allergen may cause reactions at several sites; thus a patient allergic to a certain food may develop stomach symptoms, a rash and wheezing. Allergens may affect the body through the skin (e.g. contact dermatitis due to cosmetics), in the food (e.g. allergy to strawberries), by inhalation (e.g. hayfever and asthma due to grass pollens), and by injections (e.g. insect bites and allergy to anti-tetanus serum). The resulting reactions may appear as skin rashes; swelling of the eyelids, face, lips and throat (angioedema); as abdominal symptoms (vomiting, diarrhoea and colic); or commonly as hayfever (itching eyes, running nose and sore throat), or as wheezing (asthma). Allergic reactions may be sudden and transient, e.g. sneezing, or last for years, e.g. eczema. They may be trivial, or so serious as to cause sudden death from what is called anaphylactic shock – collapse of the circulation, fall in blood pressure and acute asthma. This usually occurs in patients given an injection which contains a protein to which they have already been made sensitive by a previous injection (e.g. anti-tetanus serum; bee stings). It is rare.

One of the chemicals mainly responsible for allergic reactions is **histamine**; it is present in most tissues of the body and is released when cells are injured. It causes the small vessels of the body (capillaries) to dilate, particularly those in the skin, making it hot and red. It also makes the vessels more permeable so that plasma flows from inside the blood vessels into the surrounding tissues to produce swelling (oedema). When histamine is injected into the human skin it produces what is called a triple response: (i) a localized red spot which extends within a few seconds, reaches a maximum in about a minute and then becomes bluish; (ii) a bright red 'flame' spreads out from this spot and (iii) local swelling occurs forming a weal. (This reaction is often associated with itching and pain.) Histamine also causes the blood vessels in the brain to dilate, which produces a headache. It causes a fall in blood pressure and may increase the heart rate. Large doses may produce shock (collapse). It stimulates the muscles of the small bronchial tubes to produce constriction resulting in asthma and it stimulates the production of acid in the stomach. It is released in anaphylactic shock, allergy and injury. Its concentration is particularly high in the skin, stomach lining and in the lungs.

Any chemical that causes tissue damage will cause the release of histamine but some drugs may do this with little sign of tissue damage. The allergic effects produced by drugs may vary from an itchy skin rash to death from anaphylactic shock. The release of histamine may be caused by a physical process – e.g. sunburn, cold, light and friction – as well as by drugs. Pressure on the skin may release histamine and some people can write their name on their skin (dermatographia). The juice of the stinging nettle contains histamine which produces a skin rash called urticaria (nettle-rash).

Antihistamines

The conventional antihistamines block the action of histamine at peripheral (H_1) receptor sites. They stop, in varying degrees, most, but not all, of the effects produced by histamine. They may also reduce the intensity of allergic and anaphylactic reactions. They act, not by preventing the release of histamine, but by occupying its sites of action. They block its action on the muscles of the intestine and bronchial tubes, they reduce the weal produced by histamine and they reduce hayfever symptoms, itching skin rashes and swelling. They have no effect upon stomach secretions because they do not block H_2 receptors. Those antihistamines that block H_2 receptors are called H_2 receptor blockers (or **H_2 antihistamines**) and are used to treat patients suffering from peptic ulcers (see p. 97).

In addition to their actions in blocking the effects of histamine, some H_1 antihistamines produce drowsiness and they are referred to as **sedative antihistamines**. Others produce much less drowsiness because they do not enter the brain as easily. These are referred to as **non-sedative antihistamines**. Sedative antihistamines may also be used to prevent nausea, vomiting and dizziness (see Chapter 18).

In effective dosage all antihistamines produce adverse effects, but these vary from individual to individual and from drug to drug. *For adverse effects and precautions see A–Z of Medicines.*

Antihistamines can increase the effects of alcohol and impair driving skills, particularly the sedative ones.

Antihistamines Used to Treat Allergy

> **acrivastine*** (**Benadryl Allergy Relief, Semprex**)
> **azatadine** (**Optimine**)
> **brompheniramine** (**Dimotane**)
> **cetirizine*** (**Zirtek**)
> **chlorphenamine**(chlorpheniramine) (in **Haymine**, in **Galpseud Plus**, **Piriton**)
> **clemastine** (**Tavegil**)
> **cyproheptadine** (**Periactin**)
> **desloratadine** (**Neoclarityn**)
> **fexofenadine*** (**Telfast**)
> **hydroxyzine** (**Atarax, Ucerax**)
> **loratadine*** (**Clarityn**)
> **mizolastine*** (**Mistamine, Mizollen**)
> **promethazine** (**Phenergan**)
> **terfenadine***
> **alimemazine**(trimeprazine) (**Vallergan**)
> **triprolidine** (in **Actifed** preparations, in **Sudafed Plus**)

Those antihistamines marked with an * in the above list do not enter the brain as easily as the other antihistamines and therefore produce fewer harmful effects on the brain. In particular, they produce less drowsiness. They are referred to as **non-sedative antihistamines**. The others enter the brain and may produce drowsiness, and are referred to as **sedative antihistamines**.

Use of H$_1$ Antihistamines

There are numerous antihistamines to choose from and, bearing in mind individual variations in response, it is often a matter of trial and error before you find one that will relieve your particular allergic symptoms and produce a minimum of adverse effects. The ones that produce less drowsiness are the ones to use in the daytime. For night-time, one that produces drowsiness may be helpful, e.g. promethazine or alimemazine(trimeprazine).

1 Antihistamines are useful in relieving the symptoms of seasonal hayfever, but they have no effect upon the cause.
2 They are of little benefit in treating asthma.
3 They are used intravenously to treat angioedema (see later).
4 They are used intravenously to treat severe allergic reactions (see later).
5 Some skin rashes, such as allergic nettle-rash (urticaria), respond well to antihistamines by mouth. Long-standing rashes are little affected. Antihistamines by mouth may be used to relieve itching. When applied to the skin, there is a danger of producing allergic dermatitis. Given by mouth or injection they relieve the itching and swelling produced by insect bites.
6 They are of use in relieving the rash in serum sickness (an allergic reaction following the injection of a serum), but they do little to help the fever and joint pains.
7 They are of benefit in treating blood transfusion reactions.
8 They are of no value in treating allergic reactions affecting the stomach or intestine – nausea, vomiting, diarrhoea.
9 Many drug reactions respond well to antihistamines – but do not forget to stop the drug that caused the reaction.
10 Some antihistamines are effective in preventing motion sickness.
11 Some are useful sedatives.

Because of the variations in response between individuals taking antihistamines it is often necessary to try different ones. If a drug does not relieve your symptoms within about three days it is unlikely to do so at all. If it produces drowsiness take it at bedtime. Always take antihistamines with food, because they can irritate the stomach. If you are just starting a course, try taking the first dose on a Friday and then you have the weekend to overcome or become accustomed to the adverse effects. Avoid prolonged-release preparations until you know the nature and intensity of the adverse effects caused by the antihistamine drug in question. Prolonged-release preparations are most useful taken at bedtime in order to reduce early-morning symptoms.

Warnings: *Antihistamine drugs are complex chemicals which have many actions in the body and produce numerous effects, including adverse effects ranging from loss of appetite to serious blood disorders. They may increase the effects produced by alcohol and sedative drugs and interfere with your mental function. If they make you drowsy you should not drive a motor vehicle or operate moving machinery. Overdose with these drugs is serious and difficult to treat.*

Sedative antihistamines may produce alarming reactions in some children (stimulation, fever and convulsions).

Sodium Cromoglycate

This is a *non-steroidal anti-inflammatory drug* that works on the surface of certain cells (mast cells) to prevent the release of histamine and other chemicals that produce the allergic reaction and trigger inflammation. It may be inhaled to prevent asthma (**Aerocrom, Cromogen, Intal**) applied to the eyes to prevent allergic reactions in the eyes (**Hay-Crom, Opticrom, Vividrin**) and applied up the nose to prevent hayfever (**Rynacrom, Rynacrom Compound, Vividrin**) and by mouth to treat food allergy (**Nalcrom**).

Ketotifen

Ketotifen (**Zaditen**) produces similar effects to sodium cromoglycate but also possesses some antihistamine activity. It is taken by mouth.

Desensitization (Hyposensitization or Immunotherapy)

Hayfever, urticaria, allergic asthma, contact dermatitis and other allergic disorders are due to allergy to certain agents, e.g. foods, pollens, fur, feathers, dust, hair, mites and cosmetics. Contact dermatitis of the skin may occur due to drugs (e.g. streptomycin), metals (e.g. nickel buttons on jeans), plants (e.g. primula), paint, resins and cosmetics. Most people get to know what they are sensitive to and can avoid that substance in future. In some cases it is not possible to identify or to avoid a particular substance, e.g. hayfever. Therefore, skin tests to certain allergens may be carried out, although the results of these tests are often difficult to assess.

Desensitization (injections of an allergen under the skin at intervals using gradually increasing strengths) may be beneficial to patients who have suffered a severe allergic reaction to a wasp or bee sting. Desensitization to grass pollen may occasionally help some people who suffer from hayfever providing they do not suffer from asthma. Multiple desensitization is not recommended since it may precipitate an acute allergic reaction, particularly in children.

Patients undergoing desensitization are at risk of developing a severe allergic reaction and therefore treatment should only be given where there are adequate facilities to provide resuscitation. People with asthma are at particular risk.

Allergic Emergencies*

In addition to securing the airway and giving oxygen the following drugs are used in an allergic emergency (anaphylactic shock) and to treat angioedema (swelling of the mouth and throat):

1 **Adrenaline**(epinephrine) – intramuscularly in a dose of 0.5–1.0 mg (0.5–1 ml of 1 in 1,000 adrenaline(epinephrine) solution). Repeat every ten minutes according to pulse rate, blood pressure and improvement. If the patient is taking non-selective beta-blockers, **salbutamol** should be given by slow intravenous injection.

2 **Chlorphenamine**(chlorpheniramine) – 10–20 mg by slow intravenous infusion for 24–48 hours to prevent relapse.

3 **Hydrocortisone** (sodium succinate or sodium phosphate) 100–300 mg by slow intravenous injection – slow to work, but may prevent deterioration.

Drugs Used to Treat Hayfever

Hayfever (allergic rhinitis) is either *seasonal,* caused by allergy to, for example, grass pollen, or *perennial* (all the year round) and caused by allergy to, for example, house-dust mites or animal fur.

The most effective treatment of hayfever is to try to avoid or reduce contact with the allergen. Drug treatment aimed at *preventing* or *relieving* hayfever includes the use of:

Antihistamines by mouth (see earlier).

Antihistamine nose drops or sprays, e.g. **azelastine (Rhinolast), levocabastine (Livostin).**

Corticosteroid nasal applications, e.g. **beclometasone (Beconase** preparations, **Beclo-aqua, Nasobec), betamethasone (Betnesol, Vista-Methasone** drops), **budesonide (Rhinocort Aqua), dexamethasone** (in **Dexa-Rhinaspray Duo), flunisolide (Syntaris), fluticasone (Flixonase Nasule), mometasone (Nasonex)** and **triamcinolone (Nasacort).**

---

* Individuals at risk of allergic shock (e.g. allergy to bee or wasp stings or to peanuts) should carry adrenaline(epinephrine) with them at all times. Special kits are available containing a pre-filled syringe of adrenaline(epinephrine) (e.g. **Anapen, Ana-Guard, Epipen, Min-I-Jet**). **Ana-Kit** contains a pre-filled syringe of adrenaline(epinephrine) plus chewable tablets of chlorphenamine(chlorpheniramine) (an antihistamine).

Corticosteroids by mouth or injection (see Chapter 37) may be used if the symptoms of seasonal hayfever are severe.

Sodium cromoglycate nasal applications (**Rynacrom**, **Vividrin**) to relieve inflammation.

Anti-allergy eye drop preparations include **azelastine** (**Optilast**), **emedastine** (**Emadine**), **lodoxamide** (**Alomide**) and **levocabastine** (**Livostin**).

Anti-inflammatory eye drops include **sodium cromoglycate** (**Clariteyes**, **Hay-Crom**, **Opticrom**, **Viz-on**, **Vividrin**) or **nedocromil sodium** (**Rapitil**) may help.

A *combined antihistamine/decongestant* eye preparation may help allergy affecting the eyes, e.g. **Otrivine-Antistin** (**antazoline and xylometazoline**).

Ipratropium (**Rinatec** spray) is an anticholinergic drug (see p. 36) that may be beneficial to people suffering from a runny nose caused by perennial hayfever.

- *Treatment Plan for Allergic Rhinitis*

  If *mild*   Try an antihistamine by mouth or an antihistamine nasal application when necessary. If no improvement, add a corticosteroid spray or a sodium cromoglycate spray and use regularly.

  If *moderate*   Use a corticosteroid or sodium cromoglycate nasal application regularly. If no improvement, add an antihistamine by mouth or use an antihistamine nasal application regularly when needed.

  If *severe*   Use a corticosteroid by mouth for two weeks plus corticosteroid drops up the nose. If no improvement, maintain treatment with a local corticosteroid with or without an antihistamine by mouth or nasal applications regularly when needed.

  If *watery nose* Use local anticholinergic, e.g. **ipratropium** (**Rinatec**).

  If *nose blocked* Use local sympathomimetic decongestants, e.g. **xylometazoline** (**Afrazine, Dristan, Otradrops, Otraspray, Otrivine, Vicks Sinex**).

Drugs that Suppress the Immune System

In certain medical conditions it is necessary to dampen down (suppress) the activities of the immune system by using drugs. The drugs used for this purpose are referred to as immunosuppressive drugs. Immunosuppression is needed in treating auto-immune diseases in which the immune system attacks normal body tissues. This attack may be local as in Hashimoto's disease of the thyroid gland, or it may be general and affect many organs and tissues, for example, lupus erythematosus. Suppression of the immune system is also necessary in treating patients who have had an organ transplant, otherwise the immune system would cause rejection of the transplanted organ.

The production of antibodies and the cells involved in the immune system are dependent upon the production and multiplication of lymphocytes. Therefore any drug that interferes with the production or multiplication of lymphocytes will suppress the immune system.

The risk of immunosuppressive drugs is that by suppressing immunity (the body's resistance to infection) they throw the patient open to the risk of infection from various bacteria, fungi and viruses. Also, because lymphocytes prevent the multiplication of abnormal cells there is an increased risk of developing certain types of cancer.

Immunosuppressive Drugs

Azathioprine (**Azamune, Immunoprin, Imuran, Oprisine**) is an anti-cancer drug that helps the survival and functions of transplanted organs. It is also of benefit to some patients suffering from rheumatoid arthritis and other auto-immune disorders, usually when corticosteroids have failed to control the symptoms.

Mycophenolate mofetil (**Cellcept**) is an immunosuppressive used to prevent kidney transplant rejection. It is used in combination with ciclosporin and corticosteroids.

Chlorambucil (**Leukeran**) and **cyclophosphamide** (**Endoxana**) are used to treat certain cancers. They are also used to reduce the immune response in patients suffering from rheumatoid arthritis and other auto-immune disorders.

Corticosteroids suppress the immune reaction. They are used to prevent transplant rejection.

Ciclosporin (**Neoral, Sandimmun, SangCya**) is a powerful immunosuppressive drug and is the principal drug used to reduce the risk of rejection of transplanted organs.

Tacrolimus (**Prograf**) produces similar effects to ciclosporin although it is not related to it.

Sirolimus (**Rapamune**), **etanercept** (**Enbrel**) and **infliximab** (**Remicade**) are selective immunosuppressants which inhibit the activity of tumour necrosis factor. They are used for the treatment of rheumatoid arthritis.

Basiliximab (**Simulect**) and **daclizumab** (**Zenapax**) are monoclonal antibodies that are used for the prophylaxis of acute rejection in renal transplantation.

18

Drugs Used to Treat Nausea, Vomiting and Motion Sickness

Nausea and vomiting are symptoms. These symptoms may occur with all kinds of physical disorders, some of which are quite simple and short-lived, such as food poisoning, and some very serious and long-lasting, such as cancer of the stomach or a brain tumour. Drugs often cause nausea and vomiting (e.g. morphine, anti-cancer drugs, oestrogens) and so may motion, pregnancy and emotion (e.g. the sight of a severely injured road-accident victim). Nausea and vomiting may serve a useful purpose – as in food poisoning – but usually they are distressing symptoms which need relieving.

There is a vomiting centre in the brain which responds to stimulations from the stomach and intestine and also from the organ of balance. Another part of the brain seems to respond to chemical stimulation. It is referred to as the chemoreceptor trigger zone. It is thought that this area is stimulated by certain drugs (e.g. morphine) and also by chemicals produced in the body (e.g. in diabetes or kidney failure).

Motion Sickness

Movement can affect the organ of balance, which has associations with the vomiting centre. For example, motion produced by travelling in a car, on a boat or on a roundabout stimulates the organ of balance. This stimulates the vomiting centre, resulting in the feeling of nausea (sweating, salivation, rapid beating of the heart and the feeling you are going to vomit) and vomiting. Motion sickness is more common in children. Certain movements, e.g. swinging, will make some people sick, while others who are not made sick by swinging may become sick at sea. There are numerous physical, social and psychological factors involved in motion sickness; fortunately tolerance to motion develops over a period of several days.

Drugs Used to Treat Motion Sickness

The aim of drug use should be to try to *prevent* an attack of motion sickness developing. A short-acting drug should be taken before a short journey and a long-acting one before a long journey. Several drugs are effective, provided the right dose is taken at the right time.

Antimuscarinic drugs. These drugs may produce blurred vision, dry mouth, difficulty passing urine, constipation, drowsiness and confusion. They should not be used in patients with glaucoma or in those patients who may develop retention of urine (e.g. men with enlarged prostate glands). They are short-acting and are therefore useful for relieving motion sickness on short journeys (up to half a day). Their prolonged use for this purpose is not satisfactory because of troublesome adverse effects. The most commonly used antimuscarinic is **hyoscine** (**scopolamine; Joy-rides**, **Kwells**, **Scopoderm** adhesive skin patches). *Alcohol should be avoided. The drugs may interfere with your ability to drive a motor vehicle.*

Sedative antihistamine drugs. There is a marked variation between individuals in their response to sedative antihistamines. *The most common adverse effect is drowsiness, but in infants and young children antihistamines may produce stimulation, making them nervous and unable to sleep. Do not drink alcohol on the same day that you have taken an antihistamine drug. They may interfere with your ability to drive a motor vehicle and they may increase the effects of other depressant drugs such as sedatives, tranquillizers and sleeping drugs.*

The antihistamines most often used to treat motion sickness are:

cinnarizine (**Cinaziere,** **meclozine** (**Sea-Legs**)
  Stugeron) **promethazine*** (**Avomine,**
cyclizine (**Valoid**) **Phenergan**)

* Produces more drowsiness than the others.

Vomiting in Pregnancy

Vomiting in pregnancy is probably due to hormonal changes which occur in the early months of pregnancy. In addition, there are numerous psychological, social and dietary factors. Excessive vomiting may lead to an alteration in blood chemistry, which then causes further vomiting.

The main considerations should be: how much distress is being caused by the vomiting and what effects may drug treatment for the vomiting have upon the unborn child.

A decision in the light of these considerations is not easy. Vomiting in pregnancy is extremely distressing, and the patient needs sound advice, understanding and careful support. *Drugs should rarely be used.*

An antihistamine drug may be used occasionally, e.g. **promethazine** (**Avomine**).

Nausea and Vomiting Caused by Drugs

Anti-cancer drugs, morphine and related drugs and general anaesthetics can cause severe and persistent nausea and vomiting which needs relieving. The drugs used to produce relief include:

Dopamine blockers are effective anti-nauseant and anti-vomiting drugs, but they can produce movement disorders, particularly in children and young adults, and parkinsonism in the elderly (see p. 79). These include phenothiazine drugs such as **prochlorperazine** (**Buccastem**, **Proziere**, **Stemetil**), **perphenazine** (**Fentazin**) and **chlorpromazine** (**Largactil**), which act on the brain; **metoclopramide** (**Gastrobid Continus**, **Gastroflux**, **Maxolon**, **Primperan**) which acts on the brain and the gut; and **domperidone** (**Motilium**) which works like metoclopramide but produces fewer adverse effects on the brain and therefore less sedation and movement disorders than metoclopramide or the phenothiazines.

Although **antihistamines** may help in the above disorders they are seldom used. **Nabilone** is a synthetic cannabis-type drug which may help some people. The **5HT blockers granisetron** (**Kytril**), **ondansetron** (**Zofran**) and **tropisetron** (**Navoban**) work on the brain and gut and are equally effective. They do not block dopamine and do not cause movement disorders.

Use of Anti-vomiting Drugs

Antihistamines – to reduce nausea and vomiting caused by morphine-related drugs.

Domperidone – to reduce nausea and vomiting caused by anti-cancer drugs; may also be used to treat nausea and vomiting caused by levodopa or bromocriptine in the treatment of parkinsonism.

Metoclopramide – to reduce nausea and vomiting caused by anti-cancer drugs.

Nabilone – to reduce nausea and vomiting caused by anti-cancer drugs.

5HT blockers – to reduce nausea and vomiting caused by anti-cancer drugs.

Antipsychotic drugs – to reduce nausea and vomiting caused by morphine-related drugs and anti-cancer drugs. Prochlorperazine (a phenothiazine) or haloperidol may be helpful in nausea and vomiting caused by advanced cancer and in the initial stages of morphine treatment.

Vomiting after an anaesthetic is best treated with a phenothiazine drug or with metoclopramide.

Nausea and vomiting produced by radiation treatment for cancer are helped by phenothiazine drugs, metoclopramide, domperidone and particularly by a 5HT blocker such as **ondansetron** (**Zofran**).

Nausea and Vomiting Caused by Disease

All of the above drugs may be tried. **Metoclopramide** and **domperidone** are useful for treating nausea and vomiting caused by diseases of the stomach, duodenum, liver and gall bladder.

Dizziness (Vertigo)

The term vertigo is used to describe sensations of movements within the head or in the environment. It is always accompanied by a disturbance of balance and if severe can be associated with sweating, pallor, nausea, vomiting and occasionally diarrhoea and fainting. It may be caused by disorders of the eyes, brain, organ of balance, and ears. The organ of balance may be disturbed by infections (labyrinthitis) and by drugs such as streptomycin, quinine or aspirin. Dizziness and giddiness are much more vague. They are highly subjective feelings and may be associated with all manner of disorders.

Drugs which may help include **hyoscine** (**Kwells**), antihistamines, e.g. **cinnarizine** (**Cinaziere, Stugeron**), and phenothiazines, e.g. **prochlorperazine** (**Buccastem, Proziere, Stemetil**). **Betahistine** (**Serc**) is related to histamine and may help some individuals. An acute attack of vertigo may be helped by an injection or a suppository of **cyclizine** (**Valoid**) or **prochlorperazine** (**Stemetil**).

Ménière's Disease

This is a most unpleasant disorder which is characterized by recurrent attacks of vertigo associated with noises in the ears (tinnitus) and progressive nerve deafness. It is more common in men than women, and most attacks develop between the ages of forty and sixty years of age. It is self-limiting and spontaneous recovery occurs at any stage. Patients with Ménière's disease get very anxious and depressed and therefore need sympathy and understanding.

The drug treatment of Ménière's disease is difficult. In an acute phase the patient is unwilling to move his head because he may vomit. In between attacks, any of the drugs mentioned under the treatment of dizziness may be tried.

Hyoscine, an **antihistamine** or a **phenothiazine** are useful for preventing attacks. **Betahistine** (**Serc**) and **cinnarizine** (**Stugeron**) are promoted specifically for the treatment of Ménière's disease. In an acute attack an injection or a suppository of **cyclizine** (**Valoid**) or **prochlorperazine** (**Stemetil**) may be beneficial.

19

Drugs Used to Treat Indigestion and Peptic Ulcers

The middle and upper parts of the stomach act as a reservoir for food; the part near its outlet into the duodenum contracts and relaxes to churn and mix the food. The rate of emptying of the stomach varies with the volume of contents: the greater the volume the faster the rate of emptying. A fatty meal delays emptying; so does an increase in stomach acidity. Some drugs increase and some decrease the rate of emptying of the stomach. Another important function of the stomach is to make digestive juice. This contains hydrochloric acid (about one and a half litres are produced every day), mucus which protects the surface of the stomach and an enzyme called pepsin which helps to digest protein in food.

The stomach can get 'upset' if its lining is irritated (e.g. by aspirin or alcohol), by eating too much, by eating unusual food, or by virus or bacterial infections. The lining of the stomach can also become 'inflamed' (gastritis). This may be caused or aggravated by many things; for example, certain foods (pickles, fried food), alcohol and smoking. This irritation or inflammation may produce symptoms such as discomfort, nausea, pain and loss of appetite. These symptoms are usually referred to as indigestion or dyspepsia. Sometimes the surface of the stomach may become eroded to produce a peptic ulcer. A peptic ulcer may occur in the oesophagus (gullet), stomach (where it may be called a gastric ulcer) and in the duodenum (duodenal ulcer).

Relatively little is known about the factors which cause peptic ulcers, but there is evidence that acid and pepsin are partly responsible. However, 'normal' stomachs do not develop ulcers. Therefore, the 'normal' lining of the stomach must be protective, and it may be something affecting this protection that causes ulcers. This may be related to the mucus that covers the surface, the ability of the mucous cells to renew themselves every few days, the nutrition of the stomach itself, its blood supply, and various chemical factors. There are other factors such as heredity (there is often a family history), seasonal factors, diet, smoking, alcohol, and particularly, worry and stress.

The symptoms of peptic ulcer usually start with 'indigestion' but may start with acute pain, or bleeding or perforation. Indigestion going on for more than several days may be due to a peptic ulcer, particularly if the episodes keep recurring and if accompanied by pain rather than 'discomfort'. Pain from a duodenal ulcer often comes on when you are hungry and it wakes you in the night; whereas a gastric ulcer pain may come on fairly soon after food. Food, antacids or vomiting may relieve peptic ulcer pains.

You should consult your doctor if you have indigestion lasting more than a few weeks or recurring at intervals – you may have a peptic ulcer. The treatment of a peptic ulcer includes advice on diet – which means taking a well-balanced diet and frequent, regular, small meals. You should avoid alcohol and any foods which you know give you pain. You should stop taking coffee and avoid any drugs known to irritate the stomach; for example, aspirin, and most drugs used to treat rheumatism and arthritis. You should also stop smoking. There is no point in filling yourself full of indigestion mixture while continuing to smoke and drink alcohol. If you are worried, anxious or tense then you need help and advice on sorting out the stresses which are affecting you.

The main drugs used to treat peptic ulcers fall into three groups – drugs which neutralize the acid in the stomach (antacids), drugs which reduce the production of acid by the stomach cells and drugs which help to protect the stomach lining.

> **Note:** *Eradication of H. pylori infection should be considered in all patients with peptic ulcers (see p. 99).*

1 Drugs which Neutralize the Acid in the Stomach

Antacids neutralize the acid in the stomach contents and this relieves indigestion and the pain of a peptic ulcer. They consist of mixtures of various **base salts of sodium**, **magnesium**, **calcium**, **aluminium** and **bismuth**. The amount needed to neutralize stomach acid depends upon the rate of acid production by the stomach, the presence or absence of food, and upon the rate of emptying of the stomach. Antacids may be absorbed into the bloodstream and produce changes in the chemistry of the blood. This effect is often of no consequence, because the kidneys quickly restore the chemical balance. However, in patients with impaired kidney function this may be dangerous.

Sodium bicarbonate relieves pain rapidly, but its effects quickly wear off and it may cause changes in the blood chemistry. It releases carbon dioxide gas into the stomach which causes belching (this makes some people think it is working effectively) but it may also cause distension of the stomach, which is unpleasant. It is useful for quick relief but there is nothing to recommend its continued use. Patients with impaired heart or kidney functions should not use it because of the high sodium content. Also, it should not be used by patients with fluid retention (oedema) or raised blood pressure because it increases the blood salt level and may cause further retention of water by the kidneys.

Magnesium salts act slowly. They may cause diarrhoea and some magnesium may be absorbed into the bloodstream – they should not be used in patients with impaired kidney function.

Calcium carbonate acts quickly and effectively. Some calcium is absorbed into the bloodstream. If patients with peptic ulcers take a milk diet (which is high in calcium) and calcium carbonate regularly for long periods of time they may develop a high level of blood calcium, which may cause a group of symptoms – loss of appetite, nausea, vomiting, headache, weakness, abdominal pains, constipation and thirst. This is often called the milk-alkali syndrome ('syndrome' being the term used to indicate a group of signs and symptoms). Temporary or permanent kidney damage may occur. **Calcium salts** tend to constipate; they are, therefore, often given mixed with magnesium salts.

Aluminium hydroxide is slow to act. It does not alter the blood chemistry because it forms insoluble complexes in the stomach. **Aluminium hydroxide** and other **aluminium compounds** constipate.

Bismuth salts are not very effective as antacids and may produce toxic effects when absorbed, particularly in patients with impaired kidney function.

The Use of Antacids

Antacids relieve the symptoms of indigestion whether due to an ulcer or not (non-ulcer dyspepsia). They are also useful in relieving the pain caused by inflammation of the gullet (oesophagitis). None of the available antacids is ideal. They vary in their rate and duration of action and in the amounts required to neutralize the acid contents of the stomach. Liquid preparations and powders mixed with water are more effective than tablets. Tablets should be sucked slowly between meals; their routine use after meals to prevent symptoms is of no use. Because no specific antacid can be recommended, mixtures are generally used. Mixtures also help to avoid bowel complications such as diarrhoea from magnesium salts and constipation from calcium or aluminium salts.

Antacids interfere with the absorption of many drugs, eg. iron, vitamin supplements, aspirin, tetracycline antibiotics and cimetidine. Some have a high sodium content (salt) and should not be used by patients having treatment for raised blood pressure, heart failure, liver failure or in pregnancy – *always check with your pharmacist or doctor.*

Combined Formulations

Some antacid mixtures contain drugs which disperse wind (e.g. **activated dimeticone**) and drugs which spread the antacid over the surface of the stomach contents to form an alkaline raft which provides a 'mechanical' barrier to protect the lower end of the oesophagus from acid reflux. These latter include **co-dried gels** and **complexes of silicates and alginic acid**. They are useful in the treatment of heartburn.

For repeated use, soluble antacids such as sodium bicarbonate should be avoided. Comparable antacid preparations are not necessarily equivalent in their ability to neutralize the acid. Do not forget that the speed of action of antacids depends upon their ability to neutralize the acid in the stomach. This depends principally upon the speed with which they dissolve and the rate of emptying of the stomach. The choice is really what suits you and the right dose is what relieves *your* symptoms. The most expensive are not necessarily the best.

2 Drugs which Reduce Acid Production by the Stomach

H₂-receptor Blockers

H_2 antihistamine drugs block the histamine receptors in the stomach (see Chapter 17). This results in a reduction in both the volume and acidity of the gastric juice, which encourages healing of peptic ulcers and reduces the risk of reflux.

The H_2 antihistamines, for example **cimetidine** (**Acitak, Dyspamet, Galenamet, Peptimax, Phimetin, Tagamet, Ultec, Zita**), **famotidine** (**Pepcid**), **nizatidine** (**Axid, Zinga**) and **ranitidine** (in **Pylorid, Rantec, Ranitic, Zaedoc, Zantac**), heal peptic ulcers, particularly duodenal ulcers. They are also of use in oesophagitis, acid reflux and non-ulcer dyspepsia.

Initial treatment of peptic ulcer should preferably last for four–six weeks. A daily maintenance of half the treatment dose will prevent relapse but do not forget that they do not cure; after stopping them, ulcers may recur. Daily doses should be reduced in patients with impaired kidney function. High doses in the elderly may cause dizziness, tiredness, and, rarely, confusion. Cimetidine, nizatidine or ranitidine may cause breast enlargement in men (gynacomastia).

Proton-pump Blockers

Esomeprazole (**Nexium**), **lansoprazole** (in **Heliclear, Zoton**), **omeprazole** (**Losec**), **pantoprazole** (**Protium**) and **rabeprazole** (**Pariet**) block the production of acid in the stomach and are useful for treating peptic ulcers and acid reflux, and also ulcers caused by non-steroidal anti-inflammatory drugs. They are the treatment of choice for gastro-oesophageal reflux disease (GORD). They produce more rapid ulcer healing than the H_2 blockers and are more effective in GORD and reflux oesophagitis. They may cause diarrhoea, skin rash and headache.

3 Drugs which Protect the Stomach Lining

Liquorice wood has been used in various herbal indigestion mixtures for centuries. But when in 1948 crude powdered liquorice extract was tried in patients suffering from peptic ulcers it was found that one in five developed serious adverse effects which included high blood pressure, irregular heartbeats and muscle weakness.

Carbenoxolone improves mucosal defence. It is a less toxic derivative of liquorice and is combined with antacids in **Pyrogastrone** to treat oesophagitis and GORD. It may cause salt and water retention, and a reduction in blood potassium level. This may result in weight gain and swollen ankles, a rise in blood pressure, and heart failure. The low blood potassium may cause muscle weakness. It should not be given to elderly patients or to those with impaired heart, liver or kidney function or raised blood pressure, or to children.

Bismuth chelate (**tripotassium dicitratobismuthate**, **De-Noltab**). This is a complex bismuth preparation (not a salt) which forms a protective layer over the ulcer lining. It is active only when the stomach contents are acid. It is effective in treating stomach and duodenal ulcers. Ulcer healing may be helped by elimination of bacteria that are associated with peptic ulcers (*Helicobacter pylori*). It has an ulcer healing rate similar to cimetidine with a lower relapse rate. However, it causes darkening of the tongue, nausea and vomiting, and should not be used as long-term treatment. It should not be used in pregnancy or in patients with impaired kidney function.

Sucralfate (**Antepsin**) protects the ulcer lining from acid and pepsin attack. It is a complex of aluminium hydroxide and sulphated sucrose. It is effective in treating stomach and duodenal ulcers. It also stimulates production of mucus, bicarbonate and prostoglandins to help ulcer healing. Long-term use may be associated with the absorption of aluminium into the blood. It should be used with caution in patients with impaired kidney function.

Misoprostol (**Cytotec**) is a synthetic prostaglandin that works by stimulating the production of mucus which protects the surface of the stomach, and by stimulating the production of sodium bicarbonate (the stomach's own antacid). It also decreases acid production and improves the blood supply to the surface of the stomach. All these effects combine to protect the stomach and it is useful for preventing ulceration caused by non-steroidal anti-inflammatory drugs (NSAIDs), used in the treatment of arthritis and joint pain. It is as effective as H_2 blockers in healing duodenal ulcers but less effective in healing gastric ulcers and oesophagitis. It may cause diarrhoea and causes the uterus to contract. It should not be used in pregnancy, or if trying to get pregnant.

Healing Peptic Ulcers

The following drugs heal peptic ulcers but they do not cure them. The ulcers may recur when treatment is stopped – H_2 blockers (**cimetidine, famotidine, nizatidine, ranitidine**), **bismuth chelate** or **sucralfate**, a prostaglandin analogue (**misoprostol**), or a proton-pump blocker (**esomeprazole, lansoprazole, omeprazole, pantoprazole, rabeprazole**).

Curing Peptic Ulcers by Eradicating Helicobacter Pylori

The discovery that peptic ulcers are associated with infection by the bacteria *Helicobacter pylori* has revolutionized peptic ulcer treatment. Treatment to eradicate the infection and cure peptic ulcers involves the use of an ulcer-healing drug combined with antibacterial drugs.

● *Triple Therapy* (for one week)

An ulcer-healing drug, **lansoprazole, omeprazole, pantoprazole, ranitidine bismuth citrate**, plus any two of the following antibiotics: **clarithromycin, amoxicillin, metronidazole**.

Two-week dual therapy regimens using a proton pump inhibitor and a single antibacterial are not recommended because they produce low rates of *H. pylori* eradication.

Acid Reflux, Oesophagitis, Heartburn, Gastro-Oesophageal Reflux Disease (GORD)

The washing of stomach contents which contain acid and pepsin up into the lower end of the oesophagus (gullet) may produce inflammation of the oesophagus; this is referred to as reflux oesophagitis or gastro-oesophageal reflux disease (GORD). The characteristic symptom is heartburn – a burning pain in the centre of the lower chest after eating a large meal, stooping or lying flat. Reflux oesophagitis is a major cause of indigestion and is linked to smoking, diet and being overweight.

The reflux of acid (acid regurgitation) from the stomach into the oesophagus is caused by a weakness in the circular muscles of the diaphragm that normally close off the top of the stomach from the oesophagus (the gastro-oesophageal sphincter) and prevent swallowed food and drink from coming back up – unless of course you vomit. The reflux of acid up into the oesophagus may be due to a hiatus hernia, which allows parts of the stomach to bulge upwards (herniate) into the opening (hiatus) in the diaphragm through which the oesophagus passes.

General Treatment

Reflux can be reduced by sleeping propped up in bed (use three or four pillows), by avoiding too much bending down and, where appropriate, by stopping smoking, stopping alcohol and losing weight. Regular small, non-fatty meals will help and the amount of tea and coffee drunk should be reduced.

Drug Treatment of Heartburn

● *Antacids to Neutralize Stomach Acid*

Antacids are described earlier. Effective doses will neutralize the acid in the stomach and often provide instant relief from reflux symptoms. Antacids include:

aluminium hydroxide (**Aludrox** (liquid and tablets), **Alu-Caps**, **Actal**)
aluminium hydroxide and **magnesium hydroxide** (**Altacite**, **Birley**, **Dijex**,
   Dynese, **Entrotabs**, **Gelusil**, **Maalox**, **Maalox TC**, **Maclean**, **Moorland**,
   Mucogel)
calcium salts (**Barum Antacid**, **Rap-eze**, **Remegel**, **Rennies**, **Settlers**, **Tums**)
calcium salts and **magnesium carbonate** (**Andrews Antacid**, **Bisma-Rex**,
   Boots Indigestion, **DeWitts Antacid powder** and **tablets**, **Opas**)
magnesium carbonate (**Bismag**, **Bisodol Indigestion powder** and **tablets**,
   Carbellon, **Magnatol**, **Phillip's Milk of Magnesia**, **Roter**)

● *Additives that Protect the Surface of the Oesophagus*

Additives in antacid mixtures aimed at protecting the oesophagus provide additional relief. These additives include **alginic acid** or one of its salts (**alginates**) which are obtained from algae. They work as emulsifiers and float to the top of the stomach contents to form a 'raft' containing the antacid. This helps to protect the sensitive lining of the oesophagus from the acid in the stomach.

Alginate-containing antacids (raft-floating antacids) usually contain less antacid than ordinary antacid preparations, but the raft appears to make them more effective for relieving reflux symptoms. They provide relief in some people.

Another commonly used additive is the silicone **dimeticone**, which acts as an anti-foaming agent and helps to stop the acid contents of the stomach frothing up into the oesophagus. **Activated dimeticone** is a mixture of liquid dimeticone containing finely divided silicone dioxide which increases its de-foaming properties. In some people, antacid preparations containing dimeticone provide more relief from reflux symptoms than antacids alone.

> **Warning:** *A preparation containing dimeticone should never be taken with a preparation that contains alginic acid or an alginate because their actions oppose each other and the raft provided by the latter would sink.*

● *Antacids Plus a Local Anaesthetic to Relieve Pain*

Mucaine is an antacid mixture that contains the local anaesthetic oxethazine. There is doubt about the benefits of using a local anaesthetic for this purpose but some patients experience relief from reflux symptoms.

● *Drugs that Protect the Lining of the Stomach and Oesophagus*

Carbenoxolone added to a raft-alginate antacid (e.g. **Pyrogastrone**) has not been shown to be more effective than an H$_2$ blocker. It needs to be used with caution in older people.

Sucralfate (**Antepsin**) and **bismuth chelate** (**De-Noltab**), which are effective in treating stomach and duodenal ulcers, have no special advantages when treating reflux symtoms.

● *Drugs that Block Acid Production*

H$_2$ blockers before meals and an alkali/alginic mixture after meals provide good relief from reflux symptoms, but H$_2$ blockers appear to be less effective at treating peptic ulcers in the oesophagus than in the stomach or duodenum. Treatment should continue for two months.

Proton-pump blockers (e.g. **omeprazole**) are the drugs of choice for treating severe oesophagitis (see p. 99).

● *Drugs that Affect the Gastro-oesophageal Sphincter*

Drugs that close the circular muscle (the gastro-oesophageal sphincter) will prevent the reflux of acid up into the oesophagus. The anti-dopamine drug **metoclopramide** (**Gastrobid Continus, Gastroflux, Maxolon**) is an example of these drugs, and it can work very effectively in some people.

Combined Preparations Used to Treat Heartburn

● *Antacid Preparations containing Activated Dimeticone*
   Actonorm (gel and powder)
   Altacite Plus: co-simalcite (tablets and suspension)
   Asilone (tablets, gel and suspension)
   Bisodol Wind Relief (tablets)
   Boots Double Action Indigestion
   Kolanticon (with dicyclomine)
   Maalox Plus (tablets and suspension)

Polycrol (gel and tablets)
Simeco (tablets).

- *Antacid Preparations containing Dimeticone*
Simeco (suspension)
Sovol (suspension).

- *Antacid Preparations containing Alginic Acid or an Alginate*
Algicon (tablets and suspension)
Bisodol Heartburn
Boots Heartburn Relief
Gastrocote (tablets and liquid)
Gaviscon (tablets, liquid, infant powder)
Peptac (liquid)
Topal (tablets).

- *Other Preparations*
Mucaine (suspension) – antacids with oxetacaine (a local anaesthetic)
Nulacin (tablets) – antacids with peppermint oil
Pyrogastrone (tablets and liquid) – antacids with carbenoxolone
(ulcer-healing drug) and sodium alginate.

Drugs Used to Treat Gallstones

The bile acid **ursodeoxycholic acid** (**Destolit**, **Urdox**, **Ursofalk**, **Ursogal**) is used to treat patients with mild symptoms, healthy gall-bladders, and small or medium-sized cholesterol gallstones which are radiolucent to X-rays and are not treatable by other means. Patients need to be in hospital and monitored by X-ray and ultrasound, which require hospital supervision. Gallstones recur in one in four patients within one year of stopping treatment. Ursodeoxycholic acid produces diarrhoea less frequently than chenodeoxycholic acid and liver dysfunction has been reported with chenodeoxycholic acid.

Essential oils (e.g. in **Rowachol**) are sometimes used as additional treatment to dissolve stones in the common bile duct. They claim to dissolve cholesterol stones (radiolucent stones). However, they are only suitable for small stones because they are very slow to work – it may take years to dissolve small stones.

20

Drugs Used to Treat Diarrhoea

Rehydration

The greatest risk from diarrhoea is the loss of large volumes of water containing salts of sodium and potassium. The loss of these salts and water is particularly dangerous in babies, infants and in elderly and/or debilitated people who require urgent treatment. The priority is the replacement of lost water and salts (**rehydration**).

The addition of glucose to an oral salt solution greatly improves the absorption of salts and water through the intestinal wall into the bloodstream. Therefore, it is important that rehydration fluids contain both salts and glucose.

There are several preparations of these **salt/sugar solutions** (e.g. **Dioralyte**, **Electrolade**, **Rehidrat**). These are mixtures of sodium chloride, glucose and other salts, usually available as powders for making up into solution. Oral rehydration solutions available in Britain are only suitable for treating mild or moderate diarrhoea. If the diarrhoea is severe it may be necessary to give more sodium; for example, a formulation recommended by the World Health Organization (WHO) contains sodium chloride 3·5 g, potassium chloride 1·5 g, sodium citrate 2·9 g and anhydrous glucose 20·0 g per litre.

In emergency you can make a solution up at home but you must be careful. Dissolving the sugar and the salt in the *correct* volume of water is very important since too concentrated a solution can, in infants, produce the risk of too much salt absorption leading to convulsions.

A simple sugar/salt solution contains one level teaspoonful of household salt (5 ml) and eight level teaspoonfuls of sugar in *one* litre of water, *but it is safer to use a proprietary preparation.*

Drug Treatment of Diarrhoea

The drug treatment of diarrhoea takes second place to rehydration.

Drug treatments of diarrhoea include drugs which reduce the number of bowel movements by acting on the contents of the intestine or upon the wall of the intestine, and anti-infective drugs which are used to treat bacterial or amoebic infections.

Drugs which Alter the Bowel Contents

Inert powders are used to form bulk and carry away irritant substances. These include **hydrated aluminium silicate** (e.g. **kaolin**) and **activated attapulgite** (a hydrated magnesium aluminium silicate). However they are not recommended for the treatment of acute diarrhoea. Bulk-forming laxatives (see later) made from **starches** or **cellulose** are sometimes used in chronic diarrhoea. These bulk-forming substances (e.g. **methylcellulose, ispaghula, sterculia**) modify the frequency of the motions because they absorb water *but* they do not reduce the loss of water and salts.

Drugs which Act on the Bowel Wall (Anti-motility Drugs)

Opiate drugs (see p. 153) slow down movement of the bowel wall and may be used for treating diarrhoea and relieving painful spasms (colic) of the bowel. **Codeine** (in **Diarrest**, in **Kaodene**), **loperamide** (**Arret, Imodium, Lodiar, Diocaps, LoperaGen, Norimode, Boots Diareze capsules, Diasorb, Diocalm Ultra, Normaloe**), **morphine** (in **Diocalm**, in **Enterosan**, in **Opazimes**), and **opium** are examples. Fortunately, with these drugs, the dose to stop diarrhoea is much less than the dose which produces adverse effects.

A frequently prescribed preparation for the treatment of diarrhoea (**co-phenotrope**) contains the opiate **diphenoxylate** and a small dose of **atropine** (**Diarphen, Lomotil, Tropergen**). Diphenoxylate is related to pethidine and is used to treat diarrhoea because of its constipating effects. It should not be used in patients with impaired liver function.

> *Opiate drugs should not be given to children under four years of age.*

Antispasmodic drugs (e.g. **dicyclomine**) reduce the movements of bowel muscles and reduce spasm (which causes colic). In mild diarrhoea they may relieve pain and reduce the number of bowel movements. They are not much use in severe diarrhoea nor in the chronic diarrhoea of ulcerative colitis and similar disorders.

Antibacterial Drugs

Antibacterial drugs should be used with the utmost caution because they may alter the normal bacterial content of the intestine, which may result in a super-added fungal infection (moniliasis). With some bacterial infections, antibiotics may also prolong the period when the patient can pass on the disease as a carrier. They may also increase the risk of relapse, interfere with subsequent bacterial diagnosis and promote the development of resistant organisms and cause rashes.

Antibacterial drugs should be used to treat moderately severe and severe diarrhoeas, particularly if they are associated with chills, fever, abdominal pains and blood and/or pus in the motions. However, because of over-use in the past many bacteria are resistant to available antibiotics. Therefore, it is important that a sample of the motions is taken so that the infecting bacteria can be cultured in the laboratory and then tested for their sensitivity to selected antibiotics.

Food allergy (e.g. shellfish) can cause diarrhoea. Obviously, it is best to avoid foods to which you know you are allergic. However, should you suffer the symptoms of food allergy, **sodium cromoglicate**(cromoglycate) (**Nalcrom**) may be useful to overcome the allergic reaction.

Chronic Diarrhoea

Diarrhoea can be caused by a chronic inflammation of the bowel (e.g. ulcerative colitis, Crohn's disease). A local application of a corticosteroid can be used if the inflammation is affecting the rectum (back passage). Foams can be particularly useful (e.g. **hydrocortisone** (**Colifoam**), **prednisolone** (**Predfoam**). Prednisolone is also available in enemas (**Predenema, Predsol**) and suppositories (**Predsol**).

Certain aminosalicylates are available as enemas and suppositories: **mesalazine** (**Asacol, Pentasa, Salofalk**) and **sulfasalazine** (**Salazopyrin**).

Where the inflammation is more widespread or it does not respond to local treatment, you may take a medicine orally. These include:

- *Aminosalicylates*
  balsalazide (**Colazide**)
  mesalazine (**Asacol, Pentasa, Salofalk**)
  olsalazine (**Dipentum**)
  sulfasalazine (**Salazopyrin, Sulazine, Ucine**)

● *Corticosteroids*

hydrocortisone (**Hydrocortone**)
budesonide (**Budenofalk, Entocort CR**)
prednisolone (**Deltacortril, Precortisyl**).

Aminosalicylate should only be used with great caution in pregnancy and breastfeeding. In addition, blood disorders can occur and you should watch out for unexplained bleeding, bruising, sore throat or fever. If any of these symptoms occur you should stop taking the medicine and see your doctor immediately.

A new treatment (**infliximab** (**Remicade**)) has been introduced recently. Infliximab is a monoclonal antibody which inhibits the pro-inflammatory cytokine (the trigger mechanism for the inflammation). It is used in the treatment of severe Crohn's disease which is not responding to corticosteroid treatment. It is only used in hospital under specialist supervision.

Other drugs used to treat chronic diarrhoea (e.g. ulcerative colitis, Crohn's disease) include **azathioprine** (**Azamune, Imuran**) which is used as maintenance therapy.

Drugs used in the treatment of acute diarrhoea (e.g. **codeine, diphenoxylate, loperamide**) should be avoided as they can make diverticular disease worse.

The proper management of diet is very important in chronic diarrhoea. Some patients will require a high fibre diet while others need to avoid high fibre diets. Laxatives may be required (see Chapter 21). Diarrhoea resulting from the loss of bile-salt absorption can be treated by using **colestyramine** (**Questran, Questran Light**) which binds bile-salts.

21

Drugs Used to Treat Constipation

Drugs used to treat constipation are called laxatives. They are often misused – the result of the mistaken belief that there is some relationship between regular daily emptying of the bowels and health. It does not matter if you have your bowels opened two or three times a day or two to three times a week. It only matters if you develop a change in bowel habit; if you only go a day or two over the normal for you, this again does not matter.

We usually talk about **laxatives** when we wish to produce a soft, formed, easy-to-pass motion and a **cathartic** or **purgative** when we wish to produce a fairly quick and fluid emptying of the bowel. Most laxatives are harmless when taken infrequently, but their continued use over long periods of time may lead to complications such as fluid and salt loss. This may make you feel tired, weak and thirsty. Calcium loss may occur and lead to bone softening.

The taking of laxatives is only occasionally necessary; for example, after childbirth, after an operation for piles or some other condition around the anus, after some abdominal operations, after a coronary thrombosis and in elderly or debilitated bedridden patients. Otherwise, the use of a laxative is seldom indicated and you certainly will be no healthier if you drink a glass of health salts every morning.

The most natural treatment for simple constipation is a **high fibre diet**. This is easily achieved by eating more fruit and leafy vegetables, and wholegrain cereals, and, if necessary, by adding bran to your diet in the form of wholegrain cereal foods. In addition to diet make sure that you drink plenty of fluids, take regular exercise and develop a habit of trying to empty your bowels just after a meal when food entering the stomach stimulates the large bowel to empty its contents into the rectum, which produces the urge to go. Never neglect a feeling that you want to empty your bowels. The same advice applies if you have developed a laxative habit, but, in addition, try to reduce the dose slowly over a period of time.

Laxatives should never be taken to relieve abdominal pains, cramps, colic, nausea or any other symptom, whether associated with constipation or not. If in doubt you should always consult your doctor, particularly if you pass blood in the motions, and/or if you develop a change in bowel habits.

The occasional use of laxatives is not harmful but the danger is that you will develop the laxative habit – when you have taken one dose of laxative and it may take several days before you get the urge to go again. Unfortunately, some people cannot wait that long before taking another dose. A regular routine develops and the bowel action becomes so abnormal that it is then unable to function properly and the person will be totally reliant upon the use of these drugs. These warnings refer to all laxatives which include the old practice of taking health salts before breakfast and numerous patent health remedies.

There are four main groups of drugs used to treat constipation: stimulant, osmotic, faecal softeners and bulk-forming.

1 Stimulant Laxatives

These increase large bowel movements by irritating the lining and/or stimulating the bowel muscles to contract. They may cause cramps, increased mucus secretion and excessive fluid loss. Response to dosage varies tremendously and what may produce stomach cramps and diarrhoea in one person may have no effect in another.

Stimulant laxatives include:

bisacodyl (**Dulco-lax**)
cascara (in **Rhuaka**)
castor oil
dantron (in **co-danthramer** (**Ailax, Codalax, Danlax**), in **co-danthrusate**
   (**Capsuvac, Normax**))
docusate sodium (**Dioctyl, Docusol**)
senna (in **Boots Compound Laxative Syrup of Figs**, **Boots Senna tablets**, in
   Califig, Ex-lax Senna, in **Fam-Lax Senna**, in **Manevac**, in **Nylax with
   Senna**, in **Potter's Cleansing Herb**, in **Rhuaka, Senokot**)
sodium picosulfate (**Laxoberal**, in **Picolax**)

Senna, **cascara** and **dantron** may colour the urine red, cause excessive loss of fluids and potassium and if taken regularly may cause patchy pigmentation of part of the bowel (colon). This is not serious and is reversible on stopping the drug. Long-term high-dose administration of dantron is associated with the development of cancer in the intestine and liver of rodents. There is no evidence that dantron produces cancer in humans. It is present with polaxamer 188 in **co-danthramer** (**Ailax, Codalax, Danlax**) and with docusate sodium in **co-danthrusate** (**Capsuvac, Duco-lax, Normax**).

Phenolphthalein was used as a laxative but it caused allergic skin rashes and coloured the urine pink. **Bisacodyl** (**Dulco-lax**) is related to phenolphthalein. It may be used as a suppository as well as taken by mouth.

Castor oil differs from the other stimulant laxatives because it works on the small bowel and therefore produces an effect in about three hours. Other laxatives act on the large bowel and work in six–twelve hours.

Stimulant laxatives can be given by mouth or rectum. They should only be used to prepare the bowel for surgery or instrumentation or in severe constipation provided there is no evidence of obstruction. They should not be used in children or in pregnancy. Onset of action by mouth takes six–twelve hours. Senna is the least powerful, and sodium picosulfate is the most powerful.

2 Osmotic Laxatives (Saline Laxatives)

These are **salts of magnesium**, **sodium** or **potassium** in various mixtures. By mouth or by rectum they are incompletely absorbed and increase the bulk of the bowel contents by drawing liquid into the bowel (a process called osmosis). Some of them are made fizzy by adding sodium bicarbonate and fruity by adding weak acids such as citric and tartaric. These salts may take fluids from the body and cause dehydration, and should therefore be taken with large drinks of water. They include **magnesium sulphate** (**Epsom salts**, **Andrews Liver Salts**), **magnesium hydroxide** (**Phillip's Milk of Magnesia**, in **Milpar**), **sodium sulphate** (in **Klean-Prep**), **Eno** contains **sodium bicarbonate** plus citric and tartaric acid. Some of these preparations are called health salts, which is reasonable enough if health is defined as bowel movements and belching.

Osmotic laxatives containing sodium salts should never be given to patients with heart, liver or kidney failure. Likewise they should not be taken by patients on diuretic drugs since these drugs are given to get rid of salt from the body. Magnesium salts should not be given to patients with impaired kidney function; about 20 per cent of magnesium may be absorbed from the intestine and as it is excreted by the kidneys any impairment may lead to an accumulation of magnesium in the blood, resulting in magnesium intoxication.

Lactulose (**Duphalac, Lactugal, Osmolax, Regulose**) and **Lactitol** are non-absorbable synthetic disaccharide sugars. They have an osmotic action and increase the fluid bulk of the motions and lead to stimulation of bowel movements. They also affect the acidity and increase the bacterial content of the bowel. They may cause nausea, diarrhoea and wind.

Polyethylene glycol by mouth (in **Klean-Prep**, in **Movicol**) acts rapidly and clears the bowel prior to X-ray or endoscopy. It may also be used to treat chronic constipation and to treat faecal impaction. Total evacuation of the bowel is achieved within about four hours.

3 Faecal Softeners (Lubricant Laxatives)

There are two types of faecal softeners: mineral oils (e.g. **liquid paraffin**) and wetting agents such as **docusate sodium** in **co-danthrusate** (**Dioctyl, Norgalax, Normax**) and **poloxamer 188** in **co-danthramer** (**Ailax, Codalax**).

Liquid paraffin (in **Milpar**) softens and lubricates the motions. Its regular use should be avoided since it interferes with the absorption of carotene (pre-formed vitamin A), vitamin A and vitamin D. In pregnancy it may reduce the absorption of vitamin K and produce a disorder of blood clotting. Young, elderly and debilitated patients may rarely inhale a few drops into their lungs when they swallow liquid paraffin and this may cause a type of pneumonia. It may also be absorbed from the gut and cause swelling of lymph glands in the gut wall, the liver and spleen. It may also leak from the anus in the night and cause irritation (pruritus ani). It should not be used in children under three years of age. It should only be used occasionally to temporarily relieve constipation.

Docusate sodium lowers surface tension and is used in the pharmaceutical industry as an emulsifying or wetting agent. It softens the motions in twenty-four–forty-eight hours. It is also used to soften wax in the ears. **Poloxamer 188** is another surface active agent which acts as a lubricant laxative.

4 Bulk-forming Laxatives

These are substances which increase the bulk of the stools by absorbing water which stimulates the bowel muscles to become active. In addition they soften the stools. They usually take twelve–twenty-four hours to work. Some bulk-forming laxatives are naturally occurring substances such as gums, e.g. agar, tragacanth; **ispaghula husks** (**Fybogel, Isogel, Konsyl** in **Manevac, Regulan**) and **sterculia** (**Normacol**, in **Normacol Plus**) – these are present in numerous proprietary laxatives. Others are semi-synthetic, like **methylcellulose** (**Celevac**). They must be taken with plenty of fluids because of the risk of bowel obstruction in elderly or debilitated patients. Gums may cause hypersensitivity resulting in skin rashes and hayfever/asthma-like symptoms. **Bran** (present in **Trifyba**) is a by-product of the milling of wheat and contains about 20 per cent of indigestible cellulose. It is an effective bulk laxative and may also help to prevent certain bowel disorders such as diverticulitis.

Which Laxative to Take

For occasional attacks of constipation when living habits change (e.g. going on holiday), try a bulk-forming laxative – e.g. bran – and drink plenty of fluids, particularly if the climate is hot. Use a stimulant laxative (e.g. senna) only if necessary. A faecal softener (e.g. docusate sodium) may help after surgery on the anus or if you have painful piles. In pregnancy, change to a high fibre diet and drink plenty of fluids. After childbirth, try a high fibre diet and plenty of fluids. It may occasionally be necessary to use a stimulant laxative (e.g. senna) or a faecal softener (e.g. docusate sodium).

Bulk-forming laxatives (e.g. bran) are useful for treating irritable bowel syndrome and chronic diarrhoeal disorders such as ulcerative colitis. They are also useful in people with colostomies or ileostomies. Terminally ill patients, who may be taking constipating narcotic pain-relievers, may need the regular use of a mixture of laxatives, e.g. a faecal softener (co-danthramer) and/or lactulose with senna.

Bran

Bran comes from the outer layers of wheat grain and its fibre content varies from 30 to 50 per cent depending on the milling process and on the variety of wheat. It is present in such foods as wholemeal bread and certain breakfast cereals. It is useful for treating constipation, and for treating diverticulosis, and it may help patients suffering from irritable bowel syndrome. It is also of use in treating constipation associated with haemorrhoids, anal fissure and ulcerative colitis affecting the lower end of the colon. There are numerous products available to which bran has been added, for instance special breads, biscuits and cereals, or you can buy 'pure' bran to add to cereals, etc. The choice is not critical, but everyone should switch from white bread to wholemeal bread and high fibre cereals and reduce or try to stop eating sugary foods and foods made from refined flour. You must drink plenty of fluids to avoid obstruction from bran.

Rectally Administered Laxatives

When the faeces are impacted, laxatives administered rectally may be useful. (Remember in the elderly, impacted faeces due to constipation may present as diarrhoea, a watery leakage of faeces around the impaction.) Preparations available include **bisacodyl suppositories** (**Dulco-lax**), **phosphate enemas** (**Fleet**, **Fletchers'**) and suppositories (e.g. **Carbalax**), **docusate sodium** (**Fletchers' Enemette**, **Norgolax Micro-enemas**), **arachis oil** (**Fletchers'**), faecal softener/lubricant enemas: **Micolette** (sodium lauryl sulpoacetate and glycerol), **Micralax** (sodium citrate and sodium alkylsulphoacetate) and **Relaxit** (sodium lauryl sulphate and glycerol), and **glycerol** suppositories.

22

Drugs Used to Treat Angina

Angina pectoris is the term used to describe attacks of pain from the heart of short duration and without evidence of lasting damage to the heart muscle. It is caused by a disorder of the coronary arteries which supply the heart. This results in a deficient supply of blood to part of the working heart muscle causing a lack of oxygen which produces pain. *Coronary thrombosis* implies an attack of pain from the heart due to a thrombosis (a clot of blood) in a coronary artery; it may or may not be accompanied by evidence of damage to the heart muscle. This damage or scarring results from the cutting-off of the blood supply to part of the muscle and is called *myocardial infarction*.

In most patients angina occurs only on effort and goes off on resting – this is because on effort the heart has to do more work and the heart muscle requires more oxygen. If the coronary arteries are not healthy enough to supply the extra oxygen, the muscle starts to ache. As soon as the patient rests, the heart has to do less work, oxygen demand falls and the pain goes off. The aim of drug treatment is to improve the blood supply and therefore the oxygen supply to the heart muscle.

Drugs used to treat angina include those used to treat an acute attack or to prevent an attack over the short term and those used to prevent attacks over the long term. They belong to three major groups – nitrates, beta-blockers and calcium-channel blockers.

Nitrates

Nitrates have similar actions and effects. Their basic action is to relax muscles in the walls of blood vessels, especially veins. This causes the blood vessels to dilate, a process referred to as vasodilatation. Nitrates are therefore called **vasodilators**. These effects on the circulation cause a reduction in the workload on the heart and therefore less oxygen is needed. In addition, nitrates improve the coronary artery blood flow to affected areas of the heart. Anginal pain is relieved and can also be prevented. They increase the amount of exercise a patient can do before getting an attack of angina, and they relieve or prevent the attack of pain.

Proprietary preparations of glyceryl trinitrate available for treating angina include:

skin patches (**Deponit, Minitran, Nitro-Dur, Transiderm Nitro**)

oral sprays or pump sprays (**Coro-Nitro, Glytrin, Nitrolingual, Nitromin**)

ointment (**Percutol**)

injections (**Nitrocine, Nitronal**)

tablets to dissolve in the mouth (**glyceryl trinitrate, GTN 300 mcg**)

modified-release tablets (**Suscard, Sustac**)

Longer-acting nitrates by mouth may be used to prevent attacks coming on. They include:

isosorbide dinitrate (**Angitak spray, Cedocard Retard*, Isoket Retard*, Isordil, Sorbid SA***)

isosorbide mononitrate (**Chemydur 60XL*, Elantan, Elantan LA*, Imazin XL, Imdur*, Isib 60XL*, Ismo, Ismo Retard, Isodur, Isotrate, MCR-50*, Modisal XL*, Monit, Monit SR*, Monit XL*, Mono-Cedocard, Monomax SR***).

Isosorbide dinitrate is also available as a transdermal spray (**Isocard**) and injection (**Isoket**).

* These preparations are modified-release to produce prolonged effects.

Adverse effects of nitrates are related to vasodilation; they include throbbing headache, flushing, a fall in blood pressure on standing, and rapid beating of the heart. The headache may be troublesome initially but usually goes over time. Glyceryl trinitrate tablets can easily lose their effectiveness and you can tell this if they lose the burning sensation when you suck them. Ask your pharmacist how to store them correctly.

A combination product of **aspirin** and **isosorbide mononitrate** (**Imazin XL***) is also available for the prevention of angina and secondary prevention of myocardial infarction.

● *Tolerance to Nitrates*

All nitrates can induce tolerance, which is a lessened response to the effects of a drug and so a larger dose has to be given to produce a similar effect. This means that, if regular doses of a long-acting nitrate were used to prevent angina, the dose which initially produced relief may become less effective. Tolerance can occur within twenty-four–forty-eight hours of regular use unless a period of four to eight hours is allowed *without* treatment. Tolerance is more likely to develop with high doses than with low doses. A period of time when there is no nitrate in the blood will help to prevent tolerance; this can be achieved at night by not taking a dose of nitrate after about 8 p.m. or by removing transdermal patches before bedtime. Intravenous glyceryl trinitrate should not be given continuously for more than thirty-six hours. People who get angina at night and need treatment at night should allow themselves a period of no treatment in the daytime.

Beta-blockers

Many patients develop angina in response to an emotional upset. This is because the heart beats faster in response to fear, panic, tension, anxiety, excitation or aggression. This increases its workload and in the presence of a deficient coronary artery blood supply, anginal pain will develop. The rapid beating of the heart is caused by stimulation through nerve endings called beta-receptors. Beta-blockers can prevent this stimulation by blocking these receptors. This blocking will also prevent stimulation which occurs during exercise.

Beta-blockers have a marked effect when the heart is being stimulated by exercise, emotion or adrenaline(epinephrine)-like drugs. They reduce the effects of such stimulation to produce slowing of the rate and a reduction in the force of contraction of the heart. Some of them reduce the rate of conduction of impulses through the conducting system of the heart. The overall result from beta-blockers is a reduction in the volume of blood pumped out by the heart during each contraction and a decreased oxygen consumption because the heart has to do less work.

They reduce the response of the heart to stress and exercise and are used to prevent angina.

The discontinuance of beta-blockers after long-term therapy in a patient with angina must be done *gradually* and under the careful supervision of a doctor. Sudden stopping in these circumstances has caused heart attacks (myocardial infarction).

Acebutolol, **celiprolol**, **oxprenolol** and **pindolol** retain some stimulating effects in addition to their blocking effects – this is called intrinsic sympatho-mimetic activity (ISA). They tend to produce less slowing of the heart. They also produce less coldness of the hands and feet and less fatigue which are problems with some other beta-blockers.

Atenolol, **nadolol**, and **sotalol** are soluble in water and are therefore less likely to enter the brain to produce adverse effects such as poor sleep and nightmares. Fat-soluble beta-blockers can produce these effects because they enter the brain. Some beta-blockers have a short duration of effect and have to be given two to three times daily; however, these are usually available as slow-release preparations which means they need only to be taken once daily. (See those marked * on p. 115).

In patients with asthma, beta-blockers may also block the nerve endings supplying the bronchi and trigger an asthmatic attack. Some beta-blockers have less effect on beta receptors in the bronchi and a more selective effect on beta-receptors in the heart, e.g. **acebutolol, atenolol, bisoprolol, metoprolol**. They are referred to as *cardioselective*. Nonetheless, *it is safer to avoid all beta-blockers in patients with asthma or chronic obstructive airway disease.*

Beta-blockers can make disorders of the circulation worse, affect glucose levels in diabetic patients, and they can mask some of the symptoms of low blood sugar (hypoglycaemia) in patients taking anti-diabetic drugs, including insulin. Selective beta-blockers should be used in diabetic patients. Beta-blockers should not be used if attacks of hypoglycaemia are frequent.

Beta-blockers used to treat angina include:

acebutolol (**Sectral**)
atenolol (**Antipressan, Atenix, Tenif, Tenormin**)
bisoprolol (**Cardicor, Emcor, Monocor**)
carvedilol (**Eucardic**)
labetalol (**Trandate**)
metoprolol (**Betaloc, Lopresor, Mepranix**)
nadolol (**Corgard**)
oxprenolol (**Slow-Trasicor, Trasicor**)
pindolol (**Visken**)
propranolol (**Angilol, Bedranol SR*, Beta-Prograne, Inderal** preparations, **Lopranol LA*, Probeta LA*, Propanix, Propanix SR***)
timolol (**Betim**)

* These preparations are modified-release to produce prolonged effects.

In addition to their use in angina beta-blockers are also used to treat patients suffering from raised blood pressure, disorders of heart rhythm, migraine, anxiety, tremor, thyrotoxicosis and glaucoma (used topically). They are all equally effective, but there are differences between them which may affect choice in treating individual disorders and patients.

Carvedilol (**Eucardic**), **celiprolol** (**Celectol**) and **labetalol** (**Trandate**) block alpha and beta receptors producing a fall in blood pressure. They are used principally to treat raised blood pressure.

Calcium-channel Blockers (Calcium Antagonists)

Calcium-channel blockers or **antagonists** reduce the work of the heart by blocking the entry of calcium ions into the heart muscle cells and thus reducing the strength of contraction and slowing electrical conduction of impulses through the heart. They also decrease muscle contractions in veins and arteries producing vasodilation. They differ according to the three main effects they produce – i.e. vasodilator effects, reduced heart muscle contractility and reduced conduction of impulses, and may be divided into three classes:

Verapamil (**Cordilox, Securon, Verapress MR, Vertab SR, Univer**) depresses contractility of heart muscle and conduction of electrical impulses. Therefore, it may trigger heart failure if there is already some conduction defect or if taken with a beta-blocker.

Amlodipine (**Istin**), **felodipine** (**Plendil**), **isradipine** (**Prescal**), **lacidipine** (**Motens**), **lercanidipine** (**Zanidip**), **nicardipine** (**Cardene**), **nifedipine** (**Adalat, Adipine MR, Angiopine MR, Cardilate MR, Coracten, Coroday MR, Fortipine LA, Hypolar Retard, Nifedipress MR, Nifedotard MR, Nifopress Retard, Slofedipine, Slofedipine XL, Tenif, Tensipine MR**), **nimodipine** (**Nimotop**) and **nisoldipine** (**Syscor MR**) do not depress contractility of the heart muscle and do not depress conduction of electrical impulses. They may reverse some of the depressant effects of beta-blockers on the heart and therefore they may be taken together, but the combination may cause a marked fall in blood pressure.

Diltiazem (**Adizem SR, Adizem XL, Angitil SR, Angitil XL, Calcicard CR, Dilcardia SR, Dilzem SR, Dilzem XL, Optil SR, Optil XL, Slozem, Tildiem LA, Tildiem Retard, Viazem XL, Zemtard XL**) has little if any depressant effect on contractility of the heart muscle and dilates coronary arteries more than other arteries. This reduces the risk of a rise in heart rate which occurs with other calcium-channel blockers.

Calcium-channel blockers used to prevent angina decrease the workload of the heart, improve efficiency of contraction, reduce heart rate and improve coronary blood flow.

Potassium-channel Activators

Potassium-channel activators dilate both arteries and veins. The group includes **nicorandil** (**Ikorel**) which is used to treat and prevent angina. It is taken as tablets by mouth.

Drug Treatment of a Coronary Thrombosis

The blood may clot over a damaged area (e.g. a fatty deposit) in a coronary artery, producing a thrombus. This process is referred to as a *coronary thrombosis* and it may cause a blockage in the artery leading to a *myocardial infarction* – damage to the part of the heart muscle supplied by that artery. Sometimes a damaged coronary artery may go into temporary spasm and cause myocardial ischaemia – resulting in a temporary reduction in blood supply to the heart muscle but without causing lasting damage.

An acute attack of myocardial ischaemia or a myocardial infarction produce severe and persistent chest pain (angina-type pain) and are often referred to as heart attacks.

Depending upon the condition of the patient and the findings from the electrocardiograph (ECG), the **immediate drug treatment** may include some or all of the following:

- Oxygen by mask in order to improve the supply of oxygen to the heart and other organs.
- The treatment of any disorder of heart rhythm (see Chapter 24).
- The relief of pain by giving an injection of morphine; to prevent vomiting it may be necessary to give an injection of an anti-vomiting drug such as prochlorperazine (see Chapter 18).
- The relief of any spasm of the coronary arteries by giving a nitrate vasodilator intravenously.
- The use of a thrombus-dissolving drug intravenously to dissolve the thrombus and keep the blood supply flowing (see below).
- The prevention of a recurrence of the thrombosis by starting treatment with an anti-thrombotic drug such as aspirin (see below).
- The treatment of any complications such as heart failure (Chapter 23) or disorders of heart rhythm (Chapter 24).

The Use of Thrombus-dissolving Drugs (Clot-busters)

Damage to part of the heart muscle (myocardial infarction) is nearly always due to a thrombus blocking one of the coronary arteries or its branches (coronary thrombosis). Most damage occurs in the first few hours after the artery has been blocked by the thrombus.

Treatment of coronary thrombosis is aimed at dissolving this blockage *as quickly as possible* after it has occurred in order to keep the affected artery open and the blood supply flowing to the area of heart muscle supplied by that artery. This will limit the extent of the damage to the heart muscle, improve the functions of the heart, reduce the risk of heart complications (e.g. heart failure, disorders of heart rhythm) and reduce the risk of death.

Drugs used to dissolve the thrombus are fibrinolytics. They dissolve the fibrin mesh that forms a thrombus by activating the blood's own thrombus-dissolving mechanisms – the conversion of the inactive plasminogen to active plasmin. (Plasmin is an enzyme which slowly digests fibrin clots. It is present in the body in the form of plasminogen.) They include:

Streptokinase (Kabikinase, Streptase), which has to be given by infusion into a vein. It acts generally throughout the circulation and not just at the site of the coronary thrombosis – bleeding is therefore the most important harmful effect (see below).

Alteplase (Actilyse), **reteplase (Rapilysin)** and **tenecteplase (Metalyse)** are designed to prevent bleeding due to a generalized effect in the circulation. They are bio-engineered versions of the naturally occurring plasminogen activator and, unlike streptokinase, they target their effects directly on to plasminogen at the site of the thrombus and have a reduced effect in the general circulation, causing much less risk of bleeding. They have to be given by injection and then by infusion into a vein.

> *Because these drugs dissolve thrombi it is essential to give them as soon as possible after the onset of symptoms (e.g. chest pain) in order to try to prevent the affected artery from being blocked completely. Treatment should be given within twelve hours of the first symptom,* **but the sooner it is given the better***.*

The Use of Aspirin to Prevent Re-thrombosis

Once the effects of a thrombolytic drug have worn off there is a risk that further thrombosis will occur. This is because such treatment only dissolves the thrombus. Additional treatment is therefore necessary in order to prevent re-thrombosis: current management is to give a low daily dose of *aspirin* by mouth, *starting as soon as possible after the heart attack* and continuing for many years and probably for life.

Aspirin produces many effects on the body and one of these is to stop platelets from clumping together at the site of damage to an artery and thus reducing the risk of further thrombosis.

The effects of aspirin and streptokinase or anistreplase are additive. A combination of one or the other with aspirin will therefore help to reduce mortality. Heparin (an anti-coagulant, see p. 141) has to be added to treatment with alteplase to ensure maximum benefit. Because the body develops antibodies to streptokinase and anistreplase their effectiveness may be reduced. Therefore, treatment should not continue for more than four days and treatment with either of these drugs should not be repeated within five days to twelve months of the last course.

Preventing another Heart Attack (Secondary Prevention)

In a patient who survives a heart attack it is important to try to prevent a further attack because the risk of death will be increased according to how much the heart has been damaged. These attempts are referred to as *secondary prevention*.

The Use of Drugs in Secondary Prevention

● *Aspirin in Secondary Prevention*

The use of aspirin in preventing re-thrombosis following a heart attack is encouraging. Treatment should be started as soon as possible after the heart attack and continued for many years and probably for life.

Aspirin reduces the death rate following a heart attack if given in a dose of 150 mg to 300 mg daily for one month from the heart attack. The dose over the long term for preventing a further attack is 75–150 mg daily (see p. 143).

● *Beta-blockers in Secondary Prevention*

Beta-blockers appear to be beneficial in secondary prevention in some people. However, there is some controversy about who should receive beta-blocker treatment, which beta-blocker is the best, when the treatment should be started and stopped, and the doses that should be used.

Beta-blockers should not be used in anyone with pre-existing heart failure, low blood pressure, low pulse rate, asthma or other chronic obstructive airway diseases. They should not be stopped suddenly. **Acebutolol**, **metoprolol**, **propranolol** and **timolol** are all suitable and should be given for at least two years.

Although calcium-channel blockers are not usually used, they may be of benefit in patients who cannot take beta-blockers. **Verapamil** would appear to be the drug of choice.

● *ACE Inhibitors in Secondary Prevention*

ACE inhibitors improve survival in patients with failure of the left side of the heart following a myocardial infarction (heart attack) if started within three to ten days of the attack.

● *Nitrates in Secondary Prevention*

Nitrates are used for patients with angina. (See p. 112).

● *Fish Oils in Secondary Prevention*

Fish oils reduce the blood levels of cholesterol and fats (triglycerides) and help to reduce the stickiness of platelets, thus reducing the risk of thrombosis. They are a suitable addition or alternative to aspirin treatment, especially in those people who cannot take aspirin because they suffer from an active peptic ulcer.

23

Drugs Used to Treat Heart Failure

In the failing heart, the volume of blood in the heart chambers during relaxation of the heart muscle increases. This causes them to stretch, which interferes with their pumping capacity when they contract. More blood accumulates in the chambers causing a back-pressure to build up in the blood vessels returning blood to the heart. This back-pressure may cause congestion of the lungs and produce breathlessness and disorders of respiration. If the back-pressure affects the right side of the heart where blood from all over the body is returned, the pressure builds up in the veins and back to the tissues. This produces an increase of fluids in the tissues called oedema (dropsy). Heart failure with oedema is referred to as congestive heart failure.

Drugs Used to Treat Heart Failure

Digoxin and Related Drugs (Cardiac Glycosides)

They include **digoxin** (**Lanoxin**) and **digitoxin**. These drugs have been used for centuries to treat heart failure. They are called cardiac glycosides, and are found in a number of plants. **Digitoxin** is prepared from the leaves of *Digitalis purpurea* (purple foxglove). **Digoxin** is prepared from the leaves of *Digitalis lanata* (white foxglove). **Prepared digitalis** is a crude mixture obtained from powdered leaves of both types of foxglove plant. Digitoxin is slower acting than digoxin.

Digoxin and **digitoxin** are the most commonly used of this group of drugs. They have similar actions and effects, but they differ in the rate at which they start to act and in the duration of their effects. They act mainly on the heart. They increase both the force of contraction of the heart muscle and the work done by the heart without increasing its oxygen consumption.

In heart failure they cause the heart muscle to work more efficiently; this causes increased output from the heart, reduction of back-pressure, decrease in the size of the heart and a reduction in blood volume. The latter is produced by the effects of a more efficient circulation of blood to the kidneys, resulting in more urine being produced. Secondary to the circulatory improvement mentioned above, they reduce heart rate by reducing sympathetic drive to the heart (i.e. they reduce adrenaline(epinephrine)-like actions). They also make the heart sensitive to impulses from the vagus nerve, which slows the heart rate. In addition they slow down the rate at which electrical impulses pass from the heart's pacemaker (the part of the heart where electrical impulses start) to the rest of the heart.

Digoxin is almost completely excreted unchanged in the urine and should be used with caution in patients with impaired kidney function. It is slowly excreted and is accumulative.

Digoxin causes signs and symptoms of intoxication when taken in high doses. Too much at once or too much for too long can be dangerous. Cumulative effects may develop. Furthermore, the lower the level of potassium in the body, the more toxic the effects of digoxin.

Therefore, diuretics which reduce the level of potassium in the body can cause digoxin toxicity. It is important to monitor potassium levels when diuretics are used with digoxin.

Loss of appetite, nausea and vomiting are the earliest indications of overdose. Nausea is an important warning and vomiting can be most distressing to a patient with heart failure. They may also cause diarrhoea and abdominal discomfort or pain. These symptoms disappear in a few days, but they are generally avoidable. They must be distinguished from similar symptoms which occasionally develop in heart failure. Headache, fatigue and drowsiness may also occur and elderly patients may become confused.

The most frequent and well-recognized adverse effect on the heart is the appearance of extra heart beats. If these extra heart beats occur after each regular beat then you get what is called coupling – a good clue that the patient has been overdosed. Toxic amounts interfere with the passage of electrical impulses from the pacemaker down the main transmission paths between the upper and the lower chambers of the heart. This leads to missed or dropped heart beats and sometimes to partial or complete heart block, which means that the pacemaker has lost control and the upper and lower chambers of the heart are beating independently. This is a dangerous adverse effect and should be suspected if the heart rate drops below fifty beats per minute. However, an increase in rate is sometimes the first evidence of poisoning because of excitatory effects upon the heart muscle. This is a particular hazard in patients who are also receiving diuretics (these may reduce the blood potassium, which sensitizes heart muscle to the effects of digoxin). The rapid beating of the heart may become quite irregular, which if it affects the lower chambers (ventricles) may cause sudden death.

Dosage with digoxin involves two problems: the amount required to produce the desired effects as quickly as possible in someone not previously on the drug (initial digitalization) and the amount required to maintain the good effects with minimal adverse effects (maintenance dosage). There is a wide variation in individual response and therefore these two problems need skill and care. The 'right' dose for an individual patient is that which proves right for that person. Regular blood-level measurements should be carried out and the doses adjusted accordingly.

Digoxin is used to treat chronic heart failure. It is also used to treat disorders of heart rhythm affecting the upper chambers – these include supraventricular disorders of rhythm, atrial flutter and atrial fibrillation.

Diuretics (see Chapter 29)

These reverse the salt and water retention which occurs in heart failure as the body attempts to keep the blood volume raised in order to *compensate* for the failing heart. This causes an increased *pre-load* on the heart. Reduction in circulating volume with diuretics reduces the congestion in the lungs and elsewhere, reduces oedema, reduces breathlessness and reduces the workload on the heart. Initially a potent short-acting diuretic is needed (e.g. a loop diuretic such as **furosemide**(frusemide) or **bumetanide**). These may be replaced by a **thiazide** diuretic for maintenance therapy. Since loop and thiazide diuretics produce a fall in blood potassium, a diuretic which spares potassium such as **amiloride** or **triamterene** may be given with the diuretic (see p. 149).

Vasodilator Drugs

There are three main groups of vasodilators available for use in heart failure: those which principally affect the venous system and reduce *pre-load* pressure on the heart by reducing the volume of blood returning to the heart (e.g. **nitrates**), those which principally affect the arterial system and reduce the *after-load* by reducing the resistance to the flow of blood from the heart (e.g. **hydralazine**), and those which act on both the venous and arterial systems and reduce both *pre-load* and *after-load* (e.g. **prazosin**).

Nitrates act predominantly on veins, increase the pooling of venous blood and reduce the return of blood to the heart. This reduces the pressure (*pre-load*) on the heart and helps it to pump more efficiently. Nitrates cause a small fall in blood pressure, a small increase in heart rate and very little change in output. They are discussed on p. 112.

Hydralazine (**Apresoline**) works predominantly on the arterial system; it causes a fall in peripheral resistance, increased cardiac output and improves the blood flow through the kidneys. **Phentolamine** (**Rogitine**), **prazosin** (**Hypo-**

vase) and **sodium nitroprusside** have an effect on both the arterial and venous systems.

Angiotensin-converting Enzyme Inhibitors (ACE Inhibitors)

ACE inhibitors (see p. 131) block the formation of angiotensin II (see p. 128) and reverse the constriction of arteries that it produces. This produces a fall in resistance to the flow of blood, a fall in blood pressure and a reduced workload on the heart (after-load). They reduce the blood volume (and, therefore, pre-load on the heart) because they improve the blood supply to the kidneys and increase the excretion of salt and water in the urine. In addition, they stop the production of aldosterone (see p. 128) and therefore reverse the retention of salt and water caused by aldosterone. They also help to reduce pre-load by causing dilatation of veins.

Other Drugs Used to Treat Heart Failure

● *Heart Stimulants*

Dobutamine (**Dobutrex**, **Posiject**) acts on beta-receptors in heart muscle. It improves contraction of the heart but has little effect upon its rate. It is used to stimulate the heart to beat when it fails suddenly.

Dopexamine (**Dopacard**) is used to treat heart failure associated with surgery. It stimulates the heart, causes vasodilation, and improves blood flow through the kidneys.

Isoprenaline (**Saventrine**) increases both the heart rate and the contraction of the heart. It may be used to stimulate the heart in circulatory shock, and to treat slowness of the pulse rate resulting from the use of beta-blockers or disopyramide.

● *Phosphodiesterase Inhibitors*

Enoximone (**Perfan**) and **milrinone** (**Primacor**) improve the function of the heart muscle and dilate blood vessels. They both increase output from the heart and reduce after-load. They may be used in the short-term treatment of severe congestive heart failure. They block an enzyme in heart muscle (phosphodiesterase) and are referred to as phosphodiesterase inhibitors.

● *Vasoconstrictor Drugs in Heart Failure*

If the blood pressure falls suddenly and severely the heart may fail and therefore in emergencies drugs are occasionally used that raise the blood pressure by constricting arteries. They only have a transient effect and thus they should only rarely be used in an emergency while preparing for other life-saving treatments. The danger with these drugs is that the constriction, while raising blood pressure, also reduces the blood supply to vital organs such as the kidneys. Furthermore, in a patient who is shocked there is already maximum constriction of arteries and to increase constriction even further may be dangerous. It is more effective and safer to increase the blood volume by giving blood, plasma, or a plasma expander by infusion. If it is necessary to use a drug, **dobutamine** (**Dobutrex**), **dopamine** or **isoprenaline** (**Min-I-Jet Isoprenaline**, **Saventrine IV**) should be used.

Drugs that cause constriction of arteries and transiently raise blood pressure may be used to treat a sudden fall in blood pressure during spinal anaesthesia. They include **metaraminol** (**Aramine**), **methoxamine** (**Vasoxine**), **noradrenaline**(norepinephrine) and **phenylephrine**. *They should not be used to treat circulatory shock.*

24

Drugs Used to Treat Disorders of Heart Rhythm

Drugs used to treat disorders of heart rhythm show a wide variation in their chemical structure, their actions and their clinical use. In addition, some drugs have more than one action. They are called anti-arrhythmic drugs (arrhythmic means disorder of heart rhythm). They can be grouped as those that act on:

1 supraventricular arrhythmias (i.e. occurring above a ventricle) (e.g. **verapamil**);
2 supraventricular and ventricular arrhythmias (e.g. **disopyramide**);
3 ventricular arrhythmias (e.g. **lidocaine**(lignocaine)).

They can also be grouped as to how they work on the electrical behaviour of heart cells and are often grouped into four classes:

Class I contains those drugs which possess local anaesthetic properties and which affect the surfaces of the cells (membrane stabilizing properties) in the electrical conducting system causing a reduction in the triggering of spontaneous beats. Drugs in this group include **disopyramide** (**Dirythmin SA**, **Isomide CR**, **Rythmodan**, **Rythmodan Retard**), **flecainide** (**Tambocor**), **lidocaine** (lignocaine), **mexiletine** (**Mexitil**, **Mexitil PL**), **procainamide** (**Pronestyl**), **propafenone** (**Arythmol**), **quinidine** (**Kinidin Durules**).

Class II drugs reduce the potential for disordered rhythm which occurs in response to sympathetic stimulation of the heart, e.g. by noradrenaline(norepinephrine). These include the **beta adrenoreceptor blockers** (see p. 114) which block the effect of sympathetic stimulation.

Class III drugs prolong the resting phase of the heart. These include **amiodarone** (**Cordarone X**) and **bretylium** (**Min-I-Jet Bretylate Tosylate**).

Class IV drugs are calcium-channel blockers, e.g. **verapamil** (see p. 115). They depress the passage of impulses through the electrical conducting system. **Digoxin** is the drug of choice for treating a disorder of heart rhythm called atrial fibrillation (a very rapid, irregular, non-coordinated contraction of the heart). **Atropine** may be used to treat slow heart rate (bradycardia) after a myocardial infarction (heart attack), and bradycardia caused by beta-blocking drugs (see p. 114). The latter may be used to treat certain types of tachycardia (rapid heart rate).

Adenosine (**Adenocor**) is the drug of choice for stopping attacks of paroxysmal tachycardia (a sudden burst of heart beats).

The treatment of a disorder of heart rhythm (arrhythmia) requires a precise diagnosis using an electrocardiograph (ECG). According to the disorder of rhythm, one or more of the drugs listed above would be used.

25

Drugs Used to Treat Raised Blood Pressure

The blood is forced around the body under pressure from the contractions of the heart. The blood pressure depends principally upon the amount of blood being pumped out by the heart and the resistance it meets as it enters smaller and smaller blood vessels.

The range of 'normal' blood pressure varies between individuals, and at different times in the same individual. It is influenced by many factors, for example age, gender, physical exercise, food, smoking, drugs and changes in posture. Emotion may send your blood pressure up, whereas sleep sends it down. Repeated blood pressure recordings when you are up and about often give lower levels overall than just a single casual recording.

An individual is only considered to have a raised blood pressure (**hypertension**) if the pressure is consistently raised, in the absence of any factors which may cause a temporary increase during the recording. There are two groups of hypertension. One is very common and because we do not know what causes it we call it **essential** or **idiopathic hypertension**. The other group is called **secondary hypertension** because it is caused by a known disorder such as kidney disease, toxaemia of pregnancy, narrowing of the main artery from the heart or of an artery supplying a kidney, or a tumour (phaeochromocytoma) of the sympathetic nervous system found most often in the adrenal glands.

The blood pressure recording consists of two readings – the upper reading is the pressure at the point when the contractions (systole) of the heart forces the pulse wave of blood through the artery from which the pressure is being recorded (this is usually the artery at the front of the elbow). This is called the systolic blood pressure. The second reading is the pressure recorded between the pulse waves when the heart is relaxed, and filling with blood (diastole) ready for the next pumping action – this is called the diastolic blood pressure. The readings are recorded as the systolic over the diastolic pressures – e.g. 120/80.

The systolic blood pressure may be raised on its own by emotion, fever, pregnancy and old age, when the arteries harden and narrow. A raised diastolic blood pressure appears to be more related to resistance to the flow of blood caused by constriction of the peripheral arteries.

We are interested in high blood pressure because there is an increased predisposition to illness and death among people with a blood pressure raised above the 'normal'. There is an association between high blood pressure and disease of the arteries; such disease of the arteries supplying the brain may produce an increased risk of a stroke and disease of the coronary arteries may cause heart attacks. Sustained high blood pressure may also be associated with heart failure and kidney damage (which in turn causes an increase in pressure since damaged kidneys may produce a chemical which increases the blood pressure). High blood pressure may also damage arteries in the eyes.

We know very little about what causes essential hypertension. Blood pressure increases with age; in early life the pressure is higher in men than in women, but from middle age (round about forty-five years) the pressure becomes higher in women than in men. Men are much more likely than women to develop complications such as coronary artery disease, and in men the higher the pressure the higher the risk of premature death. Hereditary, dietary, environmental, psychological and racial factors have all been considered to account for the development of essential hypertension. Raised blood pressure is also related to obesity so that reduction in weight may help, although differences in thickness of the arm (at the point where the cuff is applied when measuring the blood pressure) may alter the recordings.

The arterial blood pressure is determined by the output from the heart (cardiac output) and the resistance to the flow of blood as it is pumped into smaller and smaller arteries at the periphery (peripheral resistance). This peripheral resistance varies according to the calibre (or narrowing) of the arteries and the thickness (or viscosity) of the blood. These are in turn controlled by the following mechanisms.

Special blood pressure receptors in the main arteries in the neck (baroreceptors) detect changes in blood pressure – a fall in blood pressure causes the baroreceptors to send messages to the vasomotor centre in the brain which triggers off an increase in sympathetic stimulation to the heart, causing an increase in rate and output, and to the peripheral arteries, causing them to constrict.

In addition, changes in blood flow to the kidneys affect the production of an enzyme, called renin, by the kidneys. This enzyme acts to produce an inactive protein (Angiotensin I), converted in the lungs to a very powerful vasoconstrictor (Angiotensin II) which also causes the release of aldosterone from the adrenal glands which acts on the kidneys to retain salt and water, thus increasing the blood volume. Renin release is activated by a reduced blood supply to the kidneys which can be caused by narrowing of arteries and thus a vicious circle is set up in patients with raised blood pressure because they have narrowing of the peripheral arteries.

Treatment of Raised Blood Pressure

Treatment of raised blood pressure decreases the risk of stroke, heart failure, kidney failure and heart attacks. To diagnose raised blood pressure it should be measured twice at each consultation and confirmed on at least three separate occasions over one–two weeks.

Non-drug treatment includes weight reduction if overweight, stopping smoking, reducing high alcohol and salt intake, reducing fat intake, increasing the amount of fruit and vegetables in the diet, reducing stress, learning to relax and taking regular physical exercise.

If the systolic blood pressure is 200 or over or the diastolic 110 or over drug treatment should start immediately. If the systolic is 160–199 or diastolic 90–109 treatment should start immediately if there are signs of complications affecting the heart or kidneys or if the patient is diabetic. If there are no complications but the patient is over sixty and/or has a family history of risk, drug treatment should be started. If at or below these levels the patient should be regularly monitored over time. The aim of treatment is to keep the systolic at 140 or below and the diastolic at 85 or below.

Drugs Used to Treat Raised Blood Pressure

Drugs used to treat raised blood pressure affect principally the blood volume and/or peripheral resistance.

Diuretics

Diuretics act on the kidneys to increase the removal of salt and water from the blood. This helps to reduce blood pressure because of a fall in circulating blood volume and a fall in output from the heart. However, during long-term use the blood volume returns to 'normal' and yet there is a continuing reduction in blood pressure due to a reduction in peripheral resistance. **Thiazide diuretics** (see p. 147) are the principal group of diuretics used to treat hypertension. Doses required to produce a fall in blood pressure seldom produce a troublesome fall in blood potassium and only a few patients may require potassium supplements if they are on long-term diuretic treatment for their hypertension (see p. 147).

Central Acting Alpha Stimulants

The predominant effect of these drugs is to stimulate blood pressure controlling receptors in the brain (centrally acting), decreasing the sympathetic nerve stimulation of arteries, causing them to dilate and reduce the blood pressure. They also stimulate nerves supplying arteries and the heart, causing a reduction in the release of noradrenaline(norepinephrine), which also helps to reduce blood pressure. Because their principal effect is on the brain they rarely cause postural hypotension (a sudden drop in blood pressure when standing up from a sitting or lying position), but may produce drowsiness, depression and excessive dreaming.

This group includes **methyldopa** (**Aldomet**) and **clonidine** (**Catapres**). They have gone out of fashion for general use but because methyldopa is safe in asthmatics, in pregnancy and in heart failure it is still used routinely. Clonidine is seldom used; it may cause a serious rebound rise in blood pressure if it is suddenly stopped. **Moxonidine** (**Physiotens**) is a more selective stimulant of receptors in the blood pressure control centre in the brain. Therefore, it produces fewer adverse effects such as dry mouth and sedation than other stimulants that act on the brain.

Adrenergic Neurone Blockers

These drugs prevent the release of noradrenaline(norepinephrine) from sympathetic nerve endings, producing dilatation of arteries and a fall in blood pressure. They may cause a fall in blood pressure on standing up after sitting or lying down (postural hypotension) and they do not control the lying-down blood pressure. They may occasionally be used in emergencies. They include **debrisoquine** and **guanethidine** (**Ismelin**).

Ganglion Blockers

These drugs block acetylcholine in the autonomic ganglia (rather like switchboxes), thus reducing sympathetic activity generally. This causes heart rate and peripheral resistance to fall, lowers the output from the heart and reduces the blood pressure. Their many adverse effects include rapid beating of the heart, blurred vision, dry mouth, constipation, difficulty in passing urine, impotence and failure to ejaculate. A severe adverse effect is a fall in blood on standing (postural hypotension). The only drug in this group that is now used is **trimetaphan**, which is used to keep the blood pressure low during surgery.

Vasodilators

These drugs lower both lying and standing blood pressures. They cause vasodilatation by a direct action on the muscles of the arteries, thus producing a decrease in peripheral resistance and a fall in blood pressure.

They include **diazoxide** (**Eudemine**), **hydralazine** (**Apresoline**), **sodium nitroprusside** and **minoxidil** (**Loniten**). Their use is reserved for treating patients with severe hypertension.

Alpha-blockers

These drugs block alpha receptors, producing dilatation of arteries and reducing blood pressure (see p. 39). Those that are not selective may produce tachycardia (rapid beating of the heart), a severe fall in blood pressure, and they may precipitate angina because they reduce the blood supply to the heart (see Chapter 22). They are not used in the routine management of hypertension but may be used in a crisis and in the diagnosis and pre-operative treatment of patients with a phaeochromocytoma (a tumour of the sympathetic nervous system). Non-selective alpha-blockers include **phenoxybenzamine** and **phentolamine** (**Rogitine**). Selective alpha-blockers include **doxazosin** (**Cardura**), **indoramin** (**Baratol**), **prazosin** (**Hypovase**) and **terazosin** (**Hytrin**). They produce fewer adverse effects than the non-selective ones. They lower blood fat levels and are suitable for treating patients suffering from co-existing diabetes or heart failure, and may be used in combination with a thiazide diuretic or beta-blocker.

Beta-blockers

These are discussed in detail on p. 114. They cause a fall in blood pressure but their mode of action is not understood. They are one of the most important groups of anti-blood pressure drugs.

Angiotensin-converting Enzyme Inhibitors (ACE Inhibitors)

These drugs inhibit the conversion of Angiotensin I to Angiotensin II (see p. 128), reduce constriction of arteries and reduce blood volume, causing a fall in blood pressure. Unlike the beta-blockers, they are safe to use in asthmatics and diabetics. They include **captopril** (**Acepril, Capoten, Ecopace, Kaplon, Tensopril**), **cilazapril** (**Vascace**), **enalapril*** (**Innovace**), **fosinopril** (**Staril**), **imidapril** (**Tanatril**), **lisinopril*** (**Carace, Zestril**), **moexipril** (**Perdix**), **perindopril** (**Coversyl**), **quinapril*** (**Accupro**), **ramipril** (**Tritace**), **trandolapril** (**Gopten, Odrik**). Those marked with * are also used to treat heart failure (see Chapter 23).

Angiotensin-II Receptor Blockers (Angiotensin-II Receptor Antagonists)

Losartan (**Cozaar**) blocks the effects of Angiotensin II at its receptor sites and unlike ACE inhibitors it does not increase bradykinin levels (which can cause oedema) and therefore does not produce the dry cough and allergic swelling of the mouth and throat (angioedema) that may occur with ACE inhibitors. **Valsartan** (**Diovan**) is another potent Angiotensin-II receptor blocker, which, unlike losartan, does not require prior activation by the liver to be effective. These drugs also block Angiotensin-II induced sodium retention. More recent additions to the group include **candesartan** (**Amias**), **eprosartan** (**Teveten**), **irbesartan** (**Aprovel**), **telmisartan** (**Micardis**). See A–Z of Medicines for individual entries.

Calcium-channel Blockers

These drugs reduce constriction of arteries, cause a fall in resistance to the flow of blood and reduce blood pressure. They are being used increasingly to treat raised blood pressure. They are discussed on p. 115.

Other Drugs

Metirosine (**Demser**) blocks the enzyme tyrosine hydroxylase, which is involved in the production of adrenaline(epinephrine)-like chemicals in the body and is used in the pre-operative treatment of phaeochromocytoma. It should not be used to treat essential hypertension.

26

Drugs Used to Lower Blood Cholesterol Levels and Blood Fat Levels

Atherosclerosis refers to the thickening of the walls of arteries caused by patchy deposits of fats and cholesterol. This causes the vessels to become narrow and the lining surface roughened, which may ulcerate (wear away) and cause the blood to clot around the patch (thrombosis). This narrowing produces serious impairment of blood flow. Atherosclerosis of the coronary arteries is directly related to angina and to deaths from heart attacks due to coronary thrombosis. When it affects the arteries supplying the brain it may cause impairment of mental function and thrombosis leading to a stroke. In the legs it may cause pains in the muscles on exercise, poor circulation to the skin and many other serious consequences.

There are many factors which are associated with coronary artery disease. We all know the risks of smoking, overeating and not taking enough exercise. One fairly constant factor which has been discussed is the relationship between high cholesterol and blood fat (triglyceride) levels and coronary artery disease.

In families who suffer from high cholesterol and/or triglyceride levels and in patients with such disorders as diabetes (in which these levels are increased) the incidence of coronary artery disease is markedly increased. In countries where diets are low in animal fats, it has been found that cholesterol and triglyceride levels are lower and the incidence of coronary artery disease is less.

There is evidence that the effective lowering of cholesterol and triglycerides may reduce deposits in arteries and reduce the risk of coronary artery disease. This lowering can be achieved by diet. If this fails, then diet plus treatment with drugs may be necessary.

The first and most important approach to preventing and treating high cholesterol and blood fat levels is to control the diet. This is because the type and ratio of different fats in the diet can influence these, particularly the ratio of unsaturated fatty acids (in vegetable and fish oils) to saturated fatty acids (in animal fats and dairy produce). A reduction in the overall consumption of fats, a decrease in animal fats, and a proportional increase in vegetable fats over animal fats may help to reduce the blood cholesterol and triglyceride levels.

Drugs which Lower Cholesterol and Triglyceride Levels

The *fibrate group of drugs* include **bezafibrate** (**Bezalip**), **ciprofibrate** (**Modalim**), **fenofibrate** (**Lipantil**) and **gemfibrozil** (**Lopid**). These drugs are effective in lowering cholesterol and triglycerides although their mode of action is not fully understood. Long-term use of these drugs may damage the muscles, particularly in patients with impaired kidney function.

Nicotinic acid is of limited use because of its adverse effects. It may reduce cholesterol and triglycerides but may produce flushing, headache and itching, which usually clear after a few weeks in most patients. Such large doses may, however, cause liver damage and jaundice. **Acipimox** (**Olbetam**) is related to nicotinic acid but is more active and longer-lasting.

Bile acid sequestrants include **colestyramine** (**Questran, Questran Light**) and **colestipol** (**Colestid**) and they reduce blood cholesterol levels. They work in the intestine by exchanging chloride ions for bile salts (which are formed in part from cholesterol) which the drugs bind into an insoluble complex that is excreted in the faeces, so preventing the reabsorption of bile salts and choles- terol. This causes further conversion of cholesterol to bile salts, which eventu- ally may lead to a reduction in blood cholesterol. They may also interfere with the absorption of other drugs (chlorothiazide, phenobarbitone, tetracyclines, thyroid hormones and many others). High doses interfere with the absorption of fat and fat-soluble vitamins, such as vitamins A and D; therefore, no other drug should be taken within one hour of a dose of colestyramine or colestipol. Extra vitamin A and D should be taken, of a type that can be mixed with water; patients on prolonged treatment should also take vitamin K.

The *statin group of drugs* include **atorvastatin** (**Lipitor**), **fluvastatin** (**Lescol**), **pravastatin** (**Lipostat**) and **simvastatin** (**Zocor**). They block the production of cholesterol in the liver and reduce blood levels of cholesterol and also triglycerides. Treatment with statins has been shown to reduce heart attacks and death from heart disease. They are the drugs of choice in patients with a high risk of coronary heart disease.

Fish oils (in **Maxepa**) are rich in omega-3-triglycerides and lower cholesterol and triglyceride levels.

Ispaghula husk (**Fybozest Orange**) contains both insoluble fibre and soluble fibre. The latter has been shown to reduce blood cholesterol levels by reducing the absorption of cholesterol and fatty acids from the intestine by binding bile acids resulting in their increased excretion. As a consequence, the liver has to use more cholesterol to manufacture bile salts, leading to a fall in the blood cholesterol level. However plasma triglycerides remain unchanged.

The Use of Cholesterol Lowering Drugs

The desirable level of cholesterol is 5.2 m.mol/l or below, 5.2–6.4 is borderline, 6.5–7.8 is abnormal and greater than 7.8 is high. The desirable level for blood fats (triglycerides) is 2.3 or below, 2.3–4.5 is borderline and 4.5 or over is very high. Raised levels of cholesterol and/or triglycerides present a risk particularly if they are associated with other risk factors such as smoking, raised blood pressure, diseases of the circulation, diabetes, severe obesity and/or a family history of raised blood fats and/or coronary artery disease.

Statins are the drugs of choice for treating hypercholesterolaemia, fibrates for treating hypertriglyccridaemia, and statins with fibrates can be used for mixed hyperlipidaemia. However, a combination of a statin with a fibrate increases the risk of side-effects including muscle weakness and must be used with great care.

Treatment should always start with a strict low-fat diet and drug treatment should be added if diet fails with borderline levels. Diet and drug treatment should be used if the cholesterol and/or blood fats are high, particularly if one or more of the above risk factors are present. Drugs should always be combined with a strict diet, weight reduction if overweight, reduction of blood pressure and stopping smoking.

27

Drugs Used to Treat Disorders of the Circulation

The Use of Drugs to Increase Circulation to the Limbs

The blood supply to the arms and legs may be affected by anything which obstructs the flow of blood through the arteries. This may be caused by a blockage within the artery; for example, a thrombus which if recognized very quickly may sometimes be treated by surgical removal. However, most thrombi are treated with drugs which stop the blood from clotting. The flow of blood may also be reduced by narrowing of arteries, which may be caused by hardening and loss of elasticity of the artery walls (arteriosclerosis). This process occurs with advancing age, especially in those patients with high blood pressure, where such changes may be found not only in medium-sized and large arteries but also in the smaller arteries which supply the various tissues and organs of the body. Medium and large arteries may also be affected by atherosclerosis (patchy deposits of fats and cholesterol on the inside walls of arteries). This narrows the artery and reduces the blood flow. It may affect the coronary arteries supplying the heart, the circulation to the brain or the circulation to the limbs. It is related to blood fat levels (see p. 133). The artery walls may also be affected by inflammation or by allergic reactions. An obscure disorder called Buerger's disease (thrombo-angitis-obliterans) occasionally affects the arteries of the legs in middle-aged men who are heavy smokers. The amount of blood flowing through an artery may also be reduced because its walls close up (go into spasm) due to some fault in the control mechanisms which normally govern the supply of blood to a particular tissue or organ.

Blood flow to any part of the body (e.g. skin, muscle) is controlled by a balance between the pressure of blood within the arteries and the amount of resistance the flow meets when it gets to the blood vessels which supply the tissues. This resistance can vary and is delicately controlled by the body. It is produced by controlling the degree of spasm of the terminal vessels and smaller arteries. This spasm is under continuous monitoring by nerves in the vessel walls which respond to three mechanisms. First, stimulation of the nerves releases a chemical called noradrenaline(norepinephrine) which produces constriction. Second, the muscles of these arteries have a natural tone which make them 'want' to constrict. Third, a variety of chemicals produced by the body in response to certain reactions may cause them to open up or close down.

There are two types of nerve receptors in blood vessels, which are simply called alpha-receptors and beta-receptors (see p. 38). Stimulation of alpha-receptors causes constriction and stimulation of beta-receptors causes dilation.

Drugs which improve the circulation act by blocking the stimulation of the alpha-receptors; or by stimulating the beta-receptors; or by acting directly upon muscles in the vessel walls. Unfortunately, most disorders of circulation are due to changes in the artery walls (arteriosclerosis, atherosclerosis) which make the walls harden and unresponsive to stimulation. Also, if a medium or large artery supplying an arm or leg is hardened and narrowed, the branch arteries (collateral circulation) are usually working to maximum capacity and cannot be further stimulated to dilate. In such cases the use of drugs may be harmful; for example, it may divert an already poor blood supply from the skin to the muscles instead, leading to further damage to the skin.

Drugs used to improve circulation are often referred to as **vasodilator drugs** and the patients who may benefit from the use of these drugs are those with disorders due to spasm of arteries (vasospasm). For example, there is a vasospastic disorder called Raynaud's disease which usually affects women under fifty. In these patients exposure to cold, and sometimes emotion, may cause the fingers to 'go dead'. All fingers are affected and sometimes the toes. The patient experiences pins and needles, numbness, burning and pain. The fingers go pale bluish and then red. Vasodilator drugs may benefit those patients with mild symptoms but severe and long-standing symptoms are usually associated with irreversible changes in the vessels which may make vasodilator drugs ineffective.

Vasodilator drugs are of limited value in other vasospastic disorders. They should not be used to treat chilblains and their use to prevent frostbite has been disappointing. This is because exposure to low temperatures closes up the blood vessels supplying local areas of skin and makes them unresponsive to vasodilator drugs. Other conditions such as acrocyanosis (blueness of the fingers, hands, ears and nose on exposure to cold) and erythrocyanosis (a bluish-red discoloration of the legs) are not helped by such drugs. A disorder characterized by red, burning feet (erythromelalgia) may occasionally be helped by vasodilator drugs.

In patients with disease of the artery walls (arteriosclerosis, atherosclerosis, Buerger's disease) vasodilator drugs may not work, but they may increase blood flow to the skin and be of use in treating ulcers of the skin caused by poor circulation. They may also be of use in treating gangrene.

Poor circulation may cause pain in the muscles on exercise (intermittent claudication), but unfortunately this is not much helped by vasodilator drugs. However, 'rest pains' in the limbs may be helped.

Vasodilator drugs relax the muscles in vessels either directly or indirectly through adrenergic nerves. The ones used to treat peripheral vascular disorders and disorders of cerebral arteries include alpha-adrenergic receptor blockers, beta-adrenergic stimulants and drugs which act directly on the vessels as a muscle relaxant.

Alpha-blockers (alpha-adrenergic receptor blocking drugs) block alpha-receptors which reduces the constricting effects of noradrenaline(norepinephrine) and, therefore, causes the peripheral blood vessels to dilate. Their effects are most marked in the arteries in the skin of the arms and legs. The arteries supplying muscles are much less affected. The selective alpha-blockers **prazosin** (**Hypovase**) and **moxisylyte**(thymoxamine) (**Opilon**) are used to treat Raynaud's disease. The vasodilator effects may cause a fall in blood pressure on standing up after lying down (postural hypotension) which may cause faintness and lightheadedness. They may also trigger a reflex increase in heart rate.

The **nicotinic acid derivative**, **inositol nicotinate** (**Hexopal**), causes arteries to dilate by a direct unknown action upon the artery walls. They cause vasodilation and increase the blood flow to muscles and skin. The changes in the skin circulation are more marked in the face and neck (where you blush) than in the arms and legs.

The calcium-channel blocker **nifedipine** (**Adalat**) dilates peripheral arteries and is used to treat Raynaud's disease. **Nimodipine** (**Nimotop**), another calcium-channel blocker, is used to relieve spasm of arteries in the brain following bleeding on the surface of the brain (subarachnoid haemorrhage).

The antihistamine **cinnarizine** (**Stugeron**, **Stugeron Forte**), which also has some calcium-channel blocking properties, is also beneficial in some people.

Cellular activators improve oxygen and glucose use by cells. They include **co-dergocrine** (**Hydergine**) used to treat mild dementia in elderly patients and **naftidrofuryl** (**Praxilene**) used to treat circulatory disorders in the limbs and/ or brain.

Pentoxifylline(oxpentifylline) (**Trental**) which is a xanthine derivative (see caffeine, p. 24) is used to treat disorders of the circulation in the limbs.

Drugs Used to Increase the Circulation to the Brain

No drug has a special effect upon the blood vessels which supply the brain. Those that are used are general vasodilators. Their effectiveness in treating disorders produced by changes in the arteries supplying the brain, though of help in some patients, has never been clearly evaluated because of the complexities involved. Furthermore, there are risks in the use of such drugs –

fall in blood pressure and redistribution of blood supply away from areas that may require more oxygen as the result of an already diminished blood supply.

Co-dergocrine (**Hydergine**) and **naftidrofuryl** (**Praxilene**) are principally used for this purpose.

28

Drugs Used to Prevent Blood from Clotting

Drugs used to prevent blood from clotting are called anticoagulants. We do not completely understand how these drugs work, partly because of the complexities involved in the process of clotting. There are a series of clotting factors which have been recognized as contributing to the eventual formation of a blood clot. Anticoagulant drugs interfere with this process. Thrombosis is the clotting of blood on the inside wall of a blood vessel and may be related to damage or changes in the surface lining and also to changes in the blood. The result is the formation of a clot (or thrombus) which may block the vessel.

Anticoagulants are used to treat thrombosis (e.g. deep leg-vein thrombosis) in order to *prevent* the thrombus (clot) from getting bigger. They also prevent pieces of the thrombus coming loose and being carried by the flow of blood to other organs – if these are the lungs or brain, the consequence may be serious and sometimes fatal. This process of a clot loosening and passing along the bloodstream is called embolism. The piece of clot which ends up wedged in and blocking a blood vessel is called an embolus. This process is one of the great dangers of thrombosis, particularly if the thrombosis affects the veins in the abdomen or legs after injury, surgical operations or childbirth.

Anticoagulants are more effective in preventing thrombus formation or the extension of an existing thrombus in the veins where blood flows more slowly and the thrombus consists of a fibrin web enmeshed with platelets and red blood cells. They are less effective in the arteries where the blood flows much faster and the thrombus is formed mainly of platelets with little fibrin.

Anticoagulants greatly reduce the risk of death in patients with thrombosis affecting deep veins of the legs or abdomen and in those patients who have developed an embolus in their lungs. They may also help to prevent deep-vein thrombosis, particularly in elderly patients confined to bed after a surgical operation. Anticoagulant drugs are also used to treat thrombosis of the vessels supplying the eyes and to treat a thrombus blocking an artery. They are used to treat patients with rheumatic heart disease who develop irregularities of heart rhythm and who run the risk of shooting off an embolus from the heart when the heart rate is controlled by drugs. Anticoagulants are also used to prevent thrombi forming on artificial heart valves, to prevent re-thrombosis after a coronary thrombosis and in kidney dialysis.

Anticoagulant Drugs

Anticoagulant drugs may be divided into two groups: those that act directly by interfering with the process of blood clotting and have to be given by injection (e.g. heparin, which prevents blood from clotting even in a test tube); and those that act indirectly and may be given by mouth. The latter act only inside the body by interfering with the production of factors involved in blood clotting. Those drugs which act directly like heparin are rapidly effective, whereas those that act indirectly are slow to work (up to three days).

Heparin

Standard heparin preparations for intravenous (in a vein) or subcutaneous (under the skin) use include **Monoparin**, **Monoparin Calcium**, **Multiparin** and **Pump-Hep**. For subcutaneous use only they include **Calciparine** and **Minihep**. Heparin flushes for keeping catheters and cannulas open include **Canusal**, **Hep-Flush**, **Heplok** and **Hepsal**.

   Heparin acts directly in the blood by preventing thrombin formation, inhibiting thrombin activity and reducing platelet stickiness. It does not work when given by mouth; it is best given by injection into a vein. It works immediately, but its effects quickly wear off and it has to be given every four or six hours. It may also be given by injection under the skin. The normal time taken for the blood to clot on glass (known as the clotting time) is about five–seven minutes. If heparin is to be effective the dose should be adjusted to keep the clotting time above fifteen minutes. The test usually used is the activated thromboplastin time (a measure of clotting time). Adverse effects to heparin therapy include bleeding into various sites and, in rare cases, fever and allergic reactions. Signs of overdose are nosebleeds, bruising, and red blood cells in the urine. Slight bleeding due to overdosage can usually be treated by stopping the drug. Severe bleeding may be reduced by giving a slow intravenous injection of protamine sulphate. For other adverse effects, see A–Z of Medicines.

● *Low Molecular Weight Heparins*

Dalteparin sodium (**Fragmin**), **certoparin** (**Alphaparin**), **enoxaparin** (**Clexane**), **reviparin** (**Clivarine**) and **tinzaparin** (**Innohep**) are low molecular weight heparins. They are obtained by breaking down the natural heparin molecule by partial depolymerization. These low molecular weight heparins have a greater effect against the formation of a thrombus but produce less risk of bleeding than the parent molecule of heparin. Their effects also last much longer, they need only be given once daily, and tests of blood clotting are not necessary. They are given by injection under the skin (subcutaneously) to prevent thrombosis in veins, particularly the risk of thrombosis associated with general and orthopaedic surgery. They are used intravenously to prevent thrombosis in blood circulation systems outside the body, which are used during blood dialysis and filtration. They are also used to treat deep-vein thrombosis. High doses may produce bleeding and adverse effects similar to those produced by heparin.

Danaparoid (**Orgaran**) is related to heparin and used for the prevention of deep-vein thrombosis in patients undergoing orthopaedic or general surgery. **Desirudin** (**Revasc**) and **lepirudin** (**Refludan**) are synthetic versions (recombinant hirudins) of heparin that are also used for the prevention of deep-vein thrombosis in patients undergoing orthopaedic surgery.

Indirect-acting Anticoagulants (Oral Anticoagulants, Vitamin K Antagonists)

Oral anticoagulants block the effects of vitamin K which is essential for the development of four clotting factors by cells in the liver.

Warfarin sodium (**Marevan**) works in forty-eight–seventy-two hours and its effects may last up to four–five days after stopping the drug. It is the drug of choice.

Acenocoumarol(nicoumalone) (**Sinthrome**) and **phenindione** (**Dindevan**) are seldom used. The main use of warfarin is in deep-vein thrombosis, to prevent emboli in patients with rheumatic heart disease and atrial fibrillation (see Chapter 24) and in patients with artificial heart valves. It should not be used to treat cerebral thrombosis or arterial blockage in a limb. It may be used in patients suffering from multiple minute thrombi in the brain causing transient attacks of ischaemia (reduction of blood supply).

● Controlling the Dose of Oral Anticoagulants

Maintenance doses of oral anticoagulants are calculated according to a blood-clotting test called the prothrombin-time (a ratio of patient's time over a control time – i.e. blood from a normal person) and this is reported as the INR (International Normalized Ratio). Daily estimates should be made initially and once a steady prothrombin-time is achieved the frequency of tests may be reduced. Since these drugs are accumulative, the dose should not be changed more frequently than every five or seven days. Bleeding is the commonest adverse effect (e.g. bruising, bleeding gums, blood in the urine); it may be reduced by administering vitamin K – in about four hours by intravenous injection, or by mouth in about twelve hours. Massive bleeding will require the transfusion of fresh frozen plasma.

It is important to take warfarin at the same time each day to maintain a steady level in the body.

● *Precautions on the Use of Oral Anticoagulants in Pregnancy*

Oral anticoagulants should not be used within twenty-four hours of childbirth. Because of the risk of damage to the baby they should not be taken in pregnancy, especially in the first three months, and not in the last three months because of the risk of bleeding in the baby and the placenta.

● *Warning Cards*

If you are on an oral anticoagulant drug you should carry a warning card and carefully check the list of drugs which may interact with anticoagulants, of which there are many, including alcohol, aspirin, St John's Wort, oral contraceptives, cimetidine, flu vaccine. If there is an unexpected change in your prothrombin-time, then check on any drug you have been taking to see if it interferes with the effects of the anticoagulant drug you are on.

Antiplatelet Drugs

When the lining of blood vessels (endothelium) is injured, platelets stick to the damaged wall. This stimulates them to release several chemicals which cause the platelets to stick together. This mass of sticky platelets can then stimulate the formation of a clot (thrombus). There are drugs available which help to reduce this platelet stickiness. They are used to treat thrombi in *arteries* where anticoagulants have little effect.

Aspirin in a single dose has an effect on platelet stickiness and the bleeding time for up to five days. Aspirin in small daily doses (75 mg daily or 300 mg on alternate days) may be used to prevent strokes in patients with transient reductions in blood flow to the brain (transient cerebral ischaemia), and in preventing a recurrence of coronary thrombosis (secondary prevention). It is also used in a dose of 150 mg to 300 mg daily for one month to prevent clots after a heart attack (coronary thrombosis producing myocardial ischaemia). A dose of 300 mg daily may prevent heart attacks (primary prevention) in patients with unstable angina. Low doses (75 to 150 mg daily) are also used following bypass surgery for coronary thrombosis.

Dipyridamole (**Persantin**) reduces platelet stickiness and is used with anti-coagulants to prevent thrombus formation on replacement heart valves.

Abciximab (**ReoPro**) is a monoclonal antibody that prevents platelets sticking together. It is used with heparin and aspirin to prevent clotting in the coronary arteries in patients undergoing dilatation of their coronary arteries (angioplasty).

Eptifibatide (**Integrilin**) and **tirofiban** (**Aggrastat**) work similarly. They are used with heparin and aspirin to prevent early myocardial infarction in patients with unstable angina.

Clopidogrel (**Plavix**) is used for the reduction of artherosclerotic events in patients with a history of ischaemic stroke, myocardial infarction or established peropheral artery disease.

Drugs that Dissolve Thrombi (Clot-Busters)

Drugs that dissolve thrombi are known as **thrombolytic drugs**. Those most commonly used dissolve fibrin in a thrombus and are referred to as fibrinolytics. **Alteplase** (**Actilyse**), **reteplase** (**Rapilysin**) and **streptokinase** (**Kabikinase, Streptase**) are used to dissolve thrombi in coronary arteries in patients who have suffered a coronary thrombosis (heart attack) – see p. 116. Streptokinase is also used to treat deep-vein thrombosis, pulmonary embolism, acute arterial thromboembolism and thrombosis in blood dialysis shunts.

Antifibrinolytic Drugs

An increase in the production of fibrin-dissolving substances (e.g. plasmin) may occur in the body in response to exercise, stress and drugs that produce adrenaline(epinephrine)-like effects, but this is of no significance. However, the condition may be inherited and be associated with bleeding complications in childbirth. It may also occur and cause problems in certain cancers and in severe shock from bleeding.

Bleeding due to a localized dissolving of fibrin in thrombi may occur after surgery on the prostate gland or bladder, due to the presence of urokinase in the urine. Localized dissolving of a thrombus may also occur after a subarachnoid brain haemorrhage and should be considered as a possible cause of rebleeding.

Tranexamic acid (**Cyklokapron**) acts as an antidote for an overdose of the thrombus-dissolving drug streptokinase. It is also used in people who produce too much thrombus-dissolving chemicals themselves and run the risk of bleeding spontaneously. Tranexamic acid blocks the activation of plasminogen to form the thrombus-dissolving substance plasmin. It is useful for stopping bleeding after tooth extraction in a haemophiliac patient, to treat heavy menstrual periods, and to treat bleeding after surgical removal of the prostate gland.

It may also be used to reduce bleeding caused by an intra-uterine contraceptive device which triggers bleeding due to fibrinolysis in some women.

Aprotinin (**Trasylol**) stops certain enzymes from dissolving plasmin. It is used to prevent severe bleeding in open-heart surgery and bleeding which may occur due to a rise in the blood level of plasmin in certain leukaemias and thrombolytic treatments.

Other Drugs Used to Prevent Bleeding (Haemostatics)

Etamsylate (**Dicynene**) is used to stop bleeding from very small blood vessels (capillaries). It blocks prostaglandins, improves the stickiness of platelets and affects the walls of capillaries. It may be used to reduce blood loss in women with heavy periods. It is also used to prevent bleeding around the heart in low-birthweight infants.

Vitamin K is necessary for the formation of blood-clotting factors (II and VII, IX and X). Its deficiency may occur in certain disorders of the intestine that interfere with the absorption of vitamin K, which is soluble in fat. Deficiency may also occur in liver disease and disease of the gall-bladder. These disorders are treated with a vitamin K preparation that dissolves in water and does not rely on fat for its absorption; **menadiol** by mouth is used for this purpose.

Newborn babies may develop a deficiency of vitamin K because their intestines lack the bacteria that normally manufacture vitamin K in the intestine. This deficiency is treated with **phytomenadione** (vitamin K1, **Konakion, Konakion MM**) by intramuscular injection or orally.

Overdose of oral anticoagulants that block the use of vitamin K in the production of blood-clotting factors in the liver is treated with vitamin K.

Epoprostenol (**Flolan**) is a prostaglandin used to stop the blood from clotting during kidney dialysis. It stops platelets from sticking together. It is given alone or with heparin.

● *Blood Products Used to Treat Haemophilia*

Factor VIII fraction, freeze dried (Human Antihaemophilic Fraction, Dried; **Alphanate Fanhdi, Hemofil M, Liberate, Monoclate-P, Replenate**) is prepared from human plasma. It is used to control bleeding in haemophilia A.

Kogenate, Recombinate and **Refacto** are preparations of synthetic (recombinant) human anti-haemophilic factor VIII.

Hyate C is an antihaemophilic factor VIII prepared from pigs' blood and used in patients who produce inhibitors to human factor VIII.

Factor VIII inhibitor bypassing fraction from human plasma is used to treat patients who produce factor VIII inhibitors.

Factor IX fraction, dried (**Alphanine, HT Defix, Mononine, Replenine-VF**) from human plasma is used to treat haemophilia B due to congenital deficiency of factor IX.

NovoSeven (recombinant antihaemophilic factor VIIa) is used to treat haemophiliac patients who have developed serious bleeding or who undergo surgery when they have developed inhibitors to factors VIII and IX.

Bene-Fix is a recombinant coagulation factor IX.

29

Diuretics

The term 'diuretic' refers to a drug which acts upon the kidneys to produce an increased output of sodium salt and water in the urine. These drugs are used to treat disorders of the heart, kidneys or liver which result in an excessive retention of fluids in the body, so much so that swelling may be visible – this is called oedema, or what used to be called dropsy. Swelling of the tissues is usually more obvious in the feet and ankles because of the effect of gravity. In a patient confined to bed the fluid gravitates to the lower part of the back which may then be swollen. Excessive fluid inside the abdominal cavity is called ascites. Diuretics are also used to treat disorders in which fluid accumulates in the lung tissue (pulmonary oedema) – this may be a serious medical emergency.

Some weak diuretics are used to decrease the fluid pressure inside the eyeball, as in the treatment of glaucoma, where the drainage of the eye fluid is impaired. In addition, diuretics are used to counter the salt and water retention produced by other drugs, and to treat overdose with certain drugs that are excreted by the kidneys, by increasing output of urine. However, their most common use is in the treatment of raised blood pressure.

The kidneys exercise a most delicate and complex control over the body's salt and water balance. Salt at first enters the urine but is subsequently reabsorbed into the bloodstream according to body needs. The amount of salt in the urine governs the amount of water passed out by the process known as osmosis (water moves from the weaker solution to the stronger when separated by a partially permeable membrane). The process of osmosis takes the direction from the weaker to the stronger solution so that if there is a lot of salt in the urine, a lot of water will pass out and be excreted in the urine. In addition, there are other rather complex chemical and hormonal processes which affect the amount of salt and water passed out in the urine.

The great majority of diuretics in use today act directly upon the kidneys by depressing the reabsorption of salt from the urine back into the blood-stream, thus producing an increased output of salt and water from the body (**diuresis**) – the increase in water excretion is therefore a secondary result of decreased salt reabsorption. Some diuretics as well as affecting the reabsorption of sodium also interfere with the reabsorption of potassium. This produces a low blood potassium level which may produce muscle weakness, constipation and loss of appetite; more seriously, a low blood potassium affects the heart. It also sensitizes the heart to digoxin and related drugs which are frequently used to treat heart failure and disorders of heart rhythm.

There are three main groups of diuretics – thiazides and related drugs, loop diuretics and potassium-sparing diuretics. Other diuretics include mild diuretics used to treat glaucoma, osmotic diuretics and xanthine diuretics.

Thiazide Diuretics and Related Drugs

Thiazides comprise the largest group of diuretic drugs. They act on the tubules in the kidneys (proximal segment of the distal convoluted tubule), preventing salt reabsorption. These drugs are of moderate potency and vary in their duration of effect. When used in effective diuretic dosage they all increase the excretion of potassium. They are used to treat disorders where fluid is retained in the body, as in heart failure. They are also used in low doses alone or in combination with other drugs to treat raised blood pressure (see p. 129).

Thiazide Diuretics

bendroflumethiazide(bendrofluazide) (**Aprinox, Berkozide, Neo-Bendromax, Neo-NaClex**)
benzthiazide (in **Dytide**)
chlortalidone (**Hygroton**)
clopamide (in **Viskaldix**)
cyclopenthiazide (**Navidrex**)
indapamide (**Natrilix, Nindaxa, Opumide, Natramid**)
metolazone (**Metenix**)
polythiazide (**Nephril**)
xipamide (**Diurexan**)

All thiazide diuretics produce similar effects and adverse effects, but vary in their rate of absorption from the gut, in their potency and in their duration of action. They reduce sodium, potassium and magnesium blood levels and sometimes increase blood calcium. They may send up the blood sugar and cause sugar to appear in the urine in diabetics and other susceptible individuals. They may also cause an increase in blood uric acid level and trigger an attack of gout in some people and they may cause a rise in blood fat levels.

They should be used with caution in patients with impaired kidney or liver function or with diabetes and in the elderly. They may rarely cause nausea, dizziness, weakness, numbness and pins and needles, skin rashes, allergic reactions, impotence, blood disorders and sensitivity of the skin to sunlight. *Note:* These adverse effects seldom occur with the low doses used to treat raised blood pressure.

Loop Diuretics

These include **bumetanide** (**Burinex**), **furosemide**(frusemide) (**Froop**, **Frusol**, **Lasix**, **Rusyde**) and **torasemide** (**Torem**). They inhibit salt reabsorption in the ascending limb of the loop of Henle in the kidneys and are therefore known as loop diuretics.

These are more potent than the thiazide diuretics and although they are chemically different they have similar effects. They act quickly when given by injection and the duration of their effect is short. Dosage must be controlled with caution since high doses may produce a massive output of urine leading to a fall in blood pressure, which in turn may result in a decreased production of urine by the kidneys. They may cause a fall in blood potassium, sodium, magnesium and calcium and a rise in blood glucose and uric acid. They are used to treat fluid retention due to heart, kidney or liver failure. **Furosemide** (frusemide) and **torasemide** are used in small dosages to treat raised blood pressure.

Potassium-sparing Diuretics

Aldosterone Antagonists

Aldosterone is a hormone produced by the adrenal glands. It plays a role in the body's salt- and water-balancing mechanisms. An excess of it may be produced by a tumour of the adrenal glands or in response to certain disorders such as severe congestive heart failure or cirrhosis of the liver associated with the collection of increased fluid in the abdomen (ascites). It works on the kidneys, where it increases the reabsorption of sodium and the excretion of potassium. There are drugs which block these effects, thus increasing the excretion of sodium (which takes water with it) and reducing the excretion of potassium.

Spironolactone (**Aldactone**, **Spirospare**) is an aldosterone antagonist used to treat oedema caused by cirrhosis of the liver, nephrotic syndrome, and chronic congestive heart failure.

Other Potassium-sparing Diuretics

Triamterene (**Dytac**) increases sodium excretion in the urine but reduces potassium loss. It is not a very potent diuretic and it is usually combined with a thiazide diuretic.

Amiloride (**Amilamont**, **Amilospare**) has effects and uses similar to triamterene.

The principal use of triamterene and amiloride is in combination with a thiazide diuretic in order to reduce potassium loss in the urine. Occasionally the use of such combinations, particularly in patients with impaired kidney function, can cause dangerously high blood potassium levels. Therefore, blood potassium levels should be regularly monitored in these patients.

> **Warnings:** *The doses of thiazide or loop diuretics used to treat* **heart failure** *may cause potassium loss and patients may need to take supplementary potassium daily; however, this can generally be avoided by using potassium-sparing diuretics or by combining a potassium-sparing diuretic with a thiazide or a loop diuretic.*

The small doses of thiazide or loop diuretics used to treat *raised blood pressure* seldom require supplementary potassium.

Supplementary potassium ought to be considered in elderly patients who may take a diet low in potassium; in those patients taking digoxin or a related drug or an anti-arrhythmic drug, in whom a fall in blood potassium level could be harmful; in patients suffering from chronic diarrhoea or laxative abuse in whom potassium loss may occur in the faeces; and in patients with overproduction of aldosterone (hyperaldosteroidism) due to serious heart, liver or kidney disease.

Including potassium in diuretic tablets has never been convincingly shown to be of any benefit in preventing a fall in body potassium levels. A potassium supplement is best taken on its own. Potassium chloride is the best salt to use because of the loss of chloride which diuretics produce. Effervescent **potassium chloride** tablets (**Kloref**, **Sando-K**) are satisfactory. Slow-release **potassium chloride** (**Slow-K**) tablets may, rarely, cause ulcers of the intestine. *Liquid preparations of potassium chloride are safest* (e.g. **Kay-Cee-L syrup**). Small doses should be used in patients with impaired kidney function and elderly patients because of the risk of a rise in blood potassium levels.

● *Diuretics Combined with Potassium Salt*
   Burinex K – bumetanide plus potassium
   Diumide-K Continus – furosemide(frusemide) plus potassium
   Lasikal – furosemide(frusemide) plus potassium
   Neo-NaClex-K – bendroflumethiazide(bendrofluazide) plus potassium

Combined Diuretic Preparations

Potassium-sparing Diuretics with Other Diuretics

- *Amiloride with a thiazide diuretic*

  Amil-Co – amiloride and hydrochlorothiazide
  Amilmaxco 5/50 – amiloride and hydrochlorothiazide
  co-amilozide – amiloride and hydrochlorothiazide
  Moduret 25, **Moduretic**, **Zida-Co** – amiloride and hydrochlorothiazide
  Moduretic – amiloride and hydrochlorothiazide
  Navispare – amiloride and cyclopenthiazide

- *Triamterene with a Thiazide Diuretic*

  co-triamterzide – triamterene and hydrochlorothiazide
  Dyazide – triamterene and hydrochlorothiazide
  Dytide – triamterene and benzthiazide
  Kalspare – triamterene and chlorthalidone
  TriamaxCo, **Triam-Co** – triamterene and hydrochlorothiazide

- *Amiloride with a Loop Diuretic*

  Aridil – amiloride and furosemide(frusemide)
  Burinex A – amiloride and bumetanide
  co-amilofruse – amiloride and furosemide(frusemide)
  Fru-Co – amiloride and furosemide(frusemide)
  Froop-Co, **Frumil** – amiloride and furosemide(frusemide)
  Lasoride – amiloride and furosemide(frusemide)

- *Triamterene with a Loop Diuretic*

  Frusene – triamterene and furosemide(frusemide)

- *Spironolactone with a Thiazide Diuretic*

  Aldactide – spironolactone and hydroflumethiazide

- *Spironolactone with a Loop Diuretic*

  Lasilactone – spironolactone and furosemide(frusemide)

Mild Diuretics Used to Treat Glaucoma

In the early 1950s a group of diuretics was introduced which blocked the action of an enzyme (an organic catalyst) which is involved in the kidneys' control of water and salt balance. The enzyme is responsible for exchanging hydrogen ions for sodium ions in the urine so that body sodium is conserved. The diuretics block this action and cause the sodium not to be reabsorbed. This group of drugs includes **acetazolamide** (**Diamox**).

In the treatment of glaucoma they reduce the formation of fluid inside the eye and reduce the pressure (see p. 63).

Osmotic Diuretics

Any substance which passes out of the blood in the kidneys and into the urine may interfere with salt reabsorption, resulting in an increase in urine volume and the excretion of larger amounts of sodium and potassium. The ones used for this purpose are called osmotic diuretics and they should produce no other action in the body. They include mannitol, urea, glucose and sucrose.

Mannitol is a type of alcohol which is excreted by the kidneys and because it is not reabsorbed it causes diuresis. It has to be given by intravenous injection. Glucose and sucrose are sugars and act in a similar way.

Osmotic diuretics may be used to keep urine flow going after severe injury, in order to prevent kidney damage, to eliminate certain drugs after overdose (e.g. aspirin, barbiturates) and to reduce the pressure due to fluid accumulation inside the eyes in glaucoma and inside the skull after head injury.

Xanthine Diuretics

This group includes **caffeine** and **theophylline**. They are present in tea, coffee, cola and cocoa. They are mild diuretics and work both directly and indirectly on the kidneys to produce a diuresis.

30

Morphine and Related Pain-relievers

The Relief of Pain

We all experience pain at some time or another and each of us varies in the amount of pain we can tolerate. Severe, continuous or unusual pain needs explaining and relief. If we have sprained an ankle, we can understand the cause of the pain and it is reasonable to take a pain-reliever. But all too often we take pain-relievers for pain, particularly headaches, without attempting to identify the cause. Pain is only a symptom and, therefore, you should always try to determine the cause. If you have toothache, do not just take pain-relievers – go to your dentist. If you get recurrent headaches try to think what brings them on – noise, smoking, worry, something in the diet, and so on. Very often pain produces fear and anxiety – somebody with chest pain may worry about having a bad heart and somebody with headache may worry about a brain tumour. If you have a pain that is continuous or unusual for you, or if you find yourself becoming anxious or worrying about pain, then these are sufficient reasons to consult your doctor. We are not all stoics and continuous pain can make some of us depressed and irritable. By far the most common pains are headaches and those from muscles and joints (e.g. rheumatic and arthritic disorders). Drugs which are taken to relieve the pain of such disorders are among the most frequently taken drugs.

Nerve endings, highly sensitive to pain, are widely distributed throughout various tissues of the body. The area of pain can usually be identified: in the skin or subcutaneous (under the skin) tissue, in muscles or joints, or in an internal organ, e.g. heart or lungs, gall-bladder, stomach or bowels. The relief of these pains need not necessarily rely on pain-relieving drugs – cold water applied to a skin burn may relieve the pain, heat or massage may relieve muscle pain, and an alkali mixture may relieve the pain of a peptic ulcer. It must be obvious, therefore, that the best way to treat pain is to attempt to relieve the underlying cause. Where the cause of the pain cannot be removed, then pain-relievers should be used.

There are two main types of pain-relieving drugs – those that work at the site of the pain by relieving inflammation and those that work on the brain and nervous system by acting on specific receptors (see later).

Those pain-relievers that relieve pain by relieving inflammation include aspirin (see Chapter 31) and the non-steroidal anti-inflammatory drugs (see Chapter 32). Pain-relievers that work on the brain and/or nervous system are often called **narcotics**. Some use the term narcotic when talking specifically about derivatives of opium and morphine-like drugs. Many consider the term narcotic to be equivalent to 'addiction-producing' and, legally, narcotics can cover all sorts of drugs including cocaine.

All *narcotic pain-relievers* are called **opiates**, because they are obtained from, or are related to pain-relievers obtained from opium. However, because they block specific pain receptors in the nervous system, called **opioid** receptors, they are now usually referred to as **opioid pain-relievers** (**opioids**). These receptors are part of the body's pain control system and are stimulated by the body's own pain-relievers, e.g. enkephalins and endorphins.

We feel pain much more if we are tense, anxious, worried or depressed and, of course, the reverse applies too. For these reasons, the testing of pain-relievers in animals and on volunteer 'patients' under laboratory conditions often gives only a limited indication of the pain-relieving potential of a drug on 'real' patients. The marked individual variations in response to drugs are further influenced by weight, gender, physical and psychological disorders, time of treatment and place of treatment. Further, about two in five patients can get relief of pain from placebo (dummy) tablets or injections. This is an interesting phenomenon, but the placebo effect soon wears off with repeated doses of dummy drugs. Therefore, a pain-relieving drug must be tested on patients suffering from pain. Opiates are usually tested on post-operative pain after abdominal surgery. Aspirin-like drugs and non-steroidal anti-inflammatory drugs are tested on rheumatic or arthritic pain.

Opiate (Opioid) Pain-relievers Used to Relieve Moderate to Severe and Severe Pain

alfentanil (**Rapifen**)
buprenorphine (**Temgesic**)
dextromoramide (**Palfium**)
diamorphine (**heroin**)
dihydrocodeine (**DF 118, DF 118 Forte, DHC Continus**)
dipipanone (in **Diconal**)
fentanyl (**Sublimaze, Durogesic**)
hydromorphone (**Palladone**)

meptazinol (**Meptid**)
methadone (**Physeptone**)
morphine (in **Cyclimorph, Morcap SR, Min-I-Jet Morphine Sulphate, MST Continus, MXL, Oramorph, Sevredol, Zomorph**)
nalbuphine (**Nubain**)
opium (raw opium)
oxycodone (**Oxynorm, OxyContin**)
papaveretum
pentazocine (**Fortral**)
pethidine (in **Pamergan P100**)
phenazocine (**Narphen**)
remifentanil (**Ultiva**)
tramadol (**Dromadol SR, Tramake, Zamadol, Zamadol SR, Zydol, Zydol SR, Zydol XL**)

Opium has been used since prehistoric times. It is obtained from the opium poppy and contains many drugs, called opium alkaloids. **Morphine** as a pain-reliever is the most widely used opium alkaloid. Concentrated preparations of opium alkaloids are also available (e.g. **papaveretum**) for the relief of pain.

Morphine is used to relieve severe pain. It produces its main effects upon the brain, heart and circulation, and the bowel. Its actions on the brain cause relief of pain, suppression of the cough centre and stimulation of the vomiting centre; drowsiness, a relaxed mood and sleep may occur. It may sometimes produce the opposite effect and cause mild anxiety and fear. Mental clouding with inability to concentrate may occur. It also causes constriction of the pupils and sweating. With increased doses these effects increase and the patient may develop constipation, nausea, vomiting, and depression of respiration.

Morphine has to be used with caution in patients with chest disorders such as asthma and chronic bronchitis, and after operations, because not only does it discourage deep breathing but it also suppresses coughing, with the result that the patient may get a collapsed lung through accumulation of bronchial secretions. Morphine-induced vomiting can be distressing in patients recovering from an operation on the stomach or who have just had a coronary thrombosis or a cataract operation. For this reason it is sometimes combined with the anti-vomiting drug **cyclizine** (in **Cyclimorph**). Morphine can also cause constipation which can be a problem.

Tolerance and drug dependence to morphine may develop (see p. xxviii). When it is stopped, patients may experience mild withdrawal symptoms which include sweating, nausea, weakness, headache and restlessness.

However, patients in continuous pain (e.g. those dying from cancer) should be given a sufficient dose to keep them free from pain and at regular intervals (every four hours) throughout the day and night or via a self-administration pump.

Dextromoramide is used to treat severe pain. It has a short duration of action and produces less drowsiness than morphine.

Diamorphine (**heroin**) is a powerful pain-reliever. It produces more euphoria than morphine, but less nausea, constipation and less of a fall in blood pressure.

Dihydrocodeine relieves moderate pain and suppresses coughs. It produces adverse effects like those of morphine, but these are usually less severe.

Dipipanone may be given by mouth combined with cyclizine, an anti-vomiting drug (in **Diconal**).

Fentanyl is given by injection pre-operatively.

Meptazinol causes less depression of breathing than morphine. It acts quickly and lasts for about 2–7 hours.

Methadone is a synthetic drug with actions identical to those of morphine. It is an effective drug for the relief of moderate to severe pain. It has an extended duration of action. Vomiting is as common as with morphine, but sedation is less. It is also used to suppress coughs (e.g. **Physeptone** linctus) and to treat heroin addiction (see p. xxix).

Nalbuphine is used to treat moderate to severe pain. It may cause less nausea and vomiting than morphine.

Oxycodone may be used as suppositories to relieve pain in terminal care.

Pethidine is a synthetic pain-reliever with similar effects to morphine. It does not constrict the pupils, but like morphine it may cause vomiting. Pethidine is used to relieve moderate to severe pain; it is more powerful than codeine but less powerful than morphine. It is used to relieve pain in head injury and in childbirth.

Phenazocine by mouth is an effective severe pain-reliever. It is of particular use in relief of pain from gall-bladder disease because it has less tendency to increase pressure inside the gall-bladder.

Tramadol is used to treat severe pain. It produces less constipation and depressed breathing than morphine and may be less addictive.

Opiate Antagonists (Opioid Antagonists)

In 1953 an opiate antagonist – **nalorphine** – was found to bring on acute withdrawal-like effects in patients who had been on morphine or heroin for long periods. In addition it was found to have good pain-relieving properties. However, it was unsuitable for use because of its bad effects on mood and because it also produced vivid daydreams, hallucinations, difficulty in focusing the eyes, sweating, nausea and feelings of being drunk. It is described as a partial agonist. **Naloxone** (**Narcan**) is related to nalorphine but has no respiratory depressing effects. It is now the preferred treatment for depression of respiration caused by opiate overdose. **Naltrexone** (**Nalorex**) is an opiate antagonist used in maintenance therapy in detoxified, formerly opiate-dependent adults.

The discovery of these drugs led to research for pain-relievers with a reduced risk of dependence. One of these, **pentazocine** (**Fortral**), is a partial antagonist used to relieve moderate to severe pain. It is more effective when given by injection than by mouth. It should not be used to relieve the pain of heart attack because it increases the workload of the heart. It may trigger pain and withdrawal symptoms in patients dependent on opiate pain-relievers. Cases of drug dependence of the morphine type have been reported in patients taking pentazocine over a long term, particularly by injection. It may also cause hallucinations, and thought disturbances.

Buprenorphine (**Temgesic**) has mixed opiate agonist/antagonist properties and is useful for relieving moderate to severe pain, but it may produce vomiting. It is longer-acting than morphine and may be taken under the tongue (sublingually) or by injection. Unlike most opiate drugs, its respiratory depressant effects are only partially reversed by naloxone. It may cause dependence.

Meptazinol (**Meptid**) is a partial agonist used to relieve moderate to severe pain. It produces nausea and vomiting but is claimed to produce a low incidence of respiratory depression.

Warning: Those opiates that relieve moderate to severe pain and severe pain differ markedly in structure and yet have similar actions and effects. Their adverse effects include nausea, vomiting, drowsiness, dizziness, constipation and respiratory depression. They differ in their onset and duration of action, in whether they are effective by mouth and in the way that individuals respond to them. They may all cause tolerance and physical dependence, and are potential drugs of abuse. They increase the effects of alcohol and other depressant drugs and they should not be taken by patients who drive motor vehicles and/or who operate machinery.

Nefopam (**Acupan**) is unrelated to morphine. It relieves moderate pain. It should not be used in patients taking paracetamol because of the risk of liver damage.

Opiate (Opioid) Drugs Used to Relieve Mild to Moderate Pain

Codeine is obtained from opium and is present in numerous preparations. It produces less mood change and is not as effective as morphine in relieving pain. It is used to relieve mild to moderate pain (often in combination with aspirin, paracetamol or some other pain-reliever). It causes constipation. It is also used in cough medicines and diarrhoea mixtures.

Dextropropoxyphene (**Doloxene**) has effects and uses similar to codeine. It is slightly less effective and is usually given in combination with other pain-relievers by mouth – for example, with paracetamol (as in **co-proxamol**).

Ethoheptazine is structurally related to pethidine, but it is only a mild pain-reliever.

> **Warning:** *Codeine, dextropropoxyphene and ethoheptazine may produce dependence. They are related to morphine.*
>
> *Combinations of opiate drugs with paracetamol or aspirin can be more* ***dangerous*** *in overdose than aspirin or paracetamol on their own, especially when taken with alcohol.*

31

Aspirin and Paracetamol

Aspirin

Aspirin relieves pain, particularly such pains as headache, period pains, toothache and pains in muscles, ligaments and joints caused by inflammation. Given as a single dose it relieves pain but given regularly every day it relieves inflammation and it can be classed as a non-steroidal anti-inflammatory drug (NSAID) – see Chapter 32. It also brings down the temperature and is useful for treating feverish colds in adults. Aspirin alters the blood salts (acid/base balance) and interferes with some of the processes involved in blood clotting and is used in preventing coronary thrombosis, see p. 118 and strokes, see p. 143.

Aspirin in mild overdosage may produce 'salicylism' – deafness, noises in the ears, nausea and dull headache. These are related to dose and disappear if the drug is stopped. It is irritant to the stomach lining and can cause pain, with nausea and vomiting. It also produces superficial ulcers in the stomach which may bleed and lead to iron-deficiency anaemia. This may occur without indigestion symptoms and may be a real danger in elderly patients on poor diets low in iron, in women with heavy periods, and in debilitated patients.

Aspirin should always be taken *after* food and it helps to take only the soluble form with plenty of fluids. It may also help to take a buffered or enteric-coated preparation if you are on *regular* aspirin treatment. If you have a peptic ulcer or hiatus hernia, you should *not* take aspirin.

A dose of aspirin every four–six hours is sufficient to maintain effective blood levels. It dissolves in the stomach faster and is absorbed more quickly if it is taken with large drinks of warm water or an alkali mixture (the basis of some commercial preparations which contain sodium bicarbonate and fizz in water).

Allergy to aspirin. Patients can become allergic to aspirin and develop vasomotor rhinitis (allergic runny nose), sinusitis, nasal polyps, bronchial asthma, swelling of the throat and mouth (angioedema) and nettle-rash. Low blood pressure and collapse may (rarely) occur. There is cross-allergy with tartrazine (an orange dye in food and drinks) and with indomethacin and some other NSAID drugs used to treat rheumatoid arthritis and related disorders.

> *Aspirin should not be given to children under the age of twelve years* *because of the risk of producing brain and liver damage in the child,* *resulting in severe vomiting, impaired consciousness, delirium and coma* *(Reye's Syndrome). This can occur if aspirin is used to treat a viral infection* *such as influenza or chickenpox. Fifty per cent of those affected die, and* *some survivors have brain damage.*
>
> *Aspirin overdose can be serious* – *always take the patient to the nearest* *hospital. Remember, aspirin is present in many pain-relieving preparations;* *always read the contents and note that aspirin may be called acetyl salicylic* *acid, acid acetylsal, or acetylsalicylicum.*

Paracetamol (acetominophen)

Paracetamol is present in numerous pain-relieving preparations. It is an effective mild pain-reliever and anti-pyretic (lowers a raised temperature). It has no anti-inflammatory properties and appears to block chemicals (e.g. prostaglandins) in the brain rather than in the tissues of the body. Paracetamol should not be used indiscriminately just because it produces less stomach upset than aspirin. It should not be used in patients with impaired kidney function.

Dangers of Overdose with Paracetamol

In the first twenty-four hours after taking an overdose of paracetamol the individual develops nausea, vomiting, loss of appetite and abdominal pains and looks pale. After twelve to forty-eight hours, signs of liver damage develop and there are changes in the acidity of the blood and the blood glucose level. In severe poisoning, liver failure may develop and progress to coma and death. Kidney damage may occur with or without liver damage and disorders of the heart rhythm may occur.

Liver damage is likely in adults who have taken 10 g (twenty 500 mg tablets) or more. This amount of paracetamol causes an excess of the toxic breakdown product of paracetamol to accumulate in the liver, leading to damage to the liver cells. When a normal dose of paracetamol is taken (1,000 mg in an adult) the liver can cope with the amount of the toxic breakdown product by detoxifying it with glutathione. However, when the dose is increased the liver becomes less able to cope with the increasing amount of the toxic chemical and the patient starts to show signs of liver damage.

Methionine (an amino acid) is an essential constituent of the diet which enhances the production of glutathione by the liver. It is used in paracetamol poisoning to increase the production of glutathione and reduce the risk of liver damage. **Co-methiamol** (**Paradote**) tablets contain both paracetamol and methionine. It is used where there is a risk of a patient taking an overdose.

> *Overdose with paracetamol may cause serious liver damage, which can be fatal.*

Benorilate

Benorilate (**Benoral**) is a compound of aspirin and paracetamol which, once it is absorbed into the bloodstream, is taken to the liver where it is split into aspirin and paracetamol. It thus acts as a mild to moderate pain-reliever. Because it contains aspirin, it also relieves inflammation and may be used to treat rheumatic disorders and painful menstrual periods.

Because it contains aspirin it should not be given to children under twelve years of age and the dose should be reduced in elderly people. Harmful effects and warnings listed under aspirin and paracetamol apply to benorilate; do not take any other pain-reliever that contains aspirin or paracetamol.

Aspirin or Paracetamol Combined with a Mild Opiate Pain-reliever

There are many preparations on the market that contain **aspirin** or **paracetamol** combined with the mild opiate, **codeine**, **dihydrocodeine** or **dextropropoxyphene**. Some also contain **caffeine**, which does not improve the pain-relieving effects but could irritate the stomach. Also, stopping caffeine after regular use can actually cause headaches! There is much disagreement as to whether these combined preparations work any better than aspirin or paracetamol on their own. You can become dependent on any preparation that contains codeine, dihydrocodeine or dextropropoxyphene. They should seldom be used in elderly patients. They are also more expensive and may complicate the treatment of overdose (see p. 157).

- *Compound Pain-relievers Include:*
  Co-codaprin – aspirin and codeine
  Co-codamol – paracetamol and codeine
  Co-dydramol – paracetamol and dihydrocodeine
  Co-proxamol – paracetamol and dextropropoxyphene

Non-steroidal Anti-inflammatory Drugs (NSAIDs)

These drugs are discussed in Chapter 32. In regular daily dosages they relieve pain and inflammation and are used to treat rheumatoid arthritis and other disorders. In one-off dosages they are also useful for relieving mild to moderate pain, e.g. headache, period pains, and muscle and joint pains. They also bring down a fever. Ibuprofen is an example of an NSAID widely used to treat aches, pains and fever associated with a cold. See p. 43.

32

Drugs Used to Treat Rheumatoid Arthritis and Related Disorders

There are three major groups of drugs used to treat rheumatoid arthritis and related disorders. These are:

1 Non-steroidal anti-inflammatory drugs (NSAIDs).
2 Steroidal anti-inflammatory drugs (corticosteroids).
3 Drugs which suppress the disease process (anti-rheumatic drugs).

1 Non-steroidal Anti-inflammatory Drugs (NSAIDs)

These drugs relieve pain and inflammation by blocking the production of prostaglandins (see Chapter 52).

- *Aspirin and Related Drugs*
  aspirin (**Caprin, Nu-seals aspirin**)
  benorilate(benorylate) (**Benoral**)
  diflunisal (**Dolobid**)

- *Non-aspirin Drugs*
  aceclophenac (**Preservex**)
  acemetacin (**Emflex**)
  azapropazone (**Rheumox**)
  celecoxib (**Celebrex**)
  dexketoprofen (**Keral**)
  diclofenac sodium (in **Acoflam**, in **Arthrotec, Dicloflex, Diclomax, Diclovol, Diclozip, Econac, Enzed, Flamrase SR, Lofensaid, Motifene, Volraman, Voltarol**)
  diflunisal (**Dolobid**)
  etodolac (**Lodine**)
  fenbufen (**Lederfen**)

fenoprofen (Fenopron)

flurbiprofen (Froben)

ibuprofen (Arthrofen, Brufen, in **Codafen Continus, Ebufac, Fenbid, Lidifen, Motrin, Rimafen.** Over the counter drugs include **Advil, Anadin-Ibuprofen, Anadin Ultra, Boot's Children's 6 Years Plus Fever and Pain Relief, Cuprofen, Galprofen, Hedex Ibuprofen, Ibrufhalal, Ibufem, Inoven, Librofem, Migrafen, Novaprin, Nurofen, Obifen, Pacifene, PhorPain, Proflex, Relcofen)**

indometacin (Flexin Cotinus, Indocid-R, Indolar SR, Indomax, Indomod, Pardelprin, Rheumacin LA, Rimacid, Slo-Indo)

ketoprofen (Fenoket, Jomethid XL, Ketil CR, Ketocid, Ketpron, Ketepron XL Ketotard, Ketovail, Ketozip XL, Ketozip XL, Larafen CR, Orudis, Oruvail)

mefenamic acid (Dysman, Ponstan)

meloxicam (Mobic)

nabumetone (Relifex)

naproxen (Arthrosin, Arthroxen, in **Napratec, Naprosyn, Nycopren, Synflex, Timpron)**

phenylbutazone* (Butacote)

piroxicam (Brexidol, Feldene)

rofecoxib (Vioxx)

sulindac (Clinoril)

tenoxicam (Mobiflex)

tiaprofenic acid (Surgam)

* Available only in hospitals.

Aspirin is an excellent anti-inflammatory drug but needs to be given regularly in fairly high doses to treat rheumatoid arthritis. These doses may produce adverse effects and aspirin has been replaced with non-aspirin NSAIDs. In a single dose these NSAIDs are as powerful as aspirin and paracetamol for relieving pain such as headache, painful periods and muscle and joint pains. Like aspirin and paracetamol they also bring down a raised temperature. In cancer pain they can be combined with an opioid pain-reliever (see Chapter 30) and they are useful for relieving pain associated with cancer secondaries in bone. In regular full dosage they produce lasting relief of pain and inflammation and are useful for treating rheumatoid arthritis, chronic back pain and chronic aches and pains in muscles. NSAIDs share similar adverse effects, such as stomach and bowel upsets, nausea, ulceration and bleeding from the stomach and intestine, allergic reactions, fluid retention and, very rarely, kidney damage (especially in patients with impaired kidney function) and blood disorders. They may make asthma worse. They should be used with caution in the elderly and in anyone with impaired heart, liver or kidney function or with peptic ulcers. They should preferably not be used in early pregnancy and they should be used in the minimum effective dose possible.

The choice of drug is whatever suits you because about four out of ten patients will respond to one NSAID and not another. They take about one week to relieve the pain of rheumatoid arthritis and about three weeks to relieve inflammation of the joints. The smallest effective dose should be used and they should be used with great caution in elderly people. *For adverse effects and precautions, see under relevant entry in A–Z of Medicines.*

Warning: *Patients allergic to aspirin (i.e. those patients who develop skin rashes and wheezing if they take aspirin – see p. 158) may also be allergic to any one of this group of drugs (refer to the list on pp. 162–3), and anyone allergic to one NSAID may be allergic to other NSAIDs.*

The Use of Topical Applications Containing an NSAID

Topical preparations (*anti-rheumatic rubs*) containing a non-steroidal anti-inflammatory drug (NSAID) may be useful for relieving local pain and swelling in an inflamed or injured joint, muscle or tendon. The NSAID penetrates the local tissues in a concentration sufficient to relieve local pain and inflammation, but only a small amount is absorbed into the bloodstream and so the risk of harmful effects elsewhere in the body is significantly reduced but may occur if large amounts are used, e.g. allergy, asthma.

These preparations should not be applied on broken skin, on the lips or eyes, or on sites of infection. They should not be used in people known to be allergic to aspirin or other NSAIDs.

They should not be used in children, in pregnancy or in breastfeeding mothers. They may irritate the skin and produce redness, itching and a rash. They may also discolour the skin. Rheumatic rubs containing an NSAID include **Difflam cream** (**benzydamine**), **Feldene Gel** (**piroxicam**), **Fenbid Forte Gel** (**piroxicam**), **Ibugel** (**ibuprofen**), **Ibumousse** (**ibuprofen**), **Ibuspray** (**ibuprofen**), **Oruvail gel** (**ketoprofen**), **Powergel** (**ketoprofen**), **Proflex cream** (**ibuprofen**), **Traxam gel** (**felbinac**) and **Voltarol Emulgel** (**diclofenac sodium**).

2 Steroidal Anti-Inflammatory Drugs (Corticosteroids)

Corticosteroids by mouth reduce inflammation. They should be used as reserve drugs when other treatments fail to produce relief. When the disease is very active and severe a high dose of a corticosteroid may be given by injection into a vein daily for three days. There are very important precautions which should be applied to the use of these drugs – see Chapter 37.

3 Disease Modifying Anti-rheumatic Drugs (DMARDs)

These drugs suppress the progression of the disease in joints and other tissues affected by rheumatoid arthritis and related diseases. They take four–six months to produce their maximum benefits and are used when NSAIDs have failed and there is evidence of progressive joint damage or general complications, e.g. affecting the eyes and/or skin. However, it is now suggested that they should be used earlier in the disease before such complications can take hold. If there is no improvement after six months they should be stopped. They include:

Chloroquine

Chloroquine (**Nivaquine**) is an anti-malaria drug used to treat rheumatoid arthritis. Prolonged use of high doses (more than 2.5 mg/kg of body weight/ day) may lead to the development of corneal opacities causing misty vision, and irreversible damage to the retina of the eye resulting in blindness. Symptoms may appear long after the drug has been stopped. Regular examinations of the eye by a specialist are necessary. **Hydroxychloroquine** (**Plaquenil**) is an alternative. For adverse effects, see entry in A–Z of Medicines. They should not be used to treat psoriatic arthritis.

Gold

Gold is often most effective in active, progressive rheumatoid arthritis. It is usually given by deep intramuscular injection (**sodium aurothiomalate** (**Myocrisin**)). **Auranofin** (**Ridaura**) is a gold preparation which can be taken by mouth.

For adverse effects and precautions, see relevant entry in A–Z of Medicines. Frequent medical check-ups, including blood and urine tests, are necessary because skin rashes, blood disorders and kidney damage may occur.

Penicillamine

Penicillamine (**Distamine**) aids the elimination of toxic metals from the body. It is used in lead poisoning and to treat certain disorders of copper metabolism. It may be used to treat severe rheumatoid arthritis that has not responded to other treatments. For adverse effects, see entry in A–Z of Medicines. Regular medical check-ups, including blood and urine tests, are necessary.

Sulphasalazine

Sulfasalazine (**Salazopyrin**, **Sulazine**) is used to treat ulcerative colitis and Crohn's disease. It is also of benefit in some individuals suffering from rheumatoid arthritis because of its anti-inflammatory effects. When taken by mouth it is hardly absorbed, and when it reaches the large bowel, bacteria break it down into a sulphonamide drug (sulphapyridine) and an anti-inflammatory drug (5-aminosalicyclic acid, which is related to aspirin). Only about a quarter of this aspirin-like drug is absorbed into the bloodstream, whereas sulphapyridine is well absorbed and probably accounts for the harmful effects which sulphasalazine produces. See entry in A–Z of Medicines.

Immunosuppressants

Immunosuppressants (see Chapter 17) damp down immune responses and are used to prevent rejection of transplanted organs. They are also useful for damping down the immune system in diseases thought to be due to the body reacting to its own tissues. This is called auto-immunity; rheumatoid arthritis may be an auto-immune disease. Immunosuppressants may be used in rheumatoid arthritis when gold, chloroquine, or penicillamine have failed. The ones used include **azathioprine** (**Azamune**, **Immunoprin**, **Imuran**, **Oprisine**), **chlorambucil** (**Leukeran**), **cyclophosphamide** (**Endoxana**), **ciclosporin**(cyclosporin) (**Neoral**, **Sandimmun**, **SangCya**) and **methotrexate** (**Maxtrex**). Look up each drug in the A–Z of Medicines.

Azathioprine and **methotrexate** are also used in arthritis associated with psoriasis.

Leflunomide (**Arava**) acts on the immune system and is used as a disease modifying anti-rheumatic drug. It is similar in efficacy to sulfasalazine and methotrexate, but it can be used when these drugs cannot.

The Use of Drugs in the Treatment of Rheumatoid Arthritis

Rheumatoid arthritis may affect one or more joints and be associated with other serious disorders affecting arteries and various internal organs. Therefore treatment will vary, and drugs such as corticosteroids, gold, chloroquine and penicillamine, etc., will only be used in serious cases and under specialist care.

Of the commonly used NSAIDs, the choice is a matter of balancing adverse effects of stomach irritation and bleeding with the beneficial effects. Other adverse effects such as fluid retention, bone-marrow and kidney damage, and potential risk of interaction with other drugs should be considered. See A–Z of Medicines.

Local Injections of Corticosteroids

Local injections of corticosteroids may be used to relieve pain, improve mobility and reduce deformity in one or a few joints. There is a risk of infecting the joint so full aseptic techniques should be used. Microcrystals in the corticosteroid suspension may occasionally cause inflammation.

Preparations include:

dexamethasone (dexamethasone, Decadron)

hydrocortisone acetate (Hydrocortistab)

methylprednisolone (Depo-Medrone and Depo-Medrone with Lidocaine (lignocaine) **(a local anaesthetic)**

prednisolone (Deltastab)

triamcinolone acetonide (Adcortyl Intra-articular/Intradermal, Kenalog Intra-articular/Intramuscular)

Note: Drug treatment of rheumatoid arthritis and related disorders is only a part of overall treatment which should include physiotherapy, hydrotherapy, wax baths, surgery, and splints and diet where appropriate.

33

Drugs Used to Treat Gout

Gout is a recurrent acute arthritis of peripheral joints which is caused by deposits of uric acid salts in or near joints and tendons. These deposits may cause acute pain and swelling of joints, at first affecting one joint (usually the big toe) but later many joints. The disease may become chronic and deforming and may be complicated by deposits of uric acid salts in the kidneys. In *primary* gout there is an increased production of uric acid, or a decreased excretion of uric acid, or a combination of both. *Secondary* gout can occur in certain blood disorders, in kidney failure, and can be brought on by drugs such as thiazide diuretics.

Drugs Used in the Treatment of Gout

Drugs are used to treat patients with gout in order to relieve pain and inflammation in an acute attack. They are also used to increase the elimination of urates by the kidneys or to block the production of uric acid in order to prevent attacks coming on.

Acute Attacks

Acute attacks of gout may be treated with non-steroidal anti-inflammatory drugs (NSAIDs) such as **diclofenac sodium**, **indomethacin** or **naproxen**. The choice is not critical. You should not use aspirin.

Colchicine, obtained from the autumn crocus, relieves the pain and inflammation of gout within a few hours but it may cause stomach pains, nausea, vomiting and diarrhoea. It is an alternative to NSAIDs in patients with heart failure, as it does not cause fluid retention, or who are taking anticoagulants.

Recurrent Gout

Recurrent attacks of gout can be prevented by increasing the excretion of uric acid salts (**urates**) in the urine with drugs such as **probenecid** or **sulphinpyrazone** (**Anturan**). These are called **uricosuric drugs**. Alternatively the formation of uric acid from purines can be reduced by using **allopurinol** (**Caplenal**, **Cosuric, Rimafurinol, Xanthomax, Zyloric**) which blocks the enzyme (xanthine-oxidase) responsible for this reaction. Such drugs are called **xanthine-oxidase inhibitors**.

Probenecid promotes the excretion of urates by reducing their reabsorption from the urine by the kidneys. It has no pain-relieving properties and is of no use in an acute attack of gout. It may set off an acute attack of gout in the first few weeks of treatment so the patient must be warned. **Sulphinpyrazone** (**Anturan**) causes excretion of urates. It may also trigger an acute attack of gout in the first few weeks of treatment. **Azapropazone** (**Rheumox**) is an NSAID (p. 162) which may be used to treat an acute attack of gout and also to prevent gout because it increases the excretion of urates in the urine.

> **Warning:** *Drugs which increase the excretion of uric acid (uricosuric drugs) may cause crystals of urates to form in the urine; therefore it is very important to drink plenty of fluids if you are taking these drugs.*

Allopurinol (**Caplenal, Cosuric, Rimapurinol, Xanthomax, Zyloric**) affects uric acid production and reduces the concentration of uric acid in the blood. Acute attacks of gout may be triggered in the early stages of treatment, but after a few weeks or months acute attacks stop and deposits of urates in cartilage get smaller (these are often visible in the cartilage of the ear lobes and are known as tophi). It may prevent kidney damage in gout and stops the formation of urate stones in the kidneys. Allopurinol is therefore useful for treating gout in patients with kidney disorders when other anti-gout drugs may not be effective or may not be advisable to use.

> **Note:** *Treatment with a uricosuric drug or allopurinol should not be started during an acute attack and once started is usually for an indefinite period. To prevent acute attacks of gout during initial treatment an **NSAID** or **colchicine** should be taken daily for about three months.*

34

Drugs Used to Treat Migraine

Some doctors label one-sided headache as migraine, particularly if it is accompanied by nausea and vomiting. Others look for all the classical symptoms of migraine – one-sided headache associated with nausea and vomiting and preceded by visual symptoms (e.g. flashing lights), speech disturbances, or disturbances of sensation (e.g. pins and needles in a foot or hand).

Migraine is uncommon under the age of five years and then its incidence increases with advancing age until it levels off in middle-age. The incidence declines in old age. It is commonest in women than in men and it may be associated with menstruation. There are many myths about migraine sufferers; for example, there is not sufficient evidence to indicate that they are more tense, neurotic or obsessional than non-sufferers. Nor is there evidence to suggest that more professional people suffer from migraine than other groups, or that migraine sufferers are more intelligent, that they suffer more from high blood pressure or visual disturbances, or that they are more involved in work which necessitates close vision. There is limited evidence that migraine runs in families.

An attack of migraine is associated with changes in the calibre of the blood vessels supplying the head and brain. It is thought that these changes occur in response to certain chemicals which are produced by the body and which are also present in various foods such as cheese. Underlying constitutional factors, which may be biochemical, possibly cause a predisposition to develop migraine in response to certain external factors.

Factors which may trigger off a migraine attack include:
- *Psychological* – e.g. anxiety, tension, worry, emotion, depression, shock, excitement.
- *Physical* – e.g. over-exertion, lifting, straining, bending, heading a football.
- *External factors* – e.g. sunlight, weather, travelling, change of routine, staying in bed, watching television, noise, smells, smoking, drugs.

● *Dietary* – e.g. irregular meals, fasting, certain foods, i.e. cheese, onion, cucumber, bananas, chocolate, fried foods, pastry, cured meats which contain sodium nitrates and nitrites (hot dogs, ham, bacon), alcohol.

Treatment of Migraine

The most important part of treatment is to try to prevent an attack starting. This means attempting to identify the trigger factors that bring on your attack (see, for example, the list above). If you develop migraine always go through a check-list of trigger factors – cross off the ones which you cannot directly relate to your attack. Try to avoid obvious trigger factors – it may be something simple like having to avoid cheese, or it may be very difficult like trying not to get tense or anxious and learning to relax. This will take time and patience but it will be worth it. Some migraine clinics teach relaxation and other useful methods of preventing an attack, but on the whole the vast majority of sufferers manage very well, without ever seeing a doctor. Many learn how to cope with an attack, but they should also try to prevent attacks coming on.

Drugs

Drug Treatment of an Acute Attack

The principle is to anticipate the onset of an attack and to take medication as soon as there is any indication that an attack is pending.

Aspirin or **paracetamol** may be all that is needed. Codeine may be useful in patients who get diarrhoea during an attack. However, in migraine the emptying of the stomach may be slowed down and this may interfere with absorption of the pain-reliever. Soluble preparations should therefore be used but if they do not work it may help if **metoclopramide** (10 mg) is taken by mouth at the first sign of an attack, followed by a dose of aspirin or paracetamol in about ten minutes. The metoclopramide relieves nausea and vomiting and promotes emptying of the stomach which improves absorption of the pain-reliever. In severe cases, particularly if there is vomiting, metoclopramide may be given by injection. An alternative is to use a suppository of **prochlorperazine** (**Stemetil**).

Combined preparations of pain-reliever plus an anti-vomiting drug include **Domperamol** (paracetamol and domperidone), **MigraMax** (aspirin and metoclopramide), **Paramax** (paracetamol and metoclopramide), and **Migraleve** (codeine, paracetamol and buclizine). Buclizine blocks H_1 Distamine receptors and may reduce nausea and vomiting and calm the individual.

If pain-relievers do not work, **ergotamine** may help; it causes constriction of the arteries. Tablets may be dissolved in the mouth (**Lingraine**), taken by mouth and swallowed (**Cafergot**), or applied as a suppository (**Cafergot**). Ergotamine will relieve the headache but it does not relieve eye symptoms. It may make nausea and vomiting worse and an anti-vomiting drug may be required. **Migril** contains ergotamine, caffeine and the anti-vomiting drug cyclizine.

Regular use of ergotamine, particularly in high doses, may cause headache, hallucinations, cold fingers and toes (there is a risk of gangrene), and reliance upon the drug. Suddenly stopping it may produce withdrawal headache. *The maximum safe dose is 6–8 mg during an attack and it should not be used more than twice a month.* It should *never* be used to prevent attacks of migraine.

Isometheptene (**Midrid**) is an alternative to ergotamine and a non-steroidal anti-inflammatory drug such as **mefenamic acid** (**Ponstan**) or **tolfenamic acid** (**Clotam Rapid**) may provide relief for some sufferers.

Sumatriptan (**Imigran**) is a serotonin blocker which may be given by mouth or by injection under the skin or by nasal spray. It can be very effective if given early in an attack. **Almotriptan** (**Almogran**), naratriptan (**Naramig**), **rizatriptan** (**Maxalt**) and **zolmitriptan** (**Zomig**) are newer versions; rizatriptan may be slightly faster working than sumatriptan.

> **Warning:** *For important adverse effects and precautions in the use of these drugs see under each drug in A–Z of Medicines.*

Prevention of Attacks

If migraine attacks are occurring frequently (e.g. one or more attacks every month), then it is helpful to try to prevent these attacks by taking a suitable drug regularly, but only for a few months at a time and providing general measures have also been taken (see earlier).

Drugs used to prevent migraine include: **Beta-blockers** (e.g. **metoprolol**, **nadolol**, **propranolol** and **timolol**) are the drugs of choice. They must not be taken with ergotamine because they may increase the risk of cold fingers and toes.

Cyproheptadine (**Periactin**) is an antihistamine that is also a serotonin blocker. It may be beneficial in some people.

Clonidine (**Dixarit**) may help sufferers sensitive to chemicals in the diet although some experts regard it as no better than a placebo.

Methysergide (**Deseril**) is a serotonin blocker that may produce serious adverse effects and should be used under hospital supervision to treat severe recurrent migraine only when all other treatments have failed.

Pizotifen (**Sanomigran**) is an antihistamine that also blocks serotonin. It may cause drowsiness and weight gain.

Read up about the adverse effects and precautions of each drug in the A–Z of Medicines.

35

Iron and Erythropoietin

Iron is necessary for the manufacture of blood; its deficiency leads to anaemia. There are many causes for anaemia other than iron deficiency, but it is by far the commonest cause and the easiest to treat. Iron-deficiency anaemia is not uncommon in women, infants and elderly people. The deficiency may be caused by a poor diet lacking foods rich in iron — these include liver, meat, eggs, wholemeal cereals, oatmeal, peas, beans and lentils. Poor iron intake is likely to occur because of faulty feeding in babies and infants, and in the elderly who live alone. However *blood loss is a principal cause of iron-deficiency anaemia*, e.g. menstruation (particularly at the menopause when menstruation may be heavy and frequent), bleeding from a peptic ulcer, bleeding from the stomach due to the regular taking of aspirin or other anti-rheumatic drugs, and bleeding at childbirth. Worm infections of the gut may produce iron deficiency, as may disorders of the stomach (e.g. surgical removal of part of the stomach in the treatment of duodenal ulcer) and intestine (e.g. ulcerative colitis). Thus treatment will require special attention to the cause of the iron-deficiency anaemia as well as the giving of iron. For this reason you should not diagnose iron deficiency just by your appearance or your symptoms. It really is quite impossible to estimate the degree and type of anaemia without special blood tests.

The symptoms produced by anaemia may be produced by many disorders – some physical, some psychological, some mild and some serious. If you develop symptoms (e.g. tiredness, breathlessness and weakness) then consult your doctor.

Iron is essential for the formation of the pigment in red blood cells called haemoglobin, which is responsible for carrying oxygen to the tissues from the lungs and carbon dioxide from the tissues back to the lungs. Two-thirds of the body's iron is present in the haemoglobin of the red blood cells. The rest is stored in the bone marrow, spleen and muscles. Absorption of iron from food takes place principally through the duodenum and the upper part of the small intestine. Its absorption is helped by acid from the stomach and it is more easily absorbed in the inorganic ferrous state. Only a small proportion of iron in food is absorbed. Even so, the iron content of the average diet in the Western world is sufficient for our needs. Obviously, you will need more if you are pregnant, breastfeeding or having heavy periods. The mechanisms for controlling the body's iron content exercise a careful control over the absorption of iron from the intestine – if you are iron deficient, absorption is increased. If you are not, then absorption is decreased. Because of menstruation women need to absorb about twice as much iron as men each day.

Iron Treatment

Iron-deficiency anaemia responds well to iron treatment but, as stated earlier, the underlying cause must be diagnosed and treated, and of course this must include advice on diet. In iron deficiency, absorption is increased but in order to produce a suitable response it is necessary to take a large amount of iron each day – about 200 mg. A good response will increase the haemoglobin level (an indication of the degree of anaemia) by about 1 per cent per day. However, in order to ensure a satisfactory level and to replenish the body's stores, treatment should continue for at least three to six months. Remember, it is no use being told that you have got iron-deficiency anaemia and then only remembering to take the tablets for a few weeks.

Iron may be given by mouth or by injection into a vein or muscle. Iron by mouth may irritate the stomach and intestine to produce nausea, vomiting, diarrhoea or constipation and abdominal pains.

There are numerous oral iron preparations on the market; the cheapest effective preparations are **ferrous sulphate** (**Feospan**, **Ferrograd**, **Slow-Fe**), **ferrous gluconate** and **ferrous fumarate** (**Fersaday**, **Fersamal**, **Galfer**). Stomach upset or diarrhoea may be reduced by taking the drug with meals (although absorption is not as good as if it is taken before meals) and by starting on a small dose – one tablet daily – and then increasing the daily dose up to two or three tablets over a period of one to two weeks. Vitamin C may increase the absorption of iron from some oral iron preparations.

Modified release tablets or capsules of iron are designed to release iron slowly, but before they release their iron they may pass through the first part of the duodenum, where iron absorption is good, and down into a lower part of the intestine where iron absorption is poor. They are less effective than ordinary iron tablets.

Liquid forms of iron include **ferrous glycine sulphate** (**Plesmet Syrup**), **polysaccharide-iron complex** (**Niferex Elixir**) and **sodium feredetate** (**Sytron Elixir**).

The regular (prophylactic) use of iron supplements may be valuable in women with heavy periods (menorrhagia), pregnancy, pre-term and low-weight babies, infants born by caesarian section, and in patients who have had surgical removal of the stomach or have malabsorption symptoms.

Iron Injections

Injections of iron (**Cosmofer, Venofer**) may occasionally be necessary if iron cannot be absorbed from the intestine, or if oral iron produces severe stomach and bowel upsets. Response to injected iron takes about fourteen days and the dose and interval between doses should be calculated from the patient's haemoglobin level and body weight. However, it is important to remember that the speed of response is no faster after injected iron than after oral iron in the individual who can absorb iron from the intestine. Because of the risks, it should only be used where absolutely necessary.

Iron sorbitol citric acid complex (**Jectofer**) is an iron sorbitol citric acid complex which is given by deep intramuscular injection. Injections can be painful, cause temporary staining of the skin at the site, and occasionally cause disorders of heart rhythm. They may cause headache, blurred vision, painful muscles, disorientation, flushing, nausea and vomiting, a metallic taste in the mouth and loss of taste. About 30 per cent of the dose is excreted by the kidneys, turning the urine black on standing, and some appears in the saliva, producing a metallic taste in the mouth. Intramuscular iron sorbitol injections should not be given to patients with kidney disorders or infections.

> **Warning:** *Iron is a drug which may produce adverse effects. Overdose may cause liver and kidney damage, collapse and death. Iron preparations, like any drug, must be kept out of reach of children.*

Iron and Folic Acid Preparations

A combination of **iron** and **folic acid** should be used to prevent iron and folic acid deficiency in *pregnancy*. Several preparations are available which contain the equivalent of about 100 mg of iron and 200–500 micrograms of folic acid, *but see the effects of folic acid in preventing spina bifida, p. 179.*

Preparations include **Fefol, Ferfolic SV, Ferrograd Folic, Galfer FA, Lexpec with Iron, Lexpec with Iron-M, Pregaday, Slow-Fe Folic.**

Erythropoietin (EPT, Epoetin Alpha and Beta)

Epoetin alpha and **beta** are bio-engineered erythropoietins. Their clinical effectiveness is the same and they are interchangeable. They are used to treat anaemia associated with chronic kidney failure before or during kidney dialysis. Erythropoietin is a hormone, principally formed by the kidneys, that regulates the production of red blood cells by the bone marrow, a process known as erythropoiesis. The kidneys trigger the production of erythropoietin if the oxygen level in the kidney tissues falls. Kidney disease resulting in failure of the kidneys to produce erythropoietin will cause anaemia, which can now be successfully treated with epoetin. Other factors which contribute to anaemia in kidney failure such as iron or folic acid deficiency should also be treated. Aluminium toxicity from dialysis infections and/or inflammatory diseases may impair the effectiveness of epoetin. It is also used to treat premature babies under thirty-four weeks of age.

Preparations include **Eprex** injections (epoetin alfa) and **NeoRecormon** (epoetin beta) injections. For Adverse Effects and Precautions see A–Z of Medicines.

36

Vitamins

Vitamins are substances which are essential for the maintenance of normal body function but they are not manufactured by the body. Therefore we have to rely upon an outside source, which in a healthy individual is found in a normal well-balanced diet.

When vitamins are taken, not as part of a well-balanced diet, but in highly concentrated forms, they must be regarded as drugs and as such they may produce adverse drug effects. Those vitamins that are soluble in water (the B vitamins and vitamin C), if taken in excess of the body's requirements, are quickly excreted. They rarely do harm, but their use is often unnecessary and wasteful. However, the fat-soluble vitamins (vitamins A, D, K and E) if taken in excess of daily requirements become stored in the body fat, where they may accumulate until toxic concentrations are reached.

Vitamins may be used to treat recognized disorders produced by vitamin deficiencies, and in such cases doctors often use very high doses. They are also used to prevent vitamin-deficiency disorders developing – as supplements to the individual's diet. Much confusion has arisen between the doses used to treat established vitamin-deficiency disorders and the doses used in supplementary treatment. Supplementary dosage need only be at the level of recommended daily intake and there is no merit in taking in more than this. Unfortunately, many over-the-counter preparations contain vitamins and these are the subject of intense marketing. The clear, but wrong and misleading, message which is being given by the manufacturers and promoters is that if 100 units of a vitamin do you good then 1,000 units will do you even more good. They are promoted as giving you vitality and zest – you don't really 'live' until you take added vitamins. Yet most people who take supplementary vitamins can afford a well-balanced diet and therefore do not need added vitamins. Still, if people think they will feel better then they probably will, but they ought to know the hazards of overdosage.

Supplementary vitamins may be of great value to those people whose diet is inadequate, e.g. those who are poor, isolated, elderly, or debilitated; those who are faddy about their food; those on diets, e.g. slimming diets; and alcoholics and others who take in too little food. Similarly, some disorders of the stomach and intestine may produce inadequate vitamin intake and people with such disorders will require supplementary vitamins. Pregnant women and women who are breastfeeding may need supplementary vitamins, and so may babies, infants, and children at puberty; they may also be needed during a debilitating illness. But, of course, there is no substitute for a good nutritious diet. After all, vitamins are only a small part of food. There is no evidence that minor deficiencies of vitamins cause debility or increased risk of getting colds and other infections.

Since deficiency of a single vitamin is rarely encountered, it is best to supplement with several vitamins in doses not larger than the recommended daily requirements which are contained in a 'normal' diet.

Vitamin A

Carotene (pro-vitamin A) and vitamin A are present in dairy produce (milk, eggs, butter, cheese), in green vegetables and carrots, in liver and fish-liver oils. Margarine has added vitamin A. Deficiency causes defective vision in dim light and thickening and hardening of the skin (hyperkeratosis) – this also affects the cornea of the eye. It is fat soluble and if large amounts are taken adverse effects are produced which include loss of appetite, itching, skin disorders, loss of weight, enlargement of the liver and spleen, debility and painful swellings of bones and joints.

> *Vitamin A may cause birth defects and women who are pregnant should not take vitamin A supplements or eat foods that have a high vitamin A content, e.g. liver and liver products.*

Vitamin B Complex

This includes:
vitamin B_1 – thiamine, aneurine
vitamin B_2 – riboflavin
vitamin B_6 – pyridoxine
nicotinamide – nicotinic acid (niacin) nicotinic acid amide, niacinamide
   folic acid – pteroylglutamic acid vitamin B_{12} – cyanocobalamin

Vitamin B_1 (thiamine, aneurine). Vitamin B_1 is present in wheatgerm, eggs, liver, peas, beans and other vegetables. Deficiency causes inflammation of nerves (peripheral neuritis), heart failure, oedema, nausea and vomiting. This group of disorders is known as beri-beri. Vitamin B_1 deficiency may also damage the brain (Werniche's encephalopathy) and cause mental confusion (Korsakow's syndrome). These disorders may occur· in alcoholics on poor diets deficient in vitamins.

Vitamin B_2 (riboflavin). Vitamin B_2 is present in yeast, milk, liver and green vegetables. Deficiency produces sore lips (angular stomatitis), ulcers of the mouth, a sore magenta-coloured tongue, skin rashes (seborrhoeic dermatitis) and blood vessels on the cornea of the eye (vascularization of the cornea).

Vitamin B_6 (pyridoxine). Vitamin B_6 is present in liver, yeasts and cereals. Deficiency may produce anaemia, nerve damage and skin disorders.

Nicotinamide. Nicotinamide and nicotinic acid (which is converted into nicotinamide in the body) are present in liver, yeast, milk, vegetables and unpolished rice. Deficiency produces pellagra (which affects the mouth, stomach and intestine, producing a sore tongue, stomatitis, gastritis and diarrhoea), the brain (causing dementia) and the skin (producing dermatitis).

Folic acid (pteroylglutamic acid). Folic acid is present in green vegetables, yeast and liver. Deficiency produces anaemia and nerve damage and may be caused by poor diet, disorders of the intestine which interfere with the absorption of folic acid from the small intestine, and by pregnancy. Anticonvulsant drugs (e.g. phenytoin, primidone, phenobarbitone) may produce anaemia which responds to folic acid. Antimalarial drugs and nitrofurantoin may also cause anaemia by interfering with folic acid metabolism.

Note: *If you are pregnant, or trying to get pregnant and wish to prevent spina bifida or other nerve damage in your baby you should take 400 micrograms daily while trying to get pregnant and for the first twelve weeks of pregnancy. To prevent recurrence you should take folic acid (4–5 mg) daily for the first twelve weeks of pregnancy.*

Vitamin B_{12} (cyanocobalamin). Vitamin B_{12} is present in meat, milk and eggs. To be absorbed into the bloodstream it has to combine with a substance secreted by the stomach known as the intrinsic factor. Vitamin B_{12} is known as the extrinsic factor and the combination of intrinsic with extrinsic factor is absorbed through the small intestine. Vitamin B_{12} is stored in the liver. Deficiency may produce nerve damage and megaloblastic anaemia because large (megalo-) primitive (-blastic) cells appear in the bloodstream. Pernicious anaemia is a B_{12} deficient anaemia due to a lack of the intrinsic factor in the stomach. Other B_{12} deficient anaemias may be produced after surgical removal of large parts of the stomach, in disorders of the small intestine and, rarely, by dietary deficiency of vitamin B_{12} in strict vegetarians or in those living in the tropics.

Vitamin C (Ascorbic Acid)

Vitamin C is present in citrus fruits, rose hips and green vegetables. Cooking reduces the vitamin C content of food. Deficiency causes scurvy – anaemia, haemorrhage into the skin and gums, bruising and bone pains. In children, vitamin C deficiency may delay bone growth.

Vitamin D

Vitamin D is present in dairy produce and fish oils. It is also produced by the skin after exposure to sunshine. Deficiency may occur in the elderly and housebound and in Asian women whose clothes cut out the sun, particularly if they live in Northern latitudes. Vitamin D deficiency produces rickets in children and osteomalacia (bone softening) in adults by interfering with calcium absorption. Excessive dosage produces a rise in blood calcium which causes debility, drowsiness, nausea, abdominal pains, thirst, constipation, loss of appetite, deposits of calcium in various tissues and organs, kidney damage and kidney stones.

Vitamin K

Vitamin K1 is present in greens and vegetables, and vitamin K_2 is produced by bacteria in the intestine. Vitamin K is necessary for the production of various blood-clotting factors by the liver. Vitamin K1 is fat soluble and requires the bile salts for its absorption from the intestine. Deficiency of vitamin K causes a reduction in blood-clotting factors, resulting in bleeding and delayed blood clotting. It may be caused by disorders of the intestine which interfere with its absorption; obstruction to the passage of bile (obstructive jaundice); and by some drugs (e.g. sulphonamides and tetracyclines) which affect vitamin K producing bacteria in the intestine. Vitamin K is given to newborn babies to prevent a low blood prothrombin level which may cause bleeding (haemorrhagic disease of the newborn).

Vitamin E

Vitamin E is present in the oil from soya beans, wheat germ, rice germ, cotton seed, maize and green leaves (e.g. lettuce). It is an antioxidant (see below).

Recommended Daily Requirements

Tables of recommended daily requirements are easily found in books on nutrition, human biology, medicine and so on. However, they specifically refer to nutrition and indicate that your food should contain the stated amounts.

Unfortunately, the manufacturers give the impression that these amounts are to be *added* to a normal diet. Do not be misled: vitamins may be required to supplement an inadequate diet but never to complement a diet. High-dose vitamin preparations should be avoided – do not be attracted because they are called 'super vitamins' or any other name that indicates that the dose is above what is normally required.

A Note on Antioxidant Vitamins and Minerals

A *radical* is a group of atoms always linked together in the same way and which can act like a single atom. They can exist for a very short time on their own (i.e. they can be free) before linking up with other atoms to form a molecule. In the body, it is thought that *free radicals* may cause damage to cells and the greatest culprits are free oxygen radicals.

One suggestion is that free radicals may damage those protein molecules that are responsible for transmitting special characteristics from one generation of cells to the next. In this way the genetic coding of the cells may be damaged and as a consequence the affected cells may age prematurely and may undergo faulty cell division leading to cancer.

Another suggestion is that the polyunsaturated fatty acid molecules that form integral components of cell walls may also be damaged by free oxygen radicals. If these cells are lining the walls of arteries, then the resultant damage can lead to the deposit of fats and cholesterol at the site causing a local swelling (a plaque). The plaque can then scar and ulcerate, causing the blood passing over it to clot (to thrombose). If this happens in a coronary artery supplying the heart it is called a coronary thrombosis.

Polyunsaturated fatty acids in food are a potential source of free oxygen radicals. This is because, when heated (e.g. used as cooking oils) or exposed to daylight, oxygen can attach itself to their free bonds and during this process of oxidation, free oxygen radicals can be released. This is why it is best to keep fats and oils and their products (e.g. margarines) in a refrigerator and it is why there is much debate about the safety of reusing cooking oils that are high in polyunsaturated fatty acids. (*Note:* oxidized fats and oils are rancid.)

Defence Against Free Radicals

Cells in the lining of the stomach, intestine and lungs act as the first line of defence against the entry of free radicals into the body. The second line of defence is *antioxidants* in the bloodstream that protect cell walls against damage from free oxygen radicals.

Several minerals (e.g. selenium, manganese and zinc), vitamin C, vitamin E and beta-carotene (a precursor of vitamin A) act as antioxidants in the body and immobilize free oxygen radicals. It is interesting to note that nature knows best because natural vegetable oils contain vitamin E. Some processed oils have the vitamin E removed and this natural antidote to free oxygen radicals has to be added back to such fat products and to margarines.

Vitamin E appears to have a particularly important role in preventing the effects of free oxygen radicals and a selenium-containing enzyme helps to remove products of this reaction. Vitamin C helps to restore vitamin E to its original form. Beta-carotenes in carrots and dark green and yellow vegetables may have similar effects to vitamin C as may related substances called caretenoids which are present in red wine, tomatoes, tea and onions. Selenium, zinc and manganese-containing enzymes may help to prevent free radicals forming.

Because of the possibility that free oxygen radicals may produce premature ageing of cells (e.g. of the skin), and be involved in causing heart disease and cancer it is not surprising that antioxidants (vitamin C, vitamin E, beta-carotene and selenium) are being pushed by health food shops and the manufacturers of vitamins.

There is nothing like the promise of a reduction in premature ageing to cloud the facts and, in these days of multimedia advertising, the message is coming across that antioxidants have very special qualities. But we don't know the effects of overdosing and we don't know what dose of antioxidants we should take and how frequently we should take them. The answer is the same for all essential nutrients – they are best provided by eating a *well-balanced* diet containing a *variety* of foods especially fresh fruits, vegetables, seeds and nuts.

37

Corticosteroids

The metabolic function of the body is under the control of several glands whose internal secretions (or hormones) are released into the bloodstream to act upon various tissues and organs. These glands include the master gland (the pituitary), the thyroid and parathyroid glands, the pancreas, the adrenal glands and the sex organs (gonads) – testes or ovaries. The effect of these hormones is to stimulate certain body processes.

Under complex control from the brain, the front part (anterior lobe) of the pituitary gland exercises control over the thyroid gland, the cortical part of the adrenal glands and the sex glands. It produces stimulating hormones which act on these organs (often known as target glands) to produce their own secretion of hormones. In addition there is a feedback mechanism so that the production of a stimulating hormone by the pituitary is controlled by the circulating level of hormone from the target gland. For example, if the level of adrenal hormones increases in the blood then the adrenal stimulating hormone decreases, and vice versa.

There are two adrenal glands which lie above the upper ends of each kidney. Each consists of a centre (medulla) which produces adrenaline(epinephrine) and noradrenaline(norepinephrine) (see p. 38) and an outer layer known as the cortex. The adrenals (from now on this will be used to indicate the adrenal cortex) produce three groups of hormones (known as **adrenocortical hormones**) which are grouped according to their main function – **glucocorticoids** act on sugar, protein and calcium metabolism; **mineralocorticoids** act on salt and water metabolism; and **sex hormones**. Their production (except aldosterone) is under the control of adrenocorticotrophic hormone from the pituitary gland – this may be referred to as ACTH or corticotropin. Except for aldosterone, there is an overlap in the actions and effects produced by these hormones.

In addition to their metabolic effects the glucocorticoids reduce inflammatory reactions and suppress the immune response. They are often referred to as *corticosteroids*, and the ones used to treat inflammation are referred to as *anti-inflammatory corticosteroids* or *anti-inflammatory steroids*, or *steroidal anti-inflammatory drugs*. They may also affect water and salt metabolism, but to a much less extent than the mineralocorticoids which control retention of sodium and excretion of potassium by the kidneys. Aldosterone is discussed in the chapter on diuretics, p. 148.

The *sex hormones* produced by the adrenals include male sex hormones (androgens) and female sex hormones (oestrogens and progestogens). Before puberty the balance of the two affects the degree of femininity and masculinity of the body. Their major sources in the body after puberty are the testes and ovaries – see the chapters on female sex hormones, male sex hormones and anabolic (body-building) steroids.

Corticosteroids

The principal aim in manufacturing corticosteroids has been to try and separate the anti-inflammatory effects from their metabolic effects on sugar, protein salts and water. Modifications of the structure of the naturally occurring glucocorticoid, cortisone, have produced drugs with greatly increased anti-inflammatory properties and reduced metabolic effects. Metabolic effects are most marked with **fludrocortisone** and are too high for **hydrocortisone** (**Efcortesol, Hydrocortone, Solu-Cortef**) or **cortisone** (**Cortisyl**) to be used on a long-term basis. Metabolic effects are minimal with **betamethasone** (**Betnelan, Betnesol**) and **dexamethasone** (**Dexsol, Decadron**). They occur only slightly with **methylprednisolone** (**Medrone, Solu-Medrone, Depo-Medrone**), **prednisolone** (**Precortisyl, Precortisyl Forte, Deltacortril**) and **triamcinolone** (**Kenalog**). **Deflazacort** (**Calcort**) is derived from prednisolone and has high glucocorticoid activity.

● *Adverse Effects of Corticosteroids*

To produce desired anti-inflammatory effects, corticosteroids may have to be given in doses far in excess of the body's needs, which greatly increases the risks of adverse effects. In these doses their effects on metabolism are complex: for example, they affect salt and water balance, producing salt and water retention (causing raised blood pressure) and potassium loss; sugar and carbohydrate metabolism is affected, producing a raised blood sugar and sugar in the urine (glycosuria); protein metabolism is affected, producing muscle wasting and weakness; calcium metabolism is affected, producing softening of bones (osteoporosis); retarded bone growth in children, wasting of the skin with appearance of stripes (striae) and disordered fat metabolism, resulting in fat being laid down on the face (moon face), shoulders (buffalo hump) and on the abdomen (Cushing's Syndrome); the effect on calcium metabolism produces increased calcium excretion in the urine and the risk of kidney stones; and uric acid excretion is increased. Other effects include indigestion and aggravation of peptic ulcers; and cataracts. In addition, they reduce the inflammatory response which may mask symptoms and signs of infections, such as tuberculosis. They also reduce the allergic response, and interfere with the processes which produce immunity. They may cause mental and mood changes and suppress the complex nervous and hormonal response to stress (e.g. infection, injury, surgery).

Measles, chickenpox and shingles may be made very much worse by corticosteroids and patients on oral (or injected) corticosteroid treatment who are exposed to these diseases should be given passive immunization (see p. 298).

Hydrocortisone is the corticosteroid most commonly used for injection and **prednisolone** is the most popular preparation by mouth. Injections of hydrocortisone are used in emergencies (e.g. severe asthma attacks, status asthmaticus). Short courses of prednisolone may be given by mouth in the treatment of severe bronchial asthma, allergies and other disorders. Long-term daily maintenance doses of prednisolone by mouth may be used in rheumatic disorders, skin disease and blood disorders. Corticosteroids by inhalation are used in the treatment of asthma and by nasal spray to treat hayfever.

⬤ Precautions on the Use of Corticosteroids

In the individual with normally functioning adrenal glands the production of corticosteroid hormones is increased at times of **stress** (e.g. **injury**, **surgery** and **infections**). This problem of increased need during stress is exaggerated in patients in whom corticosteroids are being used. The amount of circulating corticosteroids in the blood suppresses the production of ACTH by the pituitary gland, which leads to 'disuse' changes in the adrenal glands and failure of the stress mechanism. If these drugs have been used daily for more than a few weeks the body will fail to react in the normal way to stress, with the result that the patient may collapse and even die. This may also occur if the drugs are stopped suddenly. For this reason their daily dose needs increasing three or fourfold during episodes of stress and *they should never be stopped suddenly*. They should be tapered off very slowly over many weeks (depending, of course, upon how long the patient has been on them). These dangers mean that every patient on corticosteroids should carry a warning card, and if they have received them for one month or more in any two-year period they should continue to carry a steroid warning card because collapse can occur during a surgical operation up to two years after stopping them.

In order to minimize adverse effects, corticosteroid preparations by mouth (e.g. **prednisolone**) should wherever possible be taken in the morning, in the smallest effective dose for the shortest period of treatment possible. Taking the drug on alternate days may help but not with asthmatic patients. Corticosteroids by mouth or injection etc. should be used with special caution in patients with thrombophlebitis, serious mental illness, osteoporosis, acute kidney disease, raised blood pressure, glaucoma, epilepsy, diabetes, under-working of the thyroid gland, cirrhosis of the liver, pregnancy, peptic ulcers, infections such as tuberculosis, virus infections (e.g. measles) or fungal infections. Patients on treatment should *avoid* contact with anyone with chickenpox or shingles and for up to three months after stopping corticosteroids. If in contact, passive immunization should be given within three days and not later than ten days after exposure.

Adrenocorticotrophic Hormone (ACTH: Corticotropin)

This is a very complex chemical produced by the anterior lobes of the pituitary gland, which respond rapidly (within minutes) to the body's requirements. The pure substance was isolated from the pituitary glands of slaughtered animals in the 1940s and it was first synthesized twenty years later. ACTH stimulates the adrenals to produce corticosteroids and to a lesser extent male sex hormones (androgens).

The principal effects produced by ACTH are those produced by corticosteroids, but it will *always* produce disturbances of salt and water balance. ACTH is inactive when given by mouth and has to be given by injection. It is no longer used because of its adverse effects, variations in response and the waning of its effects over time.

Tetracosactide (tetracosactrin, **Synacthen**, **Synacthen Depot**) is a synthetic polypeptide resembling ACTH used for diagnosing adrenal deficiency disorders.

Warning: *The long-term use of corticosteroids by mouth with doses of 7.5mg daily or above increases the risk of developing fragile bones (osteoporosis). Most bone loss occurs in the last six months of treatment, therefore patients should have a bone scan **before** treatment starts. Patients should be given advice and other treatments aimed at preventing osteoporosis.*

38

Male Sex Hormones

The development and maintenance of reproductive organs is under the control of chemicals known as steroid hormones. These hormones are produced by the male and female sex glands and the adrenal glands. The hormones concerned with the development and maintenance of the male reproductive system are called androgens. Several androgens are produced by the testes and adrenal glands. The most powerful of these is known as testosterone.

The master gland (the pituitary) produces hormones called gonadotrophins, which stimulate the testes to make these male sex hormones. At puberty they are made in sufficient amounts to produce changes usually known as secondary sexual characteristics (or masculinization effects or androgenic effects). The voice-box enlarges and the voice gets deeper, the genitals get bigger and hair begins to appear in various parts of the body. They are responsible for the growth and development of the testicles to produce sperm. At puberty there is also a spurt in growth; body protein builds up, muscles develop and bones grow. The latter effects may be separated from the effects upon the sex organs, and because they are related to protein build-up they are called anabolic effects. Male sex hormones (androgens), therefore, have two principal effects: (1) **androgenic** – they affect the development and maintenance of reproductive organs and function; (2) **anabolic** – they affect growth and muscle bulk.

However, those male sex hormones which produce predominantly androgenic effects will also produce some anabolic effects and those which have principally anabolic effects will also produce some androgenic effects. Testosterone is the natural androgenic hormone produced by the testes but there are several synthetic preparations available. Similarly, much attention has been directed to manufacturing synthetic male sex hormones that produce predominantly anabolic effects (anabolic steroids, see next chapter).

Available preparations with marked androgenic properties include:

mesterolone (**Pro-Viron**), **testosterone** (**Andropatch**, **Primoteston Depot**, **Restandol**, **Sustanon**, **Testoderm**, **Virormone**).

Androgenic male sex hormones are used principally to treat disorders produced by failure of the testes to make these hormones. This failure may be primary, due to the lack of development or underdevelopment of the testes, or secondary, due to failure of the pituitary gland to produce sufficient gonadotrophins. In underdevelopment, or if used in adolescent males, they produce development of the secondary sexual characteristics. They stimulate growth, but may produce stunting of growth because they also close off the growing ends of the long bones.

In small doses they stimulate the production of sperm but in high doses they suppress the production of gonadotrophins by the pituitary, thus causing suppression of sperm production.

Male sex hormones are given as replacement treatment in castrated males and to treat underdeveloped testes. When given to patients with underworking of the pituitary gland they cause normal sexual development but have no effect on fertility. If this is required, pituitary hormones (gonadotrophins) should be given to stimulate the testes to develop, produce sperm and male sex hormones. They are of no use in treating impotency. Testosterone in a self-adhesive skin patch (**Andropatch**, **Testoderm**) is used as hormone replacement therapy (HRT) in males who suffer from a deficiency of or absent production of testosterone by the testes.

● *Adverse Effects and Precautions*

The adverse effects produced by testosterone and other androgens may be related to their androgenic and anabolic effects. They include increase in skeletal weight, salt and water retention, oedema, increased number of blood vessels in the skin, increased blood calcium levels and increased bone growth. In women they may affect gonadotrophin production by the pituitary and lead to suppression of the ovaries and menstruation. Large and continued doses cause masculinization in women – deep voice, acne, the male patterns of baldness and hair growth, shrinking of the breasts, increase in size of the clitoris and an increase in libido (sexual drive). They should not be given to patients with cancer of the prostate gland or liver or untreated heart failure and they should not be used in pregnancy because the unborn baby may be affected. They should be used with caution by patients who would be made worse by salt and water retention, e.g. patients with treated heart failure, impaired kidney function, migraine, raised blood pressure or epilepsy. Isolated cases of cancer of the liver have been reported for certain anabolic and androgenic steroids used for prolonged periods.

Drugs that Stop the Production of Testosterone

Buserelin (Suprefact), **leuprorelin (Prostap SR)**, **goserelin (Zoladex)** and **tripto-relin (De-capeptyl SR)** are gonadotrophin-releasing hormone analogues that initially stimulate the release of gonadotrophins by the pituitary gland. This stimulates the testes to produce testosterone, and as the blood level of testosterone rises, the release of gonadotrophins is stopped, and the testes stop producing testosterone. They are used to treat cancer of the prostate gland that depends upon testosterone for its growth and they are as effective as castration for this disorder.

Drugs that Block the Effects of Testosterone

Finasteride (Proscar) blocks the effects of testosterone on the prostate gland and helps to shrink it. This improves the flow of urine in men with an enlarged prostate gland (causing obstruction to the outlet of urine from the bladder). It is an alternative to alpha-blockers (see p. 284) in the treatment of an enlarged prostate (benign prostatic hypertrophy: BPH).

Anti-male Sex Hormone Drugs (Anti-androgens)

An anti-androgenic drug, **cyproterone**, is used as **Androcur** to treat severe hypersexuality and sexual deviation in males. It inhibits sperm production and produces reversible infertility (chemical castration). Cyproterone is included with a female sex hormone (ethinylestradiol) in **Dianette** and used to treat severe acne in women because blocking male sex hormones helps to reduce sebum production in hair follicles. This preparation is also used to treat severe and excessive hair growth (hirsutism) in women.

Bicalutamide (Casodex), **cyproterone (Cyprostat)** and **flutamide (Drogenil)** are anti-androgens used in the treatment of cancer of the prostate gland that depends on testosterone for growth.

Anti-impotence Drugs

Failure to produce an erection can be caused by a number of factors including drugs. Erectile disorders can be treated either by local or by oral administration. Drugs used include **alprostadil** and **sildenafil**.

Alprostadil (Caverject, MUSE, Viridal Duo) is a prostaglandin (see Chapter 52) given by intracavernous injection (Caverject, Viridal Duo) or intraurethral administration (MUSE). It has vasoactive properties which cause an erection by acting on the blood vessels in the corpora cavernosa.

Apomorphine (Uprima) is taken as a tablet under the tongue. It is a selective dopamine antagonist and causes smooth muscle relaxation in the corpora cavernosa which leads to engorgement and erection.

Sildenafil (**Viagra**) is given orally and it prevents the breakdown of the smooth muscle relaxant, increasing blood flow into the penis and so enhancing the erectile response to sexual stimulation.

39

Anabolic (Body-building) Steroids

Male sex hormones produce two main effects – *androgenic* (development and maintenance of sexual function) and *anabolic* (body-building function). Those male sex hormones marketed as 'body-builders' produce some effects on sexual function (androgenic) in males, but when used in women they cause less masculinization than those male hormones that produce predominantly androgenic effects in males.

Masculinization means the development of male characteristics in women – deep voice, acne, male patterns of baldness and hair growth, shrinking of the breasts, increase in size of the clitoris and increase in libido (sexual drive).

The male sex hormones that are marketed as body-builders are often referred to as *anabolic steroids*. Anabolism means making living tissue from nutrients in food and steroid refers to a group of organic chemicals related to cholesterol. All anabolic steroids are derivatives of testosterone, the principal male sex hormone made by the testes. They include: **nandrolone** (**Deca-Durabolin**) and **stanozolol** (**Stromba**).

The use of anabolic steroids to 'build up' patients recovering from injury, surgery and acute illnesses has not been shown to be of benefit. Also, in chronically ill patients who have lost weight due to protein breakdown, anabolic steroids have not been shown to be effective.

Nandrolone may be used as part of the treatment of patients suffering from aplastic anaemia and **stanozolol** is used to treat Behçet's disease and hereditary angioedema. Nandrolene may be used to treat post-menopausal osteoporosis and stanozolol can be used in elderly patients suffering from osteoporosis, to reduce the risk of fracture.

Dangers of Using Anabolic Steroids in Children

The use of anabolic steroids to increase height in underdeveloped children may actually stunt growth because they stop the growth of long bones by prematurely closing the growing ends of the bones. They may produce masculinization in female children.

The Misuse of Anabolic Steroids in Sport

Anabolic steroids have been used for many years by weight-lifters to increase their muscle bulk and hopefully their strength; by body-builders to increase their muscle bulk, and by shot-putters, javelin-throwers and others to improve the strength of their throw. In more recent years some track and other athletes have used anabolic steroids to increase the duration and intensity of their training and hopefully to increase their competition performances.

The willingness of some athletes to use anabolic steroids illegally is a matter of concern and their willingness to risk serious harmful effects, as well as the consequences of their illegal actions, is of interest because we lack convincing evidence from adequate and well-controlled studies that anabolic steroids actually improve competitive performance in, for example, track athletes. However, they increase aggressiveness – and therefore competitiveness – and they increase muscle bulk, and the mystique that surrounds their use may add to any perceived benefits.

40

Female Sex Hormones

The newborn baby girl's ovaries contain thousands of eggs or ova. Each ovum is in a fluid-filled sac called a follicle. Before puberty many of these follicles enlarge but then shrink.

Puberty

At puberty the ovaries begin to undergo cyclical changes under stimulation from hormones produced by the master gland (the pituitary). The uterus and vagina enlarge, the breasts develop, fat is laid down in certain areas giving the characteristic female figure, and hair starts to grow under the arms and on the pubes.

Menstruation

The anterior pituitary gland produces two hormones which affect the growth of the ovaries. These are called gonadotrophins because they make the gonads (ovaries) grow. One is called follicle-stimulating hormone (FSH) which stimulates the development of follicles around the ova in the ovaries. This makes the follicles grow and as one of them starts to grow more than the others it starts to produce its own female sex hormones, called oestrogens. These oestrogens then start to work on the lining of the uterus, making it grow thicker. As the blood concentration of oestrogens increases the pituitary's production of FSH decreases. The other gonadotrophic hormone is called luteinizing hormone (LH) and it acts on the developed follicle, making it rupture and release the ovum. This process is known as ovulation. LH also ensures the continuing development of the follicle after it has released the ovum and converts it into a yellowish body (corpus luteum) producing a different female sex hormone called progesterone, which belongs to the group of female sex hormones known as progestogens. This also acts on the lining of the uterus, making it ready to receive a fertilized ovum.

The first change in the uterus when its lining thickens under the influence of oestrogens is called the proliferative phase (phase of growth). The subsequent phase, after ovulation, when progesterone makes it undergo special changes in preparation for receiving a fertilized egg (ovum) is called the secretory phase (because cells develop which will be ready to secrete nutritious fluids if conception occurs and the fertilized egg settles on the lining of the uterus). Doctors, by taking a scraping (or biopsy) from the lining of the uterus, are able to tell whether the lining has undergone both changes, proliferative and secretory, and so are able to tell whether the patient has ovulated. They are also able to determine whether oestrogens and progesterone have been made in sufficient quantities to produce the changes.

Progesterone inhibits the production of LH by the pituitary whereas oestrogens stimulate its production, and so it can be seen that there is a delicate balance between FSH and LH production by the pituitary gland and the production of oestrogens and progesterone by the developing follicle and the corpus luteum respectively.

Before puberty the production of FSH and LH by the pituitary is not enough to stimulate the development of a follicle around an ovum and only small quantities of oestrogens and progesterone are produced by the ovaries. Two or three years before the development of menstruation, puberty changes are already taking place. This is thought to be due to the growth and development of the pituitary gland and also part of the brain known as the hypothalamus which exerts control over the nervous and hormonal activity in the body. As the pituitary gland develops it starts to increase its production of FSH and LH. These get to work on the ovaries and cause groups of follicles to develop. As they grow they start to produce more and more oestrogens. These oestrogens work on various tissues in the body producing the secondary sexual characteristics; in addition, the lining of the uterus starts to thicken and the first menstrual period develops (the menarche).

During the time after the first menstrual period the pituitary and hypothalamus are also developing and at times they produce too little gonadotrophic hormones to affect the production of oestrogens by the ovaries. Thus the lining of the uterus does not thicken and a young girl may go several months without a period or have irregular periods. As the pituitary settles down the periods will become more regular and menstruation will start to occur approximately every twenty-eight days.

During these first few months, ovulation does not usually occur because the pituitary does not produce sufficient LH. But as the cycles without ovulation continue (usually known as anovulatory cycles) more and more oestrogens are produced by the follicles and LH production increases, eventually causing ovulation (release of the ovum).

At the time of ovulation, the lining of the uterus is ready to receive the ovum, which after ovulation leaves the ovary and passes down a fallopian tube into the cavity of the uterus. If the ovum is not fertilized by a male sperm (and this often takes place as the ovum passes down the tube) it slowly disintegrates as it passes down the cavity of the uterus.

If the ovum is not fertilized, LH production falls and the corpus luteum shrinks, resulting in a decreasing production of progesterone and oestrogens. As the level drops the blood vessels supplying the lining of the uterus close off, the lining disintegrates and menstrual bleeding starts. When progesterone production by the shrinking corpus luteum declines, the pituitary responds by producing more LH. In response to a decreased production of oestrogens the pituitary starts to produce more FSH and the cycle starts all over again. The increase of FSH and LH starts to work on the ovaries, a new group of follicles starts to develop and the whole sequence of changes is repeated.

Pregnancy

If the ovum is fertilized it burrows into the lining of the uterus and becomes anchored. It develops a layer of cells around it (the trophoblast) which multiply and eventually form the placenta (afterbirth). At this early stage the trophoblast cells surrounding the developing fertilized ovum (now called an embryo) start to produce chorionic gonadotrophin hormone (chorionic because it is produced by the cells which go to form part of the placenta called the chorion, and gonadotrophin because it works on the gonads, or ovaries). Chorionic gonadotrophin, like LH, works on the corpus luteum in the ovary and maintains its development. This results in an increased production of progesterone by the corpus luteum, despite the fall-off in LH production by the pituitary.

Under stimulation from progesterone, the lining of the uterus continues to provide nutrition for the developing embryo until the placenta is developed. This then takes over essential duties – supplying nutrients, carrying away unwanted products, and supplying oxygen and other gases to the developing baby and carrying away carbon dioxide. In addition, the placenta (which links the baby's blood supply directly to the mother's) continues to produce chorionic gonadotrophin but also starts to produce its own oestrogens and progesterone.

This delicate and complex balance of hormones ensures that the pregnancy becomes established. After about twelve weeks the chorionic gonadotrophin production by the placenta starts to fall off, the corpus luteum shrinks at about sixteen to eighteen weeks, and production of chorionic gonadotrophin reaches a low level which lasts throughout the pregnancy. At the same time production of oestrogens and progesterone by the placenta continues to increase throughout the pregnancy, falling abruptly after delivery. The fall in oestrogens then stimulates the pituitary to produce FSH, a group of follicles gradually starts to develop in an ovary and the menstrual cycle is set in motion again. The high oestrogen and progesterone levels in pregnancy are responsible for breast development. Some chorionic gonadotrophin hormone is excreted in the urine and gives a positive urine pregnancy test early in pregnancy.

After childbirth the sucking of the baby at the breast stimulates production of a milk-production hormone (prolactin) by the pituitary gland. This stimulates further milk production (supply meets demand). At the same time prolactin serves a useful purpose by stopping the production of FSH by the pituitary and thus preventing the development of follicles in the ovaries. This prevents the breastfeeding mother from menstruating for several months after delivery, depending, of course, on how long she breastfeeds. However, it does not necessarily mean that a breastfeeding mother cannot get pregnant.

Menopause

As the ovaries get older the follicles start responding less and less to FSH. This results in a decreased production of oestrogens and for a time an increased production of FSH. Also LH production falls and ovulation fails to occur during some cycles. As ovarian function continues to decline, ovulation stops altogether. Oestrogen and progesterone production fall right off and eventually menstrual periods stop. The rise in FSH production may affect other pituitary hormone production, which may cause various menopausal changes; these include increase in weight, hot flushes, bone changes and psychological symptoms. The lack of oestrogens produces shrinking of the secondary sex organs – the breasts become smaller, the vulva and vagina undergo changes and the ovaries and uterus shrink.

From this brief description of the hormonal control of puberty, menstruation, pregnancy and the menopause it can be seen that there are two groups of hormones which control numerous functions in the female body – these are oestrogens and progestogens. Many synthetic preparations of these hormones are available and they are used for a wide variety of disorders.

Oestrogens

The main sources of oestrogens are the ovaries and the placenta. They are also produced in small amounts by the adrenal glands and by the testes in the male. Over twenty different oestrogens have been isolated from the urine of pregnant women. The three main oestrogens produced by the ovaries and placenta are **estrone**, **estradiol** and **estriol**. The most potent natural oestrogen is estradiol. Estriol is produced in large quantities by the placenta during pregnancy.

Oestrogen Preparations

The preparations available for use include naturally occurring oestrogens such as estradiol and synthetic oestrogens that resemble estradiol in structure. Synthetic oestrogens are broken down more slowly in the body than naturally occurring oestrogens and so their effects last for a longer time – the two main ones are semi-synthetic: **ethinylestradiol** and **mestranol**. They are present in many female hormone preparations, particularly oral contraceptive drugs. Other chemicals are available which, although not steroids, have oestrogenic effects – the main one in this group is **diethylstilbestrol**.

Oestrogen preparations include the *synthetic oestrogens*; **ethinylestradiol**, **mestranol**, and **diethylstilbestrol** and the *natural oestrogens*; **estradiol**, **estrone** and **estriol**. **Conjugated oestrogens** resemble natural oestrogens.

Many preparations of female sex hormones contain both oestrogens and progestogens (e.g. combined contraceptive pills).

Oestrogens are used as replacement treatment in patients who have deficient oestrogen production due to the underdevelopment of the ovaries, which causes delayed puberty and absence of periods (primary amenorrhoea); to treat menstrual irregularities; to treat symptoms and to prevent softening of bones (osteoporosis) in post-menopausal women (see **HRT** later) and occasionally to treat cancers of the breast or prostate in selected cases; and in oral contraceptive preparations.

Adverse effects from oestrogens include nausea and vomiting (which are directly related to dose), tenderness and enlargement of the breasts, headache, dizziness, irregular vaginal bleeding, fluid and salt retention, and growth of breasts in men. Low doses of oestrogen may stimulate growth of cancer of the breast and uterus. The oestrogens in oral contraceptive preparations may be responsible for changes in blood clotting leading, rarely, to the risk of venous thrombosis, and the use of high doses of oestrogens to stop milk production just after childbirth may be associated with an increased risk of thrombosis. They are not now used for this purpose and have been replaced by bromocriptine.

Progestogens

Following ovulation, progesterone is responsible for the secretory changes in the lining of the uterus during the last two weeks of the menstrual cycle. It is also necessary for maintaining pregnancy. In addition, it has many other effects. It plays an important role in the development of the placenta and it stops movements of the uterine muscle. It stops ovulation during pregnancy and plays a part in further breast development. It is produced by the corpus luteum and acts only on tissues which have been previously subjected to the actions of oestrogens. Progesterone increases the use of energy by the body;

the body temperature rises at ovulation and stays up until menstruation (i.e. during the secretory phase). This is a test for fertility, as it shows whether the patient ovulates. It is also a test to determine the time of ovulation – when pregnancy is more likely to occur – and from this the 'safe period' may also be worked out, that is, the time of the month when the risk of pregnancy is reduced. Progesterone also affects salt excretion by the kidneys.

Progesterone and Progestogen Preparations

The naturally occurring **progesterone** (**Cyclogest**, **Gestone**) is rapidly broken down in the liver to pregnanediol. Therefore, it is inactive by mouth and has to be given by suppository, intramuscular injection or by implanting a pellet under the skin. It is insoluble and cannot be injected into a vein.

There are two groups of synthetic progestogens: those related to progesterone, e.g. **dydrogesterone** (**Duphaston, Duphaston HRT**), **hydroxyprogesterone** (**Proluton Depot**) and **medroxyprogesterone** (**Depo-Provera, Provera**) and those related to the male sex hormone testosterone, e.g. **norethisterone** (**Micronor HRT, Primolut N, Utovlan**).

Progestogens are used in combined and progestogen-only oral contraceptives and in a variety of HRT preparations. They are also used to control heavy and/or irregular menstrual periods.

Anti-oestrogens

Clomifene (**Clomid**), **tamoxifen** (**Emblon, Fentamox, Nolvadex, Soltamox, Tamofen**) and **toremifene** (**Fareston**) block the actions of oestrogens at oestrogen receptor sites; they are referred to as anti-oestrogens.

The important action of these drugs is their ability to stimulate the production of gonadotrophins (LH and FSH) by the master gland (the pituitary). They do this by blocking oestrogen receptors so that the pituitary thinks the level of oestrogens in the body is low and stimulates the ovaries to produce more oestrogens. Therefore they are used to treat infertility caused by a failure to ovulate, and to treat people with absent periods or disorders of menstrual bleeding caused by failure to ovulate.

Anastrozole (**Arimidex**), **exemestane** (**Aromasin**) and **letrozole** (**Femara**) block the enzyme aromatase, which normally converts male sex hormones (androgens) into female sex hormones (oestrogens) in the tissues of the female body (but not in the ovaries). In post-menopausal women this helps to reduce the amount of oestrogens in the body. They are used to treat cancers of the breast that require oestrogens for growth (oestrogen-dependent breast cancer).

Some breast cancers and their secondary deposits require oestrogen for their continued growth, and an anti-oestrogen drug can produce very beneficial effects in some women. They offer effective alternatives to removal of the ovaries in pre-menopausal women and are very effective treatments in post-menopausal women who suffer from oestrogen-dependent cancer of the breast.

Dysmenorrhoea (Period Pain)

Because it stops ovulation, **the pill** (combined oestrogen/progestogen) is effective in relieving period pains. A progestogen on its own e.g. **dydroges-terone** (**Duphaston**) appears less effective.

With period pains it has been shown that prostaglandins are released (see Chapter 52) and a drug which blocks these is often helpful, e.g. **aspirin** or one of the non-steroidal anti-inflammatory drugs (NSAIDs) such as **ibuprofen**, **naproxen** or **mefenamic acid** – see p. 162.

Hormone Replacement Therapy (HRT)

Hormone replacement therapy (HRT) is treatment with female sex hormones in order to replace the deficiency which occurs following the menopause. It involves taking an oestrogen with or without a progestogen.

One major effect of taking oestrogens is that they make the lining of the womb thicker. If they are taken regularly every day the lining will overgrow and become sensitive to factors which may trigger the development of cancer.

To prevent this continuous overgrowth and reduce the risk of cancer, oestrogens are taken in cycles (three weeks on and one week off), and a progestogen is added to the treatment for the last ten–fourteen days of each cycle. The effect of this regimen is that when the oestrogen and progestogen are stopped the lining of the womb is shed. The bleeding is usually light and trouble-free. A tampon needs to be worn for about four–five days.

Note: *Women who have had a hysterectomy (surgical removal of the womb) have, of course, no risk of cancer of the womb and may be treated with oestrogen alone.*

Formulations Used in HRT

Oestrogen Formulations

All oestrogens can cause the same spectrum of harmful effects but the risk of developing these are reduced in HRT because *only small doses* are required and *natural oestrogens* (estradiol, estrone and estriol) are used. Conjugated oestrogens resemble natural oestrogens.

Natural oestrogens are less powerful than synthetic oestrogens (ethinylestradiol, mestranol and diethylstilbestrol). They are broken down more rapidly by the liver, which may result in a reduced risk of harmful effects on the liver and other tissues, but it also means that they are less effective than synthetic oestrogens by mouth. Furthermore, they may be poorly absorbed from the intestine, which is why other routes may be more reliable, for example:

Implants slowly release the oestrogen over a period of months. They are inserted into a fatty layer under the skin of the abdomen, thigh or buttocks under local anaesthetic. They may be useful for people who are forgetful. Beneficial effects may taper off at the end of the six months.

Adhesive patches. These are like a first-aid dressing and each patch contains enough oestrogen to last for three or four days (newer ones last for seven days). They are waterproof and transparent. The patch may irritate the skin in some women and it may come loose in the bath or shower.

Progestogen Formulations

Many preparations of progestogens are available to be taken by mouth. They are well absorbed from the intestine and they are reliable and effective. Their harmful effects are listed in the A–Z of Medicines.

A recommended HRT for a woman with a uterus would therefore be: An oestrogen skin patch applied to a clean, non-hairy area of skin below the waist and replaced with a new patch every three–four days, using a different site. Such a patch will release about 50–100 micrograms of oestrogen every twenty-four hours. In addition, one progestogen tablet should be taken daily from day fifteen to day twenty-six of each twenty-eight-day treatment with oestrogen. Eight patches and twelve tablets should be one month's treatment.

The Benefits of HRT

HRT relieves hot flushes and vaginal symptoms of the menopause. It should be taken for at least one year. A vaginal oestrogen cream will relieve vaginal symptoms. However, the oestrogen is absorbed, therefore in women with a uterus who are not also taking a progestogen it should only be applied for two–three weeks and then occasionally.

HRT prevents osteoporosis. Post-menopausal women at risk of developing osteoporosis should take HRT for about ten years from the onset of the menopause. At risk are thin, white or Asian women and/or women with a family history of osteoporosis, and women who take little exercise, particularly if they smoke and/or are alcoholics.

Women under forty-five years of age who have had their womb and ovaries removed or damaged by radiotherapy will develop a premature menopause and have a high risk of developing osteoporosis. They should take oestrogen-only HRT up to sixty years of age. Pre-menopausal women who have had their womb removed but not their ovaries should also take oestrogen-only HRT. Women who have a natural menopause under the age of forty-five should take HRT. If they have a womb they should take an oestrogen and progestogen. If they have no womb they should take an oestrogen-only HRT.

HRT may possibly reduce the risk of a post-menopausal woman developing a stroke or heart attack.

Tibolone (**Livial**) produces both oestrogenic and progestogenic effects and also some weak androgenic effects. It may be taken regularly every day to relieve hot flushes, without the need of a progestogen.

Clonidine (**Dixarit**, **Catapres**) is a central acting alpha stimulant (see p. 130) that may help to relieve hot flushes.

HRT to Maintain Well-being

Other uses of HRT are much more controversial and the subject of extensive discussion in the media. Supposed benefits focus on improved well-being, looks and sexuality, and are linked to claims that HRT may slow down ageing of the skin, may help the figure by producing less shrinkage of the breasts and, by its effects on the vagina, may help to reduce discomfort during sexual intercourse which may occur at the menopause, although it does not increase libido.

HRT (Hormone Replacement Therapy) – Preparations

The main aim of HRT is to restore circulating levels of oestrogen to the average level they were at before the menopause in order to relieve menopausal symptoms and reduce the risk of osteoporosis. For women with hot flushes and dry vagina the lowest effective dose should be used for about one year (but assessed after six months). To prevent osteoporosis, treatment should be continued for five–ten years and possibly indefinitely earlier.

Sequential Combined Therapy (Monthly Bleed)

This HRT is recommended for women with a uterus. In addition to a daily oestrogen, a progestogen is added for ten–fourteen days at the end of each cycle (which is usually monthly and produces a monthly bleed). This protects the uterus from the effects of unopposed oestrogen which may cause overgrowth of the lining of the uterus and a risk of cancer. Sequential Combined Therapy may be started shortly before or during the time when menopausal changes start to develop (pre-and peri-menopausal). It may also be used in post-menopausal women but the regular monthly bleed can be a nuisance at this age and therefore continuous combined HRT offers an alternative.

Another alternative is to take Sequential Combined HRT on a three-monthly cycle (e.g. Tridestra) which will produce a bleed only every three months.

Brand	Oestrogen	Progestogen
Climagest	Estradiol tabs	Norethisterone tabs
Cyclo-Progynova	Estradiol tabs	Levonorgestrel tabs
Elleste Duet	Estradiol tabs	Norethisterone tabs
Estracombi	Estradiol patches	Norethisterone patches
Estrapak	Estradiol patches	Norethisterone tabs
Evorel Patches	Estradiol patches	Norethisterone tabs
Femapak	Estradiol patches	Dydrogesterone tabs
Femoston	Estradiol tabs	Dydrogesterone tabs
Kliovance	Estradiol tabs	Norethisterone tabs
Nuvelle	Estradiol tabs	Levonorgestrel tabs
Premique	Conj. oestrogens tabs	Medroxyprogesterone tabs
Prempak-C	Conj. oestrogens tabs	Norgestrel tabs
Tridestra*	Estradiol tabs	Medroxyprogesterone tabs
Trisequens	Estradiol/estriol tabs	Norethisterone tabs

* *Quarterly bleed*

Continuous Combined Therapy (No Monthly Bleeding)

This HRT is for post-menopausal women with a uterus who have not had a natural period for at least one year. It provides a daily dose of oestrogen *and* progestogen. During the first six months some bleeding or spotting may occur, but after about six months no periods or bleeding will occur. It is beneficial to the bones and blood fat levels, also PMS side-effects of HRT are reduced. Patients may be switched from Sequential Combined HRT to Continuous Combined HRT if they have received Sequential Combined HRT for one to two years, if they have not had a period for several months before they started Sequential Combined HRT or if they are over fifty-four years of age.

Brand	Oestrogen	Progestogen
Climesse	Estradiol tabs	Norethisterone tabs
Kliofem	Estradiol tabs	Norethisterone tabs
Premique	Conj. oestrogens tabs	Medroprogesterone tabs

Continuous Oestrogen-only Therapy (For Women Without a Uterus)

Brand	Oestrogen
Climaval	Estradiol tabs
Dermestril	Estradiol patches
Elleste Solo	Estradiol tabs
Estraderm TTS	Estradiol patches
Estraderm MX	
Evorel	Estradiol patches
Fematrix	Estradiol patches
FemSeven	Estradiol patches
Harmogen	Estrone tabs
Hormonin	Estriol/estradiol/estrone tabs
Menorest	Estradiol patches
Oestrogel	Estradiol gel
Ovestin	Estradiol tabs
Premarin	Conj. oestrogens tabs
Progynova	Estradiol tabs
Progynova TS	Estradiol patches
Sandrena	Estradiol gel
Zumenon	Estradiol tabs

Tibolone (**Livial**) tablets are used to relieve hot flushes in post-menopausal women who have not had a natural period for at least one year. It does not affect the lining of the uterus so that bleeding does not occur. It is given continuously *without* a progestogen. At present it is not approved for preventing osteoporosis.

Raloxifene (**Evista**) is used for the treatment and prevention of post-menopausal osteoporosis.

Progestogen replacement preparations include **Duphaston HRT** (dydrogesterone) tablets and **Micronor HRT** (norethisterone) tablets.

Oestrogen Vaginal Applications

Preparation	Drug	Drug Group	Dosage Form
Estring	estradiol	natural oestrogen	vaginal ring
Ortho-Gynest	estriol	natural oestrogen	cream or pessary
Ovestin	estriol	natural oestrogen	cream

Premarin vaginal cream	conjugated oestrogens	natural oestrogen	cream
Tampovagan	diethylstilbestrol and lactic acid	progestogen	pessary
Vagifem	estradiol	natural oestrogen	vaginal tablets

Premenstrual Syndrome (PMS)

Synthetic progestogens have long been tried in this disorder without much success, and it is now argued by some that natural **progesterone** should be used. In premenstrual syndrome, cyclical, physical and mental symptoms occur in relationship to times of periods and it is suggested that in this disorder the body fails to produce sufficient progesterone in the last two weeks of the menstrual cycle (the luteal phase) and therefore the treatment is to give naturally occurring progesterone. As stated earlier, because progesterone is rapidly absorbed from the intestine and broken down in the liver it has to be given by a route which avoids this 'first pass' through the liver. The routes available are by injection (**Gestone**), by suppository or vaginal pessary (**Cyclogest**), or by implant. However, there is no convincing evidence of the benefits of progesterone in PMS or its analogue, **dydrogesterone** (**Duphaston**), which can be taken by mouth. **Oral contraceptives** may relieve PMS in some women but make it worse in others.

Pyridoxine (Vitamin B$_6$)

Pyridoxine (vitamin B$_6$) is discussed in Chapter 36. It acts as a co-enzyme, the non-protein part of certain enzymes which act as catalysts for various chemical reactions in the body. Our requirements for pyridoxine increase with the amount of protein in our diet and we generally require about 2 mg daily.

With regard to PMS, claims and counter-claims for the benefits of pyridoxine are frequently made, but there is no convincing evidence of its benefits. Regular use of high doses (500 mg daily) has been associated with nerve damage, and regular daily use of 200 mg or more may produce withdrawal symptoms if the drug is stopped suddenly. The daily dose should not exceed 50 mg.

Oil of Evening Primrose, Magnesium

There is no convincing evidence from adequate and well-controlled studies that Oil of Evening Primrose or magnesium are of benefit in women with PMS.

41

Oral Contraceptive Drugs

To understand the use of oral contraceptives, read the chapter on female sex hormones. It is most important that you should understand the hormonal control of the menstrual cycle and in particular the parts played by the female sex hormones, oestrogens and progestogens.

There are three types of oral contraceptives: combined oestrogen/progestogen preparations (usually known as 'the pill'), phasic preparations containing oestrogens and progestogens and progestogen-only preparations.

The **progestogens** used in oral contraceptives make the mucus at the entrance to the womb sticky (the 'mucus plug') which prevents sperm from entering. They also help to stop ovulation by blocking LH production and they alter the lining of the womb.

The **oestrogens** used in oral contraceptives are the semi-synthetic oestrogens **ethinylestradiol** and **mestranol**. Mestranol is converted into ethinylestradiol in the body (i.e. it is a precursor of ethinylestradiol), so when we talk about oestrogens in oral contraceptives we are usually talking about ethinylestradiol. Oestrogens stop the production of FSH and therefore the follicle does not develop and ovulation is prevented.

The combined effects of an oestrogen and a progestogen are to prevent ovulation, thin the lining of the womb, block the neck of the womb with mucus and decrease the motility and secretions in the Fallopian tubes.

The Combined Oestrogen/Progestogen Oral Contraceptive – 'The Pill'

In these, the dose of **oestrogen** is usually below 0.05 mg.* Many go below this to 0.03 mg. With low-dose oestrogen pills the margin of protection is reduced and it is very important not to miss one. The dose of **progestogen** also varies but there is a much wider margin of protection.

Phasic Combined Oral Contraceptives

Instead of a fixed dose of oestrogen and progestogen to be taken each day, phasic pills contain varying doses according to the time of the month. The doses are arranged to 'mimic' the pattern of oestrogen and progestogen production by the body throughout the menstrual cycle. The pills must be taken in strict order. The dose of progestogen may vary twice in the month (biphasic) or three times (triphasic).

Progestogen-only Preparations

These are an alternative to the combined pill in women over thirty-five years who smoke and for those with raised blood pressure, valvular disease of the heart, diabetes or migraine. There is a higher failure rate than with the combined pill and menstrual irregularities are commoner. They may be used before major surgery.

How to Take Progestogen-only Preparations

These are started on the first day of the cycle and then taken at the same time (preferably several hours *before* intercourse) every day right through without missing a day.

● *Missed Pill*

If you go over you are at risk. Take the missed pill as soon as you remember and carry on with the next pill at the *right* time. If three hours' delay or over you should avoid getting pregnant by using a condom or other method for the next seven days.

● *After Childbirth*

They may be started three weeks after delivery without affecting breastfeeding.

---

* 1.0 mg = 1,000 micrograms (0.05 mg = 50 micrograms).

● *Diarrhoea and Vomiting*

You will have reduced protection. Continue the pill but use a condom or other method of contraception during and for *seven days* after you have recovered.

● *Switching from a Combined Pill to a Progestogen-only Pill*

Start straight after you finish the course – do not have a break. With ED pills (everyday preparations, see p. 208)), miss out the dummy pills.

Depot Progestogen Preparations

Medroxyprogesterone: Depo-Provera is a long-acting progestogen preparation given by intramuscular injection. One injection (150 mg/ml) provides contraception for three months. It produces similar problems to oral preparations, particularly irregular and sometimes heavy periods, and transient infertility or irregular periods after stopping treatment. It may cause heavy periods after childbirth so it should not be started for five–six weeks after delivery.

Norethisterone enantate (**Noristerat**) is a long-acting progestogen that lasts up to eight weeks. It is given in a dose of 200 mg/ml as an oily injection deep into a muscle.

Levonorgestrel intra-uterine system (**Mirena**) contains 52 mg of levonorgestrel. It lasts up to three years.

> *For adverse effects and precautions on progestogens see under progestogens in A–Z of Medicines.*

Morning-after Pills*

There are two methods of post-coital contraception: hormone pills or intra-uterine devices.

To be effective, hormonal therapy should be started within seventy-two hours of unprotected intercourse; thereafter the failure rate rises substantially above the claimed 1 per cent. Current methods involve the use of an **oestrogen/progestogen** preparation (**Schering PC4**) to be taken in two doses. (Two pills are taken immediately and two in *exactly* twelve hours.) Nausea occurs in 50–60 per cent and vomiting in 30 per cent but these symptoms are short-lived and rarely severe. Other adverse side-effects such as headaches, dizziness, breast tenderness and withdrawal bleeding may occur.

* For **abortion pill**, see mifepristone in A–Z of Medicines.

> **Note:** *If this method fails, there is a slight risk that the baby will be damaged.*

The pills must be taken *within* the first seventy-two hours (i.e. before implantation of the fertilized ovum) and a condom should be used until the next period (which may start earlier or later than expected). See your doctor after three weeks for a check-up.

If the morning-after pill (post-coital pill) is contra-indicated, then the insertion of an intra-uterine device (IUD) within the first seventy-two hours is an alternative. With post-coital IUDs, pain and abnormal bleeding may occur and there is always a risk of infection. They should not be used in young women who have not had a baby.

How to Take the Combined Oestrogen/Progestogen Oral Contraceptive ('The Pill')

● *Starting the Pill*

For convenience, the term 'the pill' refers only to the most commonly used oral contraceptive – the oestrogen/progestogen combination. The first course may be started on the first or fifth day of the menstrual period, taking the day that the period started as the first day. You then take a pill daily for twenty-one days according to the instructions on the packet, preferably at the same time each day. When you have finished the first month's course of twenty-one days you will have seven days off the pill during which time you will have a period. You then start the next course.

The packets are push-out types and the days of the week are marked so that it is easy for you to remember when you stopped and need to restart. If you have not got a good memory there are preparations available which contain seven dummy tablets. The dummy tablets are a different colour from the contraceptive pills but all you have to do, having started the first course, is to take one pill every day – you do not have to remember when to stop and when to start. They are called ED preparations (everyday preparations). If you start an ED preparation on the fifth day avoid risk of getting pregnant for fourteen days.

● *If You Miss a Pill*

If you miss a pill at the end or at the beginning of the twenty-one days you will lengthen the number of days you are not on the pill and this will reduce your protection. If you forget a pill, take it as soon as you remember and the next one at your normal time. If you are twelve or more hours late with any pill, continue normal pill-taking as soon as you remember but you must take other precautions (e.g. condom) for the next *seven days*. If these seven days run beyond the end of your packet, start the next packet – do *not* leave a gap between packets. It doesn't matter if you don't have a period until you have finished the second packet. You may also get some bleeding on the pill-taking days but don't worry. If you are on an ED packet skip the seven dummy tablets.

● If You Get Diarrhoea and Vomiting

Diarrhoea and vomiting may interfere with the absorption of the pill and reduce its effectiveness. Therefore, continue with the pill as normal *but* take other precautions (e.g. condom) during and for *seven* days after you have got better. If the diarrhoea and vomiting occur in the last seven days of your course, go straight on with your next packet (don't stop for seven days) and with ED preparations skip the seven dummy tablets.

● If You Have Surgery

The combined pill should be stopped four weeks before major surgery and all surgery on the legs. Restart *two weeks after* you are up and about. For emergency surgery you may need an anticoagulant (heparin) protection. There is no problem with progestogen-only pills.

If You Change from a High to a Low-dose Oestrogen Pill

Start immediately after you finish your packet of high-dose oestrogen pills. In other words, skip the seven days without a pill.

● If You Change from a Lower or Same-dose Oestrogen Pill

Finish your packet, have seven pill-free days and then start new packet.

● If You Want to Change from a Combined Pill to a Progestogen-only Pill

See under progestogen-only preparations.

● If You Miss a Period and are Not Pregnant

Start any day but avoid risk of getting pregnant for seven days.

● After Childbirth if You are Not Breastfeeding

Start the pill not sooner than three weeks *after* your baby was born.

● After Childbirth if You are Breastfeeding

Do not use the combined contraceptive pill (the pill). You may use a progestogen-only pill but not sooner than three weeks after your baby was born.

● If You are Taking any Other Drug

The effectiveness of both combined oral contraceptive pills (the pill) and progestogen-only pills may be *reduced* by drugs that affect the way the liver breaks down the oestrogens and progestogens in the pills. These drugs include the anti-epileptic drugs **carbamazepine**, **phenytoin**, **phenobarbitone** and **primidone**, the antifungal drug **griseofulvin** and the antibacterial drug **rifampicin**.

If you are put on a *short course* of one of these drugs, continue the pill *but* take additional contraceptive precautions (e.g. abstain or use a condom) during treatment and for seven days after treatment is stopped. If these seven days go beyond the end of the packet, start your new one the next day (skip the seven days off the pill). With ED pills skip the days you are on dummy tablets and start the active pill the day after you finished your last packet. With **rifampicin** you should avoid the risk of getting pregnant for *four weeks* after stopping, even if the course lasted for less than seven days.

If you are on long-term treatment with any of the above drugs try a high-dose oestrogen pill (e.g. ethinylestradiol 50 micrograms or more) but take it *every day* for three months without a break and then have four days' break and start again for three months. With **rifampicin** use another method of contraception. After stopping long-term treatment with any of the above drugs use alternative contraceptive methods for four to eight weeks.

Broad spectrum antibiotics (e.g. ampicillin) may reduce the effectiveness of the combined pill by knocking out bacteria in the bowel that recycle the oestrogen (ethinylestradiol). Therefore, if you are put on a short course of a broad spectrum antibiotic you should use extra contraceptive precautions (e.g. condom) while on treatment and for seven days after stopping the treatment. If these seven days go beyond the end of your packet skip the seven pill-free days and go straight on to your next packet. In the case of ED pills, skip the seven dummy tablets and start the next packet immediately. If the course of broad spectrum antibiotics lasts for two weeks or more the bacteria in the bowel become resistant to the antibiotic so you need only follow the above directions.

● Switching to Brands that Contain a Different Progestogen

When changing from a twenty-one-day pill to a twenty-one-day pill that contains a different progestogen, continue your present pill until you have taken the last tablet and then on the *next* day start your new course of pills. Take it for twenty-one days and stop for seven days, and then start the next twenty-one-day course and so on. By doing this you will not affect the contraceptive effectiveness of the pill but you may get some breakthrough bleeding in the first month on the new pill.

If you stop your twenty-one-day pill and have seven pill-free days before starting the new twenty-one-day pill containing a different progestogen you lessen the contraceptive effectiveness of the new pill in the first seven days of taking it. Therefore use *additional* precautions against getting pregnant (e.g. condom) during these seven days on the new twenty-one-day pill.

When switching from a twenty-eight-day pill (an ED brand) to a twenty-one-day pill, all the dummy pills in the red section and the last two pills of the white section (those immediately *before* the red section) of the ED brand should be omitted and the new twenty-one-day pill started *without* a break.

Contraception will not be interrupted if you do this. If you have already started taking the dummy tablets you should continue to the *end* of the twenty-eight-day course of the ED brand and the next day you should start the new twenty-one-day pill. This lessens the contraceptive effectiveness of the new pill in the first seven days of taking it, therefore use *additional* precautions (e.g. condom) during the first seven days on the new pill. If you are changing from one twenty-eight-day pill to a new twenty-eight-day pill, contraceptive effectiveness may be lessened for fourteen days therefore take *additional* precautions (e.g. condom) for fourteen days (during the seven days on the dummy tablets of the old twenty-eight-day pill and during the first seven days of the new twenty-eight-day pill).

● *Missed Periods*

If you do not have a period, carry on as normal. If you miss two periods, stop the pill and have a urine pregnancy test done. If you have been on the pill for some time and then get breakthrough bleeding between periods, stop the pill and consult your doctor.

The Pill and Thrombosis

The greatest risk from the pill is the development of a thrombosis in a vein and the shooting off of part of this clot into the lungs, leading to death. This process is called *thromboembolism* and the thrombosis usually occurs in the *deep veins* of the legs or pelvis. It may also occur in the vessels supplying the brain (cerebral thrombosis), producing a stroke.

This *very rare* risk of thrombosis is not related to how long you have been on the pill, but it is thought to be roughly proportional to the dose of synthetic oestrogen in a preparation. There is no obvious difference between mestranol and ethinylestradiol. The safety level for oestrogen appears to be about 0.05 mg and the majority of pills do not now go above this level. There is also a very slight increase in risk for women taking pills that contain the newer progestogens, **gestodene** and **desogestrel** (30 per 100,000 women per year compared with 15 per 100,000 per year for other brands). But see precautions later.

There may be an added risk in high-risk patients. See below.

Other Adverse Effects of the Pill

The pill may cause enlargement of the breasts, fluid retention, a bloated feeling, cramps and pains in the legs, depression, headache, nausea, vomiting, weight gain, loss of libido, and raised blood pressure. Contact lenses may irritate. Use of the pill may predispose to infections of the cervix, particularly by thrush (candida), and cause loss of periods in someone who has previously had irregular or scanty periods. Reduced menstrual loss may occur and 'spotting' early in the cycle. Itching vagina (pruritus vulvae) may be produced by the pill; vaginal discharge and pruritus vulvae are more likely to occur if you are given a tetracycline or other such broad-spectrum antibiotic as well, for some other infection (e.g. bronchitis). Itching of the skin may occur and some women get a brownish colour on their face (chloasma, as seen in pregnancy). Sensitivity of the skin to the sun's rays and a blistering skin rash (porphyria) on exposure to the sun may rarely occur, and some women's hair goes thin for a few months after stopping the pill. Impaired liver function and liver tumour may occur very rarely.

After stopping the pill some women fail to have a period. This is more common in women with late puberty who previously had irregular periods. It is caused by failure of the pituitary gland to recover from its suppression by the high blood levels of oestrogens and progestogens while on the pill. The hypothalamus may also not recover its full function. The lining of the uterus in these women may not respond to oestrogens produced by their own ovaries because they have been under daily influence for many months of the oestrogen and progestogen in the pill they have been taking. Loss of periods does not appear to be harmful and if a woman does not want to get pregnant there is no need to give a drug to stimulate ovulation. Remember also that after being on the pill it may take some women a few months to get pregnant, but this is not related to the length of time they were taking the pill.

The possible long-term risk of cancer of the breast, uterus, cervix or vagina needs to be considered. The study of these risks is made more difficult by the frequently prolonged delay in the development of cancer and the complicating socio-economic factors known to influence the incidence of cancers of this kind. Women taking oral contraceptives should have regular medical examinations.

Precautions

- *To reduce the risk of thrombosis do not take the pill if two or more of the following known risk factors apply to you:* smoking (avoid if over thirty-five), raised blood pressure, 50 per cent overweight, diabetes (avoid if damage to eyes or nerves), family history of stroke or heart attack particularly in a close relative under forty-five years, varicose veins (avoid if thrombosed), severe depression, long-term immobilization, sickle cell disease, inflammatory bowel disease (e.g. Crohn's). Pills containing **gestodene** or **desogestrel** should not be used in any woman at risk of developing thrombosis.
- It is best not to use the pill if you have a high blood cholesterol level (>6.5).

- You should not take the pill if you have had a previous vein or arterial thrombosis or embolism. Previous superficial thrombophlebitis is not a reason for not taking the pill, but regular medical supervision is necessary.
- Do not take the pill if you have had an attack of severe itching of the skin and/or jaundice during pregnancy.
- Do not take the pill if you have had cancer of the breast.
- Do not take the pill if you have had an acute or severe long-standing liver disorder, if you have angina or have had a heart attack or stroke, if you have porphyria, serious valvular heart disease or gallstones.
- Do not take the pill if you have attacks of severe migraine (e.g. associated with pins and needles in the hands and/or feet). An increase in the frequency or severity of headaches on the pill indicates that a medical examination is required.
- Do not take the pill if you have undiagnosed vaginal bleeding, if you are pregnant, if you have cancer that is dependent on oestrogens (e.g. some breast cancers), or if you have chorea or otosclerosis (if getting worse).
- If you are at the menopause (and being on the pill will not affect your symptoms), stop the pill for two or three months to see if a period comes on, and if it does, go back on the pill for two or three months. If you do not have a period, do not go back on the pill. But take alternative contraceptive precautions for two years if you are under fifty years of age, for one year if you are over fifty.
- If you have a family history of diabetes, then you should be cautious. But having diabetes need not stop you going on the pill, unless you have diabetic nerve or eye damage.
- If you are due for a thyroid test then stop the pill for two months before – it interferes with tests for thyroid functions.
- Be cautious when using corticosteroids (e.g. prednisolone) – they may send your blood pressure up.
- Remember that certain drugs can speed up the breakdown of the pill in the liver, see earlier.
- If you are ever in doubt, always continue to take the pill as directed but take additional precautions until the end of the month.
- Varicose veins are not considered to be a reason for not taking the pill unless thrombosis is present or during sclerosing treatment of the veins.
- Piles (haemorrhoids) are not a reason for not taking the pill.
- If you have mild or moderate raised blood pressure, your doctor should keep you under regular observation, and also if you have epilepsy, asthma, Raynaud's disease, severe depression, chronic kidney disease, multiple sclerosis, or any disease which is likely to get worse during pregnancy. If you have severe raised blood pressure do not take the pill.

- It may be best not to take the pill if you have had previous episodes of severe mental depression, but discuss this with your doctor.
- Read about breakthrough bleeding, spotting, and scanty or absent periods.
- Read what to do if you forget to take a pill.
- Check when to avoid the risk of getting pregnant.
- Young girls (under sixteen years of age) should not go on the pill until their periods have started and are occurring regularly.
- Young girls on the pill for more than nine months should stop their pill for one month and have their daily temperatures checked to see if they are ovulating. If they are, then carry on with the pill. If they are not ovulating, then they should not be on the pill and should be referred to a gynaecologist.

When to Stop the Pill Immediately

- If you get pregnant.
- If your blood pressure rises.
- Stop six weeks before a major surgical operation or when confined to bed after an accident or illness. Start two weeks after you become fully mobile.
- If you get jaundice.
- At the first signs of a thrombosis and/or embolism, e.g. sudden severe chest pain, sudden breathlessness, coughing up blood, severe pain in the calf of one leg, severe pain in the abdomen.
- If you get a migraine or severe headaches and have never previously had an attack, especially if associated with visual disturbances, vertigo, fainting, numbness and pins and needles down one side of the body.
- If you have had a migraine before and develop very severe attacks.
- If you develop severe or unusual headaches.
- If you develop acute disturbances of vision.

Changes in Menstruation

Spotting, which is a very slight show of blood between periods, is usually of no significance. Carry on with the pill since it usually clears up. If it recurs the next month consult your doctor.

Breakthrough bleeding, which is bleeding between periods like a small period, may be stopped by taking two pills a day for two or three days and then going back on the normal course. Alternatively you may continue the course and see how things are with the next month's course. If it recurs, consult your doctor. Another way is to stop the pill for seven days and then re-start another course. Whichever you choose, if breakthrough bleeding occurs two months running you must see your doctor and have a gynaecological examination which will usually include a cervical smear test. Such an examination is also necessary if spotting or breakthrough bleeding occurs for the first time after prolonged use of the pill or if it recurs at irregular intervals.

Decreased menstrual flow is nothing to worry about.

The Choice of Pill

Progestogens act on the uterus which has been subjected (primed) to the effects of **oestrogens**. Various preparations may therefore be compared by how long they can delay a period when given in equally effective doses. In this way oestrogens may also be compared and from such studies we have learnt that ethinylestradiol is about twice as potent as mestranol. Similarly, the progestogens can be ranked in order of potency (from strongest to the weakest): **norgestrel**, **etynodiol**, **norethisterone**, **megestrol**. What is more, different chemical structures of the same drug can vary; for example, levonorgestrel is about twice as potent as norgestrel.

In the body the ratio of oestrogens to progesterone is delicately balanced to produce optimum chances of getting pregnant. Some women may produce too much oestrogen and therefore have heavy, frequent periods whereas others may produce too much progesterone and suffer from scanty and irregular periods. Both these groups of women do not produce the ideal balance of hormones to encourage conception and they may therefore be sub-fertile. It follows, therefore, that if an oestrogen is given to some women it may produce heavier periods whereas progestogens, in some women, may produce scanty periods or even absent periods if given in sufficient dosage (the principle of preparations used to delay the onset of menstruation). When the drugs are stopped, withdrawal bleeding will occur. Now it can be seen that the effects produced by oestrogens can be balanced by adding progestogens. As the doses of these increase, the risk of pregnancy gets less. But, unfortunately, adverse effects start to increase. High doses of oestrogens will produce the adverse effects mentioned earlier, as will increasing the dosage of progestogens. Thus there is a spectrum of effects and adverse effects produced by the various combination oestrogen/progestogen pills. Therefore, a pill should be chosen for you which takes into account how heavy and regular your periods were and its potential for producing adverse effects in *you*. Reread this chapter and the section on female hormones and make a note of the facts which apply particularly to *you*; for example, whether you previously had scanty periods or heavy periods, whether you are overweight or smoke, whether you have had a previous thrombosis, whether you have previously had some episodes of depressed mood, what adverse effects you have felt on certain contraceptive preparations, and so on. Remember, you may be on the pill for many years; it is most important for you and your doctor to choose the pill which suits *you* and it is no use your doctor fixing his mind on one particular brand-named product and prescribing it for everybody who wishes to take an oral contraceptive.

Abortion Pill

See under **mifepristone** in A–Z of Medicines.

Oral Contraceptive Drugs

Combined Oestrogen and Progestogen Pills – Fixed Doses

Name	Oestrogen: Dose		Progestogen: Dose	
Norinyl-1	mestranol	(0·05 mg)	norethisterone	(1·0 mg)
Ovran	ethinylestradiol	(0·05 mg)	levonorgestrel	(0·25 mg)
Brevinor	ethinylestradiol	(0·035 mg)	norethisterone	(0·5 mg)
Cilest	ethinylestradiol	(0·035 mg)	norgestimate	(0·25 mg)
Norimin	ethinylestradiol	(0·035 mg)	norethisterone	(1·0 mg)
Ovysmen	ethinylestradiol	(0·035 mg)	norethisterone	(0·5 mg)
Eugynon 30	ethinylestradiol	(0·03 mg)	levonorgestrel	(0·25 mg)
Femodene*	ethinylestradiol	(0·03 mg)	gestodene	(0·075 mg)
Loestrin 30	ethinylestradiol	(0·03 mg)	norethisterone	(1·5 mg)
Marvelon	ethinylestradiol	(0·03 mg)	desogestrel	(0·15 mg)
Microgynon 30*	ethinylestradiol	(0·03 mg)	levonorgestrel	(0·15 mg)
Minulet	ethinylestradiol	(0·03 mg)	gestodene	(0·075 mg)
Ovran 30	ethinylestradiol	(0·03 mg)	levonorgestrel	(0·25 mg)
Ovranette	ethinylestradiol	(0·03 mg)	levonorgestrel	(0·15 mg)
Femodette	ethinylestradiol	(0·02 mg)	gestodene	(0·075 mg)
Loestrin 20	ethinylestradiol	(0·02 mg)	norethisterone	(1·0 mg)
Mercilon	ethinylestradiol	(0·02 mg)	desogestrel	(0·15 mg)

*Femodene ED as for Femodene and Microgynon 30 ED – twenty-one active tablets plus seven dummy tablets – take one every day for twenty-eight days.

> *Note: Pills containing the newer progestogens, **desogestrel**, and **gestodene** increase the risk of venous thrombosis from fifteen cases per 100,000 women per year to thirty cases per 100,000 women per year. The pills that contain one or other of these are **Femodene**, **Marvelon**, **Minulet**, **Mercilon** and **Triadene**.*

Combined Oestrogen and Progestogen Pills – Biphasic and Triphasic Doses

Name	Oestrogen: Dose	Progestogen:Dose
BiNovum	ethinylestradiol 0·035 mg	norethisterone 0·500 mg – 7 tablets
	0·035 mg	norethisterone 1·000 mg – 14 tablets
Logynon*	ethinylestradiol 0·030 mg	levonorgestrel 0·050 mg – 6 tablets
	0·040 mg	levonorgestrel 0·075 mg – 5 tablets
	0·030 mg	levonorgestrel 0·125 mg – 10 tablets
Synphase	ethinylestradiol 0·035 mg	norethisterone 0·500 mg – 7 tablets
	0·035 mg	norethisterone 1·000 mg – 9 tablets
	0·035 mg	norethisterone 0·500 mg – 5 tablets
Tri-Minulet	ethinylestradiol 0·030 mg	gestodene 0·050 mg – 6 tablets
	0·040 mg	gestodene 0·070 mg – 5 tablets
	0·030 mg	gestodene 0·100 mg – 10 tablets
Triadene	ethinylestradiol 0·030 mg	gestodene 0·050 mg – 6 tablets
	0·040 mg	gestodene 0·070 mg – 5 tablets
	0·030 mg	gestodene 0·100 mg 10 tablets
Trinordiol	ethinylestradiol 0·030 mg	levonorgestrel 0·050 mg – 6 tablets
	0·040 mg	levonorgestrel 0·075 mg – 5 tablets
	0·030 mg	levonorgestrel 0·125 mg – 10 tablets
TriNovum	ethinylestradiol 0·035 mg	norethisterone 0·500 mg – 7 tablets
	0·035 mg	norethisterone 0·750 mg – 7 tablets
	0·035 mg	norethisterone 1·000 mg – 7 tablets

* Logynon ED as for Logynon and Trinovum ED as for Trinovum – twenty-one active tablets plus seven dummy tablets – take one each day for twenty-eight days.

Progestogen-only Preparations

Name	Progestogen	Dose
Depo-Provera	medroxyprogesterone	50 mg and 150 mg/1 ml (depot injection)
Femulen	etynodiol	0·5 mg tablets
Implanon	etonogestrel	68 mg implant
Micronor	norethisterone	0·35 mg tablets
Microval	levonorgestrel	0·03 mg tablets
Mirena	levonorgestrel intra-uterine system	52 mg/system

Neogest	norgestrel	0·075 mg tablets
Norgeston	levonorgestrel	0·03 mg tablets
Noriday	norethisterone	0·35 mg tablets
Noristerat	norethisterone	200 mg/1 ml (depot injection)

Warning: *There has been reported a possible association between the progestogen content of the combined pill ('the pill') and cancer of the breast and cancer of the cervix.*

42

Drugs Used to Treat Diabetes

Diabetes is the term used to refer to diabetes mellitus, which is a disorder characterized by a deficiency or diminished effectiveness of insulin, a hormone produced by the pancreas and responsible for lowering the blood glucose level by encouraging the take-up of glucose into cells to produce energy. Insulin also stimulates the conversion of glucose into a substance called glycogen for storage in muscles and in the liver for future use, and the storage of fat in fat tissue. It also influences the body's use of protein.

There are many factors which contribute to these processes but, very simply, diabetes may be regarded as either a disorder which results in too little insulin production by the pancreas for the body's requirements or a disorder in which the insulin it produces is not effective in carrying out these processes, or both. The results are that glucose removal from the blood is reduced and the release of glucose into the blood by the liver is increased. Thus, glucose is over-produced and under-used, resulting in a high blood glucose level – hyperglycaemia.

High blood glucose levels may result in glucose appearing in the urine because the kidneys cannot cope with the high concentrations; this results in an increased volume of urine leading to salt and water loss and thirst. Because the diabetic patient is unable to use the glucose in the blood, fat is mobilized and used for energy. This results in an increased amount of fat breakdown products accumulating in the blood, producing what is called ketosis and an alteration in the acidity of the blood. These chemical changes may cause coma and death if untreated. In addition, protein is also broken down, which produces wasting of muscles and loss of weight.

Many factors influence the development and progress of diabetes; for example, hereditary factors, age, gender, weight, infections, stress and physical disorders. Its treatment is difficult but rewarding and should always be in the hands of experts. Successful treatment of diabetes should be a joint effort between doctor and patient; this gives a good example of how important it is for the patient to know what is wrong, to know about the drugs prescribed, to know the effects and adverse effects of these drugs, to know when to adjust the dosage, and to know what other drugs to take and not to take.

Diabetes may be separated into two general disease syndromes (a syndrome being a group of signs and symptoms caused by a disease).

Type I or insulin-dependent diabetes mellitus (IDDM) occurs in people with little or no ability to produce insulin. These individuals develop high blood glucose levels and other chemical changes that produce severe symptoms unless they are treated with insulin. They are absolutely dependent upon insulin treatment for their survival. This most severe form of the disease usually appears in people under thirty-five years of age, particularly between childhood and adulthood (ten–sixteen years of age).

Type II or non-insulin-dependent diabetes mellitus (NIDDM) occurs mostly in people over forty years of age whose pancreas still has the ability to make insulin, but they appear to be resistant to insulin and they have a reduced ability to burn off calories, which predisposes them to become overweight. Insulin treatment is not essential for their survival and they do not develop the serious chemical changes which develop in insulin-dependent patients.

The Drug Treatment of Diabetes

In addition to diet, there are two main approaches to the treatment of diabetes – insulin by injection or blood glucose lowering drugs by mouth. The latter are called oral anti-diabetic drugs or oral hypoglycaemic drugs (hypoglycaemia meaning low blood glucose).

Insulin

Preparations of insulin must be given by injection because it is inactivated when given by mouth. In everyday treatment it is injected under the skin (into different sites). Insulin pumps are available to provide continuous subcutaneous (under the skin) injections. In an emergency (e.g. diabetic coma) insulin is injected into a vein or muscle. An enzyme called insulinase, found mainly in the liver, is responsible for its breakdown in the body.

Insulin production by the pancreas is principally regulated by the blood glucose level but many other factors may also affect its production and breakdown.

Insulin is used to treat *insulin-dependent diabetes*. It may also be used to treat *non-insulin-dependent diabetes* in individuals in whom no improvement has been obtained in response to diet control and oral anti-diabetic drugs. Insulin by injection will also be necessary in pregnancy and in non-insulin-dependent patients when they have a severe infection or are undergoing surgery. At these times – during infections, injury or surgery – the body normally requires more insulin.

Initial treatment with insulin should always be carried out in hospital, where repeated estimations of blood sugar levels may be made. Where appropriate, patients are shown how to give themselves their own injections of insulin and they should be allowed to experience the effects of an underdose and overdose and how to correct these. This process is known as stabilization: it is most important and should not be hurried. The patient is ready for discharge when the most appropriate dosage regimen of insulin for controlling the symptoms, blood sugar levels and the amount of sugar in the urine has been worked out. But patients should not be discharged until they understand their diet, how to give themselves their injection (if appropriate), test the blood and/or urine for sugar and when and how to increase the dose as required.

The choice of insulin preparation will depend on many factors and in particular on the duration of action of the various preparations available.

Injected insulin is rapidly inactivated by the liver, and therefore much work has gone into making insulin injections long-acting by ensuring their slow absorption into the bloodstream from their injection sites.

A large number of insulin preparations are available. They include extracts from the pancreatic glands of cows (*beef insulins*) and from pigs (*pork insulins*), and synthetic (*human insulins*) which are chemically modified pork insulins or are bio-engineered using DNA technology.

In addition to being grouped according to their origin, insulins may also be grouped according to their duration of action – *short-acting* (e.g. acid and neutral soluble insulins), *intermediate-acting* (e.g. insulin zinc suspension and isophane insulin) and *long-acting* (e.g. Human Ultratard). *Biphasic preparations* are also available which contain stable mixtures of a short-acting and an intermediate or long-acting preparation.

● *Intermediate and Long-acting Insulin Preparations*

By altering the acidity and adding zinc to insulin suspensions the zinc combines with the insulin to produce larger particles which, after injection, act as a depot to produce a slow release of insulin. These preparations are called **insulin zinc suspensions (IZS)** or **lente insulins** (*lente* meaning 'slow'). The size of particles determines the speed of action. **Amorphous IZS** has an intermediate duration of action (**semi-lente**). **Crystalline IZS** has a prolonged duration of action (**ultra-lente**). When the two types are mixed a preparation with an intermediate duration of action is produced (**lente insulin**).

Another method of making insulin act over a longer period is to add protamine (a protein obtained from fish sperm) to a suspension of insulin. The protamine and insulin form a complex which is much less soluble and from which insulin is slowly released after injection. The duration of action of this complex may be further prolonged by adding zinc to form **Protamine**

Zinc Insulin (PZI). However, its use is complicated by the hazard that if the blood glucose is controlled through the daytime it may fall too low during the night and early morning. Attempts to balance this effect lead to the combined use of PZI and soluble insulin. The combined effects provide sufficient cover during the day without too high a dose of Protamine Zinc Insulin working on through the night. They should not be mixed in the same syringe because excess protamine in the PZI may attach itself to the soluble insulin. Such a combination is still needed in some severe diabetics but its use has generally been replaced by the lente insulins. Some patients may be allergic to protamine and an alternative protein preparation is available – **Globin Zinc Suspension** – but this also causes allergic reactions. A preparation containing less protamine and zinc called **Isophane Insulin** is also available.

By means of chromatographical separation, impurities from the pancreas are removed from insulin preparations, thus reducing the risk of antibody formation against the insulin which has hitherto greatly impaired its effectiveness. These are called **highly purified insulins**.

Human Insulins

Human insulins are not obtained from humans, they are manufactured in laboratories by using enzymes to modify the protein structure of pork insulin (enzyme-modified pork insulins: emp); by genetic engineering using pork insulins (pork recombinant insulin: prb); and by genetic engineering using yeast cells and pork insulin (pyr). Like beef and pork insulins, human insulin preparations may be short-acting (about eight hours with a peak at one–two hours) and include both neutral and acid formulations. When formulated with zinc and/or protamine, preparations of human insulin may be intermediate or long-acting (up to thirty-five hours with an onset of action in one–four hours). In addition, mixtures are available containing neutral human insulin and isophane insulins which give a two-stage response (biphasic response).

It is important to note that all insulin preparations, whether pork, beef or human, can very rarely produce allergic reactions, and human insulin appears to be no safer in this respect than pork insulins. The risk is greatest with beef insulins.

> **Warning:** Care should be taken when changing a patient from animal insulins to human insulins, *because there is usually a reduced insulin need, and therefore an increased risk of hypoglycaemia. Furthermore, the early warning signs of a 'hypo' attack may not be as evident.*

In treating diabetes expert advice is needed on the choice of insulin preparation, the dose and timing of injections, and the time of meals. In addition a patient needs expert advice on diet, weight, smoking and exercise.

● Adverse Effects of Insulin

The commonest adverse effect of insulin treatment is hypoglycaemia or low blood sugar. This happens when a patient receives too much insulin. This may occasionally occur if a patient misses out a meal or eats a diet lacking sufficient carbohydrates. The early symptoms are weakness, giddiness, pallor, sweating, increased production of saliva in the mouth, sinking feeling in the stomach, palpitations, irritability and trembling. If these are not immediately relieved by taking a glucose sweet or sugar the patient may develop changes in mood, be unable to concentrate, lack judgement and lose self-control. Loss of memory, paralysis, double vision, pins and needles in the hands and feet, unconsciousness, convulsions and death may occur. Every diabetic patient should be allowed to experience the early warning effects of hypoglycaemia and then be taught the correct treatment to prevent an attack coming on. If a patient is unable to understand these instructions, then the nearest relative or friend should be instructed.

Local reactions may occur at the site of injections, resulting in wasting of the fatty tissue under the skin; alternatively, fatty swellings (lipomata) may rarely occur. Rotation of injection sites can help prevent these complications.

An immune reaction to insulin may rarely occur, resulting in a dramatic increase in the amount of insulin required. The insulin becomes 'neutralized' and less effective. This reaction is commoner with beef insulin than with pork insulin. Certain glandular disorders may increase sensitivity to insulin (e.g. underworking of the pituitary gland or adrenal gland), resulting in low blood glucose level.

● Interaction with Other Drugs

Oral contraceptives, diuretics, corticosteroids, MAOI antidepressants, beta-blockers and alcohol may affect the control of the blood sugar level. Beta-blockers may also *mask* the early symptoms of hypoglycaemia.

If you are on insulin you should carry a warning card saying that you are a diabetic and giving the name and dose of the insulin preparation you are taking. The card should state that if you are found behaving strangely you should be given sugar by mouth.

● Short-acting Insulins

Humalog (insulin lispro)
NovoRapid (insulin aspart)
Neutral Insulins (soluble insulins)
Human Actrapid and **Human Actrapid Penfill** (human, highly purified)
Human Velosulin (human, highly purified)
Humulin S (human, highly purified)
Insuman Rapid (human, highly purified)
Hypurin Bovine Neutral (beef, highly purified)

Hypurin Porcine Neutral (pork, highly purified)
Pork Actrapid (pork, highly purified)

● *Biphasic Insulins*
Human Mixtard preparations (human, highly purified: neutral soluble and isophane insulins in varying concentrations)
Insuman Comb (human, highly purified: neutral soluble and isophane insulins in varying concentrations)
Humulin preparations (human, highly purified: soluble and isophane insulins in varying concentrations)
Pork Mixtard 30 (isophane insulin; pork, highly purified 70%, neutral insulin; pork, highly purified 30%)

● *Intermediate and Long-acting Insulins*
Insulin Zinc Suspension (mixed)
    Insulin Zinc Suspension; mixed; IZS Lente (beef, highly purified)
    Human Monotard (human, highly purified)
    Humulin Lente (human, highly purified)
    Hypurin Bovine Lente (beef, highly purified)
    Lentard MC (beef (30%) and pork (70%), highly purified)
Insulin Zinc Suspension (crystalline)
    Human Ultratard (human, highly purified)
    Human Zn (human, highly purified)
    Hypurin Porcine Biphasic Isophane (isophane insulin; pork, highly purified 70%, neutral insulin; pork, highly purified 30%)
Isophane insulins
    Isophane (beef, highly purified)
    Human Insulatard (human, highly purified)
    Humulin I (human, highly purified)
    Insuman Basal (human, highly purified)
    Hypurin Bovine Isophane (beef, highly purified)
    Hypurin Porcine Isophane (pork, highly purified)
    Pork Insulatard (pork, highly purified)
Protamine Zinc Insulin
    Hypurin Bovine Protamine Zinc (beef, highly purified)

Oral Hypoglycaemic Drugs

Oral hypoglycaemic drugs are taken by mouth to produce a fall in blood glucose. They are used to treat non-insulin-dependent diabetes when strict dieting for at least three months has failed to control the blood glucose level. They should be used along with a strict diet and not in place of a diet. They include:

The Sulphonylureas and Related Drugs

It is thought that these drugs lower blood glucose levels by acting on the pancreas to secrete more insulin. They also have a direct effect upon the liver and potentiate the action of insulin throughout the body. They are only effective in the presence of some pancreatic function and they do not affect the take-up and release of glucose by muscles. But their action may be much more complicated than is generally thought. Their rate of breakdown in the body varies and this affects their duration of action.

The sulphonylureas include **chlorpropamide**, **glibenclamide** (**Daonil, Diabet-amide, Euglucon, Gliken, Semi-Daonil**), **gliclazide** (**Diamicron, DIAGLYK**), **glimepiride** (**Amaryl**), **glipizide** (**Glibenese, Minodiab**), **gliquidone** (**Glurenorm**) and **tolbutamide**. There is no evidence of differences in their effectiveness and all of them may produce hypoglycaemia (fall in blood glucose), particularly in the elderly and those with impaired kidney or liver function. Some patients taking chlorpropamide suffer from facial burning and flushing very shortly after drinking alcohol. This reaction to alcohol may be inherited. It also occurs with tolbutamide and rarely with glibenclamide.

Sulphonylureas tend to encourage an increase in weight. They should not be used in obese diabetics unless they have been on a strict diet and lost weight nearly down to the normal weight for their gender and age (at least within 15 per cent of that weight). Those sulphonylureas that are principally broken down in the liver should be used in patients with impaired kidney function, e.g. gliquidone, gliclazide or a short-acting one such as tolbutamide. These should also be used in elderly patients.

Biguanides

The only available biguanide is **metformin** (**Glucamet, Glucophage**). It only works if some insulin is being produced by the pancreas. It increases glucose uptake by cells in the presence of insulin and it reduces the release of glucose by the liver. It may reduce absorption of carbohydrates from the intestine and it also produces a loss of weight in overweight diabetics.

Metformin should not be given to patients with congestive heart failure or to those patients with impaired kidney or liver function. It should not be used in pregnancy. Alcohol should be used with caution by patients taking metformin. Changes in the acidity of the blood (lactic acidosis) may be produced by metformin in patients with impaired function of their kidneys, by whom it should not be used. Hypoglycaemia is not usually a problem with metformin and weight gain occurs less frequently than with the sulphonylureas.

> **Warnings:** *The blood sugar lowering effects of oral hypoglycaemic drugs may be increased by alcohol, aspirin, phenylbutazone, sulphonamides and monoamine oxidase inhibitors. Corticosteroid drugs may increase blood sugar levels, so may oral contraceptive drugs and thiazide diuretics. Therefore, caution is necessary when using these drugs in patients who are receiving oral hypoglycaemic drugs.*
>
> *In patients taking oral hypoglycaemic drugs insulin should be used during acute injury, infection or surgery and during pregnancy.*
>
> *Oral hypoglycaemic drugs should not be used to treat diabetic emergencies (ketoacidosis).*

Guar Gum

Guar gum (**Guarem**) if taken in large enough quantities can result in some reduction of blood glucose levels after meals. It probably works by retarding carbohydrate absorption from the gastro-intestinal tract. It may cause a lot of wind and it is important to maintain an adequate intake of fluid.

Other Anti-diabetic Drugs

Acarbose (**Glucobay**) blocks a digestive enzyme and delays the absorption of sugars from carbohydrates in the intestine. This prevents the rise in blood sugar level that occurs after a carbohydrate meal.

Repaglinide (**Novonorm**) stimulates the release of insulin. It acts fast and has a short duration of activity. It should be taken shortly before a meal.

Nateglinide (**Starlix**) is used in combination with metformin in Type II diabetes inadequately controlled by metformin alone.

Rosiglitazone (**Avandia**) and **pioglitazone** (**Actos**) are used in combination with metformin or with a sulphonylurea for type II diabetes mellitus not controlled by metformin or a sulphonylurea alone.

> *Adverse effects and precautions of oral anti-diabetic drugs are listed in the A–Z of Medicines.*

43

Drugs Used to Treat Thyroid Disorders

Functions of the Thyroid Gland

The thyroid gland lies in the neck in front of and on both sides of the wind-pipe (trachea). It produces two hormones called levothyroxine(thyroxine) and tri-iodothyronine. These hormones are responsible for controlling the metabolism (use of energy) of the cells in the body. The thyroid gland is under control of the master gland (pituitary gland) which produces a thyroid-stimulating hormone (thyrotropic hormone). If there is a deficiency of thyroid hormones in the blood, the pituitary increases its stimulation of the thyroid gland. The reverse happens if there is an increase of thyroid hormones in the blood.

Disorders of the Thyroid Gland

Goitre

A simple enlargement of the thyroid gland is called a goitre and it is the body's response to a deficiency of thyroid hormone production. This deficiency, as stated previously, results in the pituitary gland producing an increased amount of thyroid-stimulating hormone which causes the thyroid gland to enlarge in an attempt to produce more hormone. Because iodine is necessary for the production of thyroid hormones, enlargement (goitre) may occur if the diet is deficient in iodine. This condition may occur in certain areas well away from the sea, where water supplies lack iodine and sea foods rich in iodine are scarce. Some drugs may interfere with thyroid hormone production, e.g. para-amino-salicylic acid and sulphonamides. Iodine mixtures taken for coughs may produce thyroid enlargement and the gland may enlarge during certain periods of increased demand, e.g. puberty, pregnancy, breastfeeding.

Whatever the cause of simple goitre, the deficiency of thyroid hormone leads to an increase in size of the gland.

The treatment of goitre is to give a synthetic thyroid hormone in order to reduce the amount of thyroid-stimulating hormone being produced by the pituitary, and therefore to reduce the size of the gland.

Underworking of the Thyroid Gland

Underworking of the thyroid gland or hypothyroidism may be congenital. The baby is born with some defect of the thyroid gland and the lack of thyroid hormones affects the baby's mental and physical development, producing a group of characteristics called cretinism. Rarely, underworking of the thyroid gland may occur during childhood; more frequently it occurs in adult life, particularly in patients who have received treatment for an over-active gland. Hypothyroidism results in a slowing-down of all metabolic processes in the body. It may be associated with a thick, pale swelling of the skin which is called myxoedema.

Disorders of the thyroid gland associated with under-production of thyroid hormones include cretinism, juvenile myxoedema, adult hypothyroidism, adult myxoedema. The treatment of these disorders is to give synthetic thyroid hormones in order to replace the hormones which the gland is incapable of producing.

Synthetic Thyroid Hormones

Levothyroxine(thyroxine) Sodium (Eltroxin)

The sodium salt of levothyroxine(thyroxine) is soluble and may be given by mouth. It is considered to be the drug of choice in most thyroid deficiency disorders. Because of its delayed effects, the starting dose must be small and the dose then slowly increased at two-weekly intervals until the required response is obtained. At the start of treatment levothyroxine(thyroxine) may produce rapid beating of the heart, anginal pain in patients with coronary artery disease, and muscle cramps. Too large a dose may cause restlessness, excitement, irregular heart rhythm, headache, flushing, sweating, diarrhoea, excessive loss of weight and muscle weakness, and may affect the heart. These symptoms are usually temporary and related to dose. Levothyroxine(thyroxine) should be used with caution in patients with heart disease and in elderly patients.

Liothyronine Sodium (Tertroxin, Tri-iodothyronine)

This produces similar effects to levothyroxine(thyroxine) but it is not so long-acting. It is used when a more rapid effect is required. It should not be given to patients with angina or heart disorders. In emergencies it can be given by intravenous injection.

Overworking of the Thyroid Gland (Hyperthyroidism, Thyrotoxicosis)

This occurs more frequently in women than in men, and usually in early adult life. But it is not uncommon in later life when its features differ from those seen in the younger person. The cause is unknown. It produces many symptoms which include nervousness, tiredness, sweating, trembling, diarrhoea, breathlessness, enlargement of the thyroid gland in some patients but not in others, prominence of the eyes, heart disorders, increase of appetite and yet loss of weight.

The treatment is to give anti-thyroid drugs, or to remove part of the gland by surgery, or to knock it out by using radioactive iodine. None of these treatments has any effect upon the underlying cause of the disorder, but they do effectively prevent the consequences of overstimulation of the gland (and therefore the body) until a natural remission occurs.

Anti-thyroid Drugs

Anti-thyroid drugs are of particular use in children, young adults, pregnant women and patients with mild overworking of their thyroid glands. Treatment should continue for up to two years and there is a need for constant supervision by a specialist in thyroid disorders.

Anti-thyroid drugs interfere with the production of thyroid hormones by the thyroid gland and control may be achieved by observing changes in the patient's symptoms and by measuring the pulse rate and body weight. It is customary to start with high doses and then slowly reduce the daily dose to a satisfactory maintenance level. There are two drugs used to suppress thyroid function: **carbimazole** (**Neo-Mercazole**) and **propylthiouracil**.

Cross-allergy between the two drugs is uncommon so that one of them may be substituted for the other if the patient develops a skin rash and/or itching. They may very rarely knock out production of white blood cells and an early warning of this complication is a sore throat and fever. This is more common in the first few weeks of treatment. If these symptoms develop, a white blood count should be carried out and if low the drug should be stopped.

The dose of anti-thyroid drugs should be given once daily. It takes up to two months before the patient feels the benefit of treatment. In too large a dose they can produce hypothyroidism which may cause enlargement of the gland. They also increase the blood supply to the gland, which may produce problems if the gland is surgically removed.

Anti-thyroid drugs do not alter the disease process, they simply control symptoms until natural remission occurs. They may be combined with a small dose of levothyroxine(thyroxine), which is called blocking-replacement treatment.

Anti-thyroid drugs can be used in *pregnancy* but they may cause goitre or underworking of the thyroid gland in the baby. *Breastfeeding* mothers may take anti-thyroid drugs but they enter the breast milk and therefore the baby must be carefully monitored.

Beta-blockers (e.g. **propranolol**) are of value in relieving the symptoms of thyrotoxicosis (tremor, rapid heart beat, etc.) in preparation for surgery, while awaiting the effects of anti-thyroid drugs or radioactive iodine therapy, and in the treatment of thyrotoxic crises when a beta-blocker may be given intravenously with hydrocortisone and iodine and an anti-thyroid drug by mouth.

Iodine and **iodides** cause shrinking of overworking goitres (toxic goitres), but this effect is transient and is only used before surgery and in emergencies.

Radioactive Iodine Therapy

When given in a solution by mouth **radioactive iodine** is absorbed from the intestine and concentrates in the thyroid gland where it emits primary beta radiation causing local destruction of the thyroid gland. It is the treatment of choice in patients over about forty-five years of age, although it is increasingly being used to treat patients of all ages. It is also used to treat patients who have relapsed after surgery, and in those patients in whom the prolonged use of anti-thyroid drugs is contra-indicated, e.g. patients with heart disease. It should not be used in pregnancy, for the treatment of children and women of childbearing age. There is no evidence of an increased risk of thyroid cancer or leukaemia after radioactive iodine therapy. The dose is difficult to predict, response is variable, and there is a high incidence of hypothyroidism (underworking) produced by treatment.

Surgery (Partial Thyroidectomy)

Indications for surgery vary between countries and between individual doctors. It is the treatment of choice for a toxic nodular goitre, a large goitre, and in patients under the age of forty-five who relapse after drug therapy. Patients should receive a course of anti-thyroid drugs and beta-blockers to prepare them for surgery.

44

Local Anaesthetics

Local anaesthetics are drugs which block the transmission of sensory impulses in nerve tissues when applied locally in appropriate concentrations. Their effects are reversible and they are used to produce loss of pain without loss of nervous control – they could be called local pain-relievers. However, they can produce loss of nervous control (paralysis) if injected directly into a nerve fibre. Those local anaesthetics in common use have been selected because they do not irritate the tissues to which they are applied and they cause no permanent nerve damage. They are soluble in water and the solutions can be sterilized. Their choice depends upon the speed with which they work, their duration of action and their potential adverse effects when absorbed into the bloodstream. The latter is important since they may affect all nervous tissues including the brain.

Local anaesthetics block the physio-chemical processes which are responsible for nerve impulses developing and passing along nerves to the brain. Their effects quickly wear off when removed from their site of action and most of them cause dilation of blood vessels. Therefore, it is customary to mix a local anaesthetic with a drug which closes off the blood supply (vaso-constrictor drug), thus delaying the 'washing' of the local anaesthetic into the bloodstream. The drug used for this purpose is adrenaline(epinephrine). Its use is not without danger; for example, if the mixture is used to block pain in a finger, the constriction of blood vessels may so affect the circulation as to cause gangrene. Therefore, local anaesthetic preparations that contain adrenaline(epinephrine) should not be used near terminal arteries as in the fingers, toes, ears, nose and penis.

Adverse Effects and Precautions

Local anaesthetics are absorbed into the bloodstream and high blood levels may produce stimulation and then depression of the brain. This may cause anxiety, restlessness, yawning, nausea, vomiting, twitching, convulsions, coma and death. Pallor, sweating, a fall in blood pressure, irregular heart rhythm, heart failure and respiratory failure may also occur, producing sudden collapse and death. Repeated local use of some local anaesthetics (e.g. amethocaine, benzocaine, cocaine, procaine) may cause allergic reactions such as skin rashes, asthma and anaphylactic shock. They should be given with utmost caution to patients with impaired heart or liver function. Adverse effects are reduced by adding vasoconstrictor drugs. When applied to the eye, the protective blink reflex is lost and particles blown into the eye can damage the cornea; therefore a protection (for half a day) should always be worn over an eye that has had anaesthetic drops applied. They should not be injected into inflamed or infected tissues.

Local anaesthetics may be administered in several different ways according to the drug being used. *Surface* or *topical anaesthesia* (as a solution, jelly or lozenge) blocks pain in nerve endings in the skin or mucous membranes and to do this the local anaesthetic must have good powers of penetration.

Local or *infiltration anaesthesia* is produced by *injection* into the area. To be effective the drug must not be absorbed too quickly into the bloodstream, otherwise its effects wear off.

Injections of local anaesthetics are also used to produce *regional nerve block* to cut off pain sensation in an area, e.g. a *nerve block* as used by dentists.

Epidural anaesthesia is a nerve block produced by injecting the anaesthetic into the space between the lining membranes of the spinal cord (used in childbirth).

Caudal anaesthesia is an injection into the space between the lining membranes at the lower end of the spinal cord where the main nerves from the spinal cord run together before leaving the spine to supply the pelvis and legs.

Spinal anaesthesia is produced by injecting the local anaesthetic inside the covering membrane of the spinal cord, causing temporary paralysis of the nerves with which it comes into contact. The area affected is determined by the specific gravity of the drug (i.e. the rate at which it drops down the fluid inside the spinal cord) and by tipping the patient up or down according to the area which is to be anaesthetized. It can be used in patients who are not suitable for a general anaesthetic.

The choice of local anaesthetic depends upon many factors, but in particular upon the risk of absorption and the production of dangerous adverse effects.

Examples of the Use of Local Anaesthetics

Injectable local anaesthetics in common use include **bupivacaine** (**Marcain**), **levobupivacaine** (**Chirocaine**), **lidocaine**(lignocaine) (**Xylocaine**), **prilocaine** (**Citanest**) and **ropivacaine** (**Naropin**). **Procaine** is seldom used. **Tetracaine** (amethocaine) (**Ametop**) is principally used as a surface anaesthetic in solution (e.g. eye drops) and in lozenges to relieve a sore throat. **Benzocaine** is used in lozenges for sore throats and in ointments used to treat haemorrhoids. **Cocaine** solutions are used for application to the nose, throat, eyes and larynx before local surgery. Other local anaesthetics included in eye drops are **lidocaine** (lignocaine), **oxybuprocaine** and **proxymetacaine**.

45

Drugs Used to Treat Skin Disorders

Drugs Used in Skin Applications

We know surprisingly little about the causes of many common skin disorders, for example eczema and psoriasis. Against such a background of ignorance it is not surprising that there are many myths about treatment and where there are many claimed treatments for a particular disorder there often is no specific treatment – otherwise we would all know about it and use it. This applies particularly to skin disorders.

However, we have seen great advances in the specific and effective cure of many infective skin disorders (see antibiotic and antifungal drugs). We have also seen the introduction of the corticosteroids, which have revolutionized the relief of many skin disorders. Other old-fashioned treatments continue, for example tar and dithranol, etc., and others such as the antihistamines have not produced the results hoped for, except in their specific and effective use by mouth in allergic rashes, particularly those due to drugs. Many skin treatments remain non-specific and at the very least they should not make the disorder worse. Yet the widespread use of antihistamines, local anaesthetics, antibiotics and antiseptics in skin applications have led to the production of allergic rashes, and the inappropriate use of corticosteroids has led to other problems (p. 241).

In the treatment of skin disorders the danger is that skin preparations containing potent drugs may be applied in too large a quantity to too large an area too often and over too long a period of time. You should be as sensible about applying drugs to the skin as you should be about taking drugs by mouth. Know what you are treating, know what you are applying and know the benefits and risks.

There are numerous skin applications available – creams, ointments, lotions, dusting powders, sprays, pastes. They are used for treating skin disorders in different stages of severity and in different areas of the body. For example, *lotions* (watery solutions) are used in acute skin conditions and where the skin is unbroken. Watery lotions act by evaporation and cool the skin. When used, they should be applied frequently. The addition of alcohol to a skin lotion increases its cooling effects. Lotions are useful for applying a drug in a thin layer over a large surface or on hairy areas of the skin. When the skin is broken an *astringent* (p. 247) may be included, as it helps to seal the weeping surface of the skin. *Shake lotions* are used for scabbed and dried skin disorders. They cool by evaporation and deposit a powder on the surface. *Dusting powders* (e.g. talc) are useful for treating skin disorders which affect skin folds – under the arms, in the groin, under the breasts. *Creams* moisten the skin more than ointments and cosmetically are more acceptable. *Ointments* are greasy and give more covering than creams; this occlusiveness helps to maintain the hydration of the skin. Ointments are more suitable for chronic, dry, scaly lesions. *Pastes* are stiff preparations and are useful for dry scaly patches.

The choice of the base for creams and ointments and other skin applications is often of equal importance to the choice of 'active' drug in the preparations. The base of a skin application (vehicle) can affect the degree of hydration of the skin and the ability of the active drug to penetrate the skin. Because of the complexity of formulation of many skin preparations it is important to be most careful about dilution which affects not only the effectiveness of a preparation but also its shelf-life.

The groups of drugs most frequently included in skin applications and which are discussed in this chapter are.

1 Soothing skin applications – demulcents and emollients. These usually form the base or vehicle in which other drugs are included
2 Protective skin applications
3 Sunscreen and anti-sunburn skin applications
4 Corticosteroid skin applications
5 Antibacterial skin applications
6 Antifungal skin applications
7 Antiseptics and disinfectants
8 Anti-itching skin applications and drugs
9 Antihistamine skin applications
10 Local anaesthetic skin applications
11 Caustic and keratolytic skin applications
12 Astringent skin applications
13 Anti-perspirant skin applications
14 Deodorant skin applications
15 Other drugs used in skin applications.

1 Soothing Skin Applications

Demulcents

These are usually gums from stems, roots and branches of various plants, for example gum arabic, gum tragacanth, liquorice root, agar and sodium alginate (from algae). Synthetic drugs like methylcellulose are also used. **Glycerin** is a common constituent of skin applications and mixed with starch it forms a jelly base called starch glycerite. Glycerin should only be used in low concentrations because it can be irritant. Propylene glycol is related to glycerin and is used in lotions and ointments because it mixes with water (hydrophilic) and also dissolves in oils. Many other glycols are used to make water-soluble bases for ointments.

Demulcents are soothing because they coat the surface of the skin or mucous membranes (mouth, gums and throat) and protect the underlying area from the air and other irritating agents.

Emollients

Emollients are fats and oils which are soothing when applied to the skin. They soften the skin and are chiefly used as a base to which other active drugs (e.g. antibiotics) are added. They soften the skin by forming an oily film over the surface of the skin, thus preventing water from evaporating from the surface cells and so keeping them moist.

Emollient skin applications contain vegetable oils, animal fats, paraffin and related chemicals, and waxes.

The vegetable oils are usually cotton-seed oil, corn oil, peanut oil, almond oil and cocoa-bean oil. Animal fats are wool fats from the wool of sheep. These are of two types – wool fat (**anhydrous lanolin**) and hydrous wool fat (known just as **lanolin**) which is wool fat mixed with 20 to 30 per cent of water. Wool fat can produce skin allergies. It is not used as often as it used to be and yet the message is still given that there is something magical about preparations that contain lanolin.

Paraffin-related preparations include mineral oil (**liquid paraffin**), white petroleum, and yellow petroleum (e.g. **Vaseline** is a brand preparation of white and yellow petroleum jellies). Waxes are principally obtained from beeswax (yellow wax). White wax is bleached beeswax. **Spermaceti** is a waxy substance from the head of the sperm whale which was used to raise the melting point of ointments to stop them melting too easily when applied to warm skin (**cold creams**), particularly in hot climates. It was replaced by **jojoba oil** in 1982 in most countries. Jojoba oil comes from the beans of the jojoba bush, a native of Northern Mexico and Southern California.

2 Protective Skin Applications

Protectives are applications used to cover the skin and mucous membranes, in order to protect them from contact with an irritating agent. They are by definition insoluble and inactive and cover the skin physically rather than having any chemical effect. They include *dusting powders* which are used to protect the skin in certain areas (e.g. skin folds) and on the surfaces of ulcers and wounds. They are smooth and prevent friction, and some absorb moisture from the surface of the area to which they are applied (for example, ones containing **zinc oxide** or **starch**). On open wounds they make a crust and those containing starch have to have an antiseptic added to stop the starch fermenting. Dusting powders often contain **talc** (which is mainly magnesium silicate) and of course talc is widely available as talcum powders.

Mechanical protectives such as **collodion** were used to close off small wounds but it is now considered better to let the air get to a wound. **Petroleum gauze** and **gauzes impregnated with antibiotics** are useful as protective dressings to wounds although the tendency now is to use dry non-adherent dressings. **Barrier creams** are used to protect the skin against irritants which are water-soluble. They usually contain **dimethicone** (**silicone**) or a related silicone. These adhere to the skin and have water-repellent properties. They are available as ointments and sprays as well as creams. They provide protection against the irritating effects of soap, water, skin-cleansing agents and breakdown products from urine. They may be useful in preventing bedsores and nappy rash. They should not be used on inflamed or damaged skin, or near the eyes, because they may produce irritation. They may produce allergic skin reactions.

3 Sunscreen and Anti-sunburn Skin Applications

The health-promoting properties of sunlight have long been recognized but it is only in the past fifty years that sunbathing for cosmetic reasons has become fashionable. And it is only in more recent years that the harmful effects of solar radiation and ultraviolet light from artificial sources have become recognized. Excessive exposure to the sun's rays without appropriate protection is harmful: it causes burning and ageing of the skin, cancer of the skin, and cataracts.

Sunburn and suntan are caused by ultraviolet rays (UVR). The shorter ultraviolet waves (UVB) cause the burning and contribute to long-term changes in the skin that cause cancer and ageing. The longer waves (UVA) cause the tanning. They do not cause sunburn but they are involved in allergic reactions to the sun's rays and also in long-term damage to the skin which is associated with ageing and skin cancer.

Tanning results from migration of the brown pigment, **melanin**, from the base layer of the skin up into the surface cells. This provides some protection against sunburn but the main protection comes from a thickening of the surface layer of cells.

The acute effects (sunburn) and the chronic effects of the sun's rays on the skin are directly related to the total dose of UVR received by the skin, i.e. by the intensity, duration and frequency of exposure. Protection is offered by the melanin content of the skin and the capacity of the skin to produce new protective melanin on the skin surface (i.e. to tan).

Sunscreen Preparations

Sunscreen preparations have an important function in so far as they can protect the structure and function of the skin from damaging rays. They are chemicals in the form of clear or milky solutions, gels, creams or ointments which reduce (filter out) the harmful rays. They work by absorbing, reflecting or scattering the rays. The selection of a skin application should depend upon your liability to sunburn and to tan.

Sunscreens for application to the skin are either **chemical sunscreens** or **physical sunscreens**. **Chemical sunscreens** contain one or more UVB absorbing chemicals which filter off the harmful rays. They are usually colourless and must be non-irritant and non-staining. Frequently used products include **aminobenzoic acid**, **padimate**, **benzyl salicylate** and **mexenone**. However, they do not protect against UVA, the long-term effects of which may take ten–twenty years to appear.

Physical sunscreens are usually opaque formulations and contain particles which reflect and scatter the harmful rays (both UVA and UVB). They include **titanium**, **talc**, **zinc oxide**, **kaolin**, **ferric chloride** and **ichthyol**. They are essential for people who are ultrasensitive to the sun's rays. Physical sunscreens tend to melt in the heat of the sun.

In recent years preparations containing **methoxypsoralen** (**bergapten**) or **bergamot oil** (which contains methoxypsoralen) have been heavily promoted. The application of these formulations actually stimulates tanning (melanogenesis) which may provide improved protection but they can produce sunlight sensitivity with subsequent pigmentation. Their association with an increased risk of skin cancer has not been proved.

Sun Protection Factor (SPF)

This is a measure of the effectiveness of a sunscreen preparation. It is the ratio of the time taken for UVB rays to produce redness of the skin through a sunscreen preparation compared with the time taken to produce redness without any sunscreen application. For example, an SPF of 6 means a person should be able to stay in the sun six times longer without burning.

Factors that Influence the Sun Protection Factor (SPF)

These include the subject (skin type, age, amount of sweating, skin site), the UV intensity (season, weather, reflection), radiation source (the sun, type and age of lamp), concentration of sunscreen application, the base (vehicle) used in the preparation, the thickness of the application, effect of water (e.g. after swimming), environment (temperature, humidity, wind) and sweating. In addition, the testing procedure is very important because the effectiveness of a sunscreen preparation out of doors may not be related to its performance indoors (i.e. under laboratory conditions).

The most important consideration when purchasing a sunscreen preparation is how *you* react to sunlight. Buy a preparation that protects against both UVA *and* UVB and that suits *your requirements* and one that is manufactured by a reputable company. Most sunscreens should be reapplied after swimming and repeatedly during prolonged sunbathing. *Avoid sunbathing at midday (11.00 a.m. to 3.00 p.m.).*

Sunscreens do not stimulate tanning. Increased tanning is caused by the activation and proliferation of the pigment cells in the skin (melanocytes). This process will be decreased by the application of effective sunscreens.

Patients suffering from sensitivity to sunlight (photosensitivity) often require combination therapy with two sunscreen preparations, the first application in an alcoholic solution which evaporates and then a second application of a cream on top.

Adverse Effects of Sunscreens

Certain sunscreen formulations containing **aminobenzoic acid** may cause selective burning (smarting) and occasionally contact or photo-dermatitis. Patients allergic to sulphonamides and certain local anaesthetics (benzocaine and procaine) may have allergic reactions to aminobenzoic acid. Patients on sulphonamides or thiazide diuretics may cross-react with aminobenzoic acid and develop dermatitis.

Categories of Sunscreen Products*	SPF (Protection against UVB)
Minimal sun protection	2–4
Moderate sun protection	4–6
Extra sun protection	6–8
Maximal sun protection	8–15
Ultra sun protection	15 and over

* Details on package should include degree of protection against both UVA and UVB rays. *Note:* 'Star' rating refers to ratio of UVA and UVB protection. Four stars indicate that the product offers a balanced amount of UVA and UVB protection. Three, two and one star indicates that the product offers proportionally more protection against UVB than UVA.

Oral Treatment of Photosensitivity (Sensitivity to Sunlight)

The effectiveness of most orally taken drugs has never been proven. They include **beta-carotene** (a precursor of vitamin A) which is a natural constituent of many plants including oranges, carrots and tomatoes; and antimalarial drugs (e.g. **chloroquine**) which have been used for many years to provide protection in patients sensitive to sunlight.

Quick-tanning Preparations

These applications, which contain drugs such as **dihydroxyacetone** (**DHA**), do not stimulate the production of the tanning pigment in the skin; rather they stain the skin yellow-brown. It offers no protection to sunlight. The dye **lawsone** is no more effective.

The use of 'tanning' tablets which contain **canthaxanthin** merely colour the skin and underlying fat orangey-brown. It is used to colour foods and medicines. All products containing canthaxanthin have been withdrawn because of the risk of eye damage.

Sunburn

There are several treatments for sunburn; among the commonest are **calamine lotion** and **zinc lotion**. Applications containing a **corticosteroid** (see pp. 241–3) can be very effective. Do not use applications containing an **antihistamine** because they may produce an allergic rash and usually in sunburn there is a fairly large area of skin to be treated.

Drug-induced Sunlight Sensitivity (Photosensitivity)

This means the skin is excessively sensitive to the sun's rays and goes red and burns very easily. It may be due to a drug; for example, a tetracycline or a sulphonamide antibiotic; griseofulvin; a phenothiazine; an oral anti-diabetic drug; a thiazide diuretic; nalidixic acid; an oral contraceptive drug; gold; diphenhydramine (an antihistamine) and, rarely, saccharin.

Drugs applied to the skin may also sensitize it to sunlight, for example, **tar** (the basis of tar and ultraviolet ray treatment of psoriasis) and **hexachloro-phene**, an antiseptic present in numerous skin applications and toiletries. Various **deodorants** may also sensitize the skin, and so too may sunscreen applications (e.g. **aminobenzoic acid**).

The important thing to remember is that if you burn more quickly than usual for you, then always think – is it a drug I am taking or a skin application I am using? Stop any of these immediately and check whether they produce sunlight sensitivity.

Some people are actually allergic to sunlight and can develop severe dermatitis on exposed parts of their skin (photodermatitis). Certain disorders may produce sunlight allergy, for example porphyria (a disorder of metabolism). If you develop a rash on the exposed parts of your skin, always consult your doctor.

4 Corticosteroid Skin Applications

If you read about **corticosteroids** in Chapter 37, you will learn that they reduce inflammatory reactions. For this reason they are widely used to treat many skin disorders, in order to reduce the redness, soreness, swelling, pain and irritation which often characterize such conditions. Corticosteroids are present alone or in combination with other drugs in numerous skin, eye and ear applications prescribed by doctors. They are very effective. However, they do not cure but only suppress the symptoms, so that if the underlying skin disorder is not self-limiting, or if the causative agent is not removed (for example, contact dermatitis caused by an article worn on the body), it will flare up again when the corticosteroid preparation is stopped. This is known as a rebound effect.

Corticosteroids available for use on the skin vary in potency and therefore concentrations included in skin preparations vary from 0·001 per cent for triamcinolone up to 2·5 per cent for hydrocortisone. The popularity of any particular preparation may reflect more on the results of vigorous sales promotion rather than on any clear differences in effectiveness.

● Adverse Effects and Precautions

Corticosteroid skin preparations are not curative and if treatment is suddenly stopped the skin condition may flare up. They are of no use in treating nettle-rash (urticaria). Prolonged use may produce thinning of the skin particularly when used on the face, flexures (knees and elbows) and on moist parts of the skin. They may also produce soreness and irritation at the site of application, irreversible 'stretch marks', increase growth of hair, contact dermatitis, acne, mild depigmentation and sometimes a dermatitis around the mouth in young women.

They should not be used to treat acne rosacea or acne, dermatitis around the mouth, scabies, leg ulcers, TB, ringworm or viral skin disease, or untreated bacterial or fungal skin diseases. Extensive and/or prolonged use in pregnancy should be avoided. They are of no use in urticaria (nettle-rash) and generalized itching (pruritus). The more potent the corticosteroid the more risk there is of adverse effects. **Clobetasol** is very potent, **betamethasone** is potent, **clobetasone** is moderately potent and **hydrocortisone** is mild. Because of the risk of stunted growth and skin damage potent corticosteroids should not be used in children and the others should be used with utmost caution. Only a mild corticosteroid should be used on the face (1 per cent hydrocortisone) and not for more than five days. Use for no longer than five days in children. Potent corticosteroids should only be used in adults for a few weeks and then switched to mild ones. The general rule is to use the least powerful corticosteroid in the lowest strength for the shortest duration of time.

In using corticosteroid skin preparations it must be remembered that when inflammation is reduced the resistance to infection is lowered and secondary infection may occur. This is particularly likely to happen when corticosteroids are used under occlusive (e.g. plastic) dressings. This may cause boils, thrush and other infections to develop. Allergies may also occur to additives in corticosteroid applications and this should always be considered if there is a poor response to treatment.

Long-continued use of corticosteroids under plastic dressings may produce a local wasting of the deep layers of the skin to produce a flattened, depressed, stripy-looking area. This may take many years to go away. Corticosteroids applied to the skin may enter the blood circulation and produce harmful effects (see Chapter 37). This is particularly likely to happen with children (who may also lick the ointment off the skin) and in adults using very large amounts.

Do not forget also that corticosteroids can delay the healing of ulcers (e.g. leg ulcers). Finally, it is important that you should not borrow skin ointments containing a corticosteroid drug from a neighbour or friend – different disorders and different people respond differently.

Some skin disorders can get infected and become soggy with pus (e.g. infected eczema). In these infected skin disorders the use of an application containing a corticosteroid and an anti-infective drug (e.g. an antibiotic) may be very effective. Such a combination is also useful on skin rashes in areas where infection is likely to occur, for example, in the groin or around the anus. But do not forget that there is a slight risk that an anti-infective drug may produce an allergic reaction which the corticosteroid will mask. Remember this if a skin rash seems to be getting worse despite the fact that initially it improved with such a preparation.

The wrong use of such combinations in primary infective skin disorders may produce very severe effects. For example, if they are used to treat impetigo (a bacterial infection of the skin) a small localized patch may be turned into a serious widespread skin infection; a simple fungus infection (e.g. athlete's foot) may spread over a large area; and herpes simplex (cold sores) may produce nasty ulcers.

Corticosteroids mixed with an antibiotic, antifungal drug, or an antiseptic, may be used where the primary skin condition would be expected to respond to corticosteroids but where there is an added infection (e.g. infected eczema). The choice of preparation is not critical. Such simple principles as not too much for too long should apply, and if the disorder gets worse stop the treatment and see your doctor.

5 Antibacterial Skin Applications

When a skin infection is superficial (e.g. impetigo) an antibiotic skin application can be dramatically effective. If the infection is deeper in the skin surface (e.g. cellulitis), then local applications of an antibiotic will be useless and you will need an antibiotic by mouth or injection.

When the sulphonamides and penicillin were introduced, doctors used them liberally in skin applications and produced many allergic reactions in their patients. Not only were these allergic reactions inconvenient for the patients, they were positively dangerous for some. They sensitized the patient to the drug, with the consequent risk of a severe allergic reaction if that patient had to be given a sulphonamide or a penicillin by mouth for some more serious infection. Another problem was the development of resistant organisms.

To minimize these risks antibacterial drugs should be used on the skin that are not used by mouth or injection. Application to large areas of skin may produce general adverse effects, for example, neomycin, gentamicin, colistin and polymyxin B may damage hearing, particularly in children, the elderly and patients with impaired kidney function.

Antibacterial preparations only used topically include **framycetin** (**Soframycin**, **Sofra-Tulle**), **mupirocin** (**Bactroban**), **neomycin** (in **Cicatrin**, **Graneodin**), **polymyxin B** (in **Polyfax**), **colistin** (**Colomycin**) and **silver sulphadiazine** (**Flamazine**).

Antibacterials also used by mouth and injection include **chlortetracycline** (**Aureomycin**), **fusidic acid** (**sodium fusidate**, **Fucidin**), **gentamicin** (**Cidomycin**), **metronidazole** (**Anabact**, **Metrogel**, **Noritate**, **Rozex**, **Metrotop**, **Zyomet**) and **tetracycline** (**Achromycin**).

> *Antibiotic skin applications should be used for as short a period as possible over as small an area as possible, and if the disorder gets worse they should be stopped immediately.*

6 Antifungal Skin Applications

Before reading this section it is useful to read the chapter on antifungal antibiotics (Chapter 47). Here you will learn about the antifungal drugs which may be used locally and by mouth. Some of these have revolutionized the treatment of fungus and yeast infections. Rarely they may irritate the skin and cause allergic reactions.

There are many effective antifungal skin preparations and they vary only in their activity against specific fungi. They include **amorolfine** (**Loceryl**), **clotrimazole** (**Canesten, Masnoderm**), **econazole** (**Ecostatin, Pevaryl**), **ketoconazole** (**Nizoral**), **miconazole** (**Daktarin**), **sulconazole nitrate** (**Exelderm**) and **tioconazole** (**Trosyl**). Other effective antifungals include **amorolfine** (**Loceryl**), **nystatin** (**Nystaform, Nystan** in **Tinaderm-M**), **terbinafine** (**Lamisil**) and **tolnaftate** (in **Tinaderm** preparations). Other less effective antifungals include the **undecenoates** (e.g. in **Monphytol**, in **Mycil, Mycota**), **benzoic acid** (in **Whitfield's ointment**), **benzoyl peroxide** (in **Quinoped**) and **salicylic acid** (in **Phytex**).

7 Antiseptics and Disinfectants

There is quite a mix-up between the terms antiseptic and disinfectant. In general the term *antiseptic* is used to describe those drugs applied to the skin or other parts of the body in an attempt to prevent infection. The term *disinfectant* is used to describe a chemical applied to objects in order to destroy germs. However, the term disinfectant is often used to describe both uses. Antiseptic preparations applied to the skin are sometimes called *germicides*. Antiseptics may kill or prevent the growth of bacteria, fungi and viruses. Some disinfectants are used as antiseptics in reduced strengths but some are too irritant and some antiseptics are not strong enough to use as disinfectants.

Antiseptics and disinfectants belong to various chemical groups which can make the choice look very complex and confusing. In fact most doctors learn to use one or two preparations (often by their brand name). The choice is not critical and the need to use such preparations in the home is greatly over-emphasized in the advertising media.

Some Main Chemical Groups to which Antiseptics and Disinfectants Belong

Chlorine and chlorine-releasing substances. Chlorine kills germs and the most commonly used chlorine-releasing chemical is sodium hypochlorite. This is present in commonly used preparations such as **Chlorasol** and Milton. Others include **chlorinated soda solution** (**Dakin's solution**) and **chlorinated lime**.

Detergents. These include quaternary ammonia compounds such as **benzalkonium, cetrimide, cetylpyridinium** and **domiphen**. The most commonly used antiseptic detergent is **cetrimide** which is present in numerous preparations and **Drapolene** which contains benzalkonium and cetrimide. An important point to remember about these preparations is that soap can reduce their activity. They are also prescribed as shampoos by doctors for the treatment of scurfy disorders of the scalp.

Phenol and related drugs. These lose their effects fairly quickly when diluted.

They include phenol, cresol and thymol. Solutions of these should not be applied to wounds since they can be absorbed into the bloodstream and can be very toxic.

Chlorinated phenols. The two most widely used of these include a **chloroxylenol** (**Dettol**), and **hexachlorophene** (e.g. **Ster-Zac Powder**). Hexachlorophene may very rarely produce brain damage when applied extensively to the skin of premature babies. It may produce skin sensitivity and also make the skin sensitive to sunlight. **Chlorocresol** is another example of a chlorinated phenol.

Iodine compounds include **weak iodine solution, povidone-iodine** (e.g. **Betadine** and **Savlon Dry Powder**). These preparations may produce skin sensitivity and interfere with the function of the thyroid gland.

Dyes. There are two types of dyes used as antiseptics:

1 Acridines, which include **acriflavine, aminacrine** and **proflavine**. These are slow-acting but work in the presence of pus and damaged tissues, which inhibit the effects of some antiseptics. In high concentration they may delay wound healing and may produce skin sensitivity.

2 Dyes such as **brilliant green, gentian violet** and **malachite green**. These are derivatives of triphenylmethane and were widely used before the introduction of antibiotics and antifungal drugs.

Formaldehyde. **Formaldehyde** and related drugs may be used as disinfectants, but not as antiseptics because they irritate the skin.

Chlorhexidine. **Chlorhexidine** (e.g. **Hibitane**) is frequently used as an antiseptic. It may occasionally cause skin sensitivity and it is inactivated by soap and by cork (so it should not be kept in a corked bottle).

Other chemical groups. These include *alcohols* (e.g. **ethanol, benzyl alcohol, methylated spirit, surgical spirit**), *oxidizing compounds* (e.g. **benzoyl peroxide, hydrogen peroxide**), *salts of heavy metals* (e.g. **mercury** and **silver**) and *acids* (e.g. **acetic acid**).

● *Choice of Antiseptic and Disinfectant*

Chlorine-releasing substances such as sodium hypochlorite (e.g. Domestos, Milton) or chlorinated phenols (e.g. **Dettol**) are perfectly suitable as disinfectants, but do not forget that chlorine acts as a bleach (e.g. Domestos). For cleaning the skin a detergent such as cetrimide (e.g. **Tisept**) is useful and so are chlorinated phenols (e.g. Dettol, hexachlorophene (**Ster-Zac Powder**) and chlorhexidine (e.g. **Hibitane**)). Mixtures of cetrimide and chlorhexidine are also available and providone-iodone (e.g. **Betadine**) is useful. Salt solution is also useful for cleaning the skin.

8 Anti-itching Preparations

There are many causes of itching (pruritus). These may be in the skin, such as allergic skin rashes, eczema, nervous rashes, scabies and body lice. In these disorders scratching may give relief, but often leads to the skin being damaged and further itching. In elderly patients the skin may degenerate, producing itching. Some drugs, e.g. morphine, may produce itching. Kidney disorders, liver and gall-bladder disorders and diabetes may also produce itching. Therefore, it is important for you to be examined by your doctor if you have an itching disorder because it is better to treat the cause than to treat the itch. There are two main approaches to the drug treatment of itching but generally treatment is disappointing.

1 Skin Applications

These may contain **antiseptics** (see p. 244) in very low concentrations, for example, **phenol**, **benzyl alcohol**, **chlorbutanol**. However, these may irritate the skin and produce allergic rashes. **Local anaesthetics** in low concentrations are not very effective and may irritate the skin and produce skin allergies. **Antihistamine** creams (see p. 247) are useful for small areas (e.g. insect bites) but are not recommended for large areas because they too may produce allergic skin rashes. Other drugs such as menthol and camphor are also used. Emollients are useful if itching is associated with a dry skin.

   Crotamiton (**Eurax**) may be useful in some patients, but it should not be applied to broken skin. **Calamine lotion** is probably just as effective. **Corticosteroid** skin applications (see p. 241) are used to treat itching in eczema.

2 Drugs by Mouth

There are two main groups of drugs which are taken by mouth to relieve itching. These are the **antihistamines** and the **phenothiazines**. One commonly used drug from the antihistamine group is **trimeprazine** (**Vallergan**).

   The severe itching which accompanies obstructive jaundice may be relieved by a male sex hormone, for example, **testosterone**, which may also be helpful in senile pruritus. **Cholestyramine** may help in liver and gall-bladder disease because it reduces the blood level of bile salts, which is high in these disorders; it is thought that they are the cause of the itching.

   Caution should be applied to the use of antihistamines and phenothiazines in the elderly, because they can quickly become confused under an apparently 'normal' dose of any of these drugs. Simple skin applications should be tried first, such as **calamine lotion** or an emollient cream.

9 Antihistamine Skin Applications

Skin applications that contain antihistamines are sometimes of use in treating small, acute, irritating and painful skin lesions such as an insect bite or nettle-rash. Their regular use and their use on large areas should be avoided because they can produce allergic skin rashes. Antihistamine skin applications available include **diphenhydramine** (in **Caladryl**), **antazoline** (in **RBC, Wasp-Eze ointment**) and **mepyramine** (**Anthisan**, in **Wasp-Eze Spray**).

10 Local Anaesthetic Skin Applications

The widespread or regular use of skin applications containing a local anaesthetic is not recommended because of the risk of producing irritation of the skin and allergic rashes. They should not be used in young children because of the risk of absorption into the bloodstream.

Preparations available include **tetracaine**(amethocaine) (in **Anethaine**), **benzocaine** (in **Anthisan Plus**, in **BurnEze**, in **Lanacane**, in **Solarcaine**, in **Wasp-Eze Spray**) and **lidocaine**(lignocaine) (in **Dermidex**, in **Dettol Antiseptic Pain Relief Spray**, in **Vagisil Cream**).

11 Caustic and Keratolytic Skin Applications

Caustics are drugs which are used to destroy tissue at the site of application. If it causes a scab by precipitating protein from the damaged cells then it is also called a *cauterizant* or an *escharotic*. Surgeons use electric needles to burn (or cauterize) the ends of small bleeding blood vessels.

Some commonly used caustics are **acetic acid, phenol, podophyllum, trichloroacetic acid** and **silver nitrate**. They are used to treat warts and corns.

Keratolytics are included in some skin applications because they loosen the surface cells of the skin and cause them to swell and go soft so that they can easily be cut off. They are used to treat warts, corns and acne and include **benzoic acid** and **salicylic acid** and their salts, **benzoyl peroxide** and **resorcinol**.

12 Astringent Skin Applications

Astringents are drugs which act on the surface of cells to precipitate protein. They do not enter the cell and therefore they do not kill the cell but they make its surface less permeable to water, etc., and so it dries up and shrinks. They are included in skin applications and have the effect of hardening the skin, drying up soggy areas of damaged skin and reducing minor bleeding from skin abrasions. Astringents in various dilutions may be used in throat lozenges, mouthwashes, eye drops, ear drops and in preparations used to treat haemorrhoids; as caustics (for burning off dead tissue, etc.); and in the past they have been used to treat diarrhoea. They are now widely used in antiperspirant sprays and applications (see below). The main ones used are **salts of zinc and aluminium** and **tannins**.

Alum (**potassium aluminium sulphate powder**) has been used as an astringent to treat sweating sore feet, to shrink the stump of the umbilical cord and to treat skin abrasions, small cuts and ulcers. **Aluminium acetate** solution is a useful astringent lotion and is also used in ear drops. **Aluminium sulphate** is a strong astringent and may be used as a mild caustic; so may **silver nitrate**. **Hamamelis** is another astringent used to shrink haemorrhoids and **hamamelis water** (**witch hazel**) is used as a cooling application on sprains and bruises. **Krameria** is also used to shrink haemorrhoids and is included in some throat lozenges. **Zinc chloride** is used as a caustic, astringent and deodorant. **Zinc sulphate** is used as an astringent, particularly in eye drops. **Calamine** is used as a mild astringent.

Aluminium acetate and **zinc acetate** are mild astringents of choice but it really depends on what is being treated – sweating feet or a small abrasion, haemorrhoids or a leg ulcer.

13 Antiperspirant Skin Applications

These are available in every size, shape and colour of container, as pads, sprays, roll-ons and creams, with every possible smell, to be applied to an ever-increasing number of parts of our bodies (male and female).

The drugs most commonly used as antiperspirants include **salts of aluminium and zinc**. Some may stain fabric, some are acidic and irritate the skin, and some are soluble in alcohol and may be used in sprays and aerosols. Those antiperspirants which contain an aluminium salt may produce an allergic skin rash in sensitive skins. The mechanism of action of antiperspirants is unknown but they are considered by some experts to be astringents.

14 Deodorant Skin Applications

Like antiperspirants the market is flooded with deodorant preparations. They reduce the number of bacteria that live on the skin. Since these bacteria break down sweat to produce products that have an unpleasant odour, their reduction produces a reduction in body odour. **Antiseptics** such as **hexachlorophene** and **benzalkonium** are frequently used in deodorant preparations. Hexachlorophene may produce allergic skin rashes on sensitive skins, and benzalkonium and related complex ammonia compounds are inactivated by soap and can irritate the skin in concentrations above 1 per cent. Some deodorants contain **antibiotics** which can also cause allergic reactions and sensitize the individual to their future use. In addition, people may become allergic to the fragrances used in these preparations.

Remember – if you develop a rash in the areas where you apply a deodorant or antiperspirant, consider that it may be an allergic reaction and stop the application immediately.

Drugs enter the bloodstream more easily from mucous surfaces such as the vagina than they do from the skin and therefore they should be used with caution, particularly by pregnant women. Vaginal deodorants are best avoided because they may cause irritation and bladder trouble (urethritis and cystitis) – stick to water.

15 Other Drugs Used in Skin Applications

Allantoin is used in preparations to treat psoriasis; e.g. **Alphosyl** lotion contains allantoin and **coal-tar extract** in a non-greasy base.

Cade oil is used in preparations to treat eczema and psoriasis.

Calamine is used as a mild astringent in creams and lotions, and in dusting powder.

Dithranol is used in small concentrations in ointments and pastes to treat psoriasis and other long-standing skin disorders. It can burn and stain the skin brown and cause allergic rashes in sensitized patients.

Ichthammol is slightly antibacterial and it irritates the skin. It has been used in skin applications to treat chronic skin disorders (e.g. eczema), and mixed with glycerin it was often used as an application on superficial thrombophlebitis, on abscesses and in infections of the ears.

Potassium hydroxyquinoline is used to treat bacterial and fungal infections of the skin. It has been used as a deodorant and appears in **Quinoderm** cream, used to treat acne.

Salicylic acid is used to treat hardened skin and corns.

Selenium sulphide is used to treat dandruff and other scalp disorders. **Starch** is used in dusting powders.

Sulphur is a mild antiseptic and has been used to treat acne and other disorders.

Talc is used as a dusting powder.

Tar is used to treat eczema and psoriasis.

Zinc oxide is used as a mild astringent and as a soothing agent and protective.

These drugs appear in numerous proprietary preparations for the treatment of many skin disorders. Read details about them in the A–Z of Medicines.

Drug Treatment of Some Common Skin Diseases

Acne

Acne vulgaris (referred to as acne) usually starts at puberty. At this age, the oil-producing glands surrounding hair roots (sebaceous glands) become active under the influence of male sex hormones (androgens), which are produced by the testes, and the adrenal glands in both males and females. Production of these hormones increases up to about the age of twenty-five years, after which it levels out. People who get acne do not have higher levels of male sex hormones than people who do not develop acne and it may be that their sebaceous glands are more sensitive to male sex hormone stimulation.

Acne vulgaris affects the sebaceous glands in the skin of the face, neck, middle of the chest and back. These are areas where these glands are most active. Although acne is related to the production of male hormones, it occurs only slightly more commonly in males than females. We do not know why some people get acne and others do not, or why some just get mild acne and in others it is severe.

In acne, the outlets from grease glands get blocked by skin cells and debris and this forms what are called *blackheads* (or comedones). The glands then swell up and become infected and inflamed, to produce the red lumps (papules) and yellow lumps (pustules) of acne. If the outlet is blocked completely the glands may swell right up to form a cyst and some individuals may get an overgrowth of scar tissue (called keloid) which produces irregular lumps and bumps in the affected area.

Treatment of Acne

There is no specific treatment for acne and it is often best to use what suits you or to try different treatments, but do not be persuaded to use expensive preparations when the simplest and cheapest may be the best.

The important part of treatment of acne is to keep the skin free from grease by regular cleaning. Ordinary soap and water may be all that is needed. If this does not work, then a detergent solution such as **cetrimide** should be used.

● *Drying and Peeling Preparations*

In addition to keeping the skin clean and free from excess grease it may be necessary to apply preparations that dry and peel the skin and stop blackheads from forming. The most frequently used chemical is **benzoyl peroxide** which is present in many preparations. It not only dries and peels the skin, but also has antiseptic properties. **Salicylic acid** produces similar effects. **Azelaic acid** (**Skinoren**) peels the skin and has antibacterial effects. It can be used when benzoyl peroxide does not work.

● *Vitamin A Derivatives*

Isotretinoin (**Isotrex**, in **Isotrexin**) and **tretinoin** (**Acticin**, **Retin-A**) are related to vitamin A. They are applied as a cream, gel or lotion. They are useful in some patients with moderately severe acne, but may produce redness and peeling for several days. Too frequent use may cause dermatitis. They should not be applied to the eyes, up the nose or on the creases of the mouth. The acne may appear worse at first and it may take up to four weeks before improvement occurs. Isotretinoin may also be taken by mouth (see later).

Adapalene (**Differin**) is a retinoid-like drug which may be less irritant than isotretinoin or tretinoin.

● *Abrasive Preparations*

Abrasives may be used to help peeling and cleansing of the skin and some individuals may occasionally find these of benefit. They include **Brasivol** (fine particles of aluminium oxide in a paste) and **Ionax Scrub** (polyethylene granules with benzalkonium in a gel).

● *Antibacterial Preparations*

A **tetracycline antibiotic** (e.g. **tetracycline: Topicycline**) applied to the skin may help to reduce bacterial infection in the sebaceous glands and may possibly produce some anti-inflammatory effects. Other antibiotics included in acne applications include **clindamycin** (**Dalacin T solution**) and **erythromycin** (**Eryacne**, **Stiemycin**, with zinc acetate in **Zineryt**, with benzoyl peroxide in **Benzamycin**).

Because of the risk of producing bacterial resistance to antibiotics use a topical preparation for no more than ten–twelve weeks with a few weeks' rest and use a non-antibiotic (e.g. benzoyl peroxide) when possible. Alcoholic preparations of an antibiotic should not be used with benzoyl peroxide.

● *Antiseptic Preparations*

Hydroxyquinoline kills bacteria and fungi and is included in some acne preparations. It may produce irritation and redness.

Sulphur, which is used to produce peeling, also possesses some antiseptic effects. It is no longer considered beneficial in treating acne.

● *Anti-inflammatory Preparations*

A topical application of **nicotinamide** (a vitamin B compound) may help to relieve inflammation.

> **Warning:** *Greasy creams or ointments and corticosteroid applications may make acne worse.*

Drugs Taken by Mouth to Treat Acne

● *Antibiotics*

Bacteria that 'normally' live in the oil-producing glands may produce irritant substances from the oil which cause inflammation. Antibiotics (e.g. tetracyclines) which dissolve in fat can kill these bacteria and help to reduce the inflammation. Therefore, if the acne is moderate or severe, or does not respond to local applications, it is worth adding an antibacterial drug by mouth such as **doxycycline**, **minocycline**, **tetracycline**, or **erythromycin**. The antibacterial drug must be taken daily. Maximum improvement usually occurs within four–six months, but sometimes treatment has to be continued for a longer period. Oral antibiotics should not be given at the same time as a topical antibiotic because of the risk of producing bacterial resistance.

Tetracycline antibiotics should not be used in pregnancy (see p. 269), therefore women taking a tetracycline daily by mouth for the treatment of their acne should avoid getting pregnant while on treatment.

Long-term use of antibiotics applied to the skin and/or taken by mouth may cause a superinfection of the skin around the nose and central part of the face, causing redness and pustules. This superinfection is often difficult to treat, and the treatment should be based on trying to identify the infecting micro-organism, testing its sensitivity to antibiotics and using the appropriate antibiotic.

● *Hormones*

Male sex hormones are associated with the development of acne and female sex hormones (oestrogens) may therefore reduce some of their effects. Obviously oestrogens cannot be used in males, and because of the risks of oestrogens they should not be used alone in females. However, a combination of an oestrogen with a progestogen reduces the risks and therefore a combined oral contraceptive may help acne in some women, but high oestrogen-containing contraceptive pills may make acne worse.

Cyproterone is an anti-male sex hormone and combined with an oestrogen (ethinyloestradiol) it may be beneficial in women who suffer from severe acne and who wish to take an oral contraceptive. The combination product is marketed under the name of **Dianette**.

● *Vitamin A Derivatives*

Isotretinoin (**Roaccutane**), a vitamin A derivative, is effective in some patients with severe and nodular acne and may prevent scarring. It reduces oil production and helps to unblock hair follicles, alters bacterial growth in the sebaceous glands and produces peeling of the superficial layer of the skin. It is best used in individuals who have failed to respond to antibiotics by mouth and/or who have severe deep acne.

It may produce serious harmful effects and therefore any possible benefits need to be weighed against the risks. It should only be used when other treatments have failed and only under specialist supervision.

Athlete's Foot (Tinea Pedis)

Athlete's foot is ringworm of the feet. Scrapings from the infected area should be examined under the microscope in order to confirm the diagnosis of a fungus infection before treatment is started. An effective treatment is a local application of an antifungal drug such as **clotrimazole** (**Canesten**), **sulconazole nitrate** (**Exelderm**), **miconazole** (**Daktarin**), or **econazole** (**Ecostatin**) ointment. If one of these does not work and the infection is severe, **griseofulvin** (**Grisovin**) tablets by mouth should be added to the treatment and taken for six–eight weeks. Compound benzoic acid ointment (**Whitfield's ointment**) is fairly effective but messy to apply.

Baldness

Regaine is a solution of minoxidil which is used to stimulate hair growth in male-type baldness in men and in women who develop a diffuse thinning of the hair. During the first few months of treatment there is very little regrowth and it takes up to twelve months to see any benefit. Fewer than half of males and about one-third of females develop an acceptable growth of hair. Best results in men are obtained on a small patch of balding on the crown which has been present for only a few years. An important limitation of this treatment is that if daily applications are stopped the baldness becomes as extensive as if it had never been treated. The new growth of hair will be shed within two or three weeks of stopping treatment. For adverse effects, see A–Z of Medicines.

Chilblains

Chilblains are caused by cooling of the hands and feet and/or the whole of the body in susceptible individuals. They affect mainly toes and fingers and are caused by constriction of the small arteries in the fingers and toes on exposure to cold, followed by dilation of the arteries which results in swelling of the skin with itching and burning.

The best treatment for chilblains is *prevention* – central heating, warm clothes and physical exercise.

Drugs used to improve the circulation (see Chapter 27) should not be used, and any ointment that produces a redness and burning because it irritates the skin or dilates the arteries may do more harm than good. High doses of calcium or vitamin D have not been shown to be of value. No drug treatment can be recommended, whether by mouth or applied locally to the chilblains.

Try to prevent them, but if you develop chilblains just apply a simple greasy ointment (e.g. Vaseline) to protect the skin.

Dandruff

Dandruff is caused by an overgrowth of yeasts at the hair roots. It is worse at puberty. Any detergent shampoo is of use in treating dandruff. If used at least two or three times a week a detergent shampoo will keep the hair clear, but of course a detergent shampoo will not prevent the growth of yeast cells.

The scalp should be well massaged, the shampoo *left in contact with the scalp for several minutes and then thoroughly washed off*. Any shampoo left on the scalp may cause the dandruff to stick together and be even more visible. Detergents used in shampoos include **sodium lauryl sulphate**, **benzalkonium** and **cetrimide**.

Shampoos that contain drugs to treat dandruff are often referred to as *medicated shampoos*. Certain drug additives are included in shampoos because they may reduce the production of cells from the skin of the scalp, dissolve the particles of dandruff or break them up into smaller pieces, relieve itching and/or act as an antiseptic.

Pyrithione zinc has antibacterial and antifungal properties and is a useful treatment for dandruff. **Selenium sulphate** is probably no better than a detergent shampoo. It should not be applied within forty-eight hours of hair colouring or a permanent wave preparation. The antifungal drug **ketoconazole** (in **Nizoral** shampoo) will help to kill the yeast cells. Ketoconazole and zinc pyrithione are active against *pityosporum ovali*, an organism implicated in seborrhaeic dermatitis of the scalp. Topical lithium may also be beneficial.

Preparations which break up and loosen dandruff particles contain keratolytics. They dissolve the cement that holds the cells together. They include **sulphur**, **salicylic acid** and **allantoin**.

Tar products break up the dandruff but they smell and they may stain the skin and hair. They also make the skin sensitive to sunlight. They are useful for treating psoriasis of the scalp.

Cresol, thymol and phenol are commonly used anti-infective drugs included in shampoos. They may irritate the scalp and are of very doubtful benefit.

Dermatitis and Eczema

The terms dermatitis and eczema have the same meaning – a superficial non-infective inflammation of the skin which may be acute, sub-acute or long-lasting (chronic). When acute, the skin is red, swollen, blistered, weeping, crusted, scaling and often itching. Scratching and rubbing may cause bleeding and scarring. When it is chronic, the skin may be dry, thickened, scaling, itching and scarred.

In the United Kingdom the term *eczema* is used to describe dermatitis caused by a sensitivity to some factor from inside the body (for example, allergic dermatitis caused by food allergy) and the term *contact dermatitis* is used to describe dermatitis caused by contact with some factor outside the body (e.g. dermatitis to a cosmetic).

Atopic eczema (*atopic dermatitis*) is a chronic eczema that usually occurs in individuals with a family history of allergic disorders (e.g. eczema, hayfever, asthma). *Atopy* means an inherited tendency to develop eczema, asthma and/ or hayfever in response to certain substances taken into the body by mouth or breathed in. The cause is unknown but it is considered to be an abnormal allergic response.

Contact dermatitis is an acute or chronic inflammation of the skin caused by substances in contact with the skin. It often occurs in well-demarcated patches. It may be caused by a direct irritant (irritant dermatitis) or by an allergic reaction (allergic dermatitis).

The appearance of irritant and allergic contact dermatitis is very similar, but an allergic reaction may be more red and there may be more small blisters (vesicles) and swelling of the skin.

Contact with irritants may damage normal healthy skin and cause an existing dermatitis to flare up.

Allergic contact dermatitis is caused by a delayed allergic reaction to some substance. The skin first becomes sensitized by contact with the substance, which triggers off a delayed allergic response. This may not appear for days, months or even years, despite the fact that the individual's skin may have been in direct contact with the substance daily – for example, make-up, or an ointment for eczema.

Treatment of Acute Inflamed Dermatitis and Eczema

If the lesions are acute and wet, then wet soaks containing an astringent such as **aluminium acetate** may help. If there is a risk of infection, an antiseptic soak such as **potassium permanganate** may be beneficial.

To relieve the inflammation and itching a powerful **corticosteroid cream** should be used for the first few days and then a milder preparation should be substituted. Only hydrocortisone cream should be used on the face because others may cause harmful effects on the skin (see p. 241). If the condition is severe and extensive it may be necessary to add a corticosteroid by mouth for a few days. An antihistamine by mouth may help to relieve itching.

If infection is present a **combined corticosteroid/antibiotic cream** should be used. If the infection is severe it may be necessary to use an antibiotic by mouth after a swab has been taken to identify the infecting micro-organism. For very severe resistant atopic eczema an immunosuppressive drug such as **cyclosporin** (**Neoral, Sandimmun**) may help. See Chapter 17.

Treatment of Dry, Scaly Dermatitis and Eczema

Over a period of time the irritated skin becomes thick, scaly and itchy, resulting in much scratching. Dry, scaly patches are best treated with a soothing skin application (an **emollient**) which will soothe the skin and make it less dry and scaly.

A mainstay of treatment, particularly in atopic eczema, is the use of short courses of a mildly or moderately potent **corticosteroid ointment**, but see adverse effects and precautions on p. 241.

When the skin is very thick and scaly it may help to use a substance that peels the skin, such as **salicylic acid**, **coal tar** or **ichthammol**.

The essential fatty acid (gamolenic acid) in **evening primrose oil** is available in capsules (**Epogam**, **Efamast**) to treat atopic eczema. It may possibly be of benefit in some children.

Insect Bites and Stings

The area should be cleansed and cooling lotion applied (e.g. **calamine lotion**). Bee stings should be removed by scraping with a fingernail or knife before cleaning. If the reaction is fairly severe an **antihistamine** should be taken by mouth. An application containing **hydrocortisone** may be very effective in relieving the itching and soreness.

Most over-the-counter preparations used to relieve the symptoms of an insect bite or sting contain one or more of the following: a *counter-irritant* such as camphor or menthol, a *local anaesthetic* such as benzocaine, an *antihistamine*, a *skin protectant* such as zinc oxide or calamine, an *antiseptic* such as cresol. All these may possibly help, but some may irritate the skin and produce other problems.

Lice

Body Lice (Pediculosis Corporis)

These lice are spread from person to person by direct contact or by contact with clothing. Lice and eggs can be found in the clothing. The patient itches and scratches and should be bathed and given clean clothing. An aqueous solution of **malathion** or **carbaryl** should be applied all over the body, left on for twelve hours or overnight and then washed off. This treatment should be repeated after one week. **Calamine lotion with 1 per cent phenol** will reduce the itching.

Crabs (Pediculosis Pubis)

This infestation affects pubic and armpit hairs and causes severe itching. In adults it is spread by close sexual contact. The underclothes should be washed and the infected person should take a bath and then apply an *aqueous* solution of **malathion** or **carbaryl** to the affected area *and* to all parts of the body as well. The lotion should be left on for twelve hours or overnight and then washed off. This treatment should be repeated after one week.

> **Note:** *It may also be necessary to treat beards, eyelashes or moustaches if these have become infested.*

Head Lice (Pediculosis Capitis)

Head lice are spread by direct person-to-person contact and by contact with infected combs and hats. It is a common infestation among schoolchildren. Infestation may occasionally cause itching but usually all that can be seen are nits (eggs) on the hair shafts. The nits mature in about three to four days and the lice can then be found at the back of the head and behind the ears.

Treatment includes the use of preparations containing **carbaryl** (**Carylderm**), **malathion** (**Derbac-M, Prioderm, Quellada M, Suleo M**), **permethrin** (**Lyclear**), or **phenothrin** (**Full Marks**). In order to prevent resistance most Health Authorities rotate these treatments.

Lotions should be used in preference to shampoos because the latter are not in contact with the hair long enough to work properly.

Lindane is no longer used because there are now strains of treated lice which are resistant to it. However, resistance is also developing to the other agents and their use should be monitored.

> **Warning:** *Water-based (aqueous) preparations should be used in asthmatics and very young children in order to avoid alcoholic fumes given off by preparations that contain alcohol. Contact of twelve hours or overnight is needed to kill the nits.*
>
> *Daily shampooing and wet combing with a fine comb is probably as effective as using a pesticide and it is much safer.*

Psoriasis

The skin is continually being renewed and as dead cells are shed from the surface, new cells underneath take their place. This process maintains the normal surface of the skin (the epidermis). However, in psoriasis the process is disturbed and in certain areas of the skin new cells are produced at an excessive rate while the shedding of old cells remains normal and cannot keep pace with the number of new skin cells pushing out on to the surface. As a result these new cells pile up to produce patches of thickened skin covered in silvery scales. The patches heal over without producing a scar.

The spread and extent of these patches of psoriasis vary between acute and chronic attacks, and are affected by the age of the patient. Patches of psoriasis may differ in size from a fraction of an inch to large sheets affecting the skin of the whole of the trunk. Psoriasis may affect the fingernails, scalp, skin folds, elbows, knees, palms of the hands, soles of the feet, the back and the buttocks. The eyebrows and the skin around the anus, genitals and the navel may occasionally be affected. It may also be associated with arthritis affecting a few or many joints (psoriatic arthropathy).

There is no cure for psoriasis, but treatment can provide effective control by reducing the size of the patches and reducing inflammation. Treatment varies according to the severity and extent of the psoriasis and the areas affected.

Treatment of Acute Psoriasis

Acute psoriasis that comes on in childhood (acute guttate psoriasis) usually clears up on its own in two or three months and sometimes treatment may actually make it worse. All that is needed is a simple emollient cream.

Treatment of Mild to Moderate Psoriasis

For mild psoriasis a soothing ointment (**emollient**) may be all that is necessary. If it is moderately severe, then it may be worth trying a **coal tar product** at night and an emollient in the daytime. An application of **dithranol** for half-an-hour in the daytime may be added to the treatment. In addition, a **corticosteroid** application and/or an **anti-itching** application may be used. Exposure to the sun's rays may help, but sunburn should be avoided because psoriasis may develop at the site of any damage to the skin.

Skin applications work better if the thickened scales are removed first. This is often best achieved by having a daily bath containing an **oil emulsion** and then rubbing off the scales using a bland cream.

Coal tar products are antiseptic, they relieve itching and they help the loss of scales, and so does **salicylic acid**. They are useful for treating chronic patches of psoriasis. **Tazarotene** is a retinoid which causes drying and peeling of the skin and is used to treat plaque psoriasis.

Dithranol should be used with caution because it may irritate the surrounding skin. A ring of Vaseline should therefore be applied around the patch of psoriasis before applying the dithranol. It may stain the skin and clothing black. It works just as well if it is left on for about thirty–sixty minutes and then washed off or it can be left on all night. Low concentrations of dithranol should be used to start with and then the concentration gradually increased. Fair-skinned people are more sensitive to dithranol than dark-skinned people. Dithranol is messy and it is better to use a brand preparation such as **Dithrocream** or **Micanol**.

The use of both tar and dithranol on the face should be avoided because they may irritate the skin. Their use should also be avoided in skin folds because they may cause boils to develop. In these areas an emollient should be used.

Bland emollient creams are the applications of choice to stop itching. Local anaesthetics and antihistamine preparations should *not* be used because they may produce irritation and allergy.

Calcipotriol (**Dovonex**) is a synthetic vitamin D. It is used in ointment form to treat mild to moderate psoriasis. It stops the overgrowth of cells in the surface (epidermis) of the skin that occurs in psoriasis and helps to restore a normal turnover of the surface cells. It has less effect on calcium metabolism in the body than other synthetic vitamin D preparations (e.g. calcitriol) and therefore the risk of a raised blood calcium, calcium in the urine and bone softening is reduced. Unlike dithranol and tar it does not have an unpleasant smell and it does not stain the clothing.

Applications which soften the skin and help it to peel work by loosening keratin, a protein in the outer layer of the skin. They include **sulphur**, **salicylic acid**, **allantoin** and **resorcinol**. However, they are irritant and should not be applied over large areas since they may be absorbed, producing harmful effects.

Corticosteroid applications may be beneficial. However, they may lose their effectiveness if used every day for more than two or three weeks. It may therefore help to alternate treatment every one or two weeks between a corticosteroid and an emollient.

Adverse effects of corticosteroid applications on the skin are discussed earlier. They may be absorbed into the bloodstream and produce harmful effects. This is particularly likely to happen if they are applied under adhesive or plastic dressings; if they are applied to large areas of the body; if highly concentrated and/or potent forms are used, and/or if large amounts are applied at regular intervals.

The strength and number of applications of a corticosteroid should be gradually reduced as the treated patches of psoriasis improve. Hydrocortisone is the only corticosteroid that should be applied to the face. Thick patches of psoriasis which are resistant to applications may be injected under the skin with a solution of a corticosteroid such as **triamcinolone**. Such treatment should not be repeated within about three weeks in order to avoid wasting of the skin.

Severe and/or Chronic Psoriasis

The treatment of severe and/or chronic psoriasis follows fashions, but some old-fashioned treatments are still in favour – for instance local applications of **coal tar**, **dithranol** and **skin softeners** (e.g. **salicylic acid**). These are usually applied after a bath and after rubbing off the scales.

Ultraviolet B radiation is the basis of a treatment called *Ingram's method*. It consists of a warm bath containing a tar solution, a dose of ultraviolet radiation to produce redness, and then the application of **tar** or **dithranol** paste to the patches of psoriasis.

The tar and dithranol make the patches of psoriasis sensitive to the ultraviolet radiation. Repeated every day this treatment is effective, and in most patients it clears up patches well in about three to six weeks.

Methoxypsoralen and other psoralen drugs act on DNA in cells to slow down their rate of division. The drugs are activated by exposure of the skin to ultraviolet radiation. Methoxypsoralen is used in a treatment referred to as PUVA treatment (P stands for psoralens and UVA stands for ultraviolet A radiation). PUVA treatment is used to treat large chronic patches of psoriasis.

The methoxypsoralen is used as a bath solution or given by mouth and this is followed by ultraviolet treatment two hours later – timed to coincide with peak concentrations of the drug in the bloodstream. Treatments with gradually increasing doses of UVA are repeated two or three times a week until the psoriasis has cleared up. An average of about twenty treatments are usually required. The rash may not return for several months, but if necessary the skin can be kept clear with one PUVA treatment every one to three weeks.

> *Warning: PUVA must be used with caution because of the risk of burning and long-term risks of cataracts, premature ageing of the skin and skin cancer.*

Methotrexate is a drug used to treat cancer. It stops cells dividing and because of this action it has been found to be useful in some patients suffering from severe chronic psoriasis, but because of the risks it should only be used under hospital supervision to treat psoriasis that has not responded to any other treatment. Other drugs of this type that have been tried include **hydroxyurea** and **azaribine**. So has the immunosuppresant **ciclosporin** (see p. 89).

Etretinate: Although vitamin A is involved in skin development and function it has proved of no use in treating psoriasis. However, etretinate, which is related to vitamin A, reduces scaling and improves psoriasis. It slows down the rapid rate of cell division in skin cells and reduces the production of keratin – the hard protein that forms the outer layer of the skin. Unfortunately, serious risks may easily outweigh any benefits.

Acitretin (**Neotigason**) is a breakdown product of etretinate in the body and it has replaced etretinate in the treatment of psoriasis. It should not be used in pregnancy and patients should avoid getting pregnant for two years *after* treatment has stopped.

Tacalcitol (**Curatoderm**) is related to calcitrol (vitamin D_3). It binds to vitamin D_3 receptors in the keratin-making cells of the skin and slows down their division. It is used as an ointment to treat plaques of psoriasis.

Scabies

Scabies is due to an invasion of the outer layer of the skin (the epidermis) by a mite called *Sarcoptes scabiei*. The infection is spread from person to person by close skin contact (e.g. by holding hands, or sleeping together). Successful infection is caused by a fertilized female mite burrowing into the skin, where she lives for the rest of her life. As she burrows along the skin she lays her eggs every day for several weeks. The eggs hatch in a few days and the larvae leave the burrows and shelter in hair roots, where they develop into adult mites. They then mate and set the whole cycle going again, which takes about two weeks.

The mites burrow into the skin, particularly on the hands and feet, and after about a month an itchy rash develops at the infected sites because the individual has become sensitive (allergic) to the mites. The rash characteristically affects the wrists, ankles, fingers, buttocks, abdomen and genitals. It does not occur above the neck in adults. With any future infestation itching will start almost straight away because the individual has become allergic. An infected person may scratch so much that the skin is damaged and dermatitis may develop, which may also become infested.

Treatment

Drugs used include:
malathion (**Derbac M**, **Prioderm**, **Quellada M**, **Suleo-M**)
permethrin (**Lyclear**)

It is absolutely necessary to treat every member of the household who may have skin-to-skin contact, whether they are itching or not. It is also important to treat sexual partners.

After washing well, an application of **malathion** or **permethrin** should be applied all over the body from the neck downwards, preferably with a paintbrush and by some other member of the household. Particular attention should be paid to the webs of the fingers and toes and under the nails. The scalp, neck, face and ears should be treated in children under two years of age and in the elderly and those who are immune-deficient due to disease (e.g.

AIDS) or drugs (e.g. chemotherapy). Lotions and solutions are easier to apply than creams and ointments.

Washing thoroughly is now recommended in preference to a hot bath, which may increase the absorption of the drug into the bloodstream and possibly increase the risk of harmful effects. Aqueous preparations should be used because alcoholic ones may irritate scratched skin and the genitalia.

Benzyl benzoate (**Ascabiol**) is occasionally used but it is irritant and should not be used in children.

Warts

There are thirty-five types of viruses that cause warts. Warts may appear at any age but are commonest in children. They may be single or multiple. They may disappear without treatment in months or years and they may recur at the same site or at different sites. Patients who are immune-deficient due to drugs or disease (e.g. AIDS) may suffer from an extensive attack of warts.

The common types of warts often affect the hands and feet. The latter are often referred to as plantar warts or verrucae.

Most wart applications contain a caustic or keratolytic, which removes the keratin layer and destroys the underlying layer of the skin. Commonly used ones include **salicylic acid**, **formaldehyde** and **podophyllum**. Most of these preparations will irritate the surrounding skin and since warts clear up on their own it is not necessary to subject little children to such treatments. Because the 'life' of a wart is self-limiting, it also explains the success of various folk remedies and the 'charming away' of warts. Any treatment that is applied when the warts are disappearing on their own will be considered to have caused their disappearance!

Simple remedies are best (e.g. **salicylic acid** collodion (**Cuplex, Duofilm, Occlusal, Salactol, Salatac, Verrugon**). An adhesive plaster should be put over the warts after the application has dried.

Stronger preparations containing **formaldehyde** (**Veracur**) or **glutaraldehyde** (**Glutarol**) may work on some plantar warts in some people, but their effectiveness is difficult to predict. Preparations containing formaldehyde or glutaraldehyde may irritate the skin and cause allergic rashes. They also have an unpleasant smell. Formalin solution (3 per cent) used as a foot soak may help multiple plantar warts, or a tape impregnated with 40 per cent salicylic acid may be helpful if it is kept in place for several days at a time. Skin specialists may burn some warts with **liquid nitrogen**, or they may surgically remove large and ugly warts.

Podophyllum preparations are useful for treating *genital warts* but they can produce severe irritation of the skin and serious adverse effects if applied too heavily. They should not be used in pregnancy. Preparations include **podophyllin** paint compound and **podophyllotoxin** (**Condyline, Warticon**).

Imiquimod (**Aldara**) **cream** is used for the treatment of external genital warts.

Posalfilin, which contains podophyllin resin 20 per cent and salicylic acid 25 per cent, is suitable for treating plantar warts (verrucae). The application should be applied directly on to the wart or warts and contact with the surrounding skin should be avoided because it may irritate. A sticking plaster should then be applied over the treated wart and left in place until the next treatment is due – treatment is usually given once or twice daily. Dead skin should be removed with a pumice stone before the next application.

46

Antibacterial Drugs

Antibiotics

The term 'antibiotic' is applied to drugs obtained from one group of micro-organisms (e.g. bacteria, fungi) that are used to kill another group of micro-organisms. Antibiotics may be antibacterial and/or antifungal. They are chemicals which stop the growth of micro-organisms (bacteriostatic) and/or eventually kill them (bactericidal). Numerous antibiotics are available and they vary in their structure, action, effects and the type of bacteria which are sensitive to them. They are produced by various micro-organisms such as fungi and bacteria and have been obtained from moulds, soil and other sources. Those produced from moulds may be called biosynthetic and those whose structure is modified by the addition of other chemicals to the growing medium are called semi-synthetic.

An antibiotic may be tested by inoculating micro-organisms into a liquid culture medium which contains varying dilutions of the drug. Antibiotics are not effective against all micro-organisms; some are effective against bacteria, others against fungi, some against many bacteria or fungi and some against only a few. The number of types of bacteria or fungi against which a particular antibiotic is effective is called its antibacterial (or antifungal) spectrum. If it is active against many types it is called a broad-spectrum antibiotic.

Bacteria may become resistant to an antibiotic (even when it is used correctly) by several very complex mechanisms, and generally if resistance develops to one antibiotic from a group of antibiotics then there is cross-resistance to other antibiotics in that group. The use of two or more antibiotics together may help to prevent or delay the development of resistance. This is a technique frequently used in the treatment of tuberculosis but not normally recommended in treating other disorders except where two drugs act synergistically. Drug resistance may also be developed by micro-organisms because of improper treatment. This may be due to giving inappropriate doses, inappropriate intervals between doses, inadequate lengths of treatment or inappropriate antibiotic combinations.

Delay in starting antibiotics may affect response and so will the response of the body to the infecting micro-organism and to the drug. For example, pus cells may destroy the antibiotic effects, the acidity of the urine may change the effectiveness of certain antibiotics given to treat urinary infections, an abscess with tough walls will prevent antibiotics from getting into the abscess, and antibiotics may not be able to pass certain barriers (e.g. into the eye). Some may not be absorbed from the intestine and have to be given by injection.

Patient (host) factors such as age, genetic characteristics, general physical condition (e.g. liver and kidney function), pregnancy, history of allergy to drugs and the presence of other infections may also affect the choice of an antibiotic drug. Furthermore, the patient's response to treatment and in particular his or her 'defence mechanisms' against infections are very important.

Antibiotics may be used effectively to prevent the development of an infection if given just after exposure (e.g. high doses of penicillin after running the risk of getting gonorrhoea (providing tests have excluded syphilis)) or if given to prevent recurrence of infection with a particular organism (e.g. to prevent certain types of tonsillitis).

Adverse effects produced by antibiotics are on the increase. This is related to the increasing number of preparations available and the increasing number of patients being treated. Antibiotics may produce specific adverse effects (e.g. chloramphenicol may damage the bone marrow, neomycin may damage the kidneys), but in addition all antibiotics share two major adverse effects – the risk of allergic reactions and the risk of super-added infections with other micro-organisms.

Allergic reactions include anaphylactic shock, skin rashes, angioedema, fever and painful joints, bone-marrow damage and jaundice. Superinfections occur because many micro-organisms live together in a balanced community in many parts of our bodies (nose, mouth, intestine, skin, lungs, bladder, vagina). Any disturbance in this balance (i.e. an antibiotic, which may knock out one group of organisms) may lead to an overgrowth (superinfection) of other micro-organisms, for example, yeasts, fungi, and bacteria. These are usually minor but may occasionally be very serious and, rarely, fatal. They are difficult to treat and are more likely to occur with broad-spectrum antibiotics, in children under three years of age, in elderly and/or debilitated patients and in patients with disorders such as diabetes.

Remember – antibiotics are valuable drugs if used appropriately but because they are very effective in treating some infections they should not be used to treat just any infections (e.g. virus sore throats). They should not be used for minor infections. They should be used in appropriate doses at appropriate intervals and for an appropriate length of time. They should not be used just because they are new, particularly when effective established alternatives are available. Finally, they should never be taken without medical supervision. Never take antibiotics because 'there were a few left in the house', or because 'they did my neighbour good'. Unless you and your doctor have decided that treatment with an antibiotic is appropriate for you, do not take them without advice and do not always expect them from your doctor.

Penicillins

Penicillin was the first antibiotic to be produced by growing *penicillium* mould on broth. It became available for use in 1941. The original crude extracts of the fermentation of the mould contained several penicillins. By adding various chemicals to the fermentation, a number of naturally produced penicillins have been developed; for example, **benzylpenicillin** (**penicillin G**) and **phenoxymethylpenicillin** (**penicillin V**). In addition, the chemical structure of the penicillin may be altered to produce what are called semi-synthetic penicillins. They are not wholly synthetic; the basic penicillin structure is still obtained from moulds by fermentation.

Penicillins damage the developing cell walls of multiplying bacteria, making them burst. Therefore, they kill bacteria (*bactericidal*) but only when they are multiplying. Bacteria may become resistant to the effects of penicillins in two ways. They may produce enzymes which inactivate the penicillin – the best-known of these is called *penicillinase*, which disrupts the chemical structure (the beta-lactam ring) of the penicillin nucleus, making it inactive. Penicillinase may be referred to as a *beta-lactamase*.*

Some bacteria develop a tolerance to penicillin (resistance) and they just go on multiplying in the presence of doses which would previously have killed them. Development of resistance has often been related to the indiscriminate use of penicillins and it is a serious risk, particularly in surgical wards in hospital.

Allergic reactions to penicillins may occasionally occur, producing skin rashes, angioedema, fever and swollen joints. Anaphylactic shock (see p. 83), which is very rare, may be followed by death. It is more common after injections and in patients who have previously had an allergic reaction to penicillin. Penicillin allergy may be produced by skin ointments, ear drops, eye drops and throat lozenges. It may also follow the handling of penicillin (for instance in nurses drawing up injections), breathing it in and drinking milk from cows treated with penicillin for mastitis. For these reasons penicillin should not be used in topical applications and throat lozenges. The latter may

* *Note:* Penicillins and cephalosporins are referred to as beta-lactam antibiotics because they have a beta-lactam ring as part of their basic chemical structure.

produce a sore tongue, mouth and lips and also a black furring of the tongue.

Ampicillin and related penicillins may produce a skin rash in patients suffering from glandular fever or chronic lymphatic leukaemia. This is different from the usual penicillin rash. It is probably a toxic reaction and penicillins can be used in future in these patients. All penicillins may occasionally cause diarrhoea, nausea, heartburn and itching of the anus.

Apart from allergy, penicillins are very safe drugs. Adverse effects are more likely to occur because of errors in prescribing than from any other cause. Remember, cross-allergy to penicillin occurs: if you are allergic to one (say, penicillin V) you may be allergic to another (e.g. ampicillin). Skin-testing for allergy may be useful in detecting those patients who are likely to have a life-threatening anaphylactic reaction.

A rare adverse effect of the penicillins is irritation of the brain, producing disorders of brain function (encephalopathy). This occurs when very high doses are used intravenously or intramuscularly, particularly in patients with impaired kidney function. Injection of penicillin into the spinal fluid in high doses can cause convulsions and should be avoided.

Penicillins should not be taken for trivial infections or by patients who have had a previous allergic reaction. They should be taken with caution by patients who have had an allergic reaction to any other drug. They provide us with a range of very valuable antibiotics, which, if used appropriately, are very effective.

Penicillins are classified as follows:

- *Penicillinase-sensitive Penicillins*
  benzylpenicillin (penicillin G, Crystapen)
  phenoxymethylpenicillin (penicillin V, Apsin, Tenkicin)

- *Penicillinase-resistant Penicillins*
  flucloxacillin (Floxapen, Fluclomix, Galfloxin, Ladropen, Zoxin)

- *Broad-spectrum Penicillins*
  amoxicillin (Almodan, Amix, Amoram, Amoxil, Galenamox, Rimoxallin)
  ampicillin (Penbritin, Rimacillin)

- *Anti-pseudomonal Penicillins*
These are effective against severe infections caused by *pseudomonas* bacteria which are not affected by other penicillins.
  piperacillin (Pipril, in Tazocin)
  ticarcillin

- *Combined Preparations*
Co-amoxiclav (Augmentin, Augmentin-Duo) contains **amoxycillin** with a beta-lactamase inhibitor (**clavulanic acid**) which inhibits penicillinase. **Timentin** contains **ticarcillin** and **clavulanic acid**. Preparations containing a broad-spectrum

penicillin and a penicillinase-resistant penicillin include **co-fluampicil** (**Magnapen**) which contains **ampicillin** and **flucloxacillin. Tazocin** contains **piperacillin** and the beta-lactamase inhibitor **tazobactam**.

● *Mecillinams*

Pivmecillinam (**Selexid**) is hydrolysed in the body to mecillinam, which is the active drug. It is used in bacterial infections of the urinary tract.

Cephalosporins and Cephamycins

The **cephalosporins** are broad-spectrum semi-synthetic antibiotics produced from a natural mould antibiotic (cephalosporin C). They act on much the same groups of bacteria as the natural penicillins. They also act on a broad spectrum of bacteria in the same way as ampicillin and are effective against some bacteria which are resistant to ampicillin. They may produce allergic reactions, and cross-allergy may occur between cephalosporins and some penicillins in some patients. About 10 per cent of patients allergic to penicillin will be allergic to cephalosporins. Cross-resistance may be shown to cephalosporins by bacteria resistant to methicillin and cloxacillin.

The **cephalosporin group** includes **cefaclor** (**Distaclor**), **cefadroxil** (**Baxan**), **cefalexin** (**Ceporex, Keflex**), **cefamandole**(cephamandole) (**Kefadol**), **cefradine** (**Velosef**), **cefazolin** (**Kefzol**), **cefixime** (**Suprax**), **cefotaxime** (**Claforan**), **cefoxitin** (**Mefoxin**), **cefpirome** (**Cefrom**), **cefpodoxime** (**Orelox**), **cefprozil** (**Cefzil**), **ceftazidime** (**Fortum, Kefadim**), **ceftriaxone** (**Rocephin**), **and cefuroxime** (**Zinacef, Zinnat**).

Other similar antibiotics include **aztreonam** (**Azactam**) and **meropenem** (**Meronem**) which have a wide spectrum of activity against bacteria, including beta-lactamase producing bacteria and **imipenem** which is combined with **cilastatin** in **Primaxin**. It has a broad spectrum of activity. The cilastatin blocks an enzyme in the kidneys which inactivates imipenem.

Macrolide Antibiotics

This group includes **erythromycin** (**Erymax, Erythrocin, Erythroped, Rommix, Tiloryth**), **azithromycin** (**Zithromax**) and **clarithromycin** (**Klaricid**).

Erythromycin is active against a narrow group of bacteria similar to those sensitive to the natural penicillins. It is bacteriostatic. It may be of use in treating tissue infections caused by bacteria resistant to the natural penicillins or if the patient is allergic to penicillins. It has been widely used but bacteria quickly become resistant to it, especially if it is given for more than one week. Its use has been replaced by other antibiotics in many cases. It is inactivated by the acid in the stomach and has to be given in acid-resistant capsules, or specially covered tablets (enteric-coated) as one of its esters (e.g. erythromycin oleate or stearate). Erythromycin may cause liver damage with jaundice and fever if a second or subsequent course is given, particularly if it is given for more than two weeks. This is thought to be an allergic reaction and clears up when the drug is stopped.

Azithromycin and **clarithromycin** are not as easily destroyed by the acid in the stomach and can be given in much lower doses. They cause fewer stomach and bowel upsets than erythromycin.

Lincosamide Antibiotics

This group includes **clindamycin** (**Dalacin C**). It may cause severe diarrhoea, and also a potentially life-threatening inflammation of the bowel (pseudo-membranous colitis) which occurs more commonly in middle-aged and elderly women, especially following surgery. While this occurs, rarely, with other antibiotics as well, the incidence appears higher with clindamycin and its use should be restricted to the limited number of infections where it is clearly the drug of choice.

Tetracyclines

The first tetracycline to be discovered was **Aureomycin**, in 1948; it was grown from moulds. Another one, called **Terramycin**, was discovered in 1950. Two years later their chemical structure was determined and it was found to consist of a basic structure of four rings (tetra-cyclic). Therefore, the antibiotics were called tetracyclines and the generic name of chlortetracycline was given to Aureomycin and oxytetracycline to Terramycin. The names Aureomycin and Terramycin remained as brand names. **Oxytetracycline** (**Terramycin**) is also available under other brand names: **Oxymycin** and **Oxytetramix**. Since the 1950s numerous tetracyclines have been produced and tested but only a few have proved to be of value. These include **demeclocycline** (**Ledermycin**), **doxycycline** (**Vibramycin**), **lymecycline** (**Tetralysal**), **minocycline** (**Minocin**) and **tetracycline** (**Achromycin**, in **Deteclo, Economycin**).

One of the problems with the tetracyclines is that they are only partially absorbed from the intestine and enough reaches the lower bowel to affect the normal organisms which live there. This may alter the balance between bacteria and fungi and lead to a superinfection with thrush (*Candida*), which can infect the mouth, bowel, anus and vulva, producing soreness and irritation. A more serious risk is a super-added infection with resistant bacteria which may cause severe enteritis and, very rarely, death. This is more likely to follow the use of tetracycline during abdominal operations. These super-added infections may also affect the lungs. **Demeclocycline**, **doxycycline** and **minocycline** are better absorbed than the other tetracyclines and the risk of enteritis is reduced.

Absorption of tetracyclines from the intestine may be decreased by interaction with calcium (e.g. in milk), iron and magnesium salts (e.g. in antacids) when these are taken at the same time. None of these should be taken at the same time as a tetracycline or its absorption will be decreased and the desired therapeutic effects will not be achieved. Absorption is similarly reduced by food, with the exception of doxycycline and minocycline. Tetracyclines are excreted in the urine and in the bile. **Doxycycline** is excreted primarily via the bile and hence is the safest tetracycline in kidney failure. Since its excretory products are largely inactive, it has less effect on natural bowel bacteria than other tetracyclines, and accordingly a lower incidence of super-infection.

Very rarely, tetracyclines given by injection may produce severe liver damage (sometimes fatal) when given to pregnant women with infections of their kidneys. Tetracyclines are deposited in growing teeth, producing discoloration and staining in young children. It is not only the first set of teeth which is affected – the adult teeth may also be stained for life and there is an added risk of tooth decay. They are also deposited in bone and bone growth stops during tetracycline treatment. These effects on teeth and bone may occur before the baby is born (if the mother is given tetracyclines) and right on into childhood. Therefore, they should be avoided in pregnancy and preferably not given to children under twelve years of age. They may discolour nails at any age if taken over a prolonged period. **Doxycycline** is said to cause less staining than the other tetracyclines. Allergic reactions to tetracycline drugs are rare. Sensitivity of the skin to sunlight may occur in patients receiving **demeclocycline** or **doxycycline**; this is less likely with the others.

Tetracyclines (other than doxycycline and minocycline) may affect protein production in the body and also kidney function. These may be indicated by a rise in the blood levels of breakdown products of proteins (as estimated by blood urea levels, for example). Urea and other waste products are excreted by the kidneys and this may have no consequence if the kidneys are healthy. However, if their function is impaired these waste products may rise in the blood, producing loss of appetite, vomiting and weakness. This is called kidney failure and may occur unexpectedly in elderly patients who are given tetracyclines, usually for a chest infection.

Streptomycin and Other Aminoglycosides

Streptomycin was discovered in soil in 1944. Other aminoglycoside antibiotics have since been discovered. They include **amikacin** (**Amikin**), **framycetin** (**Soframycin**), **gentamicin** (**Cidomycin**, **Genticin**), **neomycin** (**Nivemycin**), **netilmicin** (**Netillin**), **tobramycin** (**Nebcin**). They are bactericidal against a wide spectrum of bacteria responsible for serious infections. Bacteria quickly develop resistance to streptomycin and less quickly to the others.

They are poorly absorbed from the intestine and have to be given by intra-muscular or intravenous injection. They are quickly excreted by the kidneys and impaired kidney function may lead to dangerously high blood levels. They are painful when given by injection and their principal adverse effects include deafness (which may be permanent) and disorders of the organ of balance due to damage to the main nerve which supplies the ear and organ of balance. They may also damage the kidneys and affect nerve-muscle junctions, producing muscle weakness and depression of respiration.

These adverse effects are more likely to occur with high doses, prolonged courses of treatment, in patients over middle-age and in patients with impaired kidney function. Allergic reactions may occur, particularly with streptomycin, which may also cause severe allergic skin reactions in those handling the drug (e.g. nurses). Anyone handling the drug should be very cautious and wear gloves. They should not be used in pregnancy since they can damage the baby's hearing. Their use along with certain diuretics which can damage hearing (e.g. frusemide, ethacrynic acid) should be avoided and their use should always be monitored using blood level measurements.

Streptomycin is principally used to treat tuberculosis in combination with other drugs such as **isoniazid**. **Neomycin** is too toxic for systematic use. It is not absorbed from the intestine and can be used to sterilize the bowel before surgery. Its main use is in applications for the skin, eyes and ears. Patients can become hypersensitive to neomycin.

Framycetin is similar to neomycin; only used in topical applications. **Gentamicin** is related to neomycin; it is active against a wide spectrum of bacteria. It is used to treat severe infections. **Tobramycin** has similar actions to gentamicin. **Amikacin** is useful against bacteria resistant to gentamicin.

Polymyxins and Related Antibiotics

The polymyxins are a group of antibiotics which include **colistimethate** (**Colomycin**). It is used in topical applications and by injection to treat very severe infections and by mouth to sterilize the bowel before bowel surgery. Polymyxins are poorly absorbed from the intestine and even with injections it is difficult to get a high blood level; therefore large doses have to be used. They may produce kidney damage and, rarely, damage to nerve-muscle junctions, producing muscle weakness and depression of respiration. **Polymyxin B** (in **Gregoderm**, in **Maxitrol**, in **Neosporin**, in **Otosporin**, in **Polyfax**, in **Polytrim**) is used externally.

Some Other Antibacterial Drugs

Chloramphenicol (**Chloromycetin**, **Kemicetine**) was the first broad-spectrum antibiotic to be discovered. It was introduced in 1947 and soon became widely promoted and prescribed. However, it may occasionally knock out red and white cell production by the bone marrow and its use is now restricted to treating typhoid fever and a certain type of meningitis. It is also used in eye and ear applications.

Sodium fusidate (**Fucidin**) is the sodium salt of *fusidic acid*. It is well absorbed from the intestine, broken down in the liver and excreted in the urine and bile. It is active against penicillinase-producing staphylococci and should be reserved specifically for treating these infections. It penetrates bone and is used to treat bone infection (osteomyelitis). Bacteria readily develop resistance. It may be given in combination with other antibiotics such as flucloxacillin.

The **rifamycins** are related to streptomycin. Several have been produced and one of them, **rifampicin** (**Rifadin, Rimactane**), is used to prevent meningococcal meningitis in contacts and to treat tuberculosis and leprosy.

Vancomycin (**Vancocin**) is a *glycopeptide* that is too toxic for routine use and should be reserved for treating infections resistant to other antibiotics or patients with colitis caused by other antibiotics. It is not absorbed from the intestine and has to be given by intravenous injections, which may be painful and produce thrombophlebitis. When given to treat pseudo-membranous colitis (a severe type of colitis produced by antibiotics) it is given by mouth, and because it is not absorbed it does not produce systemic effects. **Teicoplanin** (**Targocid**) is similar to vancomycin but has a long duration of action. It can be given by injection into a muscle as well as into a vein.

Synercid contains a combination of the streptograms **quinupristin** and **dalfopristin**. It is effective in Gram-positive bacterial infections. It is reserved for treating infections where other antibacterials have failed, e.g. methicillin resistant staphylococcus aureus (MRSA infections).

Quinolones

Quinolones are effective antibacterial drugs. **Nalidixic acid** (**Mictral, Negram, Uriben**) and **norfloxacin** (**Utinor**) are used to treat infections of the urinary tract. **Ciprofloxacin** (**Ciproxin**) and **levofloxacin** (**Tavanic**) are active against a wide range of organisms and are useful for treating bacterial diarrhoea infections, certain lung infections, gonorrhoea, urinary tract infections and certain blood poisonings (septicaemia). **Ofloxacin** (**Tarivid**) is a synthetic drug related to nalidixic acid. It is used to treat infections of the urinary tract and genital tract and chest infections.

Nitroimidazoles

Metronidazole (**Flagyl, Metrolyl, Vaginyl**) and **tinidazole** (**Fasigyn**) are active against anaerobic bacteria and protozoa. They are of particular use in preventing and treating abdominal surgical infections and in treating infections of the vagina or mouth (acute ulcerative gingivitis). They are also used to treat amoebiasis and giardiasis.

Sulphonamides

In 1935 it was found that the red dye, prontosil rubra, protected mice from streptococcal infections and that the active antibacterial agent in the body was a breakdown product of the red dye called sulphanilamide. Following this discovery hundreds of similar drugs have been produced and tested for antibacterial activity. They belong to the sulphonamide group and they stop bacteria from multiplying (bacteriostatic) by affecting (competing with) the use of a vitamin called folic acid, which is essential for their growth.

These drugs were used extensively in the past but because of increasing bacterial resistance and the availability of other more effective and less toxic antibiotics their use has significantly decreased. One use is in the treatment of urinary tract infections caused by bacteria sensitive to the sulphonamides.

Adverse effects to sulphonamide drugs are relatively common and vary according to the particular sulphonamide used and the susceptibility of the patient. Those patients who break down certain drugs slowly (slow acetylators) may be more at risk.

The sulphonamides in use include:

sulfametopyrazine (**Kelfizine W**)

sulfadiazine

Those sulphonamides that are poorly absorbed from the intestine (calcium sulphaloxate and sulphaguanidine) were previously used to treat infections of the intestine and to prepare the bowel before abdominal surgery. They should not be used for these purposes. **Silver sulfadiazine** (**Flamazine**) is used to treat infected skin burns, leg ulcers and bedsores.

Combinations of Sulphonamides with Trimethoprim (Co-trimoxazole)

Trimethoprim (**Monotrim, Trimopan**) blocks the use of folic acid by bacteria just after the stage blocked by sulphonamides. It is effective on its own in treating urinary tract infections and some chest infections. However, it is often given with a sulphonamide, when both drugs block folic acid. This is an example of one drug potentiating the action of another by acting *synergistically*. While sulphonamides alone are bacteriostatic this combination is bactericidal. **Co-trimoxazole** (**Chemotrim, Comixco, Fectrim, Septrin**) contains the sulphonamide **sulfamethoxazole** and **trimethoprim**. Trimethoprim is well absorbed when taken by mouth and sulfamethoxazole was selected because it is absorbed and excreted at a similar rate to trimethoprim, so that after a few days the ratio of the two drugs in the bloodstream and urine is kept relatively constant to produce optimal synergism (i.e. working together).

Co-trimoxazole may produce any of the adverse effects of sulphonamides and of trimethoprim. Since it contains two drugs, bacterial sensitivity to *each* drug should be tested and it should only be used if the bacteria are sensitive to *both* drugs, when it obviously has a wider spectrum of activity than sulphonamides alone.

> *Warning:* Co-trimoxazole has been over-used with the result that some patients (particularly elderly ones) have suffered severe adverse effects, e.g. blood disorders and generalized skin disorders. Its use should be **limited** to treating a type of pneumonia that occurs in AIDS patients (pneumocystis carinii pneumonia: PCP), toxoplasmosis and nocardiasis. It should only be used to treat flame-ups of chronic bronchitis or urinary infections when the infecting organisms have been shown to be sensitive to **both** drugs in co-trimoxazole. Also, it should not be used to treat acute otitis media in children unless there is some very good reason for doing so.

47

Antifungal Drugs

The extent and nature of diseases caused by fungi (mycoses) vary a great deal between different areas of the world. In some areas fungal diseases are regularly present in the community, whereas in other areas they only occur under certain circumstances, for example, in individuals who have immune deficiency and in whom resistance to infection is reduced. This may occur because of drug treatments or disease.

Fungal infections are spread by spores or hyphae. Normally they are breathed in or land on the skin to cause infection. From the skin and lungs the fungus may spread to other parts of the body. Fungal infections last a long time (they are chronic infections) and usually any drug treatment has to be prolonged in order to obtain a cure.

Local fungal infections of the skin, mouth, vagina or anus are usually associated with some local damage to the surface or to treatment with antibiotics. The latter disturbs the local balance of bacteria and fungi and makes it easier for fungus to start to grow. A common example of this is vaginal thrush in someone given antibiotics by mouth. Some patients may be allergic to fungi and develop asthma and other respiratory disorders.

Because fungi particularly attack patients who are immune-deficient it is important to treat the 'whole' patient in order to correct if possible any predisposing factors. Any anaemia, infection or other underlying disorder should be treated and the patient should be given vitamins, minerals and a nutritious diet. Also, it is important to remove any contact with an infected animal, whether it is a dog, farm animal, pigeon or even bats in a cave.

Antifungal drugs include:

amorolfine (**Loceryl Cream and Nail Laquer**)
amphotericin (**Abelcet, AmBisome, Amphocil, Fungilin, Fungizone**)
clotrimazole (in topical applications (**Canesten, Candiden**))
econazole (in topical applications (**Ecostatin, Pevaryl**))

fluconazole (**Diflucan**)
flucytosine (**Ancotil**)
griseofulvin (**Grisovin**)
itraconazole (**Sporanox**)
ketoconazole (**Nizoral** and in topical applications (**Nizoral** cream and
    shampoo))
miconazole (**Daktarin** and in topical applications (**Daktarin cream**))
nystatin (**Nystan** and in several topical applications (**Nystaform** cream,
    Nystan cream, **Tinaderm-M** cream))
terbinafine (**Lamisil** and in topical applications (**Lamisil**))
tioconazole (**Trosyl nail solution**)

Antifungal drugs may be grouped according to their chemical structure –
allylamines (terbinafine)
griseofulvin, imidazoles (e.g. clotrimazole, ketoconazole, tioconazole,
    miconazole)
polyene antibiotics (e.g. amphotericin, nystatin)
triazoles (itraconazole, fluconazole)

Uses of Antifungal Drugs

Amphotericin is an antibiotic which either kills fungi (fungicidal) or interferes
with their multiplication (fungistatic) according to the dose used and the
fungus being treated. It is active against a wide range of fungi and yeasts. Its
activity may be increased by giving it along with certain antibacterial drugs
and other antifungal drugs (e.g. flucytosine). It is an effective drug which may
be given by mouth or infusion into a vein; but it may occasionally produce
serious harmful effects. Therefore, expected benefits need to be balanced
against the risks of using this drug. See special warnings on the use of
intravenous amphotericin preparations in A–Z of Medicines.

As with the treatment of all fungal infections, treatment with amphotericin
has to be prolonged – usually about six–ten weeks, but sometimes as long as
sixteen weeks.

Clotrimazole is used only in local applications to treat vaginal thrush and
ringworm and other forms of infection of the skin.

Econazole is used only in local applications to treat vaginal thrush.

Fluconazole is active by mouth and is used to treat thrush infections of the
vagina and mouth and throat. It needs only to be given in a single dose each
day. It has less effect than ketoconazole on the breakdown of other drugs by
the liver and less effect on the manufacture of steroids.

Flucytosine is effective in the treatment of generalized (systemic) fungal infections caused by certain yeasts, for example thrush. It may be given by mouth and
by infusion into a vein. Fungi may become resistant to flucytosine so its use as a

single drug should be restricted. However, it increases the effects of amphotericin and the two are often used together for treatment of severe generalized infections.

Griseofulvin is given by mouth for the treatment of fungus infections of the nails and hair. It is only used to treat infections of the skin if applications of antifungal preparations have failed and/or if the disease is widespread over the body. It concentrates in keratin, a protein on the surface layer of the skin which also forms a major component of nails and hair. The drug is deposited in developing keratin-producing cells and makes them resistant to fungal infection; therefore any new growth of hair, nails or skin is free from the infection. The keratin containing the fungus is got rid of through the loss of scales from the skin, and by cutting the nails and the hair. The infected keratin is gradually replaced by uninfected keratin.

As with all antifungal drug treatments, griseofulvin should be continued for weeks or even months.

Itraconazole is used to treat thrush of the vagina and vulva, and fungal skin infections. It can remain in tissues (e.g. the skin) for up to four weeks. It enters infected cells in the base of the skin and as the cells work their way to the surface the infected cells are shed.

Ketoconazole is taken by mouth; it requires acid in the stomach if it is to dissolve and be absorbed into the bloodstream. Therefore, drugs which block acid production (e.g. indigestion mixtures) reduce its absorption. It may, rarely, produce serious harmful effects (e.g. liver damage) and therefore expected benefits from using it should be carefully balanced against such risks. It is useful in treating histoplasmosis and a range of other serious fungal infections. It is better for long-term treatment. In acute infections it is less useful, because its absorption from the intestine is erratic and it is slow to work. It may antagonize the effects of amphotericin. Ketoconazole affects the metabolism of several other drugs.

Miconazole is used in local applications, by mouth and by intravenous infusion. Because of its harmful effects the intravenous use of miconazole should be strictly limited to the treatment of severe, generalized fungal infections that have not responded to other treatments. The main use of miconazole is in local applications for the treatment of vaginal thrush and ringworm and other infections of the skin.

Nystatin is an antibiotic with a similar structure to amphotericin. It both kills fungi (fungicidal) and prevents them multiplying (fungistatic). It is available in ointments, creams, mouthwashes, tablets, pastilles and suspensions. It is too toxic to be given by intravenous injection but it is safe by mouth for treating fungal infections of the intestine because it is not absorbed into the bloodstream and is passed out in the motions. It is active against a number of yeasts and fungi but its main use is in treating yeast infections, particularly thrush of the mouth, skin, genitals and anus, and of the oesophagus, stomach and intestine.

There is no evidence that nystatin combined with an antibiotic (e.g. tetracycline) reduces the incidence of thrush of the mouth caused by antibiotics in patients who are prone to develop thrush because of their general condition.

Terbinafine (**Lamisil**) is used by mouth to treat fungal infections of the skin and nails. There is also a topical preparation.

Tioconazole is combined with undecenoic acid in **Trosyl** nail solution, which is used to treat fungal infections of the nails. The undecenoic acid encourages the diffusion of tioconazole into the nail tissue. It may cause local irritation. Best results are achieved if a course of griseofulvin is also given.

48

Antiviral Drugs

Fortunately most of us recover from most viral infections but these can be very serious and even fatal in some individuals, particularly those who are immune-deficient because of drug treatments (e.g. immunosuppressants) or because of diseases such as AIDS.

A number of antiviral drugs are available which are of benefit in treating various virus infections, but their benefits and risks have to be balanced for each individual being treated. Antiviral drugs include:

Aciclovir (**Zovirax**) is used by mouth or infusion and/or as a cream to treat and suppress herpes simplex, genital herpes, varicella (chickenpox) and herpes zoster (shingles), and to prevent herpes infections in individuals who are immune-deficient because of drug treatments (e.g. immunosuppressants) or disease (e.g. AIDS). Eye applications are used to treat herpes simplex infections of the eyes.

Amantadine (**Lysovir**) is used by mouth to prevent and treat patients suffering from influenza A in whom complications of influenza may be harmful. It has been used by mouth to treat herpes zoster (shingles). The use of amantadine to treat parkinsonism is discussed in Chapter 16.

Famciclovir (**Famvir**) is used by mouth to treat herpes zoster (shingles) and genital herpes.

Foscarnet (**Foscavir**) is given by infusion to treat cytomegalovirus (CMV) eye infections in individuals with AIDS in whom gancyclovir should not be used.

Ganciclovir (**Cymevene**) and **fomivirsen** (**Vitravene**) are used by injection to treat life- or sight-threatening cytomegalovirus (CMV) infections in individuals who are immune-deficient because of drug treatments (e.g. immunosuppressants) or disease (e.g. AIDS).

Idoxuridine (**Herpid** solution) is too toxic to be given by mouth or injection. It is used topically to treat herpes simplex and herpes zoster (shingles) infections of the skin and eyes.

Inosine pranobex (**Imunovir**) is used by mouth to treat genital herpes and genital warts. It is also used to treat herpes simplex infections (e.g. of the mouth). There is some doubt about its effectiveness.

Lamivudine (**Zeffix**) is used orally to treat hepatitis B.

Penciclovir (**Vectavir**) cream is used to treat herpes infections of the lips (labia) of the vagina.

Ribavirin (**Rebetol**, **Virazole**) is used by aerosol inhalation or by nebulizer to treat a severe virus infection of the lungs in children – respiratory syncytial virus (RSV) bronchiolitis. Rebetol is used orally in combination with interferon alfa-2b to treat hepatitis C and Virazole is used to treat severe syncytial (RSV) bronchiolitis.

Valaciclovir (**Valtrex**) is a precursor of aciclovir. It is used by mouth to treat cold sores (herpes simplex) and herpes zoster (shingles).

Zanamivir (**Relenza**) is used in the treatment of influenza. It must be used within forty-eight hours of onset of symptoms.

Antiviral Drugs Used to Treat HIV Infections

Zidovudine (**AZT**, **Retrovir**) is given by mouth to treat individuals suffering from AIDS and AIDS-related complex (ARC). It is also used to treat patients who are HIV positive but have no symptoms of ARC or AIDS in the hope that it may prevent or delay the onset. It is used in HIV-positive pregnant women who are over fourteen weeks pregnant in the hope that it will prevent the HIV virus spreading from the mother to the unborn baby.

Other antiviral drugs used to treat patients suffering from HIV infection include **abacavir** (**Ziagen**), **amprenavir** (**Agenerase**), **cidofovir** (**Vistide**), **didanosine** (**Videx**), **efavirenz** (**Sustiva**), **foscarnet** (**Foscavir**), **ganciclovir** (**Cymevene**), **indinavir** (**Crixivan**), **lamivudine** (**Epivir**), **lopinavir** (**Kaletra**), **nelfinavir** (**Viracept**), **nevirapine** (**Viramune**), **palivizumab** (**Synagis**), **ribavirin** (**Rebetol**, **Virazole**), **ritonavir** (**Norvir**), **saquinavir** (**Invirase**), **stavudine** (**Zerit**) and **zalcitabine** (**Hivid**).

49

Drugs Used to Treat Infections and Disorders of the Urinary System

Urinary Tract Infections

The normal urinary tract is free from bacteria except for some organisms near the outlet (the urethra) which contaminate it. *Infection of the urinary tract usually comes from the outside* and spreads upwards through the urethra into the bladder. It is often caused by bacteria which are normally present in the large bowel and which spread into the urethra from faeces which contaminate the skin around the anus and genitals. This spread of infection from the anus into the urethra and then upwards into the bladder is commoner in women because their urethras are short.

Bacteria may infect the urinary tract to produce infection of the kidneys (pyelitis), the bladder (cystitis) and the outlet from the bladder (urethritis). There is a wide range of effective drugs available to treat these infections, for example **ampicillin**, **cephalosporins**, **ciprofloxacin**, **gentamicin**, **trimethoprim**, **methenamine** (**Hiprex**), **nalidixic acid** (**Mictral**, **Negram**, **Uriben**), **nitrofurantoin** (**Furadantin**, **Macrobid**, **Macrodantin**), **norfloxacin** (**Utinor**) and **pivmecillinam** (**Selexid**).

The dose of antibacterial drug will depend on many factors: the severity of infection, the type of infecting bacteria, the condition of the patient and in particular the state of the patient's kidney function.

With urinary tract infections it helps to drink plenty of fluids (one and a half litres a day) and pass urine often. Also, the acidity of the urine may affect the effectiveness of an antibiotic. It is worth making the urine acid if you are taking tetracyclines, nitrofurantoin, sodium fusidate or semi-synthetic penicillins. It should preferably be made alkaline if you are taking, for example, erythromycin, lincomycin, gentamicin or cephalosporins. The decision to make your urine acid or alkaline (by taking certain acid or alkaline salts) depends upon how well your kidneys are functioning and this is a decision for your doctor.

Pain on passing urine can be relieved by making the urine alkaline by taking **sodium bicarbonate**, or by taking **sodium** or **potassium citrate**. However, they produce nausea and a potassium salt is dangerous in a patient with impaired kidney function.

Much trouble is caused through inadequate treatment of urinary infections. With first attacks, a full course of appropriate antibiotic should be taken after the urine has been examined. With the second and all subsequent attacks, the urine should be re-examined to determine the infecting organism and the appropriate antibiotic should be selected and taken. With recurrent attacks (chronic cystitis) full investigations are necessary, as well as eliminating obvious things like vaginal deodorants (particularly sprays) which can irritate the lining of the urethra. Infections of the urinary tract can be due to many causes including anatomical abnormalities, and surgical procedures or catheterization. They can occur in pregnancy and be symptomless and yet require treatment because the kidneys can become infected and be associated with anaemia, prematurity and stillbirth. In chronic cystitis, treatment after relief of acute symptoms should continue probably for up to three months or more.

Co-trimoxazole, quinolone antibiotics, nitrofurantoin, sulphonamides, tetracyclines and trimethoprim should not be used in pregnancy. Cephalosporins and penicillins are safe to use. Nitrofurantoin should not be used at the end of pregnancy (at term).

In kidney failure, impairment of functions can lead to high blood levels of antibiotics and adverse drug reactions. Methenamine, nitrofurantoin and tetracyclines should be avoided. Aminoglycosides should be used with caution.

Urgency and Frequency of Passing Urine

The desire to empty the bladder is caused by the increasing volume of urine stretching the bladder wall and stimulating stretch-sensitive nerves near the outlet from the bladder. This stimulation activates nerves which cause the muscle in the bladder to contract and empty the bladder. Drugs which block these effects and are used to treat urgency and frequency include:

> **flavoxate** (**Urispas**), an antispasmodic drug
> **oxybutynin** (**Cystrin, Ditropan**), an antispasmodic/antimuscarinic drug
> **profiverine** (**Detrunorm**), **tolterodine** (**Detrusitol**) and **trospiom** (**Rugurin**) are also antimuscarinic drugs which are used for urinary frequency, urgency and incontinence.

Tricyclic antidepressants (e.g. **amitriptyline, imipramine**, see Chapter 4) also produce some antimuscarinic effects and may be tried in the treatment of urgency and frequency.

Incontinence of Urine

Incontinence of urine refers to a lack of control over emptying the bladder. It may be due to several causes and drugs have a very limited part to play in its treatment. They may relieve the symptoms of incontinence but they do nothing to help the underlying disorder. It is better if possible to treat the cause. Drugs used to treat incontinence include:

Oxybutynin (**Cystrin**, **Ditropan**) an antispasmodic/antimuscarinic drug and **flavoxate** (**Urispas**) an antispasmodic.

Tolterodine (**Detrusitol**) and **propiverine** (**Detrunorm**) are also antimuscarinic drugs which are used for urinary frequency, urgency and incontinence.

Contigen is a skin collagen from cattle used as a collagen implant into the neck of the bladder. This increases its bulk and narrows the outflow from the bladder which helps to reduce incontinence.

> See **warnings** in A–Z of Medicines on the use of these drugs in patients suffering from enlargement of the prostate gland or glaucoma.

Bedwetting in Children

Bedwetting is obviously quite normal in babies and infants but becomes a problem when it persists or comes on again in older children. About 5 per cent of children still wet the bed at the age of ten years, and in some children a severe emotional upset may cause recurrence.

The best treatment is reassurance, support and counselling along with bladder training. Any form of punishment or criticism will only make the child worse. The use of an alarm system which sets a bell ringing the second a drop of urine is passed on to a pad placed beneath the bottom may be useful. The bell wakes up the child, who can then go and pass urine in the toilet. A reward system may also help, for instance a star chart whereby the child gets a star for every dry night and a present when there are a certain number of stars on the chart; however, the child must not be made to feel a failure if a star cannot be awarded.

Drug treatment should never be used in children under seven years of age and it should rarely be used in children over seven years, except when visiting a friend or going on holiday.

Drugs used to treat bedwetting in children include: **Tricyclic antidepressant drugs** that produce antimuscarinic effects (see Chapter 4) – e.g. **amitriptyline**. They counteract the effects of the nerves that cause the bladder to contract.

Tricyclic antidepressants may produce harmful effects on the heart and should not be continued for more than three months without carrying out an electrocardiograph (ECG). They may cause behaviour disorders in children. Relapse is common after stopping the drug.

Sympathomimetic drugs (e.g. **ephedrine**, see Chapter 4). These drugs cause the outlet from the bladder to contract and also lessen the depth of sleep.

Desmopressin. Desmopressin is related to vasopressin, which is a hormone produced by the posterior lobe of the pituitary gland. It works on the kidneys, making them produce less urine – it is an anti-diuretic hormone.

In some older children and in adults who regularly wet the bed there may be a possibility that they may be deficient in this hormone and it is worth trying desmopressin taken by nasal spray (**Desmospray, DDAVP Spray** or as tablets (**DDAVP, Desmotabs**)). One or two doses stop urine production for about ten–twelve hours, sufficient to allow a dry night. It should not be used in children aged five years or under, after three months' treatment it should be stopped and progress without treatment assessed.

Drugs Used to Treat Retention of Urine

Inability to pass urine causes retention of urine in the bladder. This may occur because of an obstruction to the outflow of urine from the bladder, for example, an enlarged prostate gland in an elderly man. It may also occur because of damage to the nerves supplying the bladder, for example, spinal injury.

Retention of urine may actually cause incontinence because the bladder fills up and then starts to overflow. This causes the patient to dribble all the time. It is called retention with overflow and is easily diagnosed as retention because the bladder is full and often tender.

Drugs used to treat chronic retention of urine include: **carbachol** by mouth or **bethanechol** (**Myotonine**) by mouth or injection. They act like acetylcholine, the parasympathetic neurotransmitter (see Chapter 9).

Distigmine (**Ubretid**) and **neostigmine** prolong the action of acetylcholine (see Chapter 9). They are used to treat retention of urine following surgical operation when a general anaesthetic has been used.

Enlarged Prostate Gland (Benign Prostatic Hypertrophy: BPH) causing Obstruction to the Flow of Urine

Difficulty in passing urine due to a benign enlargement of the prostate gland may be helped by taking a drug that relaxes the muscles around the prostate gland, for example, a selective alpha-blocker such as **alfuzosin** (**Xatral**), **doxazosin** (**Cardura**), **indoramin** (**Doralese**), **prazosin** (**Hypovase**) or **terazosin** (**Hytrin BPH**). **Tamsulosin** (**Flomax MR**) blocks special alpha receptors in the prostate gland and produces fewer generalized effects than selective alpha-blockers.

Gestonorone (**Gestronol**) is a progestogen given by an oily depot injection.

It counterbalances the effects of the male sex hormone (testosterone) and helps to reduce the size of the prostate gland thus helping the flow of urine.

Finasteride (**Proscar**) blocks an enzyme in the prostate gland that increases the potency of testosterone. This causes the prostate gland to shrink and helps the flow of urine.

Drugs Used to Treat Tuberculosis

Because of the very real problem that the bacteria which cause tuberculosis (mycobacterium tuberculosis) can easily develop resistance to anti-tuberculosis drugs, treatment is in two stages – the *initial phase* and the *continuation phase.*

The initial phase involves the use of at least three drugs and the continuation phase involves the use of two drugs. The latter is possible once tests have shown which two drugs are most effective against the particular organisms involved. But these tests of *sensitivity* may take up to three months and, for safety, during this period three drugs in combination are nearly always used.

Initial-phase treatment now involves the daily use of **isoniazid**, **rifampicin** (**Rifadin, Rimactane**) and **pyrazinamide** (**Zinamide**), supplemented by **ethambutol** if drug resistance is likely. **Streptomycin** may be added if the bacteria are resistant to isoniazid. These drugs should be continued for at least eight weeks and preferably until the results of the drug-sensitivity tests are available.

Continuation-phase treatment should follow the initial phase and include two drugs, **isoniazid** and **rifampicin** (**Rifadin, Rimactane**). Other drugs may be included e.g. **ethambutol** or **streptomycin** if resistance is suspected. **Pyrazinamide** (**Zinamide**) may be added in the first two months of treatment. Alternative reserve drugs include **capreomycin** (**Capastat**) or **cycloserine**. The *duration* of treatment is usually for a further four months but may go on for up to eighteen months according to the drugs used and the patient's response.

Combination products include **Rifater** (**rifampicin, isoniazid, pyrazinamide**), **Rifinah** (**rifampicin, isoniazid**), **Rimactazid** (**rifamipicin, isoniazid**).

For adverse effects of each of these drugs, see A–Z of Medicines.

Isoniazid daily for six months or isoniazid plus **rifampicin** (**Rifadin, Rimactane**) daily for three months are used to prevent tuberculosis in susceptible close contacts.

Rifabutin (**Mycobutin**), a recently introduced rifamycin, is used to prevent tuberculosis. It is also used in the treatment of pulmonary tuberculosis and non-tuberculous mycobacterial disease.

Note: *Patients with immune deficiency due to disease (e.g. AIDS) or drugs (e.g. immunosuppressants) may develop tuberculosis from a new infection or the reactivation of an old infection.*

Drugs Used to Treat Cancer

Cancer is a disorder of autonomous cell growth which may affect any tissue or organ. Treatment of cancer is aimed at reducing or stopping this disordered growth. Drugs are becoming increasingly useful for this purpose because not only is it possible to cure many patients suffering from various types of cancer, but drugs can also make life much more comfortable. Because of the many different types and stages of cancer it is difficult to generalize. Furthermore, the drugs used are very complex and treatment is always changing as different advances are made.

Chemotherapy

Drugs used to treat cancer are termed *cytotoxic* drugs because they kill cells. Anti-cancer drug therapy is usually referred to as **chemotherapy**. The majority of cytotoxic drugs interfere with cell division and will therefore damage *all* rapidly dividing cells, whether normal or cancerous. Areas of rapidly growing normal cells in the body include bone marrow, the lining of the mouth, stomach and intestine, and skin and hair. Therefore, cytotoxic drugs can produce short-term and reversible damage to these tissues, producing anaemia due to damage to red cell production; susceptibility to infection due to damage to white cell production; bleeding due to damage to platelets which produce clotting; nausea, vomiting and diarrhoea due to damage to the lining of the intestine; and loss of hair (alopecia).

Cytotoxic drugs are used to treat those primary or secondary cancers which have been shown to respond to drug therapy. They are also used as additional treatment in order to prevent relapse in patients who have had surgery and/ or radiotherapy. In addition, some are used to suppress the immune response of the body in patients suffering from auto-immune disorders (a sensitivity of the body to some of its own cells), or in patients who have had an organ transplant where there may be problems of rejection.

Different groups of cytotoxic drugs act differently upon the cellular growth cycle of cancer cells. Some may kill cells whether they are resting or multiplying, some may kill only those cells which are multiplying and some may kill only at a specific time in a particular phase of growth. These are important factors in considering treatment because the combination of drugs which act at different stages can have greater killing effect on cancer cells than drugs used alone. Therefore, important regimes of anti-cancer drug therapy include *combined* drug treatments, *intermittent* treatments and also *sequential* treatments in order to achieve a maximum killing effect on the cancer cells for minimum effects upon the normal cells in the body.

Because of the risks from treatment, special facilities for extra support may also be needed, e.g. blood transfusion if blood production is affected and special precautions against infection if the drugs being used damage the production of white blood cells which are normally involved in the body's protection against infection. This means that, in addition to anti-cancer drugs, several other drugs (e.g. antibiotics) and treatments may be used, which indicates the need for highly specialized care. There are five main groups of cytotoxic drugs.

1 Alkylating Drugs

These damage DNA and therefore interfere with the cells' ability to multiply (replicate). They may produce infertility which may be permanent. Prolonged use is associated with an increased incidence of acute non-lymphatic leukaemia

- *Alkylating drugs*
  busulfan (Myleran)
  carmustine (BiCNU)
  chlorambucil (Leukeran)
  cyclophosphamide (Endoxana)
  estramustine (Estracyt)
  ifosfamide (Mitoxana)
  lomustine
  melphalan (Alkeran)
  mitobronitol
  chlormethine(mustine)
  thiotepa
  treosulfan

2 Antimetabolites

These interfere with normal chemical processes inside dividing cells by affecting enzymes and preventing normal cellular division.

Drugs are available which stop the effect of any one of three enzymes that use folic acid, purine or pyrimidine as building blocks. They are therefore known as **folic acid antagonists, purine antagonists** and **pyrimidine antagonists**. Pyrimidine antagonists may damage the nails and the lining of the mouth, and produce loss of hair. Folic acid antagonists may interfere with the body's immune response to infection and foreign tissues (e.g. kidney transplants). They include:

    cladribine (**Leustat**)
    cytarabine (**Cytosar**)
    fludarabine (**Fludara**)
    fluorouracil
    gemcitabine (**Gemzar**)
    mercaptopurine (**Puri-Nethol**)
    methotrexate (**Maxtrex**)
    raltitrexed (**Tomudex**)
    tioguanine (**Lanvis**)

3 Cytotoxic Antibiotics

These interfere with DNA replication and protein synthesis. They mimic the effects of radiotherapy and therefore cytotoxic antibiotics should not be used with radiotherapy treatment because of an increased risk of damage to tissues. They include:

    aclarubicin
    bleomycin
    dactinomycin(actinomycin D) (**Cosmegen Lyovac**)
    daunorubicin (**DaunoXome**)
    doxorubicin (**Caelyx, Myocet**)
    epirubicin (**Pharmorubicin**)
    idarubicin (**Zavedos**)
    mitomycin (**Mitomycin C Kyowa**)
    mitoxantrone(mitozantrone) (**Novantrone**)

4 Vinca Alkaloids

These are alkaloids extracted from periwinkle (*Vinca rosea*) which stop cell division. They may cause nerve damage. They include:

    etoposide (**Etopophos, Vepesid**)
    vinblastine (**Velbe**)

vincristine (**Oncovin**)
vindesine (**Eldisine**)
vinorelbine (**Navelbine**)

5 Cytotoxic Immunosuppressants

Azathioprine (**Azamune, Immunoprin, Imuran, Oprisine**) blocks DNA synthesis and prevents the growth of cells (lymphocytes) involved in the immune system. It is therefore both cytotoxic and immunosuppressant.

Mycophenolate mofetil (**Cellcept**) has a more selective mode of action than azathioprine. However, the risk of opportunistic infections and the occurrence of blood disorders such as leucopenia may be higher.

6 A Miscellaneous Group of Cytotoxic Drugs

amsacrine (**Amsidine**) – similar actions to doxorubicin
altretamine (**Hexalen**)
carboplatin (**Paraplatin**) – a derivative of cisplatin
cisplatin – a platinum drug with an alkylating action
crisantapase (**Erwinase**) – the enzyme asparaginase, used to treat
   lymphoblastic leukaemia.
dacarbazine (**DTIC-Dome**)
docetaxel (**Taxotere**)
etoposide (**Vepesid**)
gemcitabine (**Gemzar**)
hydroxycarbamide(hydroxyurea) (**Hydrea**)
irinotecan (**Campto**)
oxaliplatin (**Eloxatin**) – a derivative of cisplatin
paclitaxel (**Taxol**)
pentostatin (**Nipent**)
procarbazine
temozolomide (**Temodal**)
topotecan (**Hycamtin**)
tretinoin (**Vesanoid**)

Precautions on Using Anti-cancer Drugs

Leakage into the tissues of some anti-cancer drugs from their site of injection may cause serious damage, therefore they must be administered with the utmost caution and the patient's injection site examined at regular intervals.

Nausea and vomiting may cause considerable distress and should be anticipated. Anti-nauseant drugs should be given (see Chapter 18).

Suppression of the bone marrow causing blood disorders usually occurs about seven–ten days after starting treatment. Blood counts should be carried out before each treatment and doses reduced or treatment delayed if the white cell count is down. This will give the bone marrow time to recover. If a patient whose white cell count is down develops a fever, a course of broad-spectrum antibiotics should be started immediately.

Impaired immune response may be caused by anti-cancer drugs and this may cause the rapid spread of infection. Patients must be carefully examined for the presence of an infection and appropriate treatment given.

Alopecia: reversible hair loss is common and there is no drug treatment to prevent it but cooling the scalp during intravenous infusion may help.

Reproductive function: patients should be advised on the risks of permanent male sterility and advice on sperm storage should be given. Women should be advised that their reproductive life may be shortened by the onset of a premature menopause.

Rise in blood uric acid levels may occur with some anti-cancer drugs (mercaptopurine, azathioprine) with the risk of kidney stones developing. Allopurinol (see gout, Chapter 33) should be given twenty-four hours before treatment and continued for seven–ten hours after treatment. Patients should drink plenty of fluids.

Interferons

For many years it had been known that infection with one virus could protect animals against infection with another virus, when it was discovered in 1957 that cells infected with a virus produce a substance which protects other cells from virus infection. These substances (highly active glyco-proteins) are known as *interferons*. They act on the surface of cells, causing the cell to produce proteins which protect the cell against damage from viruses.

Interferons act specifically on cells from a specific animal, e.g. mouse interferon is inactive in human cells. There are three major types of human interferon and they are standardized by their ability to reduce the replication of viruses in tissue culture – one unit of interferon is roughly the amount which reduces virus replications in tissue culture by half. The three sources of interferon are human white blood cells, fibroblasts and lymphocytes.

In the treatment of cancer, interferons have been shown to be of benefit in some experimental tumours in mice. They possess actions which obviously could have a beneficial effect. They can stop replication of DNA and RNA tumour viruses; they have been shown to inhibit growth of cancer cells, increase activity of protective white cells (phagocytosis), and increase the effects of killer-cells – both activities leading to destruction of cancer cells; they also affect the immune system by inhibiting (and increasing in some cases) antibody production and therefore may be able to reduce the number of tumour-protecting antibodies which are known to block the body's natural immune response to tumours.

Interferon alfa-2a (**Roferon-A**) is used to treat AIDS-related Kaposi's sarcoma, hairy-cell leukaemia, chronic myelogenous leukaemia, progressive T-cell lymphoma of the skin, chronic active hepatitis B, chronic hepatitis C, recurrent or secondary kidney cell cancer, condylomata acuminata and follicular non-Hodgkins lymphoma.

Interferon alfa-2b (**Intron A**) is used to treat hairy-cell leukaemia, chronic myelogenous leukaemia, AIDS-related Kaposi's sarcoma, non-Hodgkins lymphoma, chronic active hepatitis B, chronic hepatitis C and maintenance of remission in multiple myeloma. As **Viraferon** it is used to treat chronic active hepatitis B and chronic hepatitis C.

Interferon beta-1a (**Avonex**, **Rebif**) and **Interferon beta-1b** (**Betaferon**) are used to treat relapsing-remitting multiple sclerosis.

Interferon gamma-1b (**Immukin**) is used as an adjuvant to antibiotics to reduce the frequency of serious infections in patients with chronic granulomatous disease.

Aldesleukin (**Proleukin**) is a recombinant interleukin-2 used intravenously to treat secondary cancer of the kidney. It produces serious adverse effects such as fluid on the lungs (pulmonary oedema), a fall in blood pressure and bone marrow, liver, kidney, thyroid and nerve damage.

Trastuzumab (**Herceptin**) is a monoclonal antibody for the treatment of metastatic breast cancer.

52

Prostaglandins

Prostaglandins are made by most tissues in the body. They relax smooth muscle and are to be found in lung tissues where some of them cause constriction of the bronchi and others cause dilation. They may be involved in producing bronchoconstriction in asthma and their use in its treatment is being investigated. Prostaglandins in the kidneys can affect kidney blood flow and hence the blood pressure. They soften the cervix and cause the womb to contract.

Prostaglandins are present in the lining of the stomach and are involved in the production of mucus which provides a protective effect against stomach acid. Certain drugs (e.g. aspirin and non-steroidal anti-inflammatory drugs) block the production of prostaglandins and reduce this protective mechanism which may contribute to the development of peptic ulceration, a principal adverse effect of these drugs.

Prostaglandins are also involved in inflammation, in the body's immune response and in tissue damage – e.g. in rheumatoid arthritis. If their production is blocked then the inflammatory process is reduced, producing a relief from pain and swelling of joints or other involved tissues. This is the basis for the use of aspirin and non-steroidal anti-inflammatory drugs in the treatment of rheumatoid arthritis and related disorders (see Chapter 32).

The release of prostaglandins is also thought to contribute to vascular headaches (e.g. migraine) which explains the pain-relieving effects of aspirin, ibuprofen and other NSAIDs which block production of prostaglandin. Aspirin, ibuprofen and other NSAIDs can bring down the temperature in fever. In painful periods (spasmodic dysmenorrhoea) the release of prostaglandins in the uterus is thought to produce the painful spasms which can be relieved by a prostaglandin-blocking drug, such as aspirin, ibuprofen or other NSAIDs.

Prostaglandin Preparations

Alprostadil (**Prostin VR**) is used to keep open the shunt (ductus arteriosus) from the aorta to the pulmonary artery in newborn babies with congenital heart disease prior to surgery on the heart. The NSAID **indomethacin** (**Indocid PDA**) is a prostaglandin-blocker which may be used to help the ductus arteriosus to close.

Alprostadil (**Caverject, MUSE, Viridal**) is also used to treat men who fail to attain or maintain an erection. It is injected directly into the penis.

Carboprost (**Hemabate**) is used to treat bleeding after childbirth (postpartum haemorrhage) unresponsive to ergometrine and oxytocin.

Dinoprostone (**Propess, Prostin E2**) is used to start labour and to produce an abortion.

Epoprostenol (**Flolan**) stops platelets sticking together and is used to prevent the blood from clotting during kidney dialysis.

Gemeprost is used to produce an abortion and to soften the cervix before surgical procedures on the womb.

Misoprostol (**Cytotec**) is used to treat peptic ulcers caused by NSAIDs and to prevent NSAID-induced ulcers.

53

Vaccines

Active Immunity

Vaccines stimulate the production of protective antibodies and other mechanisms involved in the body's resistance to disease (i.e. they produce active immunity).

A vaccine may contain inactivated viruses (e.g. influenza vaccine) or inactivated bacteria (e.g. whooping cough or typhoid vaccines). It may contain a toxin produced by a micro-organism (e.g. tetanus vaccine), or it may contain attenuated (weakened) viruses (e.g. polio or measles vaccine) or attenuated bacteria (e.g. BCG vaccine used against tuberculosis).

Vaccines are usually given by injection, except poliomyelitis vaccine, which is given by mouth, and smallpox vaccine, which is injected into the skin (intradermally).

Live micro-organisms multiply in the body and produce a long-standing immunity, whereas inactivated vaccines need a series of injections initially and then booster injections at intervals.

Passive Immunity

If plasma from an individual immune to a specific disease is given to a patient who is not immune, then the plasma injected will provide the second individual with immediate protection against that disease. This is called *passive immunity*. The plasma contains *antibodies* against the disease. Another name for these antibodies from humans is *immunoglobulins*. An individual may also be given plasma containing antibodies from a horse and this is usually referred to as *anti-serum*. These preparations from horses can produce severe reactions (serum sickness) because the body reacts to foreign horse proteins in the plasma. Therefore, when possible, anti-serum from horses is not now used and most injections contain immunoglobulins which are human and which rarely produce a reaction – for example, anti-tetanus injections. Diphtheria antitoxin is still prepared in horses and can give rise to serum sickness.

Indications for Vaccination

Anthrax. Anyone exposed to infected hides and carcasses or to imported feeding-stuff, bonemeal and fishmeal.

Botulism. Antitoxin should be given to prevent botulism in someone who has been exposed to it or who is thought to be suffering from botulism.

Cholera. Consult the Department of Health about the requirements when travelling to certain countries. Provides little protection and does not control the spread of cholera. Booster injections are required every six months for those living in an area where cholera is prevalent.

Diphtheria. Vaccine prepared from toxin adsorbed on to a mineral carrier. Usually combined with tetanus and pertussis (whooping cough) vaccines – triple vaccine; see schedule, p. 301. Diphtheria antitoxin is used to provide passive immunity.

Haemophilus influenzae. Children under the age of thirteen months are at high risk of haemophilus influenzae type b infection.

Hepatitis A. Vaccine provides protection for those travelling frequently to high-risk areas and/or those who stay for three months or more. If given within two weeks of departure, immunoglobulin should be given into a different injection site.

Hepatitis B. Should be given to patients at risk, i.e. those who work in contact with human blood (blood banks, renal dialysis units, etc.) or who are in direct contact with a carrier and to IV drug users, individuals who frequently change their sexual partners, infants of mothers who have had hepatitis B during pregnancy or who are carriers, haemophiliacs who have regular blood transfusions of blood products, patients with chronic kidney failure, morticians, embalmers, staff and clients of residential homes for the mentally handicapped, people in prison etc. for more than six months and people who visit high-risk areas for several months and may need medical or dental treatment. Routes of infection include inoculation into a wound, incision, needle prick (note 'main-line' drug abuse) or abrasion. Takes up to six months to become immune and this lasts for about three to five years.

Influenza. Grown on eggs, therefore should not be given to patients allergic to eggs or feathers. Use in high-risk patients – elderly, debilitated and those with chronic heart and/or lung disease, kidney failure or diabetes. Also use in doctors, carers and nurses and residents of nursing homes etc. particularly if elderly.

Measles. Vaccine is given combined with mumps and rubella (German measles) vaccine. See *MMR vaccine*, below.

Meningitis. Vaccine is available against types A and C meningococcal meningitis caused by the bacteria *Neisseria meningitidis*. It is useful for people travelling abroad to areas such as Ethiopia, Sudan, the Middle East, India and parts of South America and Kenya. Saudi Arabia requires vaccination of pilgrims to Mecca during the Haj annual pilgrimage. A vaccine against H. influenzae meningitis type b is also available and is included in immunization schedules for children, see p. 301.

MMR vaccine – measles, mumps and rubella (MMR) vaccine. Has replaced measles vaccine in one-to two-year-olds; in order to eradicate these diseases, all eligible children will also be vaccinated at the age of four to five years before entry to primary school. Children exempt from MMR vaccination will be: those with a valid certificate of vaccination; those with laboratory evidence of antibodies to measles, mumps and rubella; children of those parents who object to the use of MMR and those children at risk from MMR, e.g. children with untreated cancer or immune deficiency due to drugs (e.g. immunosuppressants), high doses of corticosteroids, radiation treatment, or disease (e.g. AIDS); children who have had an injection of another *live* vaccine in the preceding three weeks and children with allergies to neomycin or kanomycin (used in preparing the vaccines). MMR vaccine may also be used to control outbreaks of measles and should be offered to susceptible children *within three days* of exposure to measles. *Note:* MMR will not prevent outbreaks of mumps or rubella because antibody response to these vaccines is slow. MMR vaccination should be deferred if the child has a fever.

It should not be given during pregnancy or if there is a risk of pregnancy. Pregnancy should be avoided for one month after MMR vaccination. MMR should not be given within three months of passive immunization with immunoglobulin. MMR should not be given to children who are severely allergic to eggs.

Children who suffer or who have suffered from convulsions or whose brothers and sisters have a history of idiopathic epilepsy should be given MMR, but the parents should be warned of the risk of fever and how to treat it with tepid sponging and paracetamol.

Protection against measles and rubella. In November 1994 in Great Britain MR vaccine (measles and rubella) was made available to all schoolchildren aged five to sixteen years irrespective of a history of measles and/or rubella or previous vaccination. This widespread vaccination provided a *booster* to those who had previously had MMR vaccination and it offered protection to those who had not – especially girls because of the damage that rubella can cause to the unborn child.

Mumps. Vaccine consists of a live weakened strain of virus grown in chick-embryo tissue culture. It is included in MMR vaccine.

Pertussis (whooping cough) is usually given with diphtheria and tetanus vaccines (triple vaccine). See schedule, p. 301. It may produce soreness at the injection site, a raised temperature and irritability. Screaming and collapse occurred in some infants with the vaccines used in the sixties. Convulsions and brain disorder may very rarely occur. Vaccination should be postponed if a child has an acute illness or a temperature from a respiratory or other infection. Vaccination should *not* be continued in children who have a severe local or general reaction to the first injection. It should be used with caution in children with a history of epilepsy and in children with any evidence of active disease of the nervous system. A personal or family history of allergy, idiopathic epilepsy or a stable brain and/or nerve disorder such as spina bifida or cerebral palsy are not reasons for not giving whooping cough vaccination. Nor is a minor infection with or without a fever.

A personal family history of convulsions caused by a fever (febrile convulsions) increases the risks of these occurring after pertussis vaccination and therefore patients should be aware of how to prevent fever by giving paracetamol as soon as a fever starts and repeating the dose in four–six hours (see p. 159). Where a child has an evolving brain and/or nerve disorder the vaccine should be delayed until the condition is stable.

Pneumococcal pneumonia. This is used in patients who run a risk of developing pneumococcal pneumonia, e.g. patients who have had their spleen removed, people with homozygous sickle cell anaemia, immune deficiency due to disease (e.g. AIDS) or drugs, chronic heart, lung, kidney or liver disease or diabetes. It should be given two weeks before removal of the spleen or starting a course of chemotherapy. Protection lasts for about five years. It should not be given to pregnant women, children under the age of two years, or when an infection is present. It should be given with caution to patients suffering from heart or lung disease. Allergic reactions to the vaccine may occur and second courses should not be given.

Poliomyelitis. See schedule, p. 301. There are two types – live and inactivated. Live polio vaccine is given by mouth usually at the same time as triple vaccine (see p. 301). Contacts of recently vaccinated babies should be careful to wash their hands after changing the baby's nappy. Live vaccine should not be given to anyone who has vomiting or diarrhoea or to anyone who is immune-deficient or who lives in a household with someone who is immune-deficient. *Inactivated* vaccine should be given to pregnant women and to patients who are immune-deficient because of disease (e.g. AIDS) or drugs.

Rabies. The vaccine (human diploid vaccine) has been shown to be life-saving. Advice on rabies vaccination should be obtained from the Department of Health. It should be used to prevent rabies in those at high risk (e.g. veterinary surgeons), to treat those who may be at risk (e.g. have been bitten by any animal in a country where rabies is endemic), and to staff caring for a person being treated for rabies.

Rubella (German measles). Rubella in pregnancy can result in a malformed baby. Immunization is recommended for pre-pubertal girls (age ten to thirteen years). To try to eliminate rubella it is now offered to all children – see MMR schedule, p. 301. It should not be used in early pregnancy and women of childbearing age should not become pregnant for one month after vaccination. It is also recommended for those in contact with pregnant women (doctors and nurses) and in patients who wish to become pregnant but who do not show evidence of previous infection (i.e. they do not have antibodies to the rubella virus). It should also be offered to women just after childbirth if they have no antibodies to rubella, since about 60 per cent of abnormalities in babies due to rubella occur in women who have had more than one baby. Susceptible pregnant women who are exposed to rubella may be passively immunized with immunoglobulin.

Smallpox. Worldwide eradication of smallpox has now been achieved and vaccination is not necessary except in special cases.

Tetanus. Tetanus toxoids stimulate the production of antitoxins. See vaccination schedule (p. 301). A booster injection is required for a dirty wound; with a clean wound it is not necessary unless ten years or more have expired since the last injection. An anti-tetanus immunoglobulin injection should be given for serious dirty wounds along with tetanus vaccination, particularly in the elderly who may not have been vaccinated.

Tuberculosis. BCG (Bacillus Calmette-Guérin) is a live weakened strain of tuberculosis vaccine obtained from infected cattle. It stimulates an increased immune response in humans which enables the body to attack and kill any infecting tuberculosis bacteria before they can attack the tissues of the body. This provides protection against the complications of a primary attack of tuberculosis.

BCG should be given to people who have a *negative test for tuberculosis* (Mantoux test); if they have been in contact with individuals who have active tuberculosis (newborn babies should be vaccinated without testing for tuberculosis); if their work brings them into contact with infected persons (e.g. doctors and nurses); to children between ten to fourteen years of age; to teachers and student teachers, vets, laboratory workers, and travellers to areas where there is a high incidence of tuberculosis.

Following BCG vaccination a small, red lump appears at the injection site within two–six weeks. This may develop into a small ulcer which heals in six–twelve weeks. Serious reactions to BCG are uncommon and include prolonged ulceration or abscess. These are usually due to faulty injection techniques.

Except in newborn babies a skin test for allergy to BCG should be carried out before vaccination. An interval of three months should be allowed between being vaccinated with another live vaccine and receiving BCG (except in infants). BCG should not be given to someone with a generalized septic skin disorder.

Typhoid. Sensible precautions include not eating green salads, uncooked meats, vegetables and not drinking tap-water in a country where typhoid is present. A local reaction to the vaccine consists of redness, swelling and pain which occurs in about six–eight hours and is followed by headache, fever and malaise for about forty-eight hours.

Typhus. Vaccination is only required when visiting certain countries. Seek advice from the Department of Health.

Yellow fever. This should not be given to children under nine months of age since it may cause encephalitis. It should not be given in pregnancy or to patients who are sensitive to eggs. Immunization lasts for about ten years.

Schedule of Vaccination Procedures (Children and Adults)

- *During the first year of life.* At two months, the *first dose* of diphtheria, tetanus and pertussis (triple vaccine) plus vaccine against *H. influenzae b, meningitis* should be given by injection and poliomyelitis vaccine by mouth should be given. The *second* and *third* doses should be given at intervals of four weeks.

  Note: If pertussis vaccine is contra-indicated or the parents decline, diphtheria and tetanus vaccine (adsorbed) should be given by injection in place of the triple vaccine (diphtheria, tetanus and pertussis).
- *During the second year of life (twelve–fifteen months).* Live measles, mumps and rubella vaccine (MMR) by injection.
- *At school entry or entry to nursery school.* MMR vaccine, diphtheria and tetanus vaccine (adsorbed) and poliomyelitis by mouth should be given.

  Note: MMR vaccine should not be given if there is documented evidence of previous MMR vaccination, valid contra-indications or laboratory evidence of immunity to measles, mumps and rubella. There should be an interval of at least three years after completing the basic (first) course of vaccines.
- *Between ten and fourteen years of age.* Tuberculosis vaccine (BCG) should be given to tuberculin-negative children and to tuberculin-negative contacts at any age. There should be an interval of not less than three weeks between BCG and rubella (German measles) vaccination.
- *Between ten and fourteen years of age.* All girls who have not got documented evidence of having received MMR vaccine should be given an injection of live rubella (German measles) vaccine regardless of a past history of an attack of rubella. *But see MMR vaccination programme.*
- *On leaving school, before employment, or on entering further education.* A booster dose of live poliomyelitis vaccine should be given by mouth or inactivated poliomyelitis vaccine by injection; also an injection of diphtheria and tetanus vaccine (adsorbed) should be given.
- *In adult life.* Live poliomyelitis vaccine by mouth should be given to previously unvaccinated adults. Three doses with an interval of four weeks. A course of live poliomyelitis vaccine by mouth should be offered

to travellers to countries where polio is endemic, and also to unvaccinated parents of a child being given oral vaccine.

Adult females of childbearing age should be tested for rubella antibodies and those who are negative should be offered live rubella vaccination by injection. Pregnancy must first be excluded and the patients warned not to become pregnant for one month after immunization.

A course of tetanus vaccine (adsorbed) should be offered to previously unvaccinated adults against tetanus. For adults, three doses at intervals of four weeks. For vaccinated people, a booster dose should be given every ten years.

Hepatitis A and B, influenza and pneumococcal vaccines should be offered to high-risk patients.

Fever Following Triple Vaccination in Infants

If fever develops after vaccination (e.g. triple vaccine) give a dose of paraceta-mol straight away and repeat the dose in four–six hours. For infants aged two–three months the dose is 60 mg and should be given on a syringe into the mouth. If the temperature remains up after the second dose of paracetamol contact a doctor.

Immunoglobulins

Immunoglobulins provide passive immunity (see earlier) which last for about two to three months. There are two classes of immunoglobulins – *normal* and *specific.*

Normal immunoglobulin is prepared from pooled human plasma and is used to provide protection against *hepatitis A* and *measles.* It may also be used to protect susceptible pregnant women against *rubella* (German measles).

Specific immunoglobulins are prepared from immunized donors or con-valescent patients. They are used against *hepatitis B, tetanus, herpes zoster* (shingles) and *rabies.*

Warnings about Drug Use

1 Always know the name of the drug that you are taking.
2 Always check its main effects and adverse effects.
3 Always tell the doctor about previous drug reactions and other allergies in you or in any member of your family.
4 Always take the drug according to the instructions on the container.
5 Never take a drug daily for more than one or two weeks without checking on the benefits and risks.
6 Never share prescribed drugs with other people.
7 Never use drugs from an unlabelled container.
8 Never keep unwanted or unused drugs in the house – always return them to your pharmacy for destruction.
9 Only keep a few household remedies to hand and in small quantities. Remember to check the expiry date before using them.
10 Keep all drugs in one safety cupboard out of reach of children.
11 Never mix the contents of one drug container with another.
12 Check with your pharmacist if you are not clear about:
   (a) The expiry date of a drug and where you should store it.
   (b) When you should take it (e.g. before or after meals).
   (c) How you should take it (e.g. with or without a drink of milk).
   (d) How frequently you should take it (e.g. four-hourly, six-hourly, four times in the day or four times in twenty-four hours).
   (e) For how many days you should take it (e.g. always finish a course of antibiotics).
13 Always ask the pharmacist for special-instruction leaflets when obtaining medicaments such as eye drops, nose drops, pessaries, etc.
14 Ask what the doctor means when he states 'as before', or 'as directed'. Ask about the maximum amount of one dose and the maximum allowable in twenty-four hours. Ask how often is 'when necessary'.

15 Be especially cautious when giving medicines to babies, debilitated and elderly patients, to those with impaired kidney or liver function, to patients with heart disease, chest disease, blood pressure, glaucoma, enlarged prostate gland, peptic ulcers, history of allergy or history of drug dependence.

16 If you are planning to become pregnant, or if you are or think you may be pregnant, be extremely cautious about any drugs you take, particularly from around the time of conception to about the twelfth to fourteenth week of your pregnancy.

17 If you are on corticosteroids, anticoagulants, anti-diabetic drugs, monoamine oxidase inhibitor antidepressant drugs or any other special drugs, always ask for and carry a warning card with you.

18 Consider the possibility of an adverse drug effect if a new symptom develops while taking a prescribed and/or over-the-counter drug (e.g. diarrhoea, skin rash) and consult your doctor.

19 Remember the risk of adverse drug interactions between drugs and also between drugs and certain foods – in particular remember the dangers of taking alcohol while taking a drug.

20 Remember that many drugs may affect your ability to operate moving machinery and drive a motor vehicle – always check for this risk.

21 If a patient under your supervision is confused or depressed and/or drinks alcohol regularly, sometimes to excess, then supervise the issue of tablets on a daily basis.

22 Never keep sleeping drugs at your bedside, particularly if you also drink alcohol.

A–Z of Medicines

A–Z of Medicines

AAA preparations ➤ benzocaine.

abacavir (in Trizivir, Ziagen) is used for the treatment of HIV infection. See Chapter 48. *Adverse effects* include lethargy, fever, headache, anorexia, allergic reactions: flu-like symptoms, cough, breathlessness, difficulty breathing, inflammation of the throat, fever, rash, stomach and bowel upsets, abdominal pain, severe tiredness, pain in muscles, pain in joints. *Precautions:* Do not use in patients with moderate to severe liver damage, severe kidney disease, in pregnancy or while breastfeeding.

Abelcet ➤ amphotericin.

Abidec drops are a multivitamin preparation which contains vitamins A, B group, C and D.

abciximab (ReoPro) is a monoclonal antibody used as an antiplatelet drug (see p. 143) along with heparin and aspirin to prevent heart complications in high-risk patients undergoing coronary angioplasty. It is given by intravenous injection. *Adverse effects* include bleeding, raised blood pressure, nausea, vomiting, fever, rapid beating of the heart and vascular disorders. *Precautions:* Do not use in patients allergic to murine monoclonal antibodies, who have active internal bleeding, who have had a stroke within the last two years, recent spinal or brain injury or major surgery, severe uncontrolled raised blood pressure, tumour or aneurysm in the brain, bleeding disorders, diabetic eye damage (retinopathy), severe liver or kidney failure, in pregnancy or in breastfeeding mothers. There is a risk of severe allergic reactions, and facilities for cardio-pulmonary resuscitation should be close at hand. *Interactions:* Increased effects with thrombolytics, anticoagulants and antiplatelet drugs.

abortion pill ➤ mifepristone.

ABVD is a combination of four anti-cancer drugs: doxorubicin (formerly adriamycin), bleomycin, vinblastine and dacarbazine. Read entries on each individual drug and see Drugs Used to Treat Cancer, Chapter 51.

AC Vax is a meningoccal polysaccharide A & C vaccine which provides long-term protection against meningoccal C.

acamprosate (Campral EC) is used as an adjunct to counselling to help alcoholics stay off alcohol. It affects certain chemical transmitters (neurotransmitters) in the brain which are thought to be involved in causing physical dependence to alcohol. It helps some people to keep off alcohol and it is most effective if started as soon as possible after alcohol withdrawal. It should be continued for one year, even if the patient relapses. *Adverse effects* include stomach and bowel upsets, skin rashes, fluctuations in libido. *Precautions:* Do not use in pregnancy, in breastfeeding mothers, in patients with impaired kidney function or severely impaired liver function. Do not use in the elderly or in children.

acarbose (Glucobay) is an oral anti-diabetic drug. See Chapter 42. It blocks the digestive enzyme alpha-glucosidase and delays the digestion of starch and sucrose and therefore reduces the rise in the blood glucose levels that occurs after eating a carbohydrate meal. *Adverse effects* include bloating and fullness, wind, soft stools, diarrhoea, abdominal pains and fullness after meals. Rarely it may cause jaundice, liver damage and skin rashes. *Precautions:* Do not use in pregnancy and breastfeeding mothers, in patients with chronic diarrhoeal disorders (e.g. ulcerative colitis, Crohn's disease) or with partial obstruction of the intestine. Do not use in patients with chronic digestive or absorption disorders, impaired liver function or severely impaired kidney function. Liver function should be monitored. It may increase the blood glucose lowering effects (hypoglycaemic effects) of insulin. Hypoglycaemic symptoms should be treated with glucose, not sucrose (sugar). *Interactions:* Adsorbents, pancreatic enzymes, neomycin, cholestyramine.

acaricides are drugs used to treat scabies, see p. 261.

Accolate ➤ zafirlukast.

Accupro ➤ quinapril.

Accuretic tablets contain the ACE inhibitor quinapril and the thiazide diuretic hydrochlorothiazide. They are used to treat raised blood pressure. See Chapter 25. *Adverse effects and Precautions* ➤ quinapril, thiazide diuretics.

ACE inhibitors (angiotensin-converting enzyme inhibitors) are used to treat raised blood pressure (see Chapter 25) and heart failure (see Chapter 23).

acebutolol (acebutolol hydrochloride, Secadrex, Sectral) is a selective beta-receptor blocker used to treat disorders of heart rhythm, angina and high blood pressure ➤ beta-blockers.

aceclofenac (Preservex) is a non-steroidal anti-inflammatory drug (NSAID). It is a potent pain-reliever and anti-inflammatory drug that appears to produce fewer adverse effects on the stomach and intestine than other NSAIDs ➤ non-steroidal anti-inflammatory drugs.

acemetacin (Emflex) is a non-steroidal anti-inflammatory drug (NSAID), see Chapter 32. It is an ester of indomethacin and is broken down to indomethacin in the liver. *Adverse effects* include stomach and bowel upsets, headaches, dizziness, noises in the ears (tinnitus), blurred vision, fluid retention (e.g. ankle swelling), itching, chest pain and, very rarely, blood disorders. *Precautions:* It should not be used in patients who are allergic to aspirin or other NSAIDs. It should not be used in patients with angiooedema (swelling of the mouth and throat), in pregnancy, or in breastfeeding mothers. It should be used with caution in the elderly, and in patients with psychiatric disorders, epilepsy, parkinsonism, congestive heart failure, impaired kidney or liver function, fluid or electrolyte imbalance, or sepsis. Blood, kidney and liver function tests should be carried out before and at regular intervals during treatment. Patients on long-term treatment should have an annual eye examination. *Interactions* ➤ non-steroidal anti-inflammatory drugs.

acenocoumarol(nicomualone) (Sinthrome) is an anticoagulant drug (see Chapter 28) with effects and uses similar to those described under warfarin sodium ➤ warfarin sodium. Do not use in breastfeeding mothers.

Acepril ➤ captopril.

acetaminophen ➤ paracetamol.

acetazolamide (Diamox) is a carbonic anhydrase inhibitor diuretic. It is used to reduce the pressure inside the eye in the treatment of glaucoma, see p. 64. It is also used to treat epilepsy. It is of doubtful value in the treatment of altitude sickness and pre-menstrual symptoms. It has occasionally been used to treat oedema (fluid retention) and congestive heart failure: see Chapter 29 on diuretics. *Adverse effects:* These are frequent, mild and reversible on stopping or reducing the dose. They include headache, flushing, drowsiness, numbness, and tingling of the face, hands and feet. Fatigue, excitement, thirst, and passing large volumes of urine may occur and, rarely, excitement and skin rashes. Liver, kidney and blood disorders have been reported. The water-salt balance of the body may be disturbed. *Precautions:* It should not be given to patients who are allergic to sulphonamides, have closed-angle glaucoma, a low blood potassium or sodium level, or kidney disorders. Use with caution in patients with emphysema, gout or diabetes. Patients on long-term treatment may need potassium supplements. Blood counts and tests of the chemistry of the blood should be carried out at regular intervals. Use with caution in breastfeeding mothers and do not use in pregnancy. Patients should report any unusual rashes. *Interactions:* Folic acid blocker anti-cancer drugs, anti-diabetic drugs and anti-blood clotting drugs.

Acetest tablets are used to test for ketones in the urine of patients with diabetes.

acetic acid is used in some cough linctuses, it is also used in rheumatic liniments, in skin applications, and in a concentrated form to treat warts and corns. It is used in Aci-Jel as an antiseptic to treat infections of the vagina. It may cause irritation of the skin. It is also used as an antifungal and antibacterial agent in the external ear canal (Ear Calm, in Otomize).

acetomenaphthone (in Ketovite) has vitamin K activity and has similar uses to those described under phytomenadione.

acetylcholine is a neurotransmitter in the autonomic nervous system (see p. 34).

Acetylcholine chloride (Miochol) is used in cataract surgery and other surgical procedures on the eyes that require rapid constriction of the pupil. *Adverse effects:* It is rapidly broken down in the body but it may produce nausea, vomiting, abdominal pain, runny nose, belching, sweating, flushing, salivation, watery eyes, involuntary emptying of the bowels and/or bladder, slowing of the heart rate, wheezing, fall in blood pressure and tightness in the chest.

acetylcysteine is used in Ilube eye drops to treat dry-eye syndrome associated with excessive mucus production. Do not wear contact lenses when using Ilube eye drops. Acetylcysteine by injection is used to protect the liver from damage following paracetamol overdose. Adverse effects include rashes and very rarely serious allergic reactions (anaphylactic reactions).

acetylsalicylic acid ➤ aspirin.

Acezide tablets contain hydrochlorothiazide (a thiazide diuretic) and captopril (an ACE inhibitor). It is used to treat raised blood pressure. *Adverse effects and Precautions* ➤ thiazide diuretics, captopril.

Achromycin ➤ tetracycline.

aciclovir (acyclovir, Zovirax) is an antiviral drug. See Chapter 48. It is used by mouth or intravenous infusion to treat herpes simplex, chickenpox and herpes zoster (shingles) infections. *Adverse effects* include stomach and bowel upsets, changes in liver and kidney function tests, headache, dizziness and fatigue. Intravenous infusion may cause inflammation and tissue damage at site of injection; rashes, confusion, hallucinations, agitation, tremors, sleepiness, psychosis, convulsions and coma may occur. *Precautions:* Patient must be kept well hydrated. Use with caution in patients with impaired kidney function and in breast-feeding mothers. *Interactions:* Probenecid. Aciclovir (Boots Avert, Herpetad, Soothelip, Viralief, Virasorb, Zovirax cream) is applied topically to treat initial and recurrent oral and genital herpes simplex infections. Treatment by mouth should be used for infections of the mouth and vagina. May cause transient irritation, mild dryness and flaking of the skin. Use with caution in patients with severely impaired kidney function. Aciclovir (Zovirax eye ointment) is used to treat herpes simplex infections of the eyes. It may cause mild stinging of the eyes and damage to the cornea (punctate keratitis).

Aci-Jel contains acetic acid which acts as an antiseptic. It is used to treat vaginal infections. It may cause local irritation and inflammation.

acipimox (Olbetam) lowers blood cholesterol and fat levels (see Chapter 26). It works in the same way as nicotinic acid (➤ nicotinic acid) but it is more active and longer-acting and less likely to cause rebound effects if treatment is stopped. *Adverse effects:* Flushing, rash, redness of the face, stomach upsets, headache and generally feeling unwell. *Precautions:* Do not use in patients with peptic ulcers, in pregnancy or when breastfeeding. Use with caution in patients with impaired kidney function.

Acitak ➤ cimetidine.

acitretin (Neotigason) is used to treat severe, extensive psoriasis (see p. 257) and severe Darier's disease. It is a breakdown product of etretinate which it has replaced. It should be prescribed *only* by, or under the supervision of, a consultant dermatologist. *Adverse effects* are mainly related to the dose used, they include dryness of the lining of the mouth, skin and eyes (conjunctivae). The skin, especially on the face, can itch, scale and go red. The dryness of the eyes can affect the wearing of contact lenses. Other adverse effects include reversible thinning and loss of hair, skinning of the palms and soles, generalized itching, nose bleeds, muscle and joint pains, drowsiness, sweating, nausea, headaches and mood changes. Rarely it can cause liver damage, blood disorders, affect night vision and make the skin sensitive to the sun's rays. Long-term use can affect bone growth. *Precautions:* Do not

use if pregnant. Avoid any risk of getting pregnant for one month before starting treatment, during and for at least two years after stopping treatment. Avoid use of tetracyclines, high doses of vitamin A or keratolytics (peeling agents). Do not donate blood during and for one year after stopping treatment. Liver function, blood fat and blood glucose levels must be monitored at start of treatment and then every three months. Avoid excessive exposure to sunlight and sunray lamps. Muscle and joint aches and pains should be investigated and X-ray checks for bone damage should be carried out on patients on long-term treatment. Do not use in children, in breastfeeding mothers or in patients with impaired liver or kidney function. *Interactions:* High doses of vitamin C.

aclarubicin is an anti-cancer drug (see Chapter 51) used to treat acute nonlymphatic leukaemia in individuals who have failed to respond to first-line treatment. It is an anthracycline and produces effects similar to those of doxorubicin. *Adverse effects* include dose-related damage to bone marrow, resulting in a fall in white cells and platelets in the blood. It may cause nausea, vomiting, diarrhoea, sore mouth and changes in liver function. Rarely, it may damage the heart, cause allergic reactions and hair loss. Infusions may cause the vein to become inflamed (phlebitis) at the site of injection. *Precautions:* It should not be used in pregnancy, in breastfeeding mothers, or in individuals with severe bone-marrow impairment. It should be used with caution in people with impaired kidney, liver or heart function, or raised blood uric acid levels. Blood tests and tests of heart function should be carried out at regular intervals.

Acnecide acne gel ➤ benzoyl peroxide.

Acnisal acne solution contains salicylic acid in a detergent base ➤ salicylic acid.

Acoflam ➤ diclofenac.

acrivastine (Benadryl Allergy Relief, Semprex) is a non-sedative antihistamine. See

Chapter 17. *Adverse effects:* It may rarely cause drowsiness. *Precautions:* It should not be used in patients with kidney failure. It should be used with caution in pregnancy and in breastfeeding mothers. It may increase the effects of alcohol and other drugs that depress the brain ➤ antihistamines.

Actal antacid tablets ➤ alexitol sodium.

ACTH ➤ corticotrophin.

ACT-Hib is a haemophilus influenzae vaccine which is given by intramuscular or deep subcutaneous injection.

ACT-Hib DTP is a haemophilus influenzae vaccine combined with diphtheria, tetanus and pertussis (whooping cough) vaccine which is given by intramuscular or deep subcutaneous injection.

Acticin cream ➤ tretinoin.

Actidose-aqua ➤ activated charcoal.

Actifed Tablets and Syrup contain triprolidine and pseudoephedrine; **Actifed** Compound Linctus contains triprolidine, pseudoephedrine and dextromethorphan; **Actifed** Expectorant contains triprolidine, pseudoephedrine and guaiphenesin ➤ individual entry for each drug.

Actilyse ➤ alteplase.

Actinac is used to treat acne. It contains chloramphenicol, hydrocortisone, butoxyethyl nicotinate, allantoin and sulphur. *Adverse effects and Precautions:* See entry on each drug. It may make the skin red. Use with caution in pregnancy.

actinomycin D ➤ dactinomycin.

Actiq ➤ fentanyl.

activated charcoal can adsorb many poisons and drugs, and when given by mouth it reduces their absorption into the bloodstream. It is used to treat acute poisonings and drug overdose. It comes as an oral suspension (Actidose-aqua advance, Charcodote, Liqui-char). It is used as a powder (Carbomix) or effervescent granules (Medi-coal) which are mixed with water and taken by mouth or by intragastric tube as soon as possible after poisoning. Charcoal has been used to treat diarrhoea and wind.

activated dimethicone (Infacol) is a silicone used in antacids to disperse wind ➤ simethicone.

Actonel ➤ risedronate.

Actonorm gel is used to treat acid or wind. It contains aluminium hydroxide gel, magnesium hydroxide and activated dimethicone ➤ antacids, simethicone.

Actos ➤ pioglitazone.

Actrapid ➤ insulins.

Acular eye solution contains ketorolac trometamol, a non-steroidal anti-inflammatory drug (NSAID). The eye drops are used to relieve pain and inflammation in the eye after surgery on the eye. *Adverse effects* include transient stinging and burning, irritation of the eye and blurred vision. *Precautions:* Do not use in patients allergic to aspirin or an NSAID. Do not use in pregnancy or in breastfeeding mothers. Do not wear soft contact lenses. Use with caution in patients with bleeding disorders or peptic ulcers. *Interactions:* Anti-blood-clotting drugs, anti-platelet drugs.

Acupan ➤ nefopam.

Acuphase clopixol ➤ clopixol.

acyclovir ➤ aciclovir.

Adalat preparations ➤ nifedipine.

adapalene (Differin) is applied as a gel to treat acne. See p. 251. It is a synthetic retinoid (related to vitamin A). *Adverse effects* include skin irritation. *Precautions:* Do not use in patients with severe acne, broken skin, eczema. Use with caution in pregnancy (adequate contraception must be used) or while breastfeeding. Avoid eyes, lips, angles of nose, mucous membranes and excessive exposure to sunlight.

Adcal ➤ calcium.

Adcal-D3 ➤ calcium.

Adcortyl (triamcinolone) is a corticosteroid. It is used in an oral paste to treat mouth ulcers (Adcortyl in Orabase), in a preparation to be injected directly into a joint in rheumatoid arthritis, into an inflamed tendon, e.g. tennis elbow, or chronic skin lesions (Adcortyl injections) and in skin cream or ointment to treat eczema, dermatitis, psoriasis, insect bites and sunburn ➤ triamcinolone. *Adverse effects and Precautions* see Chapter 37 on corticosteroids and corticosteroid skin applications, p. 241. Adcortyl in Orabase should not be used on untreated mouth infections. Use with caution in pregnancy. Avoid long-term use in children. Dentures may cause more of the paste to be absorbed and increase the risk of adverse effects.

Adcortyl in Orabase contains triamcinolone (a corticosteroid) in Orabase. It is used to treat ulcers and soreness in the mouth and gums. *Adverse effects and Precautions* ➤ triamcinolone and Orabase. Use with caution in pregnancy. Avoid long-term use in children. Dentures may cause more of the paste to be absorbed and increase the risk of adverse effects. Do not use on untreated infections of the mouth or on tuberculous or viral lesions.

Addiphos is a phosphate supplement that contains potassium phosphate, sodium phosphate, potassium hydroxide and sorbitol.

Adenocor ➤ adenosine.

Adenoscan ➤ adenosine.

adenosine (Adenocor, Adenoscan) is used intravenously to stop attacks of rapid beating of the heart (paroxysmal supraventricular tachycardia). It affects adenosine receptors in the heart muscle and coronary arteries causing the heart rate to slow down to normal. *Adverse effects* include flushing of the face, breathlessness, wheezing, chest pain, nausea, light-headedness, sweating, palpitations, rapid breathing, severe slowing of the heart rate, headache, blurred vision and a burning sensation. *Precautions:* It should not be used in second- or third-degree heart block or sick sinus syndrome (except in patients with a functioning pacemaker) or in patients with asthma. It should be used with caution in patients with atrial fibrillation (irregular heart beat) and in pregnancy.

Adgyn Combi preparation contains tablets of oestradiol (an oestrogen) and norethisterone (a progesterone) used as HRT ➤ HRT.

Adgyn Estro tablets contain estradiol (an oestrogen) used as HRT ➤ HRT.

Adgyn Medro ➤ medroxyprogesterone.

ADH (antidiuretic hormone) ➤ vasopressin.

Adipine MR ➤ nifedipine.

Adizem SR and **Adizem XL** ➤ diltiazem. See Chapter 22, p. 116. *Adverse effects and Precautions* ➤ diltiazem, thiazide diuretics.

adrenaline(epinephrine) (Anapen, Ana-Guard, Ana-Kit, Epipen, Min-I-Jet adrenaline(epinephrine)), acts on the nerve endings of the sympathetic nervous system. It produces the sort of effects caused by fear or emotion: blanched skin (caused by constriction of small arteries), dilatation of the pupils, slowing of movements of the intestine and bladder and the release of glucose by the liver. In addition it increases the blood supply to muscles, stimulates the heart increasing its rate, relaxes the muscles of the uterus and relaxes bronchial muscles. Adrenaline (epinephrine) is used medically to treat asthma and to treat severe allergic reactions. Because adrenaline(epinephrine) constricts small arteries it is often mixed with injections of a local anaesthetic in order to stop the latter from getting washed away in the bloodstream too quickly, thereby prolonging its effects. *Adverse effects:* These are common and include anxiety, breathlessness, restlessness, rapid beating of the heart, trembling, weakness, dizziness, headache and coldness of the hands and feet.

These may even occur with small doses used by dentists in local anaesthetic injections. Nervous and tense individuals easily develop these symptoms when given adrenaline(epinephrine) and so do patients with overworking of their thyroid glands. Gangrene of a finger may occur after the injection of a combined solution of adrenaline(epinephrine) and local anaesthetic into the finger. *Precautions:* Adrenaline (epinephrine) should not be used in patients who have overworking of their thyroid glands, coronary artery disease, disorders of heart rhythm, high blood pressure or hardening of the arteries (arteriosclerosis). It may cause a severe irregularity of heart rhythm in patients undergoing an anaesthetic with halothane, chloroform or cyclopropane and in patients being treated with quinidine or digitalis. Dentists should use caution when giving adrenaline(epinephrine) to patients on other drugs such as antidepressants. *Interactions* ➤ sympathomimetic drugs.

adrenaline(epinephrine) eye drops (Eppy, Simplene) are used to treat open-angle glaucoma. See p. 63. *Adverse effects* include discomfort in the eye, redness of the eye (hyperaemia), headache, skin reactions and discoloration of the eye. General effects are rare ➤ adrenaline(epinephrine). *Precautions:* Do not use in patients with closed-angle glaucoma or aphakia (absence of a lens). *Interactions:* MAOIs, tricyclic antidepressants.

adrenergic blockers ➤ adrenergic neurone blockers.

adrenergic neurone blocking drugs are used to treat raised blood pressure. See Chapter 25.

adrenocorticotrophic hormone (**ACTH**) ➤ corticotrophin.

adrenoreceptor stimulants are used as bronchodilators to treat asthma. See Chapter 14.

adriamycin ➤ doxorubicin.

adsorbents such as kaolin have been used to treat diarrhoea. See Chapter 20.

Adult Meltus is a cough expectorant which contains guaifenesin, pseudoephedrine and menthol.

Advil ➤ ibuprofen.

Advil Cold and Sinus contains ibuprofen and pseudoephedrine ➤ ibuprofen, pseudoephedrine.

AeroBec preparations ➤ beclometasone.

Aerocrom aerosol inhalations used to treat asthma contain sodium cromoglycate and salbutamol ➤ sodium cromoglycate, salbutamol.

Aerodiol is an oestrogen nasal spray which is used as HRT ➤ oestradiol.

Aerolin Autohaler ➤ salbutamol.

Aerrane ➤ isoflurane.

Afrazine Nasal Spray ➤ oxymetazoline.

Agenerase ➤ amprenavir.

Aggrastat ➤ tirofiban.

Agrippal is an influenza vaccine.

Ailax and **Ailax Forte** liquid are used to treat constipation. They contain poloxamer 188 and dantron ➤ poloxamer 188, dantron.

Airomir aerosol inhalation ➤ salbutamol.

Akineton ➤ biperiden.

Aknemin ➤ minocycline.

Akenemycin Plus is a solution of erythromycin and tretinoin used in the treatment of acne ➤ erthromycin, tretinoin.

Alba preparations ➤ albumin solution.

albendazole (Eskazole) is used to treat Hydatid disease. *Adverse effects* include stomach and bowel upsets, dizziness, headaches, rarely reversible loss of hair, rash, fever, liver damage and blood disorders. *Precautions:* Do not use in pregnancy and avoid any risk of getting pregnant during and for one month after stopping treatment. Blood counts and liver function tests should be carried out at regular intervals. Use with utmost caution in breastfeeding mothers. *Interactions:* Theophylline, anti-epileptic drugs, anticoagulants, oral contraceptives and drugs used to treat diabetes.

albumin solution (human albumin solution, Alba, Albuminar-5, Albutein, Buminate, Zenalb) contains protein derived from human serum or normal placentas. At least 90% of the protein is albumin. It is used to treat patients with a very low level of proteins in their blood (hypoproteinaemia).

Albutein ➢ albumin solution.

alclometasone (in Modrasone cream and ointment) is a mildly potent corticosteroid used to treat eczema and dermatitis. See Chapter 37 on corticosteroids and corticosteroid skin preparations, p. 241.

Alcobon intravenous infusion ➢ flucytosine.

Alcoderm emollient cream and lotion contain liquid paraffin ➢ liquid paraffin.

alcohol (ethyl alcohol, ethanol) is used as a solvent and preservative in drug preparations.

Aldactide preparations contain hydroflumethiazide (a thiazide diuretic) and spironolactone (a potassium-sparing diuretic). It is used to treat congestive heart failure. *Adverse effects and Precautions* ➢ thiazide diuretics, spironolactone.

Aldactone ➢ spironolactone.

Aldara cream ➢ imiquimod.

aldesleukin (Proleukin) is interleukin-2, an interferon (see p. 293) used by intravenous infusion to treat secondary cancer of the kidney (renal metastases). *Adverse effects* can be very severe and include damage to small blood vessels (capillaries) producing a fall in blood pressure and fluid on the lung (pulmonary oedema). It may also damage bone marrow and nerve tissue and the liver, kidneys and thyroid gland. It must only be used in special cancer treatment centres.

Aldomet ➢ methyldopa.

aldosterone blockers are used as diuretics. See Chapter 29.

alemtuzumab (MabCampath) is used in the treatment of certain leukaemias where other therapies have failed. *Adverse effects* include pain, swelling and redness at the injection site, chills, fever, fatigue, anorexia, weakness, flu-like symptoms, heart disorders, nerve damage, stomach and bowel upset, psychiatric disorders, susceptibility to infection and respiratory diseases. *Precautions:* Do not use in patients with liver or kidney damage, an allergy to murine proteins, HIV and other infections affecting the whole body, secondary tumours, in pregnancy or while breastfeeding. Use with caution in patients with heart disease, angina, high blood pressure or in the elderly. Patients should use effective contraception during and for six months after therapy.

alendronate sodium (Fosamax) is used to treat osteoporosis in post-menopausal women. It stops bone being dissolved and increases new bone formation. It increases bone mass in fragile parts of the skeleton and reduces the risk of fractures. *Adverse effects* include irritation, damage and ulcers of the oesophagus (gullet), abdominal pains, indigestion, difficulty swallowing, distension of the abdomen, stomach and bowel upsets, muscle and joint pains and headache. Rarely skin rashes may occur. *Precautions:* Do not use in pregnancy or in breastfeeding mothers or in patients with moderate or severe impairment of kidney function. Any deficiency of calcium and/or vitamin D should be corrected before starting treatment and patients should maintain an adequate intake of calcium during treatment. Do not use in patients with disorders of the oesophagus or who can not stand upright for thirty minutes after swallowing the tablet. Patients should report any discomfort or difficulty in swallowing immediately. To reduce the risk of damage to the oesophagus patients should remain upright for thirty minutes after swallowing the tablets with plenty of fluid. *Interactions:* Foods and drugs can easily bind to alendronate in the stomach and intestine, it should therefore be taken in the morning, half an hour before food or any other drug, especially calcium supplements, antacids and NSAIDs.

Alendronic acid ➤ alendronate sodium.

alexitol is an aluminium compound.

alfacalcidol (Alpha-D, One-Alpha) is a vitamin D derivative used for the treatment of bone disease caused by kidney disorders and rickets. *Precautions:* It should be used with caution in breastfeeding mothers. Blood calcium levels should be checked at regular intervals. *Interactions:* Barbiturates, anticoagulants, danazol, digitalis, thiazide diuretics, antacids, mineral oils, cholestyramine, colestipol, sucralfate.

Alfa D ➤ alfacalidol.

alfentanil (alfentanil hydrochloride, Rapifen) is a short-acting opiate pain-reliever used during surgery. See Chapter 30. *Adverse effects* include respiratory depression, a fall in blood pressure (hypotension), slowing of the heart rate (bradycardia), nausea and vomiting. *Precautions:* It should be used with caution in patients with long-term respiratory disorders, myasthenia gravis (muscle weakness due to neuromuscular abnormality). A reduced dose should be used in the elderly, in patients with impaired liver function or reduced working of their thyroid gland (hypothyroidism). In childbirth it may reduce respiration in the baby.

alfuzosin (alfuzosin hydrochloride, Xatral) is a selective alpha-blocker (see p. 284) used to treat the symptoms caused by a benign enlargement of the prostate gland. Some of the difficulty in passing urine in this condition is caused by constriction of the muscles of the urethra and prostate and alfuzosin relaxes these muscles. *Adverse effects and Precautions* are similar to those listed under prazosin.

Algesal cream contains diethylamine salicylate ➤ rubefacients.

Algicon preparations contain a co-dried gel of aluminium hydroxide and magnesium carbonate, magnesium alginate, magnesium carbonate, potassium bicarbonate and sucrose. It is used to treat heartburn and acid reflux, see p. 99. Algicon contains a low amount of sodium but is high in sugar and should be used with caution in diabetes. It should not be used in children, in patients with kidney failure or who are severely debilitated.

Alginates ➤ alginic acid.

alginic acid (in Gastrocote, in Gaviscon, in Pyrogastrone, in Topal) is obtained from coastal algae. Alginates are salts of alginic acid. They are used as thickening agents in preparing creams, pastes and gels, in tablets to help them to break up when they enter the stomach and in the food industry. They are added to antacid mixtures to make the antacid float to form a raft in the treatment of heartburn due to acid reflux disorders such as hiatus hernia. See Chapter 19.

Algipan spray contains methyl nicotinate and glycol salicylate ➤ rubefacients.

alimemazine(trimeprazine) (trimeprazine tartrate, Vallergan) is an antihistamine (see Chapter 17) which is related to phenothiazine antipsychotic drugs. Its main use is in the treatment of itching (see p. 246) and nettle-rash (urticaria). It is also used as a pre-medication to provide sedation before surgery. *Adverse effects* include drowsiness, dizziness, dryness of the mouth, skin rashes, stomach and bowel upsets, changes of mood, antimuscarinic effects (➤ antimuscarinics), fall in blood pressure, depressed breathing, skin rashes. High doses may cause involuntary movements (e.g. parkinsonism) and convulsions. *Precautions:* Do not use in patients suffering from epilepsy, glaucoma, Parkinson's disease, under-active thyroid, tumour of the sympathetic nervous system (phaeochromocytoma), myasthenia gravis (muscle weakness due to neuromuscular abnormality), impaired liver or kidney function or enlarged prostate gland (may cause difficulty in passing urine). *Interactions:* Alcohol, sleeping drugs, sedatives and other drugs that depress brain function, anti-blood pressure drugs, anti-muscarinics, anti-diabetic drugs. For other potential adverse effects ➤ antipsychotic drugs.

Alka-Seltzer ➤ aspirin.

alkaloids are a group of drugs, mostly from plant origin. They are complex organic compounds, weakly alkaline in solution and forming soluble salts with acids. They are used mainly in the form of their salts. Examples include belladonna alkaloids (e.g. atropine), opium alkaloids (e.g. morphine), vinca alkaloids (e.g. vincristine), and individual drugs such as ephedrine, nicotine, pilocarpine and tubocurarine. Many of the naturally occurring alkaloids are now synthesized.

Alkeran ➤ melphalan.

alkylating drugs are used as anti-cancer drugs. See Chapter 51.

allantoin occurs in comfrey root but it is also manufactured. It has been used to encourage wound healing and it is used in skin preparations to treat psoriasis and other skin disorders.

Allegron ➤ nortriptyline.

allergen extract vaccines are used in hyposensitization (desensitization). See Chapter 17.

allopurinol (Caplenal, Cosuric, Rimapurinol, Xanthomax, Zyloric) is a xanthine oxidase inhibitor used to treat gout. See Chapter 33. It reduces the formation of uric acid and is used in the treatment of gout. In the early stages of treatment acute attacks of gout may occur but after several weeks of continuous treatment these become less frequent and stop. Allopurinol reduces the risk of patients with gout developing kidney stones and it may prevent kidney damage. Unlike other drugs used to treat gout it may

be used in the presence of kidney damage and it may also be used to prevent a rise in plasma uric acid which may occur in some patients treated with certain diuretics. It may therefore be used along with a diuretic in patients suffering from gout and congestive heart failure. It is also used to prevent the formation of kidney stones. *Adverse effects* include nausea, vomiting and diarrhoea. It may cause rashes, sometimes with fever (stop drug immediately). Rarely, headache, vertigo, disturbances of taste, generally feeling unwell, drowsiness, a rise in blood pressure, hair loss, liver damage and nerve damage may occur. *Precautions:* Do not use to treat acute attacks of gout. Colchicine or an NSAID should be given for about four weeks at the start of treatment. Drink plenty of fluids. Use with caution in patients with impaired liver function. Reduce dose in patients with impaired kidney function. Use with caution in pregnancy and the elderly. *Interactions:* Anticoagulants, chlorpropamide, mercaptopurine, azathioprine.

Almodan ➤ amoxicillin.

Almogran ➤ almotriptan.

almond oil is used as a demulcent and as an emollient.

almotriptan (Almogran) is used for acute treatment of the headache phase of migraine attacks with or without aura. See Chapter 34. *Adverse effects* include dizziness, drowsiness, stomach and bowel upsets, fatigue. *Precautions:* Do not use in patients with heart disease, severe or uncontrolled high blood pressure, previous stroke, disorder of circulation in the arms and legs or heart attack, severe liver damage, basilar, hemiplegic or ophthalmoplegic migraine. Use with caution in patients with severe kidney damage, moderate liver damage, allergy to sulphonamides, in the elderly, in pregnancy or while breastfeeding.

Alomide eye solution is used to treat allergic conjunctivitis. It contains lodoxamide (as tromethamine). It may irritate the eyes ➤ lodoxamide.

alpha-adrenoceptor blocking drugs are used to treat raised blood pressure. See Chapter 25. Some of them (alfuzosin, doxazosin, indoramin, prazosin and terazosin) are also used to relax smooth muscle in enlarged prostatic glands (benign prostatic hypertrophy: BPH). This relaxation allows the urine to flow more easily. See p. 284.

alpha-blockers ➤ alpha-adrenoceptor blocking drugs.

Alphaderm cream contains hydrocortisone and urea. See corticosteroid skin applications (p. 241).

Alphagan ➤ brimonidine.

Alpha Keri bath emollient and oil contains liquid paraffin and lanolin oil ➤ liquid paraffin, lanolin.

Alphanate Fanhdi ➤ Factor VIII.

Alphanin ➤ Factor IX fraction, dried.

Alphaparin ➤ certoparin.

alpha tocopheryl acetate ➤ tocopheryl (vitamin E).

Alphavase ➤ prazosin.

Alphosyl HC cream contains allantoin, coal tar extract and hydrocortisone (a corticosteroid). It is used to treat psoriasis. *Adverse effects and Precautions* ➤ coal tar and see corticosteroid skin applications p. 241.

Alphosyl lotion and cream contain allantoin and coal tar extract. It is used to treat psoriasis ➤ allantoin, coal tar.

Alphosyl 2 in 1 Shampoo ➤ coal tar.

alprazolam (Xanax) is a long-acting benzodiazepine anti-anxiety drug ➤ benzodiazepines.

alprostadil is prostaglandin E. See Chapter 52. It has two main uses. As Prostin VR it is given by intravenous infusion to keep the duct between the artery to the lung and the aorta (ductus arteriosus) open in babies born with heart defects, prior to heart surgery. As Caverject or Viridal Duo it is injected into the penis to produce an erection in men suffering from an inability to obtain or maintain an erection. It is also available as a direct urethral applicator stick (MUSE).

Prostin VR: *Adverse effects:* Used intravenously it may cause changes in pulse rate, a fall in blood pressure, flushing, breathing may stop and the heart may stop, it may cause fever, diarrhoea, convulsions, blood clotting, fall in blood potassium, weakening of the wall of the ductus arteriosus and blockage to the outlet of the stomach. *Precautions:* Do not use in patients with respiratory distress syndrome (hyaline membrane disease). Use with caution in babies with a history of bleeding. Monitor blood pressure. Caverject or Viridal Duo: *Adverse effects* following injection into the penis include persistent erections (priapism) and scarring (fibrosis) of the penis, bruising, redness at site of injection, pain in testicles and bottom. Faulty injection may cause a fall in blood pressure, palpitations, headache, dizziness, shock and collapse. Do not use injections more than once in twenty-four hours and no more than three times in any one week. Erections should not last for more than one hour. *Precautions:* Do not use in patients with diseases that produce prolonged erection such as sickle cell anaemia, multiple myeloma or leukaemia. Do not use in patients with tight foreskins (phimosis), with penile implants or with disorders of the penis that cause fibrosis (scarring). An erection lasting more than four hours should be reported to the doctor. Prolonged erection (priapism) should be treated within six hours by drawing blood off and injecting a sympathomimetic drug. If this doesn't work surgery will be necessary.

MUSE: *Adverse effects* include penile or testicular pain, urinary tract irritation, swelling of veins, headache, low blood pressure, dizziness. Rarely abnormal, persistent, painful erections (priapism). *Precautions:* Do not use in patients with abnormal penile anatomy, history of recurrent priapism, blood disorders, predisposition to blood clots, unstable heart conditions, inflammation of the glans penis, inflammation of the urinary tract. Use a condom if partner is pregnant.

Altacite indigestion preparations ➤ hydrotalcite.

Altacite Plus antacid suspension and tablets contain hydrotalcite and activated dimethicone ➤ antacids, activated dimethicone.

alteplase (Actilyse) is a fibrinolytic (clot buster, see p. 117). It is used in the early treatment of a heart attack due to a coronary thrombosis. *Adverse effects* include bleeding, which is usually limited to the site of injection, nausea, vomiting, allergic skin rash and fever. Rarely, bleeding into the brain may occur. *Precautions:* Do not use in patients with pancreatitis (inflammation of the pancreas), bacterial endocarditis (inflammation of the lining of the heart), disease of the arteries supplying the brain, uncontrolled raised blood pressure, bleeding disorders, active peptic ulcers or severe liver disease, within ten days of surgery or bleeding from an injury. Use with caution in patients with severe impairment of kidney function, diabetic retinopathy (damage to the retina due to diabetes) and in pregnancy. Disorders of heart rhythm may occur during intravenous infusion. *Interactions:* Anticoagulants.

altretamine (Hexalen) is used to treat advanced ovarian cancer in patients who have failed on other treatments. See Chapter 51. *Adverse effects* include damage to nerve tissue, liver and kidneys, skin rash and itching. *Precautions:* Anti-vomiting drugs are recommended before treatment starts because nausea and vomiting are common.

Alu-Cap antacid gel ➤ aluminium hydroxide. Capsules are used to bind phosphates in the gut in patients with kidney failure.

Aludrox antacid gel ➤ aluminium hydroxide.

Aludrox antacid tablets ➤ aluminium hydroxide and magnesium carbonate ➤ antacids.

aluminium acetate is used as an astringent.

aluminium chloride is an astringent and an antiperspirant. It is used to stop excessive perspiration of armpits, hands and feet. Keep away from eyes. Do not shave armpits or use hair-removing preparations for twelve hours after application.

aluminium chloride hexahydrate (Anhydrol Forte, Driclor) is used as an antiperspirant.

aluminium dihydroxyallantoinate (Zeasorb) is used as an astringent and for removing dead skin.

aluminium hydroxide (aluminium hydroxide mixture, aluminium hydroxide gel, dried aluminium hydroxide gel, aluminium hydroxide tablet, Alu-Cap, in Asilone, in Gastrocote, in Gaviscon, in Kolanticon, in Maalox, in Mucaine, in Mucogel, in Pyrogastrone, in Topal) is a useful slow-acting antacid. *Adverse effects:* It may cause constipation and it may interfere with the absorption of phosphates and vitamins. Aluminium hydroxide decreases the absorption of tetracycline antibiotics from the intestine and therefore reduces their effectiveness. These drugs should not be given together. Do not use in patients with raised blood phosphate levels and use with caution in patients with porphyria (a hereditary disorder of metabolism). Do not use in children. It is also used to treat raised blood phosphate levels.

aluminium hydroxide-magnesium carbonate (Algicon) is used as an antacid ➤ antacids.

aluminium magnesium silicate is used as a thickening agent and as a binder in various drug preparations.

aluminium oxide is used as an antacid ➤ antacids.

aluminum silicate ➤ kaolin.

Alupent preparations ➤ orciprenaline.

Alvedon suppositories ➤ paracetamol. Use

with caution in patients with impaired kidney or liver function.

Alverine (alverine citrate, in Alvercol, Spasmonal, in Spasmonal Fibre) is an antispasmodic drug used to relieve spasm of the stomach and intestine, period pain and irritable bowel syndrome. *Adverse effects* include nausea, headache, itching, rash and dizziness. *Precautions:* Do not use in pregnancy or in breastfeeding mothers. Do not use in patients with obstruction of the bowel.

Alyrane ➤ enflurane.

amantadine (Lysovir, Symmetrel) is used to protect or treat patients suffering from influenza A virus infection when complications may be harmful, e.g. in patients with chronic chest or heart diseases. It may also be used to treat herpes zoster (shingles). However, in addition to its anti-viral effects it also stimulates dopamine receptors and its main use is to treat parkinsonism (see Chapter 16). *Adverse effects* are usually related to dose; they include insomnia, dizziness, stomach and bowel upsets, loss of appetite, blood disorders, convulsions, blurred vision, nervousness, difficulty in concentrating, dry mouth, changes in mood, and very rarely, serious mental symptoms, including hallucinations and confusion (especially in patients with impaired kidney function and patients on antimuscarinic drugs), occasionally cause a blue mottling of the skin (livido reticularis) and ankle-swelling. *Precautions:* It should not be used in patients with epilepsy, stomach ulcers, or severe kidney disease. It should be used with caution in patients with heart, liver or moderate kidney disease, recurrent eczema, confusion, or serious mental illness. It should be used with caution in the elderly, in pregnancy and in breastfeeding mothers. Treatment should be stopped slowly to avoid a flare-up of parkinsonism. *Interactions:* Antimuscarinics, levodopa, CNS stimulants, CNS depressants.

Amaryl ➤ glimepiride.

AmBisome ➤ amphotericin.

amethocaine ➤ tetracaine.

Ametop aqueous gel ➤ amethocaine. It is used as pre-treatment to the skin to relieve the pain of injections.

amfebutamone (bupropion, Zyban) is used as an aid to stop smoking. *Adverse effects* include insomnia, headache, fever, dry mouth, stomach and bowel upsets, allergic reactions on the skin, taste disorders, seizures. *Precautions:* Do not use in patients with a history of seizures, mood swings or eating disorders, severe liver cirrhosis, in pregnancy or while breastfeeding. Use with caution in patients with mild to moderate liver or kidney damage, tumour of the central nervous system, alcohol abuse or diabetes, or where there is a risk of seizure in patients with head trauma. Blood pressure should be monitored weekly if nicotine patches are also being used.

amfetamine, see Chapter 6 on amfetamines.

Amias ➤ candesartan.

Amiclav ➤ co-amoxiclav.

amifostine (Ethyol) is given by intravenous infusion to protect cells and to reduce the risk of infection in patients who develop a fall in their white blood cell count while undergoing anti-cancer treatment with cyclophosphamide and cysplatin for advanced cancer of the ovaries. It is given thirty minutes before anti-cancer treatment starts. *Adverse effects* include fall in blood pressure, nausea, vomiting, dizziness, flushing, chills, sleepiness, hiccups, sneezing and rarely a fall in blood calcium levels and allergic reactions. Very occasionally shortterm loss of consciousness may occur. *Precautions:* Patient should be well hydrated and given anti-vomiting drugs before treatment starts. The blood pressure should be carefully monitored during infusion with amifostine and stopped if blood pressure goes too low. Patients receiving treatment for raised blood pressure should have their anti-blood pressure drugs stopped twenty-four hours before treatment with amifostine. Infusion should take about fifteen minutes – the longer the time taken for the infusion the greater is the risk of adverse effects. Blood calcium levels should be checked in patients at risk of developing a fall in blood calcium. Do not use in pregnancy, in breastfeeding mothers or in patients with impaired liver or kidney function. Do not use in patients who are dehydrated or have a low blood pressure. *Interactions:* Anti-blood pressure drugs.

amikacin (amikacin sulphate, Amikin) is an aminoglycoside antibiotic ➤ aminoglycoside antibiotics.

Amikin ➤ amikacin.

Amilamont ➤ amiloride.

Amil-Co (co-amilozide) is a diuretic. Each tablet contains amiloride (a potassium-sparing diuretic) and hydrochlorothiazide (a thiazide diuretic) ➤ co-amilozide.

Amilomaxco (co-amilozide) is a diuretic. Each tablet contains amiloride (a potassium-sparing diuretic) and hydrochlorothiazide (a thiazide diuretic) ➤ co-amilozide.

amiloride (Amiloride, combined with a thiazide diuretic in co-amilozide preparations and with a loop diuretic in co-amilofruse preparations, Amilamont, in Amil-Co, in Burinex A, in Fru-Co, in Frumil, in Kalten, in Lasoride, in Moducren, in Moduret 25, in Moduretic, in Navispare) is a potassium-sparing diuretic, see Chapter 29. It is used with a thiazide or a loop diuretic to help conserve potassium. *Adverse effects* include dry mouth, stomach and bowel upsets, rashes, confusion, fall in blood sodium levels, rise in blood potassium levels and fall in blood pressure on standing up after sitting or lying down. *Precautions:* Do not use in patients suffering from kidney failure or a raised blood potassium level. Use with caution in pregnancy, in elderly patients and in patients with diabetes. *Interactions:* Potassium supplements, potassium-sparing

diuretics, ACE inhibitors, lithium, NSAIDs.

Amilospare ➤ amiloride.

aminoacridine is an antimicrobial agent used in the treatment of minor infections.

aminobenzoic acid is used in sunscreen applications. It absorbs the UVB band of the sun's rays. It is used to prevent sunburn, but because it absorbs little UVA it will provide minimum protection to the skin for patients suffering from photo-sensitivity reactions to drugs (see Chapter 45). It is also used to protect the skin against radiotherapy. *Adverse effects* include contact dermatitis and allergic dermatitis to the sun's rays (photosensitivity).

aminoglutethimide (Orimeten) blocks the production of adrenal steroids by the adrenal glands and the conversion of androgens (male sex hormones) to oestrogens (female sex hormones) in the tissues. It produces effects as if the adrenal glands were not working. It is used to treat advanced cancer of the breast in post-menopausal women and in women who have had their ovaries removed. It is also used to treat advanced cancer of the prostate and Cushing's syndrome due to cancer of the adrenal glands. *Adverse effects* include drowsiness, lethargy, unsteadiness of movement (ataxia), fever, stomach and bowel upsets, and skin rashes which may be severe. These adverse effects diminish after about six–eight weeks because the body speeds up its breakdown of the drug. Very rarely, it may cause damage to the bone marrow, producing blood disorders; thyroid dysfunction, underworking of the adrenal glands, jaundice, liver damage, severe allergic reactions; virilization in females; and a fall in blood pressure on standing up after sitting or lying down (this may cause faintness and lightheadedness). It may cause allergic effects on lung tissue (allergic alveolitis). *Precautions:* It should not be used in pregnancy or in breastfeeding mothers. Supplementary corticosteroids should be given to patients being treated for cancer of the breast or prostate, and may be required in Cushing's syndrome. Mineralocorticoids may also be required. Blood pressure, thyroid function, blood counts and blood chemistry should be checked at regular intervals. Do not use in patients with porphyria (a hereditary disorder of metabolism). *Interactions:* Oral anti-diabetic drugs, synthetic cortico-steroids, anticoagulants, theophylline, med-roxyprogesterone, diuretics.

aminoglycoside antibiotics are discussed in Chapter 46. *Adverse effects* are related to the dose and duration of treatment. They occur more commonly in the elderly and in people with impaired kidney function. They should, preferably, not be used for more than seven days. High doses and/or pro-longed use, particularly in patients with a low blood potassium, may occasionally cause damage to the kidneys and damage to the nerves in the ears, producing dizziness, vertigo, noises in the ears (tinnitus), and deafness which may be reversible. Other harmful effects produced by nerve damage include numbness, tingling of the skin, muscle twitching, convulsions, lethargy and confusion. Aminoglycosides may, rarely, cause loss of appetite, loss of weight, skin rashes, itching, generalized burning, fever, headache, nausea, vomiting, allergic reac-tions, joint pains, loss of hair and sore mouth. Prolonged use may cause a fall in levels of magnesium in the blood; rarely, a severe colitis (pseudomembranous colitis) may occur. Aminoglycosides affect nerves that supply muscles, and they may produce serious muscle fatigue and difficulty with breathing in people who have myasthenia gravis (muscle weakness due to neuro-muscular abnormality). Large doses given during surgical operations may produce a temporary disorder like myasthenia gravis in which the muscles are totally fatigued. This effect may also occur if an aminoglyco-side is given to someone who has been given neuromuscular blocking drugs or a large volume of blood that has been treated with citrate to prevent it from clotting. Local applications may cause allergic rashes; if applied extensively to the skin or to burns, some of the antibiotic may be absorbed and may, rarely, produce nerve damage in the ear, resulting in deafness and vertigo. *Pre-cautions:* Aminoglycosides must not be used in patients with hearing loss, disorders of balance (e.g. vertigo), or in the blind, or in anyone who is allergic to any one of them or who suffers from myasthenia gravis. They must be used with the utmost caution in pregnancy, breastfeeding mothers, patients with parkinsonism or in anyone with impaired kidney function; impaired ex-cretion will cause a rise in the concentration of the drug in the blood, increasing the risks of toxic effects, which are mainly damage to the ears (affecting hearing and balance) and damage to the kidneys. The risk of damage to the nerves in the ears, affecting hearing and balance, is greater in people with impaired kidney function and in individuals with normal kidney function treated with high doses and/or for longer periods of time than recommended. Warnings of damage include dizziness, vertigo, noises in the ears and hearing loss. No other drug that may produce adverse effects on the nerves in the ears, or kidney damage, should be used at the same time as an aminoglycoside, whether by injection, by mouth or applied to the skin or elsewhere. These include cis-platin, the antibacterial drugs cephaloridine, colistin, polymyxin B, streptomycin and vancomycin, and the loop diuretics bumet-anide, ethacrynic acid, frusemide and piret-anide. Diuretics given intravenously may reduce the volume of fluid in the body and increase the risks of harmful effects from aminoglycosides. The risk of adverse effects is increased if the patient becomes dehy-drated; therefore plenty of fluids should be given during treatment. *Adverse effects* may be more frequent and severe in elderly people; therefore use smaller doses and/or increase the time between doses. Kidney function and hearing function should be checked regularly, and blood levels of the drug monitored. If high doses are used, blood levels should be measured one hour after each dose and just before next dose.

This also applies to treatment given for more than seven days to infants, the elderly, obese patients and patients with cystic fibrosis. Once a day dosage may help to reduce adverse effects. *Interactions:* Increased risk of kidney damage with colistin, capreomycin, vancomycin, amphotericin, cyclosporin, any anti-cancer drugs. Increased risk of damage to hearing with cisplatin, loop diuretics, capreomycin and vancomycin. Increased risk of adverse effects from botulinum toxin, muscle relaxants, neostigmine and pyridostigmine and increased risk of severe rise in blood calcium levels from biophosphonates.

aminophylline (theophylline plus ethylenediamine, Amnivent, Min-I-Jet, Norphyllin, Pecram, Phyllocontin Continus) is used to treat asthma (see Chapter 14). *Adverse effects:* ➤ theophylline. Aminophylline can irritate the lining of the stomach and cause nausea and vomiting. It is therefore given by injection or by the rectum. Rapid injection of aminophylline may cause nausea, vomiting, restlessness, dizziness, rapid heart rate, fall in blood pressure and disordered heart rhythm. Similar effects occasionally occur with suppositories which may also irritate the rectum. Allergy to ethylenediamine can cause nettle-rash (urticaria), erythema and dermatitis. *Precautions:* It should be used with caution in patients with heart or liver disease or peptic ulcers. Use with caution in pregnancy and breastfeeding mothers ➤ theophylline.

aminosalicylates (calcium, potassium, sodium) are salts of aminosalicylic acid ➤ aminosalicylic acid.

aminosalicylic acid (4-aminosalicylic acid) and its salts were widely used with isoniazid and streptomycin to treat tuberculosis. They are now seldom used. 5-*aminosalicylic acid* (mesalazine) is a component of sulphasalazine used to treat ulcerative colitis, Crohn's disease (severe diarrhoeal disorders) and rheumatoid arthritis. Sulphasalazine is broken down by bacteria in the bowel to release 5-aminosalicylic acid

(mesalazine) and the sulphonamide, sulphapyridine ➤ sulphasalazine. Mesalazine is considered the active drug in ulcerative colitis and Crohn's disease but not in rheumatoid arthritis ➤ mesalazine.

amiodarone (amiodarone hydrochloride, Cordarone X) is used to treat disordered rhythms of the heart (see Chapter 24). *Adverse effects:* Patients on continuous therapy may develop micro-deposits in the cornea of their eyes; these can be identified on slit-lamp examination. Nerve damage, myasthenia gravis (muscle weakness due to neuromuscular abnormality) and parkinsonism may also develop. These complications disappear when the drug is stopped. It may cause sensitivity of the skin to sunlight and occasionally the skin turns a slate-grey colour. Dose-related symptoms include nausea, headache, vomiting, metallic taste in the mouth, nightmares, sleeplessness, fatigue and vertigo. Rarely thyroid, lung, liver and blood disorders, unsteadiness of movement (ataxia), skin rashes and allergic reactions may occur. *Precautions:* It should not be used in patients with thyroid dysfunction, heart block or severe slowing of the heart rate. It should not be used in pregnancy, in breastfeeding mothers or in patients sensitive to iodine. Use with caution in heart failure, impaired kidney function, the elderly and porphyria (a hereditary disorder of metabolism). The eyes should be examined regularly and tests of thyroid, lung and liver function should be carried out at regular intervals. Intravenous amiodarone should not be used in patients suffering from severe respiratory failure, shock, severe low blood pressure in the arteries or congestive heart failure. Treatment must be started in hospital under specialist supervision. *Interactions:* Calcium-channel blockers, oral anticoagulants, anti-arrhythmics, anaesthetics, beta-blockers, digoxin, phenytoin, diuretics, oral anticoagulants, digoxin, phenytoin, anti-arrhythmic drugs, erythromycin, cotrimoxazole, pentamide, antipsychotics, lithium, tricyclic antidepressants, antihistamines, anti-malarial drugs, beta-blockers, calcium-channel blockers, diuretics, corticosteroids, tetracosactrin, amphotericin, anaesthesia, ciclosporin.

amisulpride (Solian) is used to treat acute and chronic schizophrenia in which positive and/or negative symptoms are prominent. See Chapter 3. *Adverse effects* include insomnia, anxiety, agitation, drowsiness, stomach and bowel upsets, raised serum prolactin, weight gain, muscle disorders, slowness of movement. Rarely low blood pressure, slow heart beat, allergic reactions, risk of neuroleptic malignant syndrome (for symptoms ➤ antipsychotic drugs). *Precautions:* Do not use in patients with prolactin-dependent tumours, tumour of the sympathetic nervous system (phaeochromocytoma), in pregnancy (adequate contraception must be used) or while breastfeeding. Use with caution in patients with kidney damage, epilepsy, Parkinson's disease or in the elderly.

amitriptyline (amitriptyline embonate, amitriptyline hydrochloride, Elavil, Lentizol, in Triptafen) is a tricyclic antidepressant drug ➤ tricyclic antidepressants.

Amix ➤ amoxicillin.

amlodipine (amlodipine bisylate, Istin) is a calcium-channel blocker used to treat raised blood pressure (see Chapter 25) and angina (see Chapter 22). *Adverse effects* include headache, sleepiness, palpitations, abdominal pains, blood disorders, overgrowth of gums, oedema (e.g. swelling of the ankles), nausea, fatigue, dizziness and flushing. *Precautions:* It should be used with caution in patients with impaired liver function, in pregnancy and in breastfeeding mothers.

Ammonaps ➤ sodium phenylbutyrate.

ammonia (strong ammonia solution, aromatic ammonia solution) is used in smelling salts and rheumatic liniments. It is very irritant to the skin and its use in cosmetics is restricted. It is said to be useful in relieving stings from Portuguese men-of-war.

Ammonia and ipecacuanha mixture is a cough expectorant which contains ammonium bicarbonate, liquorice, ipecacuanha, camphor water, anise water and chloroform water.

Amnivent ➤ aminophylline.

amobarbital ➤ amylobarbitone.

amoebicides (e.g. diloxanide furoate, metranidazole and tinidazole) are used to treat amoebic infections.

Amoram ➤ amoxicillin.

amorolfine (Loceryl) cream and nail lacquer is used to treat fungal, mould and yeast infections of the skin and nails. They are effective against a wide range of fungi, moulds and yeasts. *Adverse effects:* It may rarely produce itching, redness and transient burning of the skin. *Precautions:* Do not use in pregnancy or in breastfeeding mothers. Avoid contact with eyes, ears, and mucous membranes. Do not use in children.

amoxapine (Asendis) is a tricyclic antidepressant ➤ tricyclic antidepressants.

Amoxil ➤ amoxicillin.

amoxicillin (amoxycillin, Almodan, Amix, Amoram, Amoxil, in Augmentin, Galenamox, in Heliclear) is a broad-spectrum penicillin ➤ penicillins and see Chapter 46.

amoxycillin ➤ amoxicillin

Amphocil ➤ amphotericin.

amphotericin (Abelcet, Ambisome, Amphocil, Fungilin, Fungizone) is an antifungal drug (see Chapter 47). *Adverse effects:* When given by infusion it may cause nausea, vomiting, loss of appetite, diarrhoea, pains in the stomach, headache, chills, fever, muscle and joint pains, and generally feeling unwell. It may occasionally cause changes in blood pressure, disorders of heart rhythm, skin rashes, blurred vision, noises in the ears (tinnitus), nerve damage, convulsions, kidney damage, allergic reactions, blood disorders and liver damage. It may cause pain and thrombophlebitis (inflammation of a vein) at the site of injection. When applied to the skin it may cause irritation, itching and rashes. *Precautions:* When given by infusion, adverse effects are common. Careful monitoring of the patient is necessary, including regular blood counts, tests of liver and kidney function and blood electrolytes. Use with caution in pregnancy and breastfeeding mothers. Abelcet, Ambisome and Amphocil are special formulations designed to reduce adverse effects especially on the kidney. *Interactions:* aminoglycosides, miconazole, digoxin and related drugs, cyclosporin, loop diuretics, thiazide diuretics.

ampicillin (Amfipen, in Ampiclox, in Magnapen, Penbritin, Rimacillin, Vidopen) is a broad spectrum penicillin ➤ penicillins and see Chapter 46.

amprenavir (Agenerase) is used in combination with other antiviral drugs in the treatment of HIV. See Chapter 48. *Adverse effects* include rashes, nausea, vomiting, diarrhoea, flatulence, abdominal discomfort, indigestion, headache, sleep disturbances, tremor, abnormal sensations in the mouth, fatigue, depression. *Precautions:* Do not use in patients with liver damage, diabetes, haemophilia or in pregnancy; avoid vitamin E supplements.

amsacrine (Amsidine) is an anti-cancer drug (see Chapter 51). *Adverse effects* include damage to the bone marrow, producing blood disorders, mild nausea and/or vomiting and sore mouth. Very rarely, it may cause convulsions and damage the liver, kidneys and heart, skin rashes and loss of hair. It may cause irritation and damage to the tissues at the site of injection. *Precautions:* See Chapter 51 on anti-cancer drugs.

Amsidine ➤ amsacrine.

amylmetacresol is an antiseptic which is used as an ingredient of lozenges in the treatment of minor infections of the mouth and throat.

amylobarbitone (Amytal, Sodium Amytal, Tuinal) is an intermediate-acting barbitu-

rate used as a sedative and hypnotic ➤ phenobarbitone.

Amytal ➤ amylobarbitone.

Anabact gel ➤ metronidazole. It is used to deodorize foul-smelling tumours.

anabolic steroids, see Chapter 39.

Anacal preparations used to treat haemorrhoids contain heparinoid and lauromacrogol ➤ heparinoid, lauromacrogol.

Anadin and **Anadin Maximum Strength** contain aspirin and caffeine; **Anadin Extra Soluble** contains aspirin, paracetamol and caffeine; **Anadin Paracetamol** contains paracetamol; **Anadin Cold Control** contains paracetamol, caffeine and phenylephrine; **Anadin Ibuprofen** contains ibuprofen; **Anadin Ultra** contains ibuprofen ➤ individual entry for each drug.

anaesthetics, local, see Chapter 44.

Anaflex cream ➤ polynoxylin.

Anafranil preparations ➤ clomipramine.

Ana-Guard pre-filled syringes contain adrenaline(epinephrine) for subcutaneous or intramuscular injection. It is used for self-treatment by patients at risk of developing a life-threatening allergic reaction. See p. 87. *Adverse effects and Precautions* ➤ adrenaline(epinephrine).

Ana-Kit contains pre-filled syringe of adrenaline(epinephrine), two chewable tablets of the antihistamine chlorpheniramine, two sterile pads and a tourniquet. It is used for self-treatment by patients at risk of developing a life-threatening allergic reaction. See p. 87. *Adverse effects and Precautions* ➤ adrenaline, chlorpheniramine.

analgesics (pain-relievers). See morphine and related pain-relievers (Chapter 30), aspirin and paracetamol (Chapter 31), and non-steroid anti-inflammatory drugs (Chapter 32).

Anapen Adult and **Junior** pre-filled syringes contain adrenaline(epinephrine) for intramuscular injection. They are used for self-treatment by patients at risk of developing a life-threatening allergic reaction. See p. 87. *Adverse effects and Precautions* ➤ adrenaline(epinephrine).

anastrozole (Arimidex) blocks the enzyme (aromatase) that normally converts male sex hormones (androgens) into female sex hormones (oestrogens) in the tissues of the female body (but not in the ovaries). In post-menopausal women this helps to reduce the amount of oestrogens in the body and is used to treat cancers of the breast that require oestrogens for growth (oestrogen-dependent breast cancers). *Adverse effects* include hot flushes, sweating, vaginal irritation, thinning of the hair, stomach and bowel upsets, rash, headache, sleepiness and weakness. *Precautions:* Do not use in pregnancy, in breastfeeding mothers, in pre-menopausal women, in women with severe impairment of kidney function or moderate or severe impairment of liver function. *Interactions:* Oestrogens.

Anbesol liquid contains cetylpyridinum, chlorocresol and lidocaine(lignocaine) ➤ individual entry for each drug.

Ancotil ➤ flucytosine.

Andrews Antacid contains calcium and magnesium.

Andrews Liver Salts is a laxative which contains citric acid, magnesium sulphate and sodium bicarbonate, see Chapter 21.

Androcur ➤ cyproterone.

androgens (male sex hormones), see Chapter 38.

Andropatch ➤ testosterone. It is a self-adhesive patch containing testosterone dissolved in a gel. The testosterone is slowly released over twenty-four hours. It is used as HRT in males (testosterone replacement therapy) in conditions where there is a deficient or absent production of testosterone by the testes.

Anectine ➤ suxamethonium.

Anethaine cream ➤ tetracaine.

aneurine is vitamin B1, see Chapter 36.

Anexate for injection ➤ flumazenil.

Angettes tablets ➤ aspirin.

Angeze ➤ isosorbide mononitrate.

Angilol ➤ propranolol.

Angiopine and **Angiopine MR** ➤ nifedipine.

angiotensin-converting enzyme inhibitors ➤ ACE inhibitors.

angiotensin-II receptor antagonists ➤ angiotensin-II receptor blockers.

angiotensin-II receptor blockers are used to treat raised blood pressure. See Chapter 25.

Angiozem ➤ diltiazem.

Angitak Spray ➤ isosorbide dinitrate.

Angitil and **Angitil SR** ➤ diltiazem.

Anhydrol Forte ➤ aluminium chloride.

anise oil (anisi oil) is pale yellow oil from anise (aniseed). It is used as a flavouring agent and is included in cough remedies. It is also used to treat wind (carminative).

Anodesyn preparations contain ephedrine, lidocaine(lignocaine) and allantoin. It is used to treat piles.

Anquil ➤ benperidol.

Antabuse ➤ disulfiram.

antacids are discussed in Chapter 19. *Adverse effects:* Aluminium salts may constipate and magnesium salts may cause diarrhoea. This is why they are often mixed together in antacid preparations. Calcium carbonate (chalk) may constipate. Sodium bicarbonate, calcium carbonate and magnesium carbonate may cause wind and stomach discomfort because of the release of carbon dioxide. Excessive dosages of antacids, especially in patients with impaired kidney function may produce toxic effects from the absorbed minerals, calcium carbonate and aluminium hydroxide.

Interactions: Antacids reduce the absorption of fosinopril, diflunisal, some antibacterial drugs (azithromycin, cefpodoxime, ciprofloxacin, isoniazid, nitrofurantoin, norfloxacin, ofloxacin, pivampicillin, rifampicin, and most tetracyclines), gabepentin, phenytoin, itraconazole, ketoconazole, chloroquine, hydroxychloroquine, phenothiazines, biophosphonates, penicillamine and oral iron (absorption reduced by magnesium tricylicate). Sodium bicarbonate increases absorption of lithium. Antacids increase the excretion in the urine of aspirin and quinidine.

antazoline (antazoline phosphate, antazoline sulphate, Optilast, in Otrivine-Antistin) is an antihistamine ➤ antihistamines.

Antepsin ➤ sucralfate.

anthelmintic drugs are used to treat worm infections, e.g. threadworm, roundworm, tapeworm. They include piperazine, mebendazole, niclosamide and thiabendazole.

Anthisan cream ➤ mepyramine.

Anthisan Plus cream ➤ mepyramine, benzocaine.

Anthracyclines are cytotoxic antibiotics which are used in the treatment of cancer. See Chapter 51.

anthraquinone glycosides are obtained from plants and are used as stimulant laxatives. See Chapter 21. They include cascara, frangula and senna.

anti-allergic drugs, see Chapter 17.

anti-androgens, see p. 189.

anti-arrhythmic drugs, see Chapter 24.

anti-angina drugs, see Chapter 22.

anti-anxiety drugs, see Chapter 2.

antibacterial drugs, see Chapter 46.

antibacterial skin applications, see p. 243.

antibiotics, see Chapter 46.

anticholinesterases, see p. 35.

anticoagulants, see Chapter 28.

anticonvulsants ➤ anti-epileptic drugs.

anti-D (Rho) immunoglobulin (Partobulin) is used to prevent rhesus-negative mothers from forming antibodies to their unborn babies' rhesus positive red blood cells which may pass into the mother's bloodstream during childbirth or abortion. It should be injected within seventy-two hours of the birth or the abortion. The aim is to prevent the mother forming antibodies which would damage the red blood cells of any subsequent baby causing it to develop haemolytic anaemia.

antidepressants, see Chapter 4.

antidiabetic drugs, see Chapter 42.

antidiarrhoeal drugs, see Chapter 20.

antidiuretic hormone ➤ vasopressin.

antidiuretic hormone blockers: demeclocycline (a tetracycline antibiotic) blocks the effects of antidiuretic hormone on the kidneys and raises the blood sodium level.

anti-emetics (anti-vomiting drugs), see Chapter 18.

anti-epileptic drugs, see Chapter 15.

antifibrinolytic drugs, see p. 144.

antifungal drugs, see Chapter 47.

antifungal skin applications, see p. 243.

anti-giardial drugs are used to treat giardiasis. They include metronidazole, tinidazole and mepacrine.

anti-hepatitis B immunoglobulin ➤ hepatitis B immunoglubulin.

antihistamines are discussed in Chapter 17. *Adverse effects* of antihistamines that produce drowsiness (**sedative antihistamines**) include sweating, chills; dry mouth, nose and throat; allergic skin rashes, severe allergic reactions, sensitivity of the skin to sunlight; fall in blood pressure, headaches, palpitations, rapid beating of the heart, extra heart beats; blood disorders, including damage to circulating red blood cells; sedation, sleepiness, dizziness, disturbed coordination leading to clumsiness; fatigue, confusion, restlessness, excitement, nervousness, tremors, irritability, insomnia, feeling of well-being (euphoria), heaviness and weakness of the hands and feet, blurred vision, double vision, vertigo, noises in the ears, convulsions, stomach upset, nausea, vomiting, diarrhoea, constipation, frequency of passing urine, difficulty in passing urine, liver disorders, depression, hair loss, impotence, painful muscles, fall in blood pressure, early menstrual periods, thickening of the phlegm, tightness of the chest, wheezing. Children and elderly people are usually more sensitive to the adverse effects of antihistamines. *Precautions:* Antihistamines should not be used by patients who are allergic to them or in patients with porphyria (a hereditary disorder of metabolism). Because of their antimuscarinic effects they should be used with utmost caution in patients with epilepsy, glaucoma, narrowing of the outlet from the stomach (pyloric stenosis), enlarged prostate gland, or any obstruction to the outflow of urine from the bladder. They should be used with caution by patients who suffer from asthma, over-active thyroid gland, liver disease, or raised blood pressure. Antihistamines may produce excitement instead of drowsiness, particularly in young children; overdose in children may, very rarely, cause hallucinations, convulsions and death. Antihistamines reduce allergic reactions and therefore interfere with skin tests for allergies. They should be stopped at least one week before such a test. In elderly people adverse effects may be more frequent and severe, particularly dizziness, feeling faint, drowsiness, difficulty in passing urine, dry mouth, nose and throat, nightmares, excitement, nervousness, restlessness, constipation. They should be used with caution. Antihistamines may cause drowsiness and affect the ability to drive a motor vehicle or operate moving machinery. They increase the effects of alcohol. Antihistamines that produce little drowsiness (**non-sedative antihistamines**) do not easily enter the brain; therefore they produce less drowsiness and other effects on the brain, and fewer antimuscarinic effects (e.g. dry mouth, blurred vision, constipation). They include acrivastine (Semprex), astemizole (Hismanal), cetirizine (Zirtek) and loratadine (Clarityn) ➤ entries on each drug. *Interactions:* Alcohol, sleeping drugs, sedatives, anti-anxiety drugs (increased sedative effects with sedative antihistamines); astemizole and terfenadine increase the risk of disorders of heart rhythm with antiarrhythmic drugs, erythromycin and related drugs (macrolides), the antifungal drugs itraconazole, ketoconazole and possible other imidazoles. Triazoles block metabolism of astemizole and terfenadine producing risk of serious disorders of heart rhythm; antimuscarinic effects and sedative effects of antihistamines are increased by MAOIs and tricyclic antidepressants also increase risk of serious disorders of heart rhythm with astemizole and terfenadine; ketotifen with oral anti-diabetic drugs can cause depressed platelet count and bleeding; astemizole when used with terfenadine may cause serious disorders of heart rhythm; halofantrine, antipsychotic drugs, betablockers and diuretics increase the risk of serious disorders of heart rhythm from astemizole and terfenadine. Antihistamines increase the effects of antimuscarinic drugs.

antihistamine skin applications, see p. 247.

antihypertensive drugs (drugs used to lower a raised blood pressure), see Chapter 25.

anti-inflammatory pain-relievers (anti-inflammatory analgesics) ➤ nonsteroidal anti-inflammatory drugs (NSAID).

anti-itching skin applications and drugs by mouth, see p. 246.

anti-leprotic drugs are used to treat leprosy. They include dapsone, clofazimine and rifampicin.

anti-manic drugs include antipsychotic

drugs (see Chapter 3) and lithium (see Chapter 4).

antimetabolites are used as anti-cancer drugs. See Chapter 51.

anti-migraine drugs, see Chapter 34.

antimotility drugs are used to treat acute diarrhoea, see p. 104.

antimuscarinic drugs are discussed in Chapter 9. *Adverse effects* include dryness of the mouth and difficulty in swallowing, dryness of the nose and throat, blurred vision, flushing and dryness of the skin, slowing followed by quickening of the heart rate, palpitations, disorders of heart rhythm, desire to pass urine but with an inability to do so, constipation, giddiness, confusion, vomiting, unsteadiness, and pain in the chest due to acid reflux from the stomach up into the oesophagus. High doses cause rapid beating of the heart, high temperature, restlessness, confusion, excitement, mania, delirium, hallucinations, and a rash on the face and chest. *Precautions:* Antimuscarinic drugs should not be used in men with enlarged prostate glands, in people with paralysis of the intestine, narrowing of the outlet from the stomach (pyloric stenosis), acid reflux up the oesophagus, or closed-angle glaucoma. Do not use when the environmental temperature is high, particularly in children. They should be used with caution in elderly men and in anyone with a fever, a rapid pulse rate (e.g. due to overworking of the thyroid gland), or heart failure, or during heart surgery. Reduced bronchial secretions caused by antimuscarinic drugs may make it difficult for people with bronchitis to cough up phlegm, which may accumulate and cause a blockage. People with Down's syndrome are sensitive to the effects of antimuscarinic drugs, whereas albinos appear to be resistant. Harmful effects may be more frequent and severe in the elderly; therefore use with caution. *Interactions:* Alcohol (sedative effects of hyoscine increased), nefopam, disopyramide, tricyclic antidepressants, MAOIs, ketoconazole (delayed absorption), anti-

histamines, phenothiazines, cisapride (antagonizes effects on gut), domperidone and metoclopramide (effects on gut antagonized by propantheline), amantadine, nitrates (dry mouth affects dissolving of nitrate tablets), mexiletine (atropine delays absorption).

antineoplastic drugs, see Chapter 51 on anti-cancer drugs.

anti-oestrogens, see p. 198.

antiperspirants, see p. 248.

antiplatelet drugs, see p. 143.

Antipressan ➤ atenolol.

antiprotozoal drugs include antimalarials, amoebicides, triclomonacides, antigiardial drugs, Leishmaniacides, drugs used to treat toxoplasmosis and drugs used to treat pneumocystis pneumonia (PCP).

antipruritic drugs (anti-itching drugs), see p. 246.

antipsychotic drugs are discussed in Chapter 3. *Adverse effects:* Not all of the following harmful effects have been reported with every antipsychotic drug, but they have been reported with one or more of them, and should be borne in mind whenever these drugs are used: dry mouth, blocked nose, blurred vision, headache, nausea, constipation, drowsiness, apathy, pallor, depression, hypothermia, agitation, painful erection of the penis (priapism), inhibition of ejaculation, difficulty in passing urine, flare-up of mental illness, fall in blood pressure (sometimes fatal), disorders of heart rhythm, abnormalities on electrical tracings of the heart (ECG) and blood disorders. Rarely, there may be liver damage including jaundice, production of milk from the breasts and enlargement of the breasts in both men and women, irregular menstrual periods, sensitivity of the skin to sunlight, allergic reactions, skin rashes, asthma, mild fever, increased appetite and increased weight. Prolonged use of high doses may cause opacities in the lens and cornea of the eyes, and purplish pigmentation of the skin, cornea, conjunctiva and retina. Injections may cause pain and local swelling (nodules), a sudden fall in blood pressure and rapid beating of the heart. A particular problem with antipsychotic drugs is the occasional development of abnormal involuntary movements. These include restless movements (inability to keep still, jitteriness, agitation, difficulty in sleeping), dystonias (spasm of muscles, producing abnormal involuntary movements of the face, neck, back, arms and hands, difficulty in swallowing, protrusion of the tongue and abnormal movements of the eyes), parkinsonism (mask-like face, drooling, shaking (tremors), rigid muscles and shuffling walk), tardive dyskinesia (rhythmical involuntary movements of the face, tongue, mouth and jaw – e.g. puffing of the cheeks, puckering of the mouth, protrusion of the tongue, chewing movements – and sometimes these movements are associated with abnormal involuntary movements of the arms and legs). Very rarely, patients treated with an antipsychotic drug may develop a high body temperature (hyperthermia), varying levels of unconsciousness, rigidity of the muscles, paleness (pallor), rapid beating of the heart, changes in blood pressure and sweating, and the individual may be incontinent of urine. This group of signs and symptoms is known as the 'neuroleptic malignant syndrome', and it may be fatal. It has been reported with chlorpromazine, flupenthixol and haloperidol. Any antipsychotic drug being taken should be stopped at the earliest sign of this syndrome. There is no effective treatment and it usually lasts for about five–ten days after stopping the drug. The symptoms may be very prolonged if the patient has been receiving a depot injection of an antipsychotic drug. *Precautions:* Antipsychotic drugs should not be used in patients who are comatose, who are severely depressed or have impaired bone-marrow function. They should be used with caution in patients with diseases of the circulation affecting the heart or brain, chronic chest diseases, tumour of the sympathetic nervous system (phaeochromocytoma), epilepsy, parkinsonism, a history of jaundice, acute infections, underactive thyroid, myasthenia gravis (muscle weakness due to neuromuscular abnormality), enlarged prostate glands; and in pregnancy, in breastfeeding mothers, in the elderly in very hot or cold weather. Initial sedation may affect the ability to drive a motor vehicle or operate moving machinery, and they increase the effects of alcohol. Regular eye examinations should be carried out and the skin should be examined for patches of pigmentation. Withdrawal after long-term use should be gradual. *Interactions:* Chlorpromazine and possibly other phenothiazines cause a severe fall in blood pressure on standing up after sitting or lying (postural hypotension) when given with an ACE inhibitor; blood pressure lowering effects increased with general anaesthetics; increased sedative and blood pressure lowering effects with morphine and related drugs (opiates); antacids reduce the absorption of phenothiazines; rifampicin reduces blood levels of haloperidol; blood levels and antimuscarinic effects of tricyclic antidepressants increased by phenothiazines; fluoextine increases blood level of haloperidol; oxypertine causes excitation and raised blood pressure with MAOIs; antipsychotics reduce effectiveness of anti-epileptic drugs; carbamazepine reduces blood levels of haloperidol; phenytoin speeds up metabolism of clozapine; increased risk of serious disorders of heart rhythm with astemizole and terfenadine; increases blood pressure lowering effects of anti-blood pressure drugs; increased movement disorders with methyldopa and metrosine; increased risk of serious disorders of heart rhythm with halofantrine; antimuscarinic drugs increase antimuscarinic effects produced by phenothiazines but blood levels of phenothiazines are reduced; increased sedative effects with sleeping drugs, sedatives and anti-anxiety drugs; phenothiazines increase the risk of disorders of heart rhythm with sotalol; propranolol increases blood levels of chlorpromazine; increased blood pressure lowering effects with calcium-channel blockers; diuretics increase risk of disorders of heart rhythm with pimozide; increased risk of movement disorders with metoclopramide; blocks blood prolactin lowering effects and anti-parkinsonism effects of bromocriptine; antagonizes effects of apomorphine, levodopa, lysuride and pergolide used to treat parkinsonism; increased risk of movement disorders and nerve damage when lithium is given with clozapine, haloperidol or phenothiazines; vasoconstrictor effects of sympathomimetic drugs blocked by antipsychotic drugs. The dose of antipsychotic drug by mouth should be increased slowly, no more than once a week. Patients should have their pulse rate, blood pressure, temperature, fluid intake and electrocardiograph monitored at regular intervals. High doses should only be used for a short period of time (no more than three months). When patient is stabilized the daily dose can be given in just one dose. *Depot injections* should be used with caution and the patient carefully monitored for movement disorders and mood changes. When transferring from oral to depot injections the dose by mouth should be gradually reduced and then stopped. Do not use depot injections in children, or in patients who are confused or in coma caused by drugs that depress brain function. Do not use in patients with parkinsonism or who are intolerant to antipsychotic drugs.

antipyretic drugs (drugs used to bring down a raised temperature) include aspirin, paracetamol and ibuprofen.

antiseptics, see p. 244.

antispasmodics are used to relax the smooth muscles of the stomach and intestine and relieve colicky pains. They include antimuscarinic drugs (e.g. atropine, dicyclomine, hyoscine butylbromide, poldine and propantheline) and other drugs such as alverine, mebeverine and peppermint oil.

antithyroid drugs (thyroid blockers), see Chapter 43.

antituberculous drugs, see Chapter 50.

antitussives (anti-cough drugs), see Chapter 11.

antiviral drugs, see Chapter 48.

Anturan ➤ sulphinpyrazone.

Anugesic-HC preparations contain hydrocortisone (a corticosteroid), and soothing antiseptic/astringent drugs (zinc oxide, bismuth oxide, benzyl benzoate and Peru balsam) and a local anaesthetic (pramocaine). They are used to treat haemorrhoids and itching anus (pruritus ani). *Adverse effects and Precautions* see Chapter 37 on corticosteroids. Avoid prolonged use. Use with caution in pregnancy. Do not use if a viral, fungal or tuberculous infection is present.

Anusol preparations contain soothing, antiseptic and astringent drugs (bismuth gallate, bismuth oxide, Peru balsam and zinc oxide). They are used to treat haemorrhoids and itching anus.

Anusol HC preparations contain hydrocortisone (a corticosteroid), and soothing, antiseptic and astringent drugs (zinc oxide, bismuth oxide, benzyl benzoate and Peru balsam) and a local anaesthetic (pramocaine). They are used to treat haemorrhoids and itching anus. *Adverse effects and Precautions* see Chapter 37 on corticosteroids. Avoid prolonged use. Use with caution in pregnancy. Do not use if a viral, fungal or tuberculous infection is present.

anxiolytics ➤ anti-anxiety drugs.

anxiolytic-sedatives ➤ anti-anxiety drugs.

APD ➤ disodium pamidronate.

APO-go ➤ apomorphine.

apomorphine (apomorphine hydrochloride, APO-go, Britaject, Uprima) is a derivative of morphine with structural similarities to dopamine ➤ dopamine. It blocks the effects of dopamine and is used to treat parkinsonism not responding to levodopa and other dopaminergic drugs. See Chapter 16. *Adverse effects:* Nausea, vomiting (which may be persistent), movement disorders (dyskinesia), unsteadiness on the feet and falls, confusion, drowsiness, euphoria, depression, restlessness, tremor, fall in blood pressure on standing up after sitting or lying down (postural hypertension), light-headedness, personality changes, blood disorders and depressed breathing. *Precautions:* Do not use in patients whose brain or breathing are depressed, who are over-sensitive to opiates, who are demented or have some neuro-psychiatric disorder. Do not use in pregnancy or in breastfeeding mothers, or in patients on levodopa who develop severe movement disorders and psychiatric problems. Use with caution in patients who tend to easily develop nausea and vomiting, who have heart or circulatory disorders, a disorder of thyroid, pituitary or adrenal function, impaired kidney function or a history of a postural hypertension. Use with caution in the elderly. Monitor blood count, kidney function, heart function and blood pressure at regular intervals. When given with levodopa a test for haemolytic anaemia should be carried out at start of treatment and then every six months. *Interactions:* May counteract the effects of anti-psychotic drugs.

APP is an antacid preparation which contains homatropine, aluminium, bismuth, calcium and magnesium.

appetite stimulants contain aromatic bitters such as alkaline gentian mixture and acid gentian mixture.

appetite suppressants (slimming drugs), see Chapter 8.

apraclonidine (Iopidine) is a derivative of clonidine. It is an alpha$_2$ stimulant (see p. 64) used as eye drops to control the pressure in the eye after laser surgery for glaucoma. It may also be used as eye drops to provide additional short-term treatment (not more than one month) for chronic glaucoma. *Adverse effects* include dry mouth, disturbances of taste, redness of the eye (hyperaemia), retraction of eye lids and blanching of conjunctiva. May be absorbed and affect the blood pressure and circulation. *Precautions:* Do not use in patients

with severe heart or circulatory disorders including raised blood pressure and history of fainting (vasovagal attacks). Do not wear soft contact lenses. Use with utmost caution in pregnancy, in breastfeeding mothers and in patients with impaired liver or kidney function. Monitor eye pressure regularly. Drowsiness may affect ability to drive. Allergy may occur to the preservative (preservative-free preparations are available). *Interactions:* Systemic sympathomimetics, tricyclic antidepressants, anti-blood pressure drugs, digoxin and related drugs (cardiac glycosides), clonidine.

Apresoline ➤ hydralazine.

Aprinox ➤ bendrofluazide.

aprotinin (Tisseel-Kit, Trasylol) is an anti-fibrinolytic drug (see Chapter 28). It is used to treat life-threatening haemorrhage due to open heart surgery and to a high level of plasmin in the blood, which may occur during surgical removal of some malignant cancers, in certain types of leukaemia and in thrombolytic treatment (thrombus-dissolving treatment, see Chapter 28). *Adverse effects:* It may cause thrombophlebitis (inflammation in the vein) at the site of injection and, occasionally, allergic reactions.

Aprovel ➤ irbesartan.

Apsin ➤ penicillin V.

Apstil ➤ stilboestrol.

Aquadrate emollient cream contains urea ➤ urea.

Aquasept solution ➤ triclosan.

aqueous cream contains emulsifying wax, white soft paraffin, liquid paraffin, phenoxyethanol and water, see emollients, p. 236.

Aqueous iodine solution (Lugol's solution) is made up of iodine, potassium iodide and water. It is used to treat patients with an overactive thyroid gland (thyrotoxicosis) prior to surgery. *Adverse effects* include cold-like symptoms, headache, watery eyes, pain in the salivary glands, laryngitis, bronchitis and rashes. Prolonged use can cause depression, insomnia, impotence and goitre in infants of mothers taking iodine. *Precautions:* Do not use if breastfeeding. Use with caution in pregnancy and in children, avoid long-term use.

arachis oil is peanut oil.

Aramine ➤ metaraminol.

Aranesp ➤ darbepoetin.

Arava ➤ leflunomide.

Aredia ➤ pamidronate.

argipressin is a synthetic vasopressin included in Pitressin injections ➤ vasopressin.

Aricept ➤ donepezil.

Aridil ➤ co-amilofruse.

Arilvax is a live yellow fever vaccine.

Arimidex ➤ anastrozole.

arnica flower (extract of) is used as a local application to bruises and sprains. It is of doubtful value. It is used in homoeopathic medicine.

Aromasin ➤ exemestane.

Arpicolin ➤ procyclidine.

Arret ➤ loperamide.

Artelac ➤ hypromellose.

Arthrofen ➤ ibuprofen.

Arthrosin ➤ naproxen.

Arthrotec preparations contain the nonsteroidal anti-inflammatory drug diclofenac sodium and misoprostol, a synthetic prostaglandin which is added to prevent diclofenac from causing ulceration of the stomach and bowel. *Adverse effects and Precautions* ➤ nonsteroidal anti-inflammatory drugs, misoprostol.

Arthroxen ➤ naproxen.

articaine (Septanest) is a local anaesthetic for dental use.

artificial saliva provides relief from a dry mouth. The composition is similar to natural saliva. Preparations include Luborant (for any disorders causing a dry mouth) and Salivace and Glandosane which are used to treat dry mouth caused by radiotherapy or sicca syndrome. Salivix pastilles stimulate production of saliva. See entry on each drug.

artificial tears are used to lubricate the eye for patients suffering from dry eye due to a lack of natural tears.

Arythmol ➤ propafenone.

5-ASA ➤ 5-aminosalicylic acid.

Asacol ➤ mesalazine.

Asasantin Retard is a combined preparation of aspirin and dipyridamole. It is an antiplatelet preparation (see p. 143) used after a heart attack to prevent further attacks ➤ aspirin, dipyridamole.

Ascabiol emulsion ➤ benzyl benzoate.

ascaricides are drugs used to treat common roundworm infections. They include mebendazole, pyrantel and piperazine.

ascorbic acid is vitamin C, see Chapter 36.

Asendis ➤ amoxapine.

Aserbine contains malic acid, benzoic acid, salicylic acid and propylene glycol. The solution and cream are used to remove dead tissue around wounds, pressure sores and varicose ulcers. Avoid contact with eyes.

Asilone suspension contains activated dimethicone, aluminium hydroxide gel and light magnesium oxide. Tablets contain activated dimethicone, aluminium hydroxide and sorbitol ➤ antacids, activated dimethicone.

Askit is a painkiller which contains aspirin and aloxiprin ➤ aspirin.

Asmabec ➤ beclometasone.

Asmasal ➤ salbutamol.

Asmaven ➤ salbutamol.

Aspav pain-relieving tablets contain

aspirin and papaveretum ➤ aspirin, papaveretum.

aspirin is an anti-inflammatory painreliever, see Chapter 31. It also stops platelets from sticking together and is used to prevent re-thrombosis in someone who has had a coronary thrombosis, and to prevent strokes (see p. 143). Available anti-platelet aspirin preparations include Angettes, Caprin and Nu-Seals. *Adverse effects:* Aspirin may produce irritation of the lining of the stomach and may cause nausea, vomiting, pain and bleeding from the stomach. This is not altered by changes in formulation and it may be unaccompanied by indigestion symptoms. Some people are allergic to aspirin and develop skin rashes and symptoms like those seen in hayfever or asthma. It increases blood-clotting time and it may produce swelling of the throat (angioneurotic oedema) and nettle-rash (urticaria). High doses produce dizziness, noises in the ear (tinnitus), sweating, nausea, vomiting, mental confusion and over-breathing. *Precautions:* Aspirin should not be taken by anyone with a stomach upset or disorder such as peptic ulcer. It should never be taken on an empty stomach or with alcohol. Always take aspirin with a long drink. Aspirin should not be given to children under twelve years because of the risk of producing brain and liver damage (see warning on p. 159). It should not be given to people who suffer from haemophilia or to people on anticoagulant drugs, or who suffer from asthma. It should be used with caution in patients with impaired kidney or liver function, who wheeze or who have suffered an allergic reaction to aspirin or an NSAID. Use with caution in pregnancy and do not use at end of pregnancy because of its effects on blood clotting. Do not use in breastfeeding mothers. *Interactions:* NSAID, anticoagulants, phenytoin, valproate, corticosteroids, methotrexate, spironolactone, diuretics, acetazolamide, metoclopramide, mifepristone, probenecid, sulphinpyrazone. Aspirin may increase the effects of drugs used to treat diabetes, it increases the toxicity of sulphonamides, and it decreases the effects of some drugs used to treat gout. It should be given with caution to the elderly and debilitated who may be anaemic and to people who are anaemic or suffer from impaired kidney function.

Aspro Clear ➤ aspirin.

astringents, see p. 247.

astringent skin applications, see p. 247.

AT 10 ➤ dihydrotachysterol.

Atarax ➤ hydroxyzine.

Atenix ➤ atenolol.

AtenixCo ➤ cotenidone.

atenolol (Antipressan, Atenix, in Beta-adalat, in Kalten, in Tenben, in Tenif, in Tenoret 50, in Tenoretic, Tenormin, Totamol) is a selective beta-receptor blocking drug used to treat hypertension, angina and disorders of heart rhythm ➤ beta-blockers. Also ➤ co-amylozide, cotenidone.

Ativan ➤ lorazepam.

atorvastatin (Lipitor) is used to lower blood cholesterol levels. See Chapter 26. *Adverse effects* include stomach and bowel upsets, headache, pain in muscles, weakness, insomnia. Like all statins it may damage muscles producing muscle pain (➤ simvastatin). *Precautions:* Do not use in patients with active liver disease or persistent raised liver enzymes. Use with caution in patients with a history of alcohol abuse or liver disease, in pregnancy (ensure adequate contraception) or while breastfeeding.

atosiban (Tractocile) is an oxytocin receptor blocker used to delay imminent preterm birth in women with regular uterine contractions and normal foetal heart rate. *Adverse effects* include nausea, headache, dizziness, vomiting, hot flushes, rapid heart beat, low blood pressure, high blood sugar levels, injection site reactions. *Precautions:* Do not use where gestation is less than twenty-four weeks or more than thirty-three weeks, in premature rupture of membranes after thirty weeks, in any condition of mother or foetus in which continuation of pregnancy is hazardous. Use with caution where the placenta is in the wrong position, or in patients with kidney or liver damage.

atovaquone (in Malarone, Wellvone) is an antiprotozoal drug used to treat mild to moderate *Pneumocystis carinii* pneumonia (PCP) in patients intolerant to cotrimoxazole. PCP is a common cause of pneumonia in AIDS patients. *Adverse effects* include headache, nausea, vomiting, diarrhoea, rash, fever, insomnia, anaemia, low blood sodium and disturbances of liver function tests. *Precautions:* Use with caution in patients suffering from diarrhoea or who have difficulty taking it with food. Do not use in breastfeeding mothers and use with caution in pregnancy, in patients with impaired kidney or liver function and in the elderly. *Interactions:* Metoclopramide, rifampicin, zidovudine.

atracurium (atracurium besylate, Tracrium) is a non-depolarizing muscle relaxant, see p. 42. It is used to relax muscles during surgery. It is inactivated by thiopentone and other alkaline solutions. It may cause a transient red rash on the chest and neck.

atropine (atropine methonitrate; atropine sulphate, in Isopto atropine, in Lomotil, Minims atropine, in Tropergen) is an antimuscarinic drug ➤ antimuscarinic drugs.

Atrovent preparations contain ipratropium ➤ ipratropium.

Audax ear drops contain choline salicylate and glycerol. They are used to relieve pain in the ear. Do not use if ear drum is perforated.

Audicort ear drops contain neomycin, undecenoic acid and triamcinolone. They are used to treat otitis externa. *Adverse effects and Precautions:* see entry on each drug. Do not use if ear drum is perforated. Use with caution in pregnancy and breastfeeding

mothers. May cause local irritation and superinfection.

Augmentin and **Augmentin-Duo** contain clavulanic acid (a betalactamase inhibitor) and amoxicillin (broad-spectrum penicillin). *Adverse effects and Precautions:* ➤ penicillins, clavulanic acid.

auranofin (Ridaura) is an orally active gold compound used to treat rheumatoid arthritis, see Chapter 32. Its effectiveness is comparable to gold injections. *Adverse effects:* Diarrhoea, nausea, abdominal pain, ulceration of the intestine, rashes, itching, soreness and ulcers in mouth (stomatitis), conjunctivitis, disturbances of taste, loss of hair, blood disorders, kidney damage, scarring of the lungs (fibrosis). *Precautions:* Do not use in patients with a history of ulceration of the intestine, fibrosis of the lungs, severe dermatitis, bone-marrow damage or severe blood disorders. Do not use in patients with severe kidney or liver disease, or in pregnancy or when breastfeeding. Use with caution in patients with impaired kidney or liver function, inflammatory bowel disease, skin rashes or history of bone-marrow disease. Blood counts and urine tests for protein should be carried out before treatment and at one-monthly intervals during treatment. Women of childbearing potential should, where appropriate, use contraceptives during and for six months after treatment.

Aureocort ointment contains triamcinolone (a corticosteroid) and chlortetracycline (a tetracycline antibiotic). *Adverse effects and Precautions:* see corticosteroid skin applications p. 241 and ➤ tetracyclines.

Aureomycin preparations ➤ chlortetracycline.

aurothiomalate ➤ sodium aurothiomalate.

Avandia ➤ rosiglitazone.

Avaxim injection is an inactivated hepatitis A vaccine.

Aveeno emollient skin applications contain colloidal oatmeal.

Avloclor ➤ chloroquine.

Avoca caustic pencil contains silver nitrate which is used for the removal of warts from the hands and feet.

Avomine ➤ promethazine.

Avonex ➤ interferon beta.

Axid ➤ nizatidine.

Axsain cream ➤ capsaicin.

Azactam ➤ aztreonam.

Azamune ➤ azathioprine.

azapropazone (Rheumox) is a non-steroidal anti-inflammatory drug (NSAID) used to treat rheumatic disorders (see Chapter 32) and also gout (see Chapter 33). *Adverse effects* include fluid retention, ulceration and bleeding from the stomach, sensitivity of the skin to sunlight, skin rashes and, rarely, inflammation of the lungs (alveolitis) and blood disorders. *Precautions:* Do not use in patients with peptic ulcers, ulcerative colitis (chronic diarrhoeal disorder), blood disorders, or severe impairment of kidney or liver function. Do not use in pregnancy or in breastfeeding mothers. Use with caution in patients with a past history of peptic ulcers, in the elderly, patients with impaired kidney function, raised blood pressure, heart failure or asthma. Do not use in patients with porphyria (a hereditary disorder of metabolism), or who are allergic to aspirin or NSAIDs. Avoid exposure to sunlight. *Interactions:* Anti-coagulants, anti-diabetic drugs, cimetidine, digoxin, lithium, methotrexate, phenytoin.

azatadine (azatadine maleate, in Congesteze, Optimine) is an antihistamine ➤ antihistamines.

azathioprine (Azamune, Immunoprin, Imuran, Oprisine) is an immunosuppressive drug (see p. 88). It is used to treat rheumatoid arthritis (see Chapter 32) and ulcerative colitis (chronic diarrhoeal dis-

order), and to prevent transplant rejection. *Adverse effects:* It may damage the bone marrow (producing blood disorders), and cause liver damage, stomach and bowel upsets, muscle wasting, skin rashes, hair loss, generally feeling unwell, dizziness, vomiting, fever, rigors, muscle aches and pains, joint pains, nausea, liver damage, jaundice, pancreatitis, disorders of heart rhythm and fall in blood pressure (if so stop immediately) and allergic reactions. *Precautions:* It should not be used in pregnancy or in patients with impaired liver function or blocked bile duct. Use with caution in patients with impaired kidney function or infection. Monitor carefully and carry out regular blood tests. Avoid undue exposure to the sun. Do not use in patients allergic to it or to mercaptopurine. *Interactions:* Allopurinol, anti-cancer drugs, muscle relaxants. *For other Adverse effects and Precautions* ➤ mercaptopurine.

azelaic acid is an antibacterial drug used in Skinoren cream to treat acne. *Adverse effects* include local irritation of the skin and rarely sensitivity of the skin to the sun's rays. *Precautions:* Avoid contact with eyes and use with caution in pregnancy and when breastfeeding.

azelastine (Rhinolast aqueous nasal spray) is a sedative antihistamine used to treat nasal allergy, e.g. hayfever. See Chapter 17. *Adverse effects* include irritation of the lining of the nose and disturbance of taste. *Precautions:* Use with caution in pregnancy and in breastfeeding mothers ➤ antihistamines. It is also used in eye drops (Optilast) to treat inflammation caused by hayfever.

azidothymidine (AZT) ➤ zidovudine.

azithromycin (Zithromax) is a macrolider-elated antibiotic (see p. 268) which is chemically related to erythromycin but has greater activity against a broader range of bacteria including some gram-negative bacteria. It is used to treat infections of the upper and lower respiratory tract, skin and soft tissues, otitis media and uncomplicated genital infections due to *Chlamydia trachomatis*. *Adverse effects* include stomach and bowel upsets, allergic reactions, sensitivity of the skin to sunlight, jaundice, impaired hearing, effects on the liver (a rise in liver enzymes) and a fall in white blood cells. *For other adverse effects* ➤ erythromycin. *Precautions:* It should not be used in patients with liver disease and it should be used with special caution in patients with moderate or severe kidney or liver impairment, in pregnancy and breastfeeding mothers. *Interactions:* ergot derivatives, antacids, cyclosporin, digoxin, warfarin.

Azopt ➤ brinzolamide.

AZT (azidothymidine) ➤ zidovudine.

aztreonam (Azactam) is a monobactam antibiotic (see p. 268) with a wide spectrum of activity against bacteria, including beta-lactamase producing bacteria. *Adverse effects* include skin rashes, itching, diarrhoea, nausea and/or vomiting, mouth ulcers, altered taste, cramps in the stomach, and pain and inflammation at the site of injection. It may very rarely produce a thrush infection, weakness, confusion, dizziness, sweating, headache, muscle aches, fever, sneezing and a blocked nose, a fall in blood pressure, breast tenderness, bad breath, blood disorders, liver damage, jaundice, and allergic reactions. *Precautions:* It should be used with caution in patients allergic to penicillins and cephalosporins. Breastfeeding mothers should not breastfeed during treatment. It should not be used in pregnancy or in patients allergic to the drug. It should be used with caution in patients with impaired kidney or liver function. *Interactions:* Anticoagulants.

Baby Meltus is a cough medicine for children which contains dilute acetic acid.

bacampicillin (bacampicillin hydrochloride, Ambaxin) is a broad spectrum penicillin ➤ penicillins and see Chapter 46.

bacillus Calmette-Guérin (BCG) (Onco-Tice) is used for the treatment of cancer of the bladder. *Adverse effects* include cystitis, pain or burning on urination, frequent need to urinate, blood in the urine, generally feeling unwell, fever, flu-like syndrome, systemic BCG infection. *Precautions:* Do not use in patients with active tuberculosis or after physical trauma caused while inserting a catheter.

bacitracin is an aminoglycoside antibiotic (see p. 243) used mainly in topical applications. It is present in Cicatrin and Polyfax. It should not be used on large areas of damaged skin because it may be absorbed and damage the nerves of hearing and balance ➤ aminoglycoside antibiotics.

baclofen (Baclospas, Balgipen, Lioresal) is a derivative of GABA, a neurotransmitter in the brain which damps down the effects of stimulant neurotransmitters. It is used as a skeletal muscle relaxant (see p. 42) in patients who suffer from strokes, cerebral palsy, meningitis, multiple sclerosis or spinal injury. *Adverse effects* include drowsiness, nausea, vomiting, confusion, fatigue and excitability. Rarely, it may cause dizziness, a fall in blood pressure, euphoria, hallucinations, depression, pins and needles, slurred speech, tremors, floppy muscles, insomnia, visual disturbances, rashes, allergic reactions, itching, noises in the ears (tinnitus), difficulty passing urine and impairment of liver function. *Precautions:* It should not be used in patients with peptic ulcers. Use with caution in patients with epilepsy, serious mental illness, diabetes, strokes or impaired heart, kidney or liver function. Use with caution in the elderly, in pregnancy and in breastfeeding mothers. Tests of kidney and liver function should be carried out before and at regular intervals during treatment. The drug should be stopped gradually to reduce the risk of withdrawal effects which may affect the ability to drive. *Interactions:* Anti blood pressure drugs, lithium, fentanyl, morphine, tricyclic antidepressants, levodopa, carbidopa, sedatives and sleeping drugs.

Baclospas ➤ baclofen.

Bactroban nasal ointment ➤ mupirocin.

Bactroban ointment ➤ mupirocin.

BAL (British Anti-Lewisite) ➤ dimercaprol.

Balgifen ➤ baclofen.

Balmosa cream is used to treat rheumatism. It contains menthol, camphor, methysalicylate and capsicum ➤ rubifacients.

balsalazide (Colazide) is a salicylate used to treat mild to moderate ulcerative colitis (chronic diarrhoeal disorder) and to prevent its recurrence. See Chapter 20. *Adverse effects* include headache, abdominal pain, stomach and bowel upsets, gallstones. *Precautions:* Do not use in patients with an allergy to salicylates, severe liver or kidney damage, in pregnancy or while breastfeeding. Use with caution in patients with asthma, bleeding disorders, ulcer, mild liver or kidney damage. Any unexplained bleeding, bruising, sore throat or generally feeling unwell should be reported.

Bambec ➤ bambuterol.

bambuterol (bambuterol hydrochloride, Bambec) is converted into terbutaline in the body. Terbutaline is a selective beta$_2$ stimulant used as a bronchodilator to treat asthma. See Chapter 14. *Adverse effects and Precautions* are similar to those listed under salbutamol.

Bansor ➤ cetrimide.

Baratol ➤ indoramin.

barbiturate drugs are derived from barbituric acid. They were previously widely used as sleeping drugs (see Chapter 1) and as sedatives (see Chapter 2). Some are used as anti-epileptic drugs (see Chapter 15). They depress brain function and are capable of producing drug dependence (see p. xxvii). *Adverse effects and Precautions* of barbiturates are listed under phenobarbitone ➤ phenobarbitone. Rapidly acting barbiturates are used intravenously as general anaesthetics. They include thiopentone sodium and methohexitone sodium.

barrier preparations usually contain water-repellent substances such as dimethicone and other silicones. They are applied as creams and ointments which also contain an oily base of white, soft paraffin or lanolin. They protect the skin from irritants, pressure, urine and faeces.

Barum antacid ➤ calcium salts.

basiliximab (Simulect) is an antibody that is used with ciclosporin and corticosteroids to prevent rejection in patients who have had a kidney transplant. *Adverse effects* include allergic reactions. *Precautions:* Do not use in patients who are pregnant or breastfeeding.

bath additives usually contain an oily base (e.g. liquid paraffin, soya oil). They are used to soften the skin to treat eczema, itching and other dry skin disorders. They may have other drugs added such as antiseptics. Coal tar derivatives are frequently used as bath additives in preparations used to treat chronic eczema and psoriasis.

Baxan ➤ cefadroxil.

BCG ➤ bacillus Calmette-Guérin.

BCG vaccine, see p. 300.

becaplermin (Regranex) is a growth hormone derived from human blood that is used to treat ulcers of the skin caused by nerve damage due to poorly controlled diabetes. *Adverse effects* include infection, ulcers, redness of the skin and pain. Rarely blisters and swelling may occur. *Precautions:* Do not use in patients with cancer at or near the ulcer site, in pregnancy or while breastfeeding. Use with caution in patients with osteomyelitis (inflammation of the marrow and hard tissue of the bone), diseases of the arteries or infected ulcers.

Beclazone ➤ beclometasone.

Beclo-aqua ➤ beclometasone.

Becloforte preparations ➤ beclometasone.

beclomethasone ➤ beclometasone.

beclometasone (beclomethasone) is a potent corticosteroid (see Chapter 37). It is used by inhalation to treat asthma (Aerobec,

Asmabec, Beclazone, Becloforte, Becodisks, Becotide, Filair, Pulvinal Beclometasone, Qvar, in Ventide preparations) see Chapter 14. It is also used to treat hayfever and perennial rhinitis (Beclo-aqua, Beconase, Care Hayfever Relief, Nasobec, Zonivent) see p. 87; and to treat skin disorders (e.g. eczema) (Propaderm) see p. 241. *Adverse effects:* see Chapter 37 on corticosteroids. *By inhalation:* May cause hoarseness and thrush of the mouth and throat. *To the skin:* see p. 241. *To the nose:* May cause irritation, nose bleeds, taste and smell disturbances. *Precautions:* Use *inhalations* with caution in patients with active or dormant tuberculosis of the lungs, in breastfeeding mothers and in pregnancy, use *nose sprays* with caution in patients with untreated infections of the nose, in pregnancy and in breastfeeding mothers. For precautions on *skin applications*, see p. 241.

Becodisks ➤ beclometasone.

Beconase preparations ➤ beclometasone.

Becotide ➤ beclometasone.

Bedranol SR ➤ propranolol.

Beechams All in One contains paracetamol, guaiphenesin and phenylephrine; **Beechams Cold and Flu**, **Beechams Flu-Plus Berry Fruits**, **Beechams Flu-Plus Powder**, **Beechams Hot Blackcurrant**, **Beechams Hot Lemon** and **Beechams Hot Lemon and Honey** contain paracetamol and phenylephrine; **Beechams Flu-Plus caplets** contain paracetamol, caffeine and phenylephrine; **Beechams Lemon tablets** contain aspirin; **Beechams Powders** and **Beechams Powders capsules** contain aspirin and caffeine; **Beechams Throat Plus** contains benzalkonium and hexylresorcinol ➤ individual entry for each drug.

Begrivac is an inactivated flu vaccine.

belladonna (belladonna extract: in Bellocarb, belladonna liquid extract) is an antimuscarinic drug ➤ antimuscarinic drugs.

Benadryl Allergy Relief ➤ acrivastine.

bendrofluazide ➤ bendroflumethiazide.

bendroflumethiazide(bendrofluazide) (Aprinox, in Centyl K, in Corgaretic, in Inderetic, in Inderex, Berkozide, Neo-Bendromax, Neo-Naclex, in Neo-Naclex-K, in Prestim, in Tenben) is a thiazide diuretic ➤ thiazide diuretics.

Bene-Fix ➤ Factor IX.

Benerva ➤ thiamine.

Benoral ➤ benorilate.

benorylate ➤ benorilate.

benorilate (benorylate, Benoral) is a paracetamol-aspirin ester. It is used as a mild pain-reliever, see Chapter 31. It is also used to treat muscle and joint pains, rheumatoid arthritis, arthritis and fever. *Adverse effects:* It may produce nausea, gastric upset, drowsiness, dizziness, noises in the ears and skin rashes. *Precautions:* Do not use in children under twelve years of age ➤ aspirin. It should be used with caution in patients with impaired kidney or liver function. It should not be given to patients who are sensitive to aspirin ➤ aspirin, paracetamol.

benoxinate ➤ oxybuprocaine.

benperidol (Anquil) is an antipsychotic drug used to control deviant and antisocial sexual behaviour. *Adverse effects and Precautions:* Do not use in patients with parkinsonism symptoms. Use with caution in pregnancy and breastfeeding mothers. Regular blood counts and tests of liver function should be carried out in patients on long-term treatment ➤ antipsychotic drugs.

benserazide (in Madopar) blocks the enzyme that breaks down levodopa to dopamine in the body (dopa-decarboxylase). It is combined with levodopa in co-beneldopa (Madopar) to treat parkinsonism (see Chapter 16). *Adverse effects and Precautions:* ➤ levodopa.

bentonite is a soapy clay used to make suspensions semi-solid. Bentonite powder is used by mouth to adsorb corrosive poisons in cases of accidental poisoning.

Benylin Chesty Cough and **Benylin Children's Night Cough** contain diphenhydramine; **Benylin Children's Chesty Cough** and **Benylin Non-Drowsy for Chesty Cough** contain guaifenesin; **Benylin Children's Cough and Colds** contains dextromethorphan and triprolidine; **Benylin Children's Dry Cough** contains pholcodine; **Benylin Cough and Congestion** contains dextromethorphan, diphenhydramine and pseudoephedrine; **Benylin Day and Night, night tablets** contain paracetamol and diphenhydramine; **Benylin Day and Night, day tablets** contain paracetamol and phenylpropanolamine; **Benylin Dry Cough** contains dextromethorphan and diphenhydramine; **Benylin 4 Flu** contains paracetamol, diphenhydramine and pseudoephrine; **Benylin Non-Drowsy for Dry Cough** contains dextromethorphan; **Benylin With Codeine** contains codeine and diphenhydramine ➤ individual entry for each drug.

benzalkonium (benzalkonium chloride) is used as an antiseptic and disinfectant. It has effects like cetrimide. It is used as a preservative in eye drops and is present in some skin applications and throat lozenges.

Benzamycin gel contains erythromycin and benzoyl peroxide. It is used to treat acne. See p. 250. *Adverse effects and Precautions* ➤ erythromycin and benzoyl peroxide. Use with caution in pregnancy and breastfeeding mothers. May produce mild irritation. Avoid contact with eyes and lining of the mouth and nose.

benzatropine (benztropine mesylate, Cogentin) is an antimuscarinic drug used to treat parkinsonism and drug-induced parkinsonism (see Chapter 16). *Adverse effects and Precautions* ➤ trihexyphenidyl (benzhexol). High doses may cause confusion, agitation and skin rashes. Rather than causing stimulation like trihexyphenidyl(benzhexol) it can produce sedation. Also see entry on antimuscarinic drugs.

benzhexol ➤ trihexyphenidyl(benzhexol).

benzocaine (ethyl aminobenzoate) is a local anaesthetic. It is available in lozenges (in Merocaine, in Tyrozets) to relieve pain in the mouth and throat and also in local applications (AAA Spray). May rarely cause allergic reactions. Avoid prolonged use. Use with caution in pregnancy and breastfeeding mothers.

benzodiazepines are discussed in Chapters 1 and 2. *Adverse effects* include drowsiness, light-headedness, fatigue, loss of control over voluntary movements (ataxia), confusion, constipation, depression, double vision or blurred vision, headache, low blood pressure, loss of memory, incontinence of urine or difficulty in passing urine, jaundice due to liver damage, changes in libido (sexual drive), altered salivation, nausea, skin rashes, slurred speech, forgetfulness, tremor, vertigo, blood disorders, depression of breathing and, with injectable preparations, thrombophlebitis (inflammation of the vein) at the site of injection. Paradoxical reactions may occur, which include talkativeness, excitement, anxiety, hallucinations, aggressiveness, antisocial behaviour, spasm of muscles, rage and disturbed sleep. Adjustment of dose up or down may make symptoms worse. In a susceptible person, benzodiazepines can trigger underlying depression and the patient may become suicidal. Harmful effects of benzodiazapines may be more frequent and severe in the elderly; the smallest dose possible should be used for the shortest duration of time. Elderly people run the risk of developing incoordination of movement, drowsiness and agitation. They may wet themselves in the night or have difficulty in passing urine, and they may become confused and forgetful. Benzodiazepines cause tolerance and dependence; see Chapter 2. *Precautions:* Do not use in patients who have difficulty breathing or who sometimes stop breathing for a moment in their sleep (sleep apnoea syndrome), with severe liver disease, myasthenia gravis (muscle weakness due to neuromuscular abnormality), phobic or obsessional states, drug or alcohol abuse, chronic psychosis, or as sole treatment for depression or anxiety depression. They should be used with caution in patients with chest disorders, porphyria (a hereditary disorder of metabolism), impaired kidney or liver function, in the elderly, in pregnancy, labour and in breastfeeding mothers. They may impair the ability to drive a motor vehicle or operate machinery, and they increase the effects of alcohol. See risks of withdrawal, p. 9. *Interactions:* Increased sedative effects with alcohol, general anaesthetics, opiate pain-relievers, antidepressants, antipsychotics, antihistamines, lofexidine, baclofen and nabilone; erythromycin blocks metabolism of midazolam and increases its blood level; isoniazid blocks metabolism of diazepam; rifampicin increases metabolism of diazepam; fluvoxamine increases blood levels of some benzodiazepines; anti-epileptics increase metabolism and reduce the effectiveness of clonazepam; phenytoin blood levels are affected by diazepam and possible other benzodiazepines; itraconazole, ketoconazole and fluconazole increase blood levels of midazolam and cause prolonged sedative effects; blood pressure lowering effects of anti-blood pressure drugs increased by benzodiazepines; increased sedation with alpha-blockers; diltiazem and verapamil block metabolism of midazolam and increase its blood level; disulfarim blocks metabolism of benzodiazepines and increases their sedative effects; benzodiazepines occasionally antagonize effects of levodopa; cimetidine blocks metabolism of benzodiazepines and increases their blood levels; and omeprazole blocks metabolism of diazepam and increases its blood level.

benzoic acid has antibacterial and antifungal properties. It is used as a preservative in medicines, foods and cosmetics. Salts of benzoic acid are more soluble in water than benzoic acid and are used as astringents. They are added to some oral preparations as a preservative. They can become oxidized and cause discoloration. Benzoic acid is applied to the skin to treat fungal infections of the skin, usually as a compound ointment

with salicylic acid. It may also be used to clean ulcers and remove dead skin from wounds (in Aserbine). *Adverse effects:* It may cause allergic reactions and large doses by mouth may irritate the stomach. It may irritate the skin, eyes and mucous membranes (e.g. lining of the mouth).

benzoic acid ointment compound contains salicylic acid and benzoic acid. It is also known as Whitfield's ointment and is used to treat patches of fungal infections affecting the skin. *Adverse effects and Precautions* ➤ benzoic acid, salicylic acid.

benzoin (sumatra benzoin, in Frador) is from a balsam resin. It is used in inhalations to treat catarrh and in skin applications as an antiseptic and protective agent.

benzoin tincture compound (Friar's Balsam) contains Sumatra benzoin, storax, aloes and alcohol. Its vapours are inhaled by adding it to boiling water and breathing in the steam. It is used in this way to relieve a blocked nose caused by a cold.

benzophenone (oxybenzone) is a sunscreen agent. Rarely, it may cause contact dermatitis and make the skin sensitive.

benzoyl peroxide (in Acnecide, in Benzamycin, in Brevoxyl, Panoxyl, in Quinoderm, in Quinoped) is an antiseptic (see p. 244) and is also used for removing dead skin (see p. 247). It is mainly used in skin applications to treat acne. *Adverse effects* include skin irritation and peeling. Occasionally it may cause contact dermatitis. *Precautions:* Avoid contact with eyes and lining of nose and mouth. May bleach fabrics. Do not use to treat acne rosacea.

benzthiazide (in Dytide) is a thiazide diuretic ➤ thiazide diuretics.

benztropine ➤ benzatropine.

benzydamine (benzydamine hydrochloride) is an anti-inflammatory drug. It is present in Difflam Oral Rinse solution and Difflam Spray to treat a sore mouth and throat. It may cause numbness of the mouth. It is also present in Difflam cream used to treat muscle and joint pains.

benzyl alcohol is used as an antiseptic, and as a weak local anaesthetic, in various skin applications.

benzyl benzoate (Ascabiol) is used to treat scabies (see p. 261) *Adverse effects:* It may irritate the skin and occasionally cause skin rashes. It can produce a burning sensation when applied to the genitals or areas of skin that have scratch marks. *Precautions:* Do not use in children. Avoid contact with eyes and mucous membranes (e.g. lining of the nose, mouth, vagina). Do not use on broken or infected skin. Use with utmost caution in pregnancy and breastfeeding mothers.

benzylpenicillin (penicillin G) ➤ crystapen.

beractant (Survanta) is used to treat respiratory distress syndrome (hyaline membrane disease) in premature babies. *Adverse effects:* Bleeding into the lungs. *Precautions:* Continuous monitoring required to avoid too much oxygen entering the bloodstream.

bergamot oil is obtained from the fresh peel of fruit of *Citrus bergamia (Rutaceae)*. It is used in perfumes and especially in hair preparations. It is also used in suntan applications, see p. 237. There is doubt that concentrations below 1% have any tanning effect and there is evidence that psoralens produce skin cancer in mice.

Berkozide ➤ bendrofluazide.

Beta-Adalat contains atenolol (a selective beta-blocker) and nifedipine, (a calcium-channel blocker). It is used to treat angina (see Chapter 22) and raised blood pressure (see Chapter 25) ➤ beta blockers, nifedipine.

beta-adrenoceptor blocking drugs ➤ beta-blockers.

beta-adrenoceptor stimulants are used as bronchodilators to treat asthma. See Chapter 14. They also relax the muscle of the uterus and are used in selected patients to stop uncomplicated premature labour in women who are twenty-four to thirty-three weeks pregnant. They delay delivery for forty-eight hours so that the mother can have appropriate treatment to improve her health. The beta-adrenoceptor stimulants used for this purpose include ritodrine, salbutamol and terbutaline. *Adverse effects and precautions* ➤ salbutamol.

beta-blockers are discussed in Chapter 22. *Adverse effects* include slowing of the heart rate, fall in blood pressure, heart block, numbness and pins and needles in the hands and feet, coldness of the fingers and toes, mental depression, tiredness on exertion, insomnia, nightmares, drowsiness, confusion, weariness, fatigue, visual disturbances and hallucinations. Beta-blockers may occasionally produce a reversible depression associated with disorientation in time and place, short-term memory loss, clouded thinking and emotional changes. They may cause nausea, vomiting, stomach upsets, bowel changes, allergic reactions, wheezing; and, very rarely, blood disorders, loss of hair, a psoriasis-like skin rash and dry eyes. *Precautions:* Beta-blockers should not be used in patients with untreated heart failure, serious heart block, serious disorders of the circulation or untreated phaeochromocytoma (tumour of the sympathetic nervous system). They should be used with caution in late pregnancy and in breastfeeding mothers, and they should be withdrawn gradually in patients with angina. *Note:* Beta-blockers that are most soluble in water are less likely to enter the brain and cause disturbed sleep and nightmares etc. than the ones that are soluble in fat (lipid soluble). They include atenolol, celiprolol, nadolol and sotalol. However, because they are water soluble they are excreted by the kidneys and they may accumulate in the blood of patients whose kidney function is impaired, lower doses should therefore be given in such patients. Some beta-blockers may be able to stimulate as well as block beta-receptors (e.g. oxprenolol, pindolol and acebutolol), they therefore cause less slowing of the heart and coldness of the fingers and toes. However, remember that all beta-blockers slow the heart rate and may precipitate heart failure in those patients prone to develop heart failure. Sotalol may cause life-threatening disorders of heart rhythm. Beta-blockers affect blood sugar control and must be used with caution in diabetics. They may also mask some of the early symptoms of hypoglycaemia (see p. 222). Selective blockers should be used in diabetics but avoided if patient has frequent attacks of hypoglycaemia. *Non-selective beta-blockers should definitely not be used in patients with asthma or obstructive airways disease and selective ones should preferably not be used.* Beta-blockers should be used with caution in patients with heart failure controlled by digoxin and diuretics, impaired kidney or liver function, thyrotoxic crisis and general anaesthesia (withdraw before elective surgery). *Interactions:* verapamil, Class I anti-arrhythmic drugs, anti-diabetic drugs, general anaesthetics, reserpine, anti-blood pressure drugs, ergot drugs, cimetidine, sedatives, sleeping drugs, sympathomimetics, indomethacin. *Note:* Sotalol should no longer be used to treat angina, raised blood pressure or over-active thyroid. It must *only* be used to treat certain disorders of heart rhythm. To change over from sotalol to another drug the dose of sotalol should be gradually reduced over one–two weeks, the patient carefully monitored (particularly those with coronary heart disease), and at the same time replacement treatment should be started.

Betacap scalp applications ➤ betamethasone.

Beta-Cardone ➤ sotalol.

Betadine ➤ povidone iodine.

Betaferon ➤ interferon.

Betagan eye drops ➤ levobunolol.

betahistine (betahistine dihydrochoride, Serc) is used to treat vertigo, noises in the ears (tinnitus) and hearing loss associated with Ménière's disease (for symptoms see p. 93). It produces effects similar to his-tamine. *Adverse effects* include flushing, tingling, chilliness, nausea, vomiting, diarrhoea, headache, rashes, itching, rapid beating of the heart, and shivering. *Precautions:* It should be given with caution to patients with asthma or peptic ulcer. It should not be given to children and should not be given with antihistamines. Use with caution in pregnancy and breastfeeding mothers.

betaine hydrochloride when dissolved in water forms hydrochloric acid. It is used to treat patients unable to produce hydrochloric acid in their stomachs. It is present in Kloref and Kloref-S used as potassium supplements.

beta-lactam antibiotics have a similar basic chemical structure – a lactam ring. They include the penicillins, cephalosporins and cephalomycins. See Chapter 46.

betalactamases are enzymes produced by certain bacteria that disrupt the chemical structure of beta-lactam antibiotics (the beta-lactam ring) thus making the antibiotics inactive, see p. 266.

Betaloc ➤ metoprolol.

Betaloc-SA ➤ metoprolol.

betamethasone is a corticosteroid, see Chapter 37 on corticosteroids. For administration by mouth betamethasone (Betnelan) and betamethasone sodium phosphate (Betnesol) are used. The latter is also used in injections of betamethasone and in eye, nose and ear drops (Betnesol and Vista-Methasone). Betamethasone valerate (Betnovate and Diprosone) is used in skin applications and as Betacap and Betta-mousse to treat the scalp. *Adverse effects and Precautions*, see Chapter 37. For scalp and skin applications ➤ corticosteroid skin applications, p. 241. *Ear drops* should not be used if patient has a perforated ear drum. Use with caution in pregnancy and avoid prolonged use in infants. *Eye drops* may cause a rise in pressure inside the eye, thinning of the cornea, cataract and fungal infections. Do not use if a viral, fungal, tuberculous or purulent bacterial infection is present. Avoid prolonged use in pregnancy and infants. Do not wear contact lenses. *Nose drops:* Use with caution in pregnancy. Do not use to treat viral, fungal or tuberculous infections.

Beta-Prograne ➤ propranolol.

betaxolol (Betoptic, Kerlone) is a selective beta-receptor blocker drug. It is used to treat raised blood pressure. See Chapter 25. *Adverse effects and Precautions:* ➤ beta-blockers. It is also used in Betoptic to treat glaucoma (see p. 63).

bethanechol (Myotonine) is a parasympathomimetic (muscarinic) drug (see Chapter 9) that produces effects similar to those produced by acetylcholine (➤ acetylcholine). However, the enzyme cholinesterase breaks it down less quickly than it breaks down acetylcholine, and therefore bethanechol acts for a longer time. It is used to treat reflux oesophagitis, absent movements of the small intestine and stomach, and retention of urine. *Adverse effects* include nausea, vomiting, abdominal cramps, frequent passing of urine, blurred vision and sweating (➤ acetylcholine). *Precautions:* Do not use in patients with asthma, over-active thyroid, obstruction to the outflow from the bladder, obstruction of the bowel, severe slow heart rate, low blood pressure, recent heart attack, epilepsy, parkinsonism, or in pregnancy.

Betim ➤ timolol.

Betnelan preparations ➤ betamethasone.

Betnesol preparations ➤ betamethasone.

Betnesol N ear, eye and nose applications contain betamethosone (a corticosteroid) and neomycin (an antibiotic). *Adverse effects and Precautions* ➤ betamethasone, neomycin. *Ear drops* may cause allergic reactions. Do not use in patients with a perforated ear drum or in patients with a viral, fungal, tuberculous or purulent bacterial infection. Avoid prolonged use in pregnancy. *Eye drops* may cause thinning of the cornea, cataract, rise in pressure inside

the eye, and allergic reactions. Do not use if patient has glaucoma, corneal ulcers, or a viral, fungal, tuberculous or purulent bacterial infection. Do not wear soft contact lenses. *Nose drops* may cause allergic reactions. Do not use in patients with a viral, fungal, tuberculous or bacterial infection. Avoid prolonged use in pregnancy.

Betnovate preparations ➤ betamethasone.

Betnovate C preparations contain betamethasone (a corticosteroid) and clioquinol (an antibacterial/antifungal). *Adverse effects and Precautions* ➤ betamethasone, clioquinol.

Betnovate N preparations contain betamethasone (a corticosteroid) with neomycin (an antibiotic). *Adverse effects and Precautions* ➤ betamethasone, neomycin.

Betoptic eye drops contain the beta-blocker drug betaxolol. They are used to treat open-angle glaucoma. *Adverse effects* include transient discomfort in the eye, and rarely redness, decreased sensitivity and damage to the cornea. *Precautions:* Do not use in patients with a slow heart rate or serious heart failure. Do not wear soft contact lenses. Use with caution in patients with asthma or obstructive airways disease, diabetes, over-working of the thyroid gland and with general anaesthetics. For general adverse effects and precautions of beta-blockers ➤ beta-blockers.

Bettamousse scalp application ➤ betamethasone.

bezafibrate (Bezagen, Bezalip, Bezalip-Mono, Zimbacol) is a fibrate drug used to reduce high blood cholesterol and fat levels (see Chapter 26). *Adverse effects:* Stomach and bowel upsets, itching, nettle-rash, impotence, headache, dizziness, vertigo, fatigue, hair loss and muscle damage, producing weakness and pain. *Precautions:* It should not be used in patients with severe liver or kidney impairment, gall-bladder disease, in pregnancy or in breastfeeding mothers. The risk of muscle damage is increased in patients with impaired kidney function and possibly underworking of the thyroid gland (see fibrates for warnings on muscle damage). Use of ciclosporin or a statin drug at the same time may increase the risks. *Interactions:* Anticoagulants, anti-diabetic drugs, MAOIs.

Bezagen ➤ bezafibrate.

Bezalip ➤ bezafibrate.

Bezalip-Mono tablets ➤ bezafibrate.

bicalutamide (Casodex) is an anti-androgen drug (see p. 189) used to treat cancer of the prostate gland. *Adverse effects* include hot flushes, weakness, itching, tenderness and swelling of the breasts and sleepiness. Rarely it may cause jaundice, liver damage, blood disorders and disorders of the heart (e.g. angina, heart failure, disorders of rhythm), stomach and bowel upsets, insomnia, dizziness, loss of appetite, dry mouth, decreased libido, impotence, sweating, rashes, breathlessness, changes in weight, fluid retention (causing swelling of the ankles), chest and abdominal pains and raised blood sugar level. Adverse effects are more likely in the elderly. *Precautions:* Use with caution in patients with impaired liver function. Liver function tests at start and during treatment should be considered. *Interactions:* Cimetidine, ketoconazole, oral anticoagulants.

BiCNU ➤ carmustine.

biguanides are a group of drugs used to treat diabetes. See Chapter 42. The only available drug in this group is *metformin*.

bile acid sequestrants, see Chapter 26.

BiNovum is a biphasic oral contraceptive. See p. 217.

Bioral gel ➤ carbenoxolone.

Biorphen ➤ orphenadrine.

biperiden (Akineton) is an antimuscarinic drug used to treat parkinsonism. See Chapter 16. *Adverse effects and Precautions* are similar to those listed under benzhexol ➤ benzhexol. Biperiden may also cause

drowsiness and a fall in blood pressure following injection. Also see antimuscarinic drugs.

biphosphonates (bisphosphonates) are used to treat bone disorders. Disodium etidronate is used to treat Paget's disease of bone. It slows down the increased rate of bone turnover that occurs in this disease. Sodium pamidronate and sodium clodronate are used to treat raised blood calcium levels in patients suffering from secondary bone cancer. Disodium etidronate is available with calcium carbonate (Didronel PMO tablets) to treat osteoporosis of the spine.

Birley is an antacid containing salts of aluminium and magnesium ➤ antacids.

bisacodyl (Dulcolax) is a stimulant laxative. See Chapter 21. It may cause abdominal cramps and suppositories may produce local rectal irritation.

Bismag is an antacid containing magnesium and sodium bicarbonate ➤ antacids.

Bisma-Rex is an antacid containing salts of bismuth, calcium and magnesium, and peppermint oil ➤ antacids.

bismuth chelate ➤ bismuth salts.

bismuth citrate ➤ De-Noltab.

bismuth salts by injection were once widely used to treat syphilis. Soluble bismuth salts are harmful because they can be absorbed into the body and they should not be used. Insoluble salts are included in some antacid mixtures and as protectives in some skin preparations, as an astringent in haemorrhoidal preparations, in suppositories and in diarrhoea mixture. Bismuth salts by mouth have occasionally caused brain damage and bone and joint disorders after prolonged use as antacids. They can make the faeces black.

bismuth subgallate ➤ bismuth salts.

bismuth subnitrate ➤ bismuth salts.

Bisodol preparations are antacids. **Bisodol**

Heartburn Relief tablets contain alginic acid, calcium and sodium bicarbonate; **Bisodol Indigestion powder and tablets** contain calcium, magnesium and sodium bicarbonate; **Bisodol Wind Relief tablets** contain calcium, magnesium, sodium bicarbonate and activated dimethicone ➤ antacids and individual entry for each constituent drug.

bisoprolol (Cardicor, Emcor, Monocor, in Monozide) is a selective beta-blocker used to treat angina (see Chapter 22) and raised blood pressure (see Chapter 25) ➤ beta-blockers.

bisphosphonates ➤ biphosphonates.

Blemix ➤ minocycline.

Bleo-Kyowa ➤ bleomycin.

bleomycin (Bleo-Kyowa) is used as an anti-cancer drug (see Chapter 51). It interferes with DNA synthesis in cancer cells inhibiting growth and cell division. *Adverse effects* include fever, anorexia, tiredness, nausea, and pain and inflammation at the injection site. Occasionally it may produce delayed effects on the lungs (interstitial pneumonia and fibrosis). Previous radiotherapy to the chest is an aggravating factor. The majority of patients may develop hard (indurated) red, tender swellings on their finger tips, ridging of the nails, lesions of the skin and mucous membranes, blisters (bullae) over pressure points and loss of hair. These usually disappear once the drug is stopped. *Precautions:* It should not be used in pregnant or breastfeeding women nor in patients with chest infections. Patients on treatment should have a chest X-ray weekly. The dose should be reduced in patients with impaired kidney function.

Bocasan antiseptic produces similar effects to hydrogen peroxide. It contains sodium perborate monohydrate and sodium hydrogen tartrate. It is used as a mouth rinse to treat gingivitis and stomatitis. Do not use in patients with impaired kidney function.

Bonefos ➤ sodium clodronate.

Bonjela gel is used to treat ulcers of the tongue and mouth. It contains choline salicylate to relieve pain, cetalkonium chloride (antiseptic), menthol, alcohol and glycerin ➤ choline salicylate, cetalkonium.

Bonjela pastilles contain aminoacridine (aminacrine) and lidocaine(lignocaine) ➤ individual entry for each drug.

Boots Avert ➤ aciclovir.

Boots Catarrh Cough Syrup contains codeine and creosote; **Boots Children's 1 year Plus Night Time Cough Syrup** contains diphenhydramine and pholcodeine; **Boots Cold and Flu Relief tablets** contain paracetamol, caffeine and phenylephrine; **Boots Cold Relief Hot Blackcurrant** and **Boots Cold Relief Hot Lemon** contain paracetamol ➤ individual entry for each drug.

Boots Children's 3 months Plus Pain Relief contains paracetamol; **Boots Children's 6 years Plus Fever and Pain Relief** contains ibuprofen ➤ individual entry for each drug.

Boots Compound Laxative Syrup of Figs is a laxative containing figs and senna ➤ senna.

Boots Diareze capsules ➤ loperamide.

Boots Double Action Indigestion is an antacid containing aluminium, magnesium and activated dimethicone; **Boots Heartburn Relief** is an antacid containing alginic acid, calcium and sodium bicarbonate; **Boots Indigestion tablets and mixture** are antacids containing calcium, magnesium and sodium bicarbonate ➤ individual entry for each drug.

Boots Senna tablets ➤ senna.

borotanic complex is a constituent of Phytex paint, which is used to treat fungus infections of the skin and nails. The borax part of the complex has antibacterial and antifungal properties and the tannic acid part acts as an astringent.

Botox ➤ botulinum toxin.

botulinum A toxin-haemagglutinin ➤ botulinum toxin.

botulinum toxin (botulinum A toxin-haemagglutinin complex, Botox, Dysport, NeuroBloc) is used to treat blepharospasm (spasm of the eyelids) and one-sided facial spasm. It is given by injection into the muscles of the upper and lower eyelids and upper facial area. *Adverse effects* include irritation and watering of the eye, drooping of the upper eyelid, double vision and other disturbances of vision, bruising and swelling of eyelids and paralysis of muscles around the eye. *Precautions:* Do not use in pregnancy or in breastfeeding mothers or in disorders such as myasthenis gravis (muscle weakness due to neuromuscular abnormality). It is also used to treat spasmodic torticollis (spasms in the neck which restrict movement).

bowel cleaning solutions are used before surgery, endoscopy and radiological examinations of the bowel to ensure that it is completely empty of solid contents. *Adverse effects* include nausea, bloating, abdominal cramps, vomiting, irritation of the anus, nettle-rash and allergic reactions. *Precautions:* Do not use in patients with an obstruction of the stomach or intestine, perforated bowel, distension or inflammation of the bowel or if weight is less than 20 kg. Use with caution in pregnancy, in patients with ulcerative colitis (chronic diarrhoeal disorder), diabetes, oesophageal reflux, impaired gag reflex and in patients who are unconscious or semiconscious. Medicines taken by mouth within one hour of taking a bowel-cleansing solution may not be absorbed and may not therefore be effective. *Preparations* include Klean-Prep.

Bradosol lozenges ➤ benzalkonium.

Bradosol Plus lozenges contain the antiseptic domiphen and the local anaesthetic lidocaine(lignocaine) ➤ domiphen, lidocaine(lignocaine).

Brasivol contains aluminium oxide in large particles and is used as an abrasive together with a cleansing base to treat acne.

bretylium (bretylium tosylate, Min-I-Jet Bretylium Tosylate) is used to treat disorders of heart rhythm (see Chapter 24). *Adverse effects:* These include fall in blood pressure and nausea, and initial worsening of the disorder. Damage to tissue at site of injection may occur. *Precautions:* Do not use in patients with phaeochromocytoma (tumour of the sympathetic nervous system). Use with caution to treat disorders of heart rhythm caused by digoxin and do not give noradrenaline(norepinephrine) or other sympathomimetic drugs.

Brevibloc ➤ esmolol.

Brevinor is a combined oral contraceptive. See p. 216.

Brevoxyl ➤ benzyl peroxide.

Brexidol ➤ piroxicam.

Bricanyl preparations ➤ terbutaline.

brimonidine (Alphagan) eye drops are used where beta-blockers are ineffective or unsuitable, or in addition to beta-blockers, in the treatment of open-angle glaucoma or high blood pressure in the eye. See Chapter 13. *Adverse effects* include swelling in the eye and distension of blood vessels in the eye (ocular hyperaemia), stinging, itching, allergic reactions, dry mouth, headache, fatigue and drowsiness. *Precautions:* Use with caution in patients with severe heart disease, depression, insufficient blood supply to the brain or heart, Raynaud's syndrome (for symptoms see p. 137), low blood pressure on standing, blood clots, kidney or liver damage, in pregnancy or while breastfeeding. Do not wear soft contact lenses.

brinzolamide (Azopt) eye drops are used where beta-blockers are ineffective or unsuitable, or in addition to beta-blockers, in the treatment of open-angle glaucoma or high blood pressure in the eye. See Chapter 13. *Adverse effects* include disturbed vision, pain in the eye, distension of blood vessels in the eye (ocular hyperaemia), unpleasant taste in the mouth, headache. *Precautions:* Do not use in patients with liver or severe kidney damage, disorders of blood chemistry, history of allergy to sulphonomides or while breastfeeding. Use with caution in patients with pseudoexfoliative, pigmentary or narrow angle glaucoma, diabetes, eye disorders, those who wear contact lenses or in pregnancy.

Britaject ➤ apomorphine.

BritLofex ➤ lofexidine.

Broflex ➤ benzhexol.

Brolene eye drops and ointment contain the antiseptic dibromopropamidine isethionate. The eye drops also contain benzalkonium as a preservative. Not suitable for people wearing contact lenses. Of little value in treating infections of the eye except for *acanthamoeba keratitis* (neomycin may be used as additional treatment).

bromazepam (Lexotan) is a benzodiazepine used to treat anxiety ➤ benzodiazepines.

bromocriptine (bromocriptine mesylate, Parlodel) stimulates dopaminergic receptors. It is used in the treatment of parkinsonism (see Chapter 16). It stops production of the milk-producing hormone prolactin, and it is used to prevent lactation after childbirth. It blocks the release of growth hormone by the pituitary gland and may be used to treat acromegaly due to overworking of the pituitary gland. It is also used to treat certain types of infertility in women, cyclical benign breast disease and severe mastalgia (painful breasts). *Adverse effects* include nausea, vomiting, dizziness, fall in blood pressure on standing up after sitting or lying down (may produce dizziness and lightheadedness), dryness of the mouth, leg cramps, headaches, nasal congestion, constipation, and sedation. Rarely, high doses may cause hallucinations, confusion, involuntary movements (dyskinesia), coldness of the fingers and toes and a scarring disorder in the abdomen (retroperitoneal fibrosis) – stop immediately if this occurs.

Precautions: Use with caution in patients with a history of psychotic illness and in patients with severe heart disease. It stimulates ovulation, therefore regular gynaecological examinations should be carried out and mechanical forms of contraception should be used if patient wishes to avoid conception. There is a risk of peptic ulcers in patients being treated for acromegaly. Do not use in patients with toxaemia of pregnancy, in women with raised blood pressure following childbirth or in patients allergic to it or to ergot drugs. *Interactions:* Alcohol, erythromycin, metoclopramide, anti-blood pressure drugs.

brompheniramine (Dimotane, in Dimotane Plus, in Dimotapp) is an antihistamine drug ➤ antihistamines.

Bronalin Decongestant Elixir contains pseudoephedrine; **Bronalin Dry Cough** contains dextromethorphen and pseudoephedrine; **Bronalin Expectorant** contains ammonium chloride and diphenhydramine; **Bronalin Junior Linctus** contains diphenhydramine ➤ individual entry for each drug.

Bronchodil ➤ reproterol.

bronchodilators are used to treat asthma. See Chapter 14.

Brufen preparations ➤ ibuprofen.

Buccastem buccal tablets contain the phenothiazine drug prochlorperazine which dissolves to a gel when sucked between the upper lip and the gums. They are used to treat nausea, vomiting, motion sickness, migraine and vertigo. See Chapter 18 ➤ prochlorperazine.

buclizine (buclizine hydrochloride, in the anti-migraine preparation Migraleve) is a sedative antihistamine drug ➤ antihistamines.

Budenofalk ➤ budesonide.

budesonide is a potent corticosteriod used in a nasal spray to treat hayfever (seasonal rhinitis and perennial allergic rhinitis), vasomotor rhinitis and nasal polyps (Rhinocort Aqua) see p. 87; by inhalation to treat asthma (Pulmicort, Symbicort) see Chapter 14; in ointments and creams to treat skin disorders such as eczema and psoriasis (Preferid) see p. 241; and used orally in chronic diarrhoea (Budenofalk, Entocort). *Adverse effects:* When applied up the nose it may cause sneezing, stinging, dryness, slight nose bleeds and rarely raised pressure in the eyes, and by inhalation from an aerosol it may cause hoarseness, thrush of the mouth and throat, rarely skin rashes and paradoxical wheezing. Inhalations should not be used in patients with active tuberculosis. Nasal sprays and inhalations should be used with caution in pregnancy and in patients with viral or fungal infections. *For general adverse effects and Precautions* see Chapter 37 on corticosteriods; for adverse effects on the skin, see corticosteroid skin applications p. 241.

bumetanide (Burinex, in Burinex A, in Burinex K) is a loop diuretic (see Chapter 29). *Adverse effects and Precautions* are similar to those listed under frusemide. Bumetanide may also cause rashes, muscle pains and thrombocytopenia.

bupivacaine (bupivacaine hydrochloride, in Marcain, in Marcain with adrenaline) is a local anaesthetic with effects and uses similar to lidocaine(lignocaine), but it works for a longer duration. Overdose may cause a fall in blood pressure, muscle twitching, depression of respiration and convulsions. Its use in childbirth may cause the baby's heart to slow down. It should be used with caution in patients with liver or heart disorders, or who are elderly and/or debilitated.

buprenorphine (Subutex, Temgesic) is an opiate pain-reliever, see Chapter 30. *Adverse effects* include drowsiness, nausea, dizziness and sweating. *Precautions:* Use with caution in patients with narcotic dependence, impaired liver function, chronic chest disorders, in pregnancy and labour. For other potential adverse effects ➤ morphine.

Interactions: MAOIs, sedatives, sleeping drugs.

Bupropion ➤ amfebutamine.

Burinex ➤ bumetanide.

Burinex A contains bumetanide (a loop diuretic) and amiloride (a potassium-sparing diuretic). See Chapter 29. *Adverse effects and Precautions* ➤ bumetanide and amiloride.

Burinex K tablets contain bumetanide (a loop diuretic) and potassium chloride (a potassium supplement). See Chapter 29. *Adverse effects and Precautions* ➤ bumetanide, potassium supplements.

BurnEze aerosol ➤ benzocaine.

Buscopan ➤ hyoscine butylbromide.

buserelin is a gonadotrophin-releasing hormone analogue which is used in Superfact nasal spray to treat cancer of the prostate dependent on male sex hormones for growth. It initially stimulates the pituitary to produce luteinising hormone (LH), but the end result is that it prevents the release of LH, causing a reduction in testosterone production by the testes. *Adverse effects* include hot flushes, irritation of the nose when nasal spray is used, loss of libido, depression, headache, dizziness, nausea, vomiting, diarrhoea, nettle-rash, and rarely swelling of the breasts. *Precautions:* Do not use if testicles have been removed, or in tumours which are not sensitive to male hormones. *Interactions:* Nasal decongestants. Buserelin is also used in Supercur nasal spray to treat endometriosis (it initially stimulates and then blocks the production of hormones by the ovaries and stops the periods). It is also used as part of infertility treatment – it desensitizes the pituitary gland prior to stimulating ovulation with gonadotrophins. *Adverse effects* include hot flushes, dry vagina, loss of libido, emotional upsets, breast tenderness and changes in size, headache, migraine, nausea, depression, abdominal pain, fatigue, weight changes, nervousness, dizziness, drowsiness, back pain, muscle pain, acne, nettle-rash, itching, constipation, vomiting, sleep disturbances, blurred vision, growth of body hair, pins and needles in the hands and feet, ovarian cysts and irritation of the nose. *Precautions:* Do not use in pregnancy and use a mechanical means of contraception if sexually active. Do not use in breast-feeding mothers, in women with undiagnosed vaginal bleeding or who are suffering from hormone dependent cancer. Use with utmost caution in patients at risk of developing osteoporosis and in patients who are depressed.

Buspar tablets ➤ buspirone.

buspirone (Buspar) is an anti-anxiety drug (see Chapter 2) not related to the benzodiazepines. *Adverse effects:* Dizziness, headache, nervousness, light-headedness, excitement and nausea. Rarely, rapid beating of the heart, chest pain, drowsiness, confusion, dry mouth, fatigue and sweating. *Precautions:* Do not use in patients with epilepsy or who suffer from severe kidney or liver impairment. Do not use in pregnancy or when breastfeeding. Use with caution in patients with impaired kidney or liver function. In order to avoid withdrawal symptoms, reduce benzodiazepines slowly over several weeks before starting a patient on buspirone. *Interactions:* MAOIs, alcohol may impair driving skills.

busulfan (Myleran) is an anti-cancer drug. See Chapter 51. *Adverse effects:* It may cause blood disorders producing haemorrhages and bone-marrow damage (this may be irreversible and come on several months after treatment is stopped). Loss of periods (amenorrhoea) may start up to six months after the drug is stopped. It may cause deep pigmentation of the skin and scarring of the lungs. *Precautions:* It should not be used in pregnancy or by breastfeeding mothers. Frequent blood counts should be carried out during and after treatment.

busulphan ➤ busulfan.

Butacote ➤ phenylbutazone.

butobarbital (butobarbitone, Soneryl) is an intermediate-acting barbiturate. It is used as a sleeping drug, (see Chapter 1). *Adverse effects and Precautions* ➤ phenobarbitone sodium.

butobarbitone ➤ butobarbital.

butoxyethyl nicotinate is used for removing dead skin (a keratolytic), see p. 247. It is present in Actinac lotion, used to treat acne.

Buttercup Honey and Lemon contains ipecacuanha and menthol; **Buttercup Syrup Traditional** contains squill ➤ individual entry for each drug.

butyrophenones are a group of antipsychotic drugs. See Chapter 3. The group includes benperidol, droperidol and haloperidol. They are likely to produce more pronounced movement disorders than other antipsychotics. Benperidol is used to treat deviant antisocial sexual behaviour. As well as being used as antipsychotics, droperidol and haloperidol are also used to treat nausea and vomiting produced by anti-cancer drugs. See Chapter 18. Haloperidol is also used to treat motor tics.

Cabaser ➤ cabergoline.

Cabdrivers is a cough medicine ➤ dextromethorphan and menthol.

cabergoline (Cabaser, Dostinex) is a dopamine-receptor stimulant used to stop milk production soon after childbirth and to suppress milk production in breastfeeding mothers. It is also used to treat disorders of the pituitary gland that cause over-production of prolactin (the milk-producing hormone) resulting in a raised level of prolactin in the blood (prolactinaemia), milk production (galactorrhoea) and menstrual disorders. *Adverse effects* include headache, vertigo, nausea, dizziness, breast pain, stomach and bowel upsets, weakness, fatigue, depression, pins and needles, hot flushes. Rarely it may cause palpitations, nose bleeds, and disturbed vision (hemianopia). *Precautions:* Do not use in children under sixteen years of age. Do not use in pregnancy and avoid the risk of getting pregnant while on treatment and for one month after treatment has stopped. Use non-hormonal contraception. Do not use in patients with severe impairment of liver function, after childbirth or in mothers with a history of depression following childbirth. Use with caution in patients with kidney, liver or heart disease, Raynaud's syndrome, stomach or bowel ulceration or bleeding, raised blood pressure or serious mental disorders. Check pituitary function before treatment and monitor blood pressure and blood prolactin levels. Stop at least one month before trying to conceive. *Interactions:* Antipsychotic drugs, ergot drugs, dopamine-blockers, macrolide antibiotics and anti-blood pressure drugs.

Cacit effervescent tablets ➤ calcium carbonate.

Cacit D3 is a calcium and vitamin D3 (colecalciferol) supplement ➤ calcium carbonate, colecalciferol and see Chapter 36 on vitamins. It is used to treat calcium/vitamin D deficiency in elderly people, as supplementary treatment in patients suffering from osteoporosis, vitamin D dependent osteomalacia (adult rickets) and in pregnancy. *Adverse effects* include constipation and wind. *Precautions:* Do not use in patients with overactive parathyroid glands, excess of calcium in the urine, severe kidney failure or decalcifying tumours (tumours that decrease calcium in the bones and cause a rise in blood calcium levels). Use with caution in patients with impaired kidney function or a history of kidney stones.

cade oil (juniper tar) is used in skin applications (e.g. Gelcotar, Polytar) to treat eczema and psoriasis, and in medicated soaps.

cadexomer iodine is a carboxymethyl ether containing iodine. It is present in Iodosorb as a powder of micro-beads containing iodine. The micro-beads absorb fluid to form a gel which releases the iodine. It is also used as a paste (Iodoflex). It is used to treat pressure sores and varicose leg ulcers. *Precautions:* Do not use in pregnancy

or breastfeeding mothers or in patients with overworking of their thyroid gland and use with caution in other thyroid disorders. *Interactions:* Lithium, sulphonylureas (oral anti-diabetic drugs).

Caelyx ➤ doxorubicin.

Cafergot tablets and suppositories contain ergotamine and caffeine. They are used to treat migraine (see Chapter 34). *Adverse effects and Precautions* ➤ ergotamine, caffeine.

caffeine has a stimulating effect upon the central nervous system and a weak diuretic effect. It is present in some over-the-counter pain-relievers, tonics and pick-me-ups. *Adverse effects and Precautions* see Chapter 5.

Caladryl cream and lotion contain calamine, diphenhydramine (an antihistamine) and camphor. They are used to treat irritation of the skin, sunburn, insect bites and stings. See warning on using skin preparations containing an antihistamine (p. 247). Do not use on broken skin, lining of the mouth, nose, vagina etc. or in chickenpox, measles or on weeping skin rashes.

calamine is a zinc salt (zinc carbonate) coloured with an iron salt (ferric oxide). It is a mild astringent and is used in various skin applications.

Calanif ➤ nifedipine.

Calceos chewable tablets are calcium and vitamin D3 (colecalciferol) supplements ➤ calcium carbonate, colecalciferol and see Chapter 36 on vitamins. They are used to treat calcium/vitamin D deficiency in elderly people, as supplementary treatment in patients suffering from osteoporosis, vitamin D dependent osteomalacia (adult rickets) and in pregnancy. *Adverse effects* include constipation and wind. *Precautions:* Do not use in patients with overactive parathyroid glands, excess of calcium in the urine, severe kidney failure or decalcifying tumours (tumours that decrease calcium in the bones and cause a rise in blood calcium levels). Use with caution in patients with impaired kidney function or a history of kidney stones.

Calcichew preparations ➤ calcium carbonate.

Calcichew D3 is a calcium and vitamin D3 (colecalciferol) supplement ➤ calcium carbonate, colecalciferol and see Chapter 36 on vitamins. It is used to treat calcium/vitamin D deficiency in elderly people, as supplementary treatment in patients suffering from osteoporosis, vitamin D dependent osteomalacia (adult rickets) and in pregnancy. *Adverse effects* include constipation and wind. *Precautions:* Do not use in patients with overactive parathyroid glands, excess of calcium in the urine, severe kidney failure or decalcifying tumours (tumours that decrease calcium in the bones and cause a rise in blood calcium levels). Use with caution in patients with impaired kidney function or a history of kidney stones.

Calcicard D3 Forte is a calcium and vitamin D3 (colecalciferol) supplement ➤ calcium carbonate, colecalciferol and see Chapter 36 on vitamins. It is used to treat calcium/vitamin D deficiency in elderly people, as supplementary treatment in patients suffering from osteoporosis, vitamin D dependent osteomalacia (adult rickets) and in pregnancy. *Adverse effects* include constipation and wind. *Precautions:* Do not use in patients with overactive parathyroid glands, excess of calcium in the urine, severe kidney failure or decalcifying tumours (tumours that decrease calcium in the bones and cause a rise in blood calcium levels). Use with caution in patients with impaired kidney function or a history of kidney stones.

Calcicard CR ➤ diltiazem.

Calcidrink ➤ calcium carbonate.

calciferol (ergocalciferol) has the same effects and uses as vitamin D. See Chapter 36. Deficiency of vitamin D causes rickets in children and osteomalacia (bone softening) in adults. *Adverse effects:* Excessive daily doses may produce loss of appetite, nausea, vomiting, diarrhoea, loss of weight, head-ache, dizziness and thirst. The amount of calcium in the urine is raised and the patient may develop kidney stones and calcification of arteries.

Calcijex ➤ calcitriol.

Calciparine (calcium heparin) ➤ heparin.

calcipotriol (Dovonex) is synthetic vitamin D. It is used as a skin cream or scalp lotion to treat mild to moderate psoriasis, see p. 259. It stops the over-growth of cells in the surface (epidermis) of the skin that occurs in psoriasis and helps to restore a normal turnover of the surface cells. It has less effect on calcium metabolism in the body than other synthetic vitamin D preparations (e.g. calcitriol) and therefore the risks of a raised blood calcium, calcium in the urine and bone softening are reduced. *Adverse effects* include transient irritation and, rarely, dermatitis of the face or around the mouth. It may also cause itching, make the psoriasis worse, sensitize the skin to sunlight and cause a rise in blood calcium levels. *Precautions:* It should not be used in patients with disorders of calcium metabolism. It should not be applied to the face, and the hands should be washed after application. It should be used with caution in pregnancy and in breastfeeding mothers. It is not recommended for children.

calcitonin is a hormone produced by the thyroid gland that works with parathyroid hormones to regulate the laying down of new bone and dissolving of old which helps to maintain the blood calcium level. It is used to lower blood calcium levels in Paget's disease and if the blood calcium is high in certain malignant cancers. *Adverse effects* include nausea, tingling of the hands, flushing, vomiting, an unpleasant taste and allergic reactions. *Precautions:* It is obtained from thyroid glands of pigs and may produce allergic reactions in susceptible individuals. Tests for allergy to it (using a skin scratch test) should be carried out in people with a history of allergy. Use with caution in pregnancy and breastfeeding mothers. *Interactions:* Digoxin and related drugs.

Note: **Synthetic salmon calcitonin** (salcatonin, Calsynar, Forcaltonin, Miacalcic) causes less allergy and is more useful for long-term treatment ➤ calcitonin (salmon).

calcitonin (salmon) (Calsynar, Forcaltonin, Miacalcic) is a synthetic salmon calcitonin ➤ calcitonin. It is used to lower a raised blood calcium level in emergencies, to treat Paget's disease of the bone, and to relieve pain associated with secondary cancer deposits in the bone. *Adverse effects* include nausea and, occasionally, vomiting, diarrhoea, dizziness, tingling of hands, unpleasant taste, slight flushing of the face and skin rashes. Rarely, severe allergic reactions may occur. Inflammation may occur at the site of injection. *Precautions:* It should not be used in breastfeeding mothers and where possible it should not be used in pregnancy or if there is a risk of pregnancy, in elderly people and in people with impaired kidney function. The blood level of alkaline phosphatase and the urinary level of hydroxyproline should be regularly monitored and the treatment adjusted accordingly. In patients with a history of allergy, a skin sensitivity test to calcitonin (salmon) should be carried out before starting treatment. Some patients may develop antibodies to salmon calcitonin but this bears no relationship to the risk of allergic reactions and does not affect response to treatment. *Interactions:* Digoxin and related drugs.

calcitriol (Calcijex, Rocaltrol) is a vitamin D derivative that is used to treat bone disease caused by kidney failure. It is also used to treat post-menopausal osteoporosis. *Adverse effects:* Increased level of calcium in the blood and in the urine. *Precautions:* Do not use in patients with raised blood calcium levels. Do not use other vitamin D preparations. Monitor blood calcium levels and use with caution in pregnancy.

calcium acetate is used as a source of calcium in solutions used for dialysing blood. The powder may be used in skin applications.

calcium alginate is a calcium salt of alginic acid. It is used in special dressings as an absorbable material to stop bleeding from wounds. Alginate dressings may be removed by applying 3% sodium citrate solution for a few minutes and washing out with sterile water.

calcium and ergocalciferol tablets contain calcium salts and ergocalciferol (calciferol, vitamin D2). They are used as a calcium supplement ➤ calcium salts and see Chapter 36 on vitamins.

calcium antagonists ➤ calcium-channel blockers.

calcium carbonate (chalk) is an antacid (in Gaviscon, in Peptac) (see Chapter 19). It may cause constipation and belching. Avoid prolonged or excessive dosage along with an increased intake of milk or cream. This may cause the milk-alkali syndrome: loss of appetite, nausea, vomiting, headache, weakness, abdominal pains, constipation and thirst associated with a high blood calcium level and changes in the acidity of the blood. It is also used to treat calcium deficiency and osteoporosis (Adcal, in Adcal D3, Cacit, in Cacit D3, in Calceos, in Calcicard D3 Forte, in Calcichew, Calcidrink, Calcium 500, in Sandocal, in Titralac). However, calcium supplements should only be taken where dietary calcium intake is lacking. The dietary requirement varies with age and can be greater in children, pregnancy, breastfeeding mothers and the elderly. In the treatment of osteoporosis, a calcium intake which is double the normal recommended amount helps to reduce the rate of bone loss.

calcium-channel blockers (calcium antagonists) see p. 115. They are used to treat angina (Chapter 22), raised blood pressure (Chapter 25), prevent migraine (Chapter 34) and to treat disorders of heart rhythm (Chapter 24).

calcium folinate is a calcium salt of folinic acid ➤ folinic acid.

calcium glubionate (in Calcium Sandoz)

is used as a source of calcium to treat and prevent calcium deficiency disorders.

calcium gluconate is used as a source of calcium to treat and prevent calcium deficiency disorders.

calcium heparin (Calciparine) ➤ heparin.

calcium lactate is used as a source of calcium to treat and prevent calcium deficiency disorders.

calcium lactobionate (in Calcium Sandoz) is used as a source of calcium to treat and prevent calcium deficiency disorders.

calcium leucovorin ➤ folinic acid.

calcium levofolinate (Isovorin) is used to enhance the effect of the anti-cancer drug 5-fluorouacil (5-FU) in cancer of the bowel. See Chapter 51. *Adverse effects* include allergic reactions, fever. *Precautions:* Do not use in pregnancy or while breastfeeding. The simultaneous administration of methotrexate should be avoided.

calcium salts. Various salts of calcium are used to supplement the diet, as antacids, in skin preparations, to treat calcium deficiency and osteoporosis. Calcium supplements to the diet are needed if dietary intake of calcium is inadequate. Requirements vary according to age; growing children need an adequate amount of calcium in their diet and so do pregnant women, breastfeeding mothers and post-menopausal women. Children on special diets (e.g. milk-free diets) will need calcium supplements and so will patients with rickets and osteomalacia in the early stages of their treatment with vitamin D. *Adverse effects:* Calcium salts by mouth can cause irritation of the stomach and bowel and constipation and wind. *Precautions:* Use with caution in patients with obstructive bowel disease, ulceration of the bowel, and kidney stones. Do not use in patients with a raised blood calcium or a raised blood uric acid level. *Interactions:* Tetracyclines.

Calcium-Sandoz syrup is used as a source of calcium to treat and prevent calcium deficiency disorders.

Calcium 500 ➤ calcium carbonate.

Calcort ➤ deflazacort.

Calgel contains lignocaine (a local anaesthetic) and cetylpyridinium (an antibacterial). It is used to treat infant teething. *Adverse effects and Precautions* ➤ lignocaine, cetylpyridinium.

Califig is a laxative containing figs and senna ➤ senna.

Calimal ➤ chlorpheniramine.

Calmurid HC cream contains Calmurid with hydrocortisone (a corticosteroid) added. *Adverse effects and Precautions* see corticosteroid skin applications p. 241.

Calmurid skin preparations contain urea (a skin softener) and lactic acid (a keratolytic, see p. 247). They are used to treat chronic dry skin.

Calpol, Calpol Fast Melts and **Calpol 6 Plus** ➤ paracetamol.

Calsalettes is a laxative containing aloin.

Calsynar ➤ calcitonin (salmon).

CAM elixir ➤ ephedrine.

Camcolit ➤ lithium.

camphor is an aromatic substance used in rheumatic liniments. It is also used to relieve itching and muscle aches. Note that camphorated oil has been withdrawn because of its toxicity. Camphor has also been used in cough medicines and to treat gripe. Camphor-related compounds (monoterpines) are occasionally used to dissolve gallstones and kidney stones. *Precautions:* It is dangerous to place a camphor preparation up the nostrils of an infant to relieve snuffles. Even a small quantity applied in this way may cause the infant to collapse.

Campral EC ➤ acamprosate calcium.

Campto ➤ irinotecan.

candesartan (Amias) is an angiotensin-II

receptor blocker used to treat high blood pressure. See Chapter 25. *Adverse effects* include upper respiratory tract infection, back pain. *Precautions:* Do not use in patients with severe liver damage, in pregnancy or while breastfeeding. Use with utmost caution in patients with obstruction to the flow of blood from the heart into the main artery (aortic stenosis), through the mitral valve (mitral stenosis) or into the main artery to a kidney (renal artery stenosis), or in patients suffering from obstructive hypertropic cardiomyopathy (enlargement of the muscles of the heart).

Candiden ➤ clotrimazole.

Canesten preparations ➤ clotrimazole.

Canesten HC cream contains hydrocortisone (a corticosteroid) and clotrimazole (an antifungal drug). *Adverse effects and Precautions:* see corticosteroid skin applications p. 241 and ➤ clotrimazole. It may produce mild burning and irritation and allergic reaction.

Canusal solution contains heparin sodium. It is used to flush catheters, canulas etc. and is not for systemic use ➤ heparin.

Capasal shampoo contains salicylic acid, coconut oil and distilled coal tar. It is used to treat dry scaly scalp conditions, for example, seborrhoeic dermatitis, psoriasis and cradle cap. Contact with the eyes should be avoided and if it irritates the scalp treatment should be stopped.

Capastat ➤ capreomycin.

capecitabine (Xeloda) is used to treat colorectal cancer. See Chapter 51. *Adverse effects* include dizziness, fatigue, stomach and bowel upsets, hair loss, skin or nail damage, fever, weakness, limb pain, headache, nerve damage, fluid retention, disorders of the blood, weight loss, dehydration, difficulty breathing, watery eyes, appetite loss and nose bleeds. *Precautions:* Do not use in patients with severe kidney or liver damage, an allergy to fluoropyramidines or fluorouracil, certain enzyme deficiencies, blood dis

orders, in pregnancy or while breastfeeding. Use with caution in patients with a history of heart disease, with calcium imbalance in the blood, moderate liver or kidney damage, diabetes, diarrhoea, abdominal pain, nausea, inflammation of soft tissues in the mouth, or in the elderly.

Caplenal ➤ allopurinol.

Capoten ➤ captopril.

Capozide tablets contain captopril (an ACE inhibitor) and hydrochlorothiazide (a thiazide diuretic). They are used to treat raised blood pressure. *Adverse effects and Precautions:* ➤ captopril, thiazide diuretics.

capreomycin (Capastat) is an antibiotic used to treat tuberculosis (see Chapter 50). It is used when other drugs have failed. It should only be used along with other anti-tuberculous drugs in order to reduce the development of resistant bacteria. It is not absorbed from the intestine and has to be given by intramuscular injection. *Adverse effects:* It may produce vertigo, noises in the ears, and disturbances of salt and water balance in the body. It may, rarely, cause irreversible deafness and also progressive kidney damage. Allergic skin rashes and fever and transient liver abnormalities have been reported. It may rarely produce blood disorders. Pain and hardness of the tissues may occur at injection sites. *Precautions:* It should be given with caution to patients with impaired hearing, impaired kidney function and to those patients with a history of allergy or liver disease. Tests of hearing and balance and tests of liver and kidney function should be carried out at regular intervals during treatment. Do not use in pregnancy. *Interactions:* Streptomycin, viomycin and any drug that is known to damage hearing, balance or the kidneys.

Caprin ➤ aspirin.

capsaicin (in Axsain, Zacin) is an extract from capsicum peppers. It is used in heat rubs ➤ rubefacients.

capsicum oleoresin (in Balmosa, in

Cremalgin) is extracted from red peppers. It is used in heat rubs ➤ rubefacients.

Capsuvac ➤ co-danthrusate.

CaptoCo is a combination of hydrochlorothiazide and captopril used in the treatment of mild to moderate hypertension ➤ captopril, hydrochlorothiazide.

captopril (Acepril, in Acezide, Capoten, in Capozide, Ecopace, Hyteneze, Kaplon, Tensopril) is an ACE inhibitor used to treat raised blood pressure (see Chapter 25) and heart failure (see Chapter 23). *Adverse effects* include fall in blood pressure, persistent dry cough, voice changes, discomfort in the throat, diarrhoea or constipation (occasionally), headache, dizziness, fatigue, weakness, nausea, vomiting (occasionally), muscle cramps, taste changes, sore mouth, indigestion, abdominal pains, impaired kidney function, raised blood potassium levels (especially in patients with impaired kidney function), allergic skin reactions (sometimes severe), rapid beating of the heart, blood disorders, heart attack, stroke, back pains, flushing, jaundice, pancreatitis, disturbed sleep, nervousness, mood changes, impotence, hair loss and serious skin disorders. The drug may cause a group of symptoms which includes fever, inflamed blood vessels (vasulitis), painful muscles and joints, rash, sensitivity of the skin to the sun's rays, other skin reactions and changes in the blood ➤ ACE inhibitors. *Precautions:* It should not be used in patients with previous allergy to captopril or other ACE inhibitors, in pregnancy, in breastfeeding mothers or in patients with aortic stenosis (obstruction to the flow of blood from the heart into the main artery). It should not be used to treat raised blood pressure caused by kidney disease. Use with caution in severe congestive heart failure and in patients with impaired kidney function. Blood tests, kidney tests, and urine tests (for protein) should be carried out at regular intervals. It may produce a marked fall in blood pressure in patients under anaesthesia for surgery and in patients who are receiving diuretic

therapy, on a low sodium diet, on dialysis or who are dehydrated. Use with caution in the elderly. *Interactions:* Potassium-sparing diuretics, potassium supplements, NSAIDs, vasodilator drugs, clonidine, allopurinol, procainamide, probenecid, immunosuppressants, lithium.

Carace ➤ lisinopril.

Carace Plus contains the ACE inhibitor lisinopril and the thiazide diuretic hydrochlorothiazide. It is used to treat raised blood pressure. *Adverse effects and Precautions* ➤ lisinopril, thiazide diuretics.

carbachol is a cholinergic drug (see Chapter 9) which shares some of the actions of acetylcholine. It is given after an abdominal operation to patients whose bowels are inactive (atony), or who cannot empty their bladders, see p. 284. It is also used in eye drops (Isopto carbachol) to reduce the pressure inside the eye in patients with glaucoma, see p. 63. *Adverse effects* when given by mouth or injection include sweating, nausea, vomiting, blurred vision, slow heart rate, intestinal colic and faintness. *Precautions:* Carbachol should not be given to patients with acute heart failure, bronchial asthma, peptic ulcer, obstruction to the passage of urine, overworking of the thyroid gland, recent heart attack, epilepsy or low blood pressure. Do not use in pregnancy. *Interactions* ➤ parasympathetic drugs. Carbachol eye drops (e.g. Isopto carbachol) should not be applied to the eye of a patient with corneal abrasions because it may be absorbed. It should not be used in patients suffering from acute iritis. Do not wear soft contact lenses.

Carbagen ➤ carbamazepine.

Carbalax suppositories contain sodium bicarbonate and sodium acid phosphate. They are used as an osmotic laxative, see Chapter 21 and ➤ sodium bicarbonate, sodium acid phosphate.

carbamazepine (Carbagen, Epimaz, Tegretol, Teril CR, Timonil Retard) is used to treat epilepsy. See Chapter 15. It is also used to treat facial pain (trigeminal neuralgia), nerve pains caused by diabetes, in the prevention of manic depressive psychosis that has not responded to lithium (see p. 22) and occasionally to treat partial pituitary diabetes insipidus. *Adverse effects* include nausea, vomiting, dizziness, headache, drowsiness, disturbed vision, loss of control over voluntary movements (ataxia), dry mouth, loss of appetite, diarrhoea and constipation. A widespread red rash may occur and elderly patients may become confused and agitated. Rarely it may cause blood disorders, liver damage, *serious* skin disorders, painful joints, fever, nerve damage, impaired kidney function, enlarged lymph nodes, heart disturbances, swelling of the breasts (in men), milk production, movement disorders (dyskinesia), depression, impotence, aggression, allergic reactions (may affect the lungs), fall in blood sodium level and fluid retention and sensitivity of the skin to the sun's rays. *Precautions:* Do not use in patients suffering from a conduction defect of their hearts unless the heart rate is controlled with a pacemaker. Do not use in patients with porphyria (a hereditary disorder of metabolism) or a history of bone-marrow depression causing blood disorders. Use with caution in patients with impaired kidney or liver function, heart disease, skin disorders or who have previously suffered blood disorders caused by other drugs. Carry out blood tests and tests of liver and kidney function at start of treatment and at regular intervals during treatment. Use with caution in pregnancy (risk of damage to spinal cord in the baby), mother should take 5 mg folic acid daily to prevent damage and tests for spinal cord damage should be carried out (alphafetoprotein test and ultrasound scan between third and sixth months of pregnancy). Use with caution in breastfeeding mothers and patients with glaucoma. Avoid suddenly stopping the drug. Watch out for early signs of blood and liver damage and skin disorders. Patient should report immediately to the doctor if he/she develops a fever, sore throat, rash, mouth ulcers, bruising or any bleeding. *Interactions:* Oral anticoagulants, MAOIs, combined oral contraceptives, erythromycin, doxycycline, isoniazid, cimetidine, dextropropoxyphene, calcium-channel blockers, viloxazine, corticosteroids, anti-epileptic drugs, lithium, benzodiazepines, methadone, theophylline, danazol, haloperidol, fluoxetine, alcohol.

carbaryl (Carylderm) is an insecticide used for treating head lice, see p. 256. *Adverse effects:* It may irritate the skin. *Precautions:* Use with utmost caution in infants under six months and in patients with asthma. Use only lotion in patients with eczema. Contact with the eyes and broken or infected skin should be avoided. Preparations containing alcohol should not be used in children, in individuals who suffer from asthma or to treat crabs. To avoid alcoholic fumes, use aqueous solutions. May cause cancer in animals, therefore a possible risk in humans. Do not use lotion more than once a week for three weeks at a time.

Carbellon is an antacid which contains magnesium, charcoal and peppermint oil.

carbenoxolone (carbenoxolone sodium) is combined with antacids in Pyrogastrone to treat oesophagitis and acid reflux (see p. 101). *Adverse effects:* Carbenoxolone may cause salt and water retention in the body, which leads to swelling (oedema) and an increase in weight and blood pressure. This may trigger heart failure in patients who have some underlying heart disorder. It also reduces the blood potassium which may produce muscle disorders ➤ potassium. *Precautions:* Do not use in patients with heart, liver or kidney disease, or low blood potassium. Do not use in elderly people or in pregnancy. Use with caution in patients in whom salt and water retention could be harmful, e.g. those with raised blood pressure. Weight, blood pressure and blood chemistry should be checked at regular intervals. Treatment should never be continued for more than four–six weeks. Potassium usually has to be added to the diet. *Interactions:* digoxin, diuretics, NSAIDs, anti-arrhythmic drugs, antibacterial drugs, anti-blood pressure drugs. Carbenoxolone is also used as a gel (Bioral) and as granules (Bioplex) to treat ulcers of the mouth, see Chapter 12.

carbidopa (in Sinemet) blocks the enzyme that breaks down levodopa in the body (dopadecarboxylase). It is combined with levodopa in co-careldopa (Sinemet) to treat parkinsonism. See Chapter 16.

carbimazole (Neomercazole) is an anti-thyroid drug, see Chapter 43. It reduces the production of thyroid hormone. *Adverse effects:* These usually occur in the first few months of treatment and include nausea, headache, skin rashes, joint pains and, rarely, jaundice, blood disorders and loss of hair. *Precautions:* Infants should not be breastfed by mothers taking carbimazole. Patients should report sore throats, skin rashes, mouth ulcers or fever immediately, since these may precede blood disorders by several days. Caution is necessary when using this drug in patients with impaired liver function, and during pregnancy. Do not use in patients with any evidence that the thyroid gland is pressing on the wind-pipe because the drug may produce enlargement of the thyroid gland in high doses. *Interactions:* Radioactive iodine.

carbocisteine (Mucodyne) is used to liquefy sputum (see p. 51) in patients who produce excessive amounts of sticky sputum. It is also used to treat glue ear in children. *Adverse effects* include stomach and bowel upsets, rash and nausea. *Precautions:* Do not use in patients with active peptic ulcer. Use with caution in pregnancy and patients with a history of peptic ulcer.

Carbo-Dome preparations contain coal tar solution. They are used to treat psoriasis ➤ coal tar.

carbomer (polyacrylic acid, Gel Tears, Viscotears liquid gel) is a synthetic acrylic polymer used as eye drops to treat dry eyes.

Carbomix is a preparation of activated charcoal used to treat acute poisoning by mouth and drug overdosage. *Interactions:* Antidotes or drugs given to produce vomiting (emetics).

carbonic anhydrase inhibitors are weak diuretics. See Chapter 29. They include acetazolamide and dichlorphenamide which are used to block the formation of fluid in the eye in the treatment of glaucoma. See p. 63. They are taken by mouth. *Dorzolamide* is a selective carbonic anhydrase inhibitor which is active when applied topically to the eye (Trusopt eye solution). The use of acetazolamide to treat mountain sickness is of doubtful value – the best treatment is to descend to a lower level and then gradually acclimatize.

carboplatin (Paraplatin) is an anti-cancer drug (see Chapter 51). *Adverse effects:* It is a derivative of cisplatin and produces fewer adverse effects such as nausea, vomiting, kidney and nerve damage or damage to hearing. However, it produces more damage to the bone marrow than cisplatin. Very rarely loss of hair, impaired liver function, fever, chill and alteration in taste and allergic reactions may occur. *Precautions:* See Chapter 51 on anti-cancer drugs.

carboprost (Hemabate) is a prostaglandin (see Chapter 52) used to treat haemorrhage after childbirth due to failure of the womb to contract. Carboprost is recommended when oxytocin combined with ergometrine has failed. *Adverse effects* include nausea, vomiting, diarrhoea, chills, sweating, headache, dizziness, high temperature, flushing and wheezing. Occasionally, it may cause a rise in blood pressure, breathlessness and fluid on the lungs (pulmonary oedema). It may cause pain and redness at the site of injection. *Precautions:* It should not be used in women with heart, lung, kidney or liver disease. It should be used with caution if the womb is scarred from previous injury, or if there is acute infection around the uterus (acute pelvic inflammatory disease). It should be used with caution in women with anaemia, asthma, diabetes, epilepsy, high or low blood pressure, glaucoma, or jaundice.

carboxymethylcellulose is used in various drug preparations as a suspending agent, dispersal agent and emulsifying agent. It is used as a bulk laxative, and is widely used in the food industry. It is also used in artificial saliva (Glandosane, Luborant).

Cardene ➤ nicardipine.

cardiac glycosides: Digoxin is the most commonly used cardiac glycoside. It is used to treat heart failure (see Chapter 23) and disorders of heart rhythm (see Chapter 24).

Cardicor ➤ bisoprolol.

Cardilate MR ➤ nifedipine.

Cardura ➤ doxazosin.

Cardura XL ➤ doxazosin.

Care Hayfever Relief ➤ beclometasone.

Carisoma ➤ carisoprodol.

carisoprodol (Carisoma) is used to relieve spasm of skeletal muscles (see p. 42). *Adverse effects* include drowsiness, nausea, headache, constipation, dizziness, lassitude, flushes and skin rashes. *Precautions:* It should not be used in patients with acute, intermittent porphyria (a hereditary disorder of metabolism), in pregnancy or in breastfeeding mothers. It should be used with caution in patients with impaired kidney or liver function, or with a history of alcoholism or drug dependence. Long-term use should be avoided and the drug should be stopped slowly by gradually reducing the daily dosage. *Interactions:* Sedatives, sleeping drugs, anticoagulants, corticosteroids, oral contraceptives, phenytoin, griseofulvin, rifampicin, phenothiazines, tricyclic antidepressants.

carmellose gelatin paste (in Orabase, in Orahesive) is used to treat painful mouth ulcers. It coats and protects the ulcer surface ➤ carmellose sodium.

carmellose sodium is used as a suspending agent in the food industry and in the preparation of gels and ointments. It acts as a protective when applied to the skin or mouth. It is also used as a lubricant in dry eye conditions (Celluvisc).

carminatives are drugs which enable you to belch gas from the stomach. The active constituent is usually a volatile oil which has a pleasant flavour. They work by producing a mild irritation of the lining of the mouth, oesophagus and stomach. This produces salivation, a feeling of warmth, and possibly relaxation of the muscle at the junction between the oesophagus and stomach, thus allowing gas to escape. The volatile oils used as carminatives include dill, peppermint, aniseed, caraway, cloves and ginger. *Adverse effects:* Essential oils are irritant and excessive use and/or high doses may cause nausea, vomiting and diarrhoea. Overdose by mouth may depress the brain and breathing, or stimulate the brain, producing convulsions. They may irritate the skin and cause contact dermatitis.

carmustine (BiCNU) is an alkylating agent used in the treatment of cancer (see Chapter 51). *Adverse effects:* These include nausea and vomiting, damage to the bone marrow producing blood disorders, burning at the site of injection and flushing of the skin. *Precautions:* See Chapter 51.

carnitine (Carnitor) is used to treat carnitine deficiency. Carnitine is present in the normal Western diet and is also manufactured in the liver from the essential amino acids methionine and lysine. It helps to transport long chain fatty acids into cells to be burned to produce energy. Deficiency may be due to a genetic defect, severe liver disease or to excessive loss in kidney dialysis. Symptoms of a low blood sugar and myasthenia gravis (muscle weakness due to neuromuscular abnormality) may occur. *Adverse effects* include nausea, vomiting, abdominal pain and diarrhoea. These may be related to the dose used. *Precautions:* Use with caution in patients with impaired kidney function, in pregnancy and in breastfeeding mothers.

Carnitor ➤ carnitine.

carteolol is a non-selective beta-blocker ➤ beta-blockers. It is used in Teoptic eye drops to treat glaucoma, see p. 64. *Adverse effects* include burning, pain and irritation of the eyes, blurred vision and redness. Rarely, it may cause inflammation of the cornea. *Precautions* ➤ beta-blockers. Do not wear soft contact lenses. *Interactions:* Beta-blockers by mouth.

carticaine ➤ articaine.

carvedilol (Eucardic) is an alpha- and beta-blocker used to treat raised blood pressure. See Chapter 25. *Adverse effects* include headache, dizziness, fatigue, fall in blood pressure on standing up after sitting or lying down, stomach and bowel upsets, slow pulse rate, cold hands and feet, dry eyes, flu-like symptoms, allergic skin rashes, stuffy nose, wheezing, depressed mood, disturbed sleep, numbness and pins and needles in hands and feet, disorders of liver function, blood disorders, angina and heart failure, heart block. *Precautions:* Do not use in patients with moderate or severe heart block, severe slowness of the pulse, uncontrolled heart failure, asthma, chronic obstructive airways disease, impaired liver function, pregnancy or breastfeeding mothers. Use with utmost caution in patients with impaired heart function, overworking of the thyroid gland or diabetes. *Interactions:* General anaesthetics, class I anti-arrhythmics, verapamil, digoxin, rifampicin.

Carylderm preparations ➤ carbaryl.

cascara (Rhuaka) is the dried bark of *Rhamnus purshiana*. It is a stimulant laxative used to treat constipation. See Chapter 21.

Casodex ➤ bicalutamide.

castor oil is used as a stimulant laxative to treat constipation. See Chapter 21. Large doses may produce nausea, vomiting, colic and severe loss of fluid with purgation. It is also used as a soothing application in eye drops and skin ointments.

Catapres ➤ clonidine.

Catarrh-EX contains paracetamol, caffeine and phenylephrine ➤ paracetamol, caffeine, phenylephrine.

Caverject ➤ alprostadil.

Ceanel Concentrate (shampoo for psoriasis) contains phenylethyl alcohol, cetrimide and undecenoic acid, see entry on each drug. Avoid contact with eyes.

Cedocard and **Cedocard Retard** ➤ isosorbide dinitrate.

cefaclor (Distaclor) is a cephalosporin antibiotic ➤ cephalosporins.

cefadroxil (Baxan) is a cephalosporin antibiotic ➤ cephalosporins.

cefalexin (Ceporex, Keflex, Kiflone, Tenorex) is a cephalosporin antibiotic ➤ cephalosporins.

cefamandole (cephamandole, Kefadol) is a cephalosporin antibiotic ➤ cephalosporins.

cefazolin (Kefzol) is a cephalosporin antibiotic ➤ cephalosporins.

cefixime (Suprax) is a cephalosporin antibiotic ➤ cephalosporins.

cefotaxime (Claforan) is a cephalosporin antibiotic ➤ cephalosporins.

cefoxitin (Mefoxin) is a cephalosporin antibiotic ➤ cephalosporins.

cefpirome (Cefrom) is a cephalosporin antibiotic ➤ cephalosporins.

cefpodoxime (Orelox) is a cephalosporin antibiotic ➤ cephalosporins.

cefprozil (Cefzil) is a cephalosporin antibiotic used to treat upper respiratory tract infections, inflammation of the middle ear (otitis media), acute exacerbation of chronic bronchitis and skin infections. See Chapter 46. *Adverse effects* include stomach and bowel upsets, dizziness, nappy rash, superinfection, genital itching, inflammation of the vagina and blood disorders. *Precautions:* Use with caution in patients with severe kidney damage, history of stomach and bowel disease (particularly colitis), phenylketonuria, an allergy to penicillins, in pregnancy or while breastfeeding ➤ cephalosporins.

cefradine (Nicef, Velosef) is a cephalosporin antibiotic ➤ cephalosporins.

Cefrom ➤ cefpirome.

ceftazidime (Fortum, Kefadim) is a cephalosporin antibiotic ➤ cephalosporins.

ceftriaxone (Rocephin) is a cephalosporin antibiotic ➤ cephalosporins.

cefuroxime (Zinacef, Zinnat) is a cephalosporin antibiotic ➤ cephalosporins.

Cefzil ➤ cefprozil.

Celance ➤ pergolide.

Celebrex ➤ celecoxib.

celecoxib (Celebrex) is a non-steroidal anti-inflammatory drug used to treat osteoarthritis and rheumatoid arthritis. See Chapter 32. *Adverse effects* include fluid retention, stomach and bowel upsets, dizziness, insomnia, upper respiratory tract disorders, skin rash. *Precautions.* Do not use in patients with a history of allergy to sulphonamides or NSAIDs, active peptic ulcer or bleeding from the stomach or bowel, inflammatory bowel disease, severe kidney or liver damage, severe congestive heart failure, in pregnancy (effective contraception must be used) or while breastfeeding. Use with caution in the elderly and black patients – use low starter doses. Also use with caution in patients with impaired kidney or liver function, a history of stomach or bowel disorders, heart failure or raised blood pressure.

Celectol ➤ celiprolol.

Celevac ➤ methylcellulose.

celiprolol (Celectol) is a selective beta-receptor blocker used to treat raised blood pressure (see Chapter 25). It has some intrinsic sympathomimetic activity at $beta_2$ receptors (see p. 114). *Adverse effects and Precautions* ➤ beta-blockers.

Cellcept ➤ mycophenolate mofetil.

cellulose is used as a bulking and suspending agent in the manufacture of tablets and liquid medicines.

Celluvisc eye drops ➤ carmellose sodium.

central nervous system stimulants ➤ stimulant drugs and see Chapters 5 and 6.

Centrapryl ➤ sclogiline.

Centyl K is a diuretic containing bendroflumethiazide and potassium chloride ➤ bendroflumethiazide and see Chapter 29.

cephalexin ➤ cefalexin.

cephalosporins are discussed in Chapter 46. *Adverse effects:* The commonest adverse effects produced by the cephalosporins are allergic reactions. Any one of the cephalosporins is likely to cause allergic reactions, which are similar to those produced by the penicillins. This may be because they share a similar chemical structure. Immediate allergic reactions may occur, causing a severe allergic emergency (anaphylaxis), wheezing and nettle-rash (urticaria). A delayed allergic reaction comes on after several days and produces a measles-like rash with fever. Swollen glands and fever may occur on their own without a rash. About 10% of patients allergic to penicillins will be allergic to the cephalosporins, but there is no skin test to predict this cross-allergy. About 5% of patients will be allergic to cephalosporins. Cephaloridine (a first-generation cephalosporin) may occasionally cause kidney damage, particularly when given in a high dose and when given with a loop diuretic drug such as frusemide or ethacrynic acid. Other cephalosporins have caused kidney damage in patients whose kidney function is already impaired. The risk of kidney damage is increased in elderly people if a cephalosporin is given with other antibiotics that may cause kidney damage, for example, gentamicin or tobramycin. Several of the cephalosporins interfere with blood clotting factors and may occasionally cause bleeding, particularly in elderly and debilitated patients. Cephalosporins may occasionally cause nausea, vomiting and diarrhoea and, very rarely, blood disorders, liver damage, skin rashes, a severe form of colitis (pseudo-membranous colitis) which is more likely to occur with higher doses, jaundice, nervousness, hyperactivity, sleep disturbances, confusion, headache, dizziness, and super-infection. Injections of cephalothin may be painful. *Precautions:* Cephalosporins should not be used in an individual who has had an allergic reaction to any of the cephalosporins. They should not be used in people who suffer from porphyria (a hereditary disorder of metabolism). They should be used with caution in anyone allergic to penicillins or who has impaired kidney function. Cephalosporins may give false positive tests for sugar in the urine and for haemolytic anaemia (Coombs' test). *Adverse effects* from cephalosporins may be more frequent and severe in elderly people because they may have impaired kidney function. They should be used with caution in pregnancy and in breastfeeding mothers. *Interactions:* aminoglycosides, loop diuretics. Antacids reduce absorption of cefpodoxime; cephamandole causes disulfiram-like reaction with alcohol; antacids reduce absorption of cefpodoxime; cephamandole increases anti-coagulant effects of warfarin and nicoumalone; H_2-blockers cause reduced absorption of cefpodoxime; probenecid reduces urinary excretion of cephalosporins causing increased blood levels.

cephamandole ➤ cefamandole.

cephazolin ➤ cefazolin.

cephradine ➤ cefradine.

Ceporex ➤ cefalexin.

Cepton ➤ chlorhexidine.

Cerebrovase ➤ dipyridamole.

Cerezyme ➤ imiglucose.

certoparin (Alphaparin) is a low molecular weight heparin (see Chapter 28) used to prevent thromboembolism during and after surgery. *Adverse effects* include minor bleeding at site of injection, reduced platelet count (thrombocytopenia), allergic reactions, changes in liver function tests and osteoporosis ➤ heparin. *Precautions:* Do not use in children. Do not use in patients allergic to heparin, with major bleeding disorders, active ulceration of the stomach or intestine, severe raised blood pressure, sub-acute bacterial endocarditis or severe impairment of liver or kidney function. Platelet counts should be monitored at frequent intervals. *Interactions:* NSAIDs, oral anticoagulants.

Cerubidin ➤ daunorubicin.

Cerumol ear drops contain paradichlorobenzene and chlorbutanol in arachis oil. It is used to dissolve ear wax (see p. 57). Do not use if ear drum is perforated or if patient has eczema or dermatitis of the ear (otitis externa).

cetalkonium (in Bonjela, in Teejel) is used as an antiseptic. It has effects like cetrimide.

Cetavlex cream ➤ cetrimide.

cetirizine (Zirtec) is a non-sedative antihistamine (see Chapter 17). *Adverse effects* include drowsiness, headache, dry mouth, stomach and bowel upsets, agitation and dizziness. *Precautions:* Do not use if breastfeeding. Use with caution in pregnancy and in patients with impaired kidney function. Increases effects of alcohol. Although it produces less drowsiness than sedative antihistamines it may still affect driving skills. For other adverse effects and precautions of antihistamines ➤ antihistamines.

cetraben is a skin softening cream containing white soft paraffin and light liquid paraffin.

cetrimide (in Ceanel Conc, Cetavlex, in Drapolene, in Hibicet Conc, Siopel, Steripod Yellow, Tisept) is a surface-active drug with antiseptic, emulsifying and detergent properties. It is used as a skin-cleansing agent in numerous preparations and also in shampoos. Some patients may develop sensitivity to cetrimide after repeated applications. It may cause the skin of the scalp to become very dry.

cetrorelix (Cetrotide) is a luteinising hormone releasing hormone (LHRH) blocker (see p. 193) used in the treatment of female infertility. It is used to prevent premature ovulation in controlled ovarian stimulation. *Adverse effects* include pain, swelling and redness at the site of injection, nausea, headache. *Precautions:* Do not use in patients with moderate or severe kidney or liver damage, patients who are post-menopausal, pregnant or breastfeeding.

Cetrotide ➤ cetrorelix.

cetyl alcohol is used in the preparation of ointments and creams.

cetylpyridinium (cetylpyridinium chloride) is used as an antiseptic. It has effects similar to those described under cetrimide. It is used in throat lozenges, gargles and teething gels.

chamomile (chamomile flowers, in Kamillosan) has a pleasant aromatic odour and appears in some cough medicines, indigestion remedies and hair preparations.

charcoal is used to absorb gases in the treatment of flatulence and distension, as a deodorant for foul-smelling wounds, and is given by mouth in the first-aid treatment of poisoning by certain drugs to delay absorption into the body ➤ activated charcoal.

Charcodote ➤ activated charcoal.

Chemotherapy, see Chapter 51.

Chemotrim ➤ co-trimoxazole.

Chemydur and **Chemydur 60XL** ➤ isosorbide mononitrate.

Chimax ➤ flutamide.

Chirocaine ➤ levobupivacaine.

chlomethiazole ➤ chlormethiazole.

Chloractil ➤ chlorpromazine.

chloral betaine ➤ cloral betaine.

chloral hydrate (Welldorm elixir) is a sleeping drug (see Chapter 1). *Adverse effects* include headache, nausea, dizziness, excitement, drowsiness, delirium, disorientation, paranoia, skin rashes and blood disorders. *Precautions:* It irritates the stomach and must be taken well diluted. Chloral hydrate should not be used in pregnancy, in breastfeeding mothers, in patients with severely impaired liver, heart or kidney function or with peptic ulcers. If a patient taking chloral hydrate regularly has a drink of alcohol there may be a fall in blood pressure causing flushing, rapid beating of the heart and faintness. It should be used with caution in patients with porphyria (a hereditary disorder of metabolism). *Drug dependence:* It produces drug dependence of the barbiturate/alcohol type and increases the effects of alcohol. It may affect the ability to drive and operate moving machinery. *Interactions:* Alcohol, sedatives, sleeping drugs, anticoagulants.

chlorambucil (Leukeran) is an anti-cancer drug (see Chapter 51). *Adverse effects:* The most frequent adverse effect is damage to the bone marrow, producing severe blood disorders. Nausea, vomiting, diarrhoea, ulceration of the mouth occur infrequently and very rarely it may cause lung damage, liver damage, fever, allergic reactions, skin rashes, nerve damage and cystitis. *Precautions:* It should not be used in pregnancy or in breastfeeding mothers or in patients with porphyria (a hereditary disorder of metabolism), or when there is a risk that bone-marrow function is decreased (e.g. within four weeks of radiotherapy or another anti-cancer drug).

chloramphenicol (Chloromycetin, Kemicetine, Minims chloramphenicol, Sno-Phenicol) is an aminoglycoside antibiotic (➤ aminoglycosides). *Adverse effects:* Chloramphenicol may cause nausea, vomiting, diarrhoea, sore mouth and tongue, severe skin rashes and damage the bone marrow, causing blood disorders which sometimes can be very serious and cause death (e.g. aplastic anaemia). The aplastic anaemia may develop weeks or months after chloramphenicol treatment was started. Occasionally it may cause haemolytic anaemia in individuals with G6PD deficiency. High doses may cause the 'grey syndrome' in premature babies – distended abdomen, vomiting, ashen-grey colour, low temperature, progressive blue coloration, difficulty in breathing, collapse of the circulation and death in a few hours or days. A similar syndrome has been reported in adults and children given high doses of chloramphenicol. Prolonged use by mouth may knock out the bacteria in the intestine that produce vitamin K, resulting in bleeding disorders. Very rarely, prolonged use may cause nerve damage and damage to nerves of the eyes, causing blindness. It may occasionally cause allergic reactions. *Precautions:* Do not use to treat trivial infections or to prevent infections. Do not use in pregnancy or in breastfeeding mothers. Blood counts should be carried out regularly during treatment. Avoid repeated courses and prolonged treatments. Reduce dose in patients with impaired liver or kidney function. *Actinac lotion* used to treat acne contains chloramphenicol. *Chloromycetin* eye ointment and *Minims Chloromycetin* eye drops are used to treat bacterial infections of the conjunctivae. *Interactions:* Anticoagulants, anti-diabetic drugs, phenytoin.

Chlorasol wound-cleaning solution ➤ sodium hypochlorite. Do not take by mouth. Avoid contact with eyes and clothing. It may irritate the skin.

chlorbutanol (chlorbutol, in Cerumol, in Frador, in Monphytol) is a mild sedative and local pain-reliever. It has been used in anti-motion sickness preparations but is of doubtful value. It also has antibacterial and antifungal properties. It is used as a preservative in some injections, eye drops and ear drops.

chlorbutol ➤ chlorbutanol.

chlordiazepoxide (chlordiazepoxide hydrochloride, Librium, Tropium) is a benzodiazepine anti-anxiety drug ➤ benzodiazepines.

chlorhexidine (Cepton) is an antiseptic/disinfectant active against a wide range of bacteria, some fungi and some viruses. *Adverse effects:* It may, rarely, cause allergic skin reactions, and strong solutions may irritate the skin and eyes. The use of mouthwashes and dental preparations that contain chlorhexidine may discolour the teeth and tongue. They may produce a transient burning sensation of the tongue and disturbances of taste. Rarely, mouthwashes may cause 'skinning' of the mouth and swollen salivary glands. *Precautions:* It should not be used on sensitive tissue (e.g. in ear drops) and it may be absorbed into contact lenses which may then irritate the eyes. Oral gel containing chlorhexidine should not be used at the same time as dentifrices.

chlormethiazole ➤ clomethiazole.

chlormethine(mustine) (mustine hydrochloride, mechlorethamine) is an anticancer drug. See Chapter 51. *Adverse effects* include nausea, vomiting, diarrhoea, peptic ulcer, drowsiness, psychosis, loss of hair, deafness and noises in the ears (tinnitus), several months without a period (amenorrhoea), reduced sperm count and skin rashes. Damage to the bone marrow may occur, leading to severe blood disorders. Injections may produce pain, irritation and inflammation of the vein at the injection site. *Precautions:* See Chapter 51 on anticancer drugs.

chlorocresol is a disinfectant and antiseptic. It is used in various preparations for disinfection of the skin and wounds. It is also used as a preservative in creams and certain injections.

chlorofluorocarbons (CFCs) are gradually being replaced by hydrofluoroalkanes (HFAs) as propellants used in pressurized (aerosol) inhalations in the treatment of asthma.

chloroform is no longer used as an inhalation anaesthetic because of its toxicity. Chloroform water and spirit are still used in some preparations to treat wind, as a flavouring agent, or as a preservative, but because chloroform may cause cancer in animals there are doubts about the safety of using it regularly for prolonged periods of time.

Chlorohex mouthwash ➤ chlorhexidine.

Chloromycetin ➤ chloramphenicol.

chloroquinaldol (in Locoid C) has antibacterial and antifungal activities and is used to treat skin infections. *Adverse effects and Precautions* ➤ clioquinol.

chloroquine (chloroquine phosphate, chloroquine sulphate, Avloclor, Nivaquine) is used to prevent and treat malaria, amoebiasis of the liver, and giardiasis. It is also used to treat rheumatoid arthritis and similar disorders (see Chapter 32). *Adverse effects* include itching (pruritus), headache, stomach and bowel upsets, skin rashes and visional disturbances. Large doses over long periods (as used to treat rheumatoid arthritis) may produce damage to the eyes (degeneration of the retina and opacities of the cornea). White patches on the skin due to loss of pigment may occur, and it may also cause whitening of the hair, thinning of the hair, blood disorders and allergic reactions. It may cause psoriasis to flare up. Convulsions and mental breakdown may, very rarely, occur. Adverse effects are rare with doses used to treat malaria. *Precautions:* Use with caution in patients with epilepsy, porphyria (a hereditary disorder of metabolism), impaired kidney or liver function, psoriasis, blood disorders, G6PD deficiency (it should not be used to treat rheumatoid arthritis in pregnancy), and in breastfeeding mothers. Eye tests should be carried out before and at regular intervals during treatment. *Interactions:* Antacids, anti-epileptic drug.

chloroxylenol (in Rinstead gel, in Zeasorb) is used as an antiseptic and disinfectant. It is less toxic than phenol. Wet dressings in contact with the skin may produce allergic reactions.

chlorphenamine (chlorpheniramine, chlorpheniramine maleate, chlorprophenpyridamine maleate, in Haymine, Piriton) is an antihistamine ➤ antihistamines.

chlorpheniramine ➤ chlorphenamine.

chlorpromazine (chlorpromazine hydrochloride, Chloractil, Largactil) is a phenothiazine antipsychotic drug (see Chapter 3). It is also used to treat nausea and vomiting (see Chapter 18) ➤ antipsychotic drugs.

chlorpropamide is a sulphonylurea oral antidiabetic drug (Chapter 42) ➤ sulphonylureas.

chlorquinaldol (in Locoid C) has antibacterial and antifungal properties and is used in the treatment of skin infections.

chlortalidone (Hygroton, in Kalspare, in Tenoret 50, in Tenoretic) is a thiazide diuretic used to treat heart failure (Chapter 23) and raised blood pressure (Chapter 25) ➤ thiazide diuretics.

chlortetracycline (chlortetracycline hydrochloride) is a tetracycline antibiotic ➤ tetracyclines. It is available as Deteclo tablets to treat general infections and acne, as Aureomycin cream and ointment to treat bacterial skin infections and as Aureomycin eye ointment to treat eye infections sensitive to chlortetracycline. It is available combined with triamcinolone (a corticosteroid) in Aureocort used to treat infected eczemas ➤ Aureocort. *Adverse effects and Precautions* ➤ tetracyclines. Aureomycin eye and skin preparations may cause superinfection. They should not be used in the last half of pregnancy or in breastfeeding mothers.

chlorthalidone ➤ chlortalidone.

chlorthymol ➤ chlorothymol.

cholestyramine ➤ colestyramine.

choline is an essential factor in nutrition but it cannot be classified as a vitamin. It is the basic constituent of lecithin. Choline functions as a methyl donor in metabolism. The daily requirement has not been established and there are no valid reports of its effectiveness in any treatment. *Adverse effects* include nausea, vomiting, diarrhoea, depression, incontinence and a fishy odour.

choline salicylate is used to relieve pain in local applications. It has effects similar to aspirin. It is used in Audax ear drops and Bonjela and Teejel to treat mouth ulcers.

cholinesterase is an enzyme which breaks down acetylcholine at parasympathetic nerve endings. See Chapter 9.

cholinesterase inhibitors ➤ anticholinesterases.

Choragon ➤ chorionic gonadotrophin.

choriogonadotropin (Ovitrelle) is used to treat infertility. *Adverse effects* include swelling and redness at site of injection, headache, tiredness, stomach and bowel upset, abdominal pain and over-stimulation of the ovaries (ovarian hyperstimulation). *Precautions:* Do not use in patients with cancer of the hypothalamus, pituitary gland, ovaries, uterus or breast, undiagnosed vaginal bleeding, ectopic pregnancy in previous three months, blood clots (thromboembolic disorders) or in post-menopausal women.

chorionic gonadotrophin (human chorionic gonadotrophin, Choragon, HCG Gonadotraphon LH, Pregnyl, Profasi) is obtained from the urine of pregnant women. It is produced by the placenta. It has effects similar to those produced by pituitary luteinizing hormone (LH). In males it is occasionally used to stimulate sperm production associated with underworking of the pituitary gland. It has also been used to treat delayed puberty but has little advantage over testosterone (➤ testosterone). In women it is used to treat a nonovulatory infertility due to an absence or reduced production of LH and FSH (follicle stimulating hormone) by the pituitary gland. Treatment with FSH (or menotrophin) to stimulate the development of follicles is followed by chorionic gonadotrophin to stimulate ovulation. It is also used to produce superovulation in women undergoing IVF. *Adverse effects* include fluid retention especially in males (reduce the dose), headache, rash, mood changes, tenderness and enlargement of the breasts in males and females. High doses may cause sexual precocity and overstimulation (hyperstimulation) of the ovaries. *Precautions:* Use with caution in patients in whom fluid retention could be harmful, e.g. those with heart, kidney or liver disease, asthma, epilepsy, migraine, or raised blood pressure. Do not use in patients with androgen-dependent cancer.

Cicatrin preparations contain the aminoglycoside antibiotics neomycin and bacitracin, and the amino acids, cysteine, glycine and threonine. They are used to treat superficial bacterial skin infections. *Adverse effects and Precautions:* Allergic reactions and damage to hearing ➤ aminoglycosides. Do not use on large areas of damaged skin because of the risk of absorption.

ciclosporin (cyclosporin) (Neoral, Sandimmun, Sang Cya) is a potent immunosuppressant (see Chapter 17). It is used to prevent rejection in tissue and organ transplants. It is also used in the treatment of severe atopic eczema, severe psoriasis and severe active rheumatoid arthritis that have not responded to conventional treatments. *Adverse effects* include impaired kidney function (in first few weeks) and occasionally structural damage to the kidneys in patients on long-term treatment. It may cause tremor, overgrowth of body hair, raised blood pressure (especially in heart transplant patients), impaired liver function, overgrowth of the gums, fatigue, burning sensations in the hands and feet (usually during first week), rash (possibly allergic), anaemia, headache, raised blood potassium levels, raised blood uric acid levels, gout, raised blood cholesterol and magnesium levels, nerve damage, weight increase, fluid retention, confusion, painful or absent periods, muscle damage, muscle cramps and weakness, inflammation of the bowel, blood disorders, malignant tumours, lymph gland abnormalities and brain malfunction (encephalopathy). When given with spironolactone, male patients may develop enlargement of the breasts. *Precautions:* Monitor kidney function, liver function, blood pressure, blood chemistry and blood cholesterol at regular intervals. Use with caution in pregnancy, in breastfeeding mothers and in patients with raised blood potassium, uric acid or cholesterol levels or with porphyria (a hereditary disorder of metabolism). If treating *rheumatoid arthritis* do not use ciclosporin in patients with impaired kidney function, raised blood pressure not under control with anti-blood pressure drugs, infections not under control or patients suffering from malignant cancers. Carry out tests of kidney function before treatment (at least twice) and monitor every two weeks for three months and then every two weeks after that. The dose of the drug should be adjusted according to the results of kidney function tests that measure creatinine clearance. Monitor blood pressure and stop treatment if it goes up and cannot be controlled by anti-blood pressure drugs. Monitor liver function if given with an NSAID. When treating *atopic eczema* or *psoriasis* precautions are as above. Avoid excessive exposure to the sun's rays and the use of UVB and PUVA. If patients with atopic eczema develop herpes simplex (cold sores) allow to clear before starting treatment and stop if it develops and is severe during treatment. *Interactions:* Systemic antibiotics, live vaccines, phenytoin, ketoconazole, fluconazole, itraconazole, erythromycin, rifampicin, carbamazepine, barbiturates, calcium-channel blockers, colchicine, oral contraceptives, propafenone, prednisolone, methyl prednisolone, potassium supplements, potassium-sparing diuretics, NSAIDs, grapefruit juice.

cidofovir (Vistide) is used in combination with probenecid in cytomegalovirus (CMV) inflammation of the retina in AIDS patients. See Chapter 48. *Adverse effects* include protein in the urine, blood disorders, weakness, creatinine increase, fever, hair loss, nausea, rash, kidney failure (sometimes fatal), hearing disturbances, inflammation of the pancreas, lack of muscle tone in the eye. *Precautions:* Do not insert into the eye or use in patients with kidney damage, in pregnancy or while breastfeeding. Use with caution in patients with diabetes.

Cidomycin preparations ➤ gentamicin.

cilastatin is combined with imipenem in Primaxin. It blocks an enzyme in the kidneys that partially breaks down imipenem ➤ Primaxin.

cilazapril (Vascace) is used to treat raised blood pressure (see Chapter 25). It is also used with digoxin and/or diuretics to treat chronic heart failure (see Chapter 23). It is an ACE inhibitor (see p. 123) which is rapidly metabolized in the lining of the stomach and intestine and in the liver to its active metabolite, cilazaprilate. *Adverse effects* include headache, dizziness, fatigue, nausea, indigestion, coughing and skin rashes. Rarely it may cause allergic reactions (angioedema) and blood disorders. *Precautions:* Do not use in patients with fluid in the abdomen (ascites), obstruction to the flow of blood from the heart into the main artery (e.g. aortic stenosis), in pregnancy or in breastfeeding mothers. Do not use in patients with hypertrophic cardiomyopathy. Use with caution in patients with impaired kidney or liver function, congestive heart failure, salt or fluid loss, during surgery or anaesthesia. Do not use in patients who have suffered from allergic reactions after previous ACE inhibitor treatment. *Interactions:* Potassium-sparing diuretics, NSAIDs, potassium supplements, anti-diabetic drugs, lithium, desensitization preparations, corticosteroids, procainamide.

Cilest is a combined oral contraceptive drug. See p. 216.

Ciloxan ➤ ciprofloxacin.

cimetidine (Acitak, in Algitec, Dyspamet, Galenamet, Tagamet, Zita) is an H_2 antihistamine blocker used to treat stomach and duodenal ulcers, including those produced by non-steroidal anti-inflammatory drugs (NSAIDs), see Chapter 19. It is also used to treat acid reflux (see p. 99) and other disorders where a reduction in stomach acid is beneficial. *Adverse effects* include diarrhoea, tiredness, dizziness. Occasionally it may cause confusion (especially in the elderly) and liver damage. Very rarely, it may cause headache, painful muscles and joints, blood disorders, changes in kidney function, pancreatic function and heart rate, heart block and loss of hair. In men, prolonged use of high doses may cause enlargement of the breasts and impotence. These feminization effects are reversible when the drug is stopped. *Precautions:* Do not use in patients who are allergic to it. Use with caution in patients with impaired liver or kidney function (reduce the dose) and exclude stomach cancer before starting treatment because the drug may mask the symptoms. Use with caution in pregnancy and in breastfeeding mothers. *Interactions:* Cimetidine affects enzymes in the liver that metabolize certain drugs. It may interact with the following drugs: oral anticoagulants, phenytoin, theophylline, lignocaine, diazepam, chlordiazepoxide, propranolol, imipramine, morphine.

Cinaziere ➤ cinnarizine.

cinchocaine (in Proctosedyl, in Scheriproct, in Ultraproct, in Uniroid HC) is a local anaesthetic.

cinnarizine (Cinaziere, Stugeron, Stugeron Forte) is an antihistamine. It is used to treat nausea, dizziness and motion sickness (see Chapter 18). In high doses it is used to treat disorders of the peripheral circulation (see Chapter 27). *Adverse effects and Precautions* ➤ antihistamines.

Cipramil ➤ citalopram.

ciprofibrate (Modalim) is a fibrate drug used to lower blood cholesterol and fat levels. See Chapter 26. *Adverse effects* include stomach and bowel upsets, vertigo, headache, hair loss, impotence, fatigue, muscle damage causing weakness and pains and rarely dizziness and drowsiness. *Precautions:* Do not use in patients with severe impairment of liver or kidney function, low blood albumin levels or gall-bladder disease, in pregnancy or in breastfeeding mothers. Use with utmost caution in patients with mild or moderate impairment of liver or kidney function or underworking of the thyroid gland. Patients should report unexplained muscle weakness or pains immediately. Periodic tests of liver function should be carried out (➤ fibrates for warnings on muscle damage). *Interactions:* Anticoagulants, oral anti-diabetic drugs, oral contraceptives, statins, fibrates.

ciprofloxacin (Cilovan eye drops, Ciproxin) is a quinoline antibacterial drug, see p. 272. *Adverse effects* include nausea, vomiting and diarrhoea, dizziness, headache, tremor, confusion, convulsions, blurred vision, joint pains, sleep disturbances, tiredness and allergic reactions (skin rashes and itching). It may affect ability to perform skilled tasks (e.g. motor driving) and, very rarely, cause disturbed liver and kidney function, sensitivity of the skin to sunlight, severe skin rashes, transient hearing loss, inflammation of a tendon (stop treatment and rest the limb), impaired taste and smell, blood disorders, Stevens-Johnson syndrome (a severe form of inflammatory skin disease), inflammation of the bowel and rapid beating of the heart. Injections may cause pain and inflammation at the site of injection. *Precautions:* It should not be used in pregnancy and breastfeeding mothers and preferably not in children or growing adolescents. It should be used with caution in patients with epilepsy or severe kidney impairments. Patients should drink plenty of fluids. It should be used with caution in patients with G6PD deficiency. *Interactions:* theophylline, cyclosporin, magnesium, aluminium or iron salts, anticoagulants, NSAIDs, glibenclamide, opiate pain-relievers, probenecid. Ciprofloxacin is included in Ciloxan eye drops used to treat corneal ulcers and bacterial infections of the eyes. *Adverse effects* include transient local irritation, bitter taste and skin rashes (stop immediately). *Precautions:* Do not wear soft contact lenses while on treatment. Use with caution in pregnancy and breastfeeding mothers.

Ciproxin ➤ ciprofloxacin.

cisatracurium (Nimbex injections) is a non-depolarizing muscle relaxant (see p. 42) used during surgery and intensive care. *Precautions:* Do not use in pregnancy. Use with caution in patients with myasthenia gravis (muscle weakness due to neuromuscular abnormality), allergy to neuromuscular blocking drugs, burns, or who have disturbances of their serum electrolytes. *Interactions:* General anaesthetics, other non-depolarizing muscle relaxants, suxamethonium, antibiotics, anti-arrhythmic drugs, diuretics, ganglion blockers, magnesium and lithium salts, phenytoin, carbamazepine.

cisplatin is an anti-cancer drug (see Chapter 51). It is of particular use in cancer of the testicles and cancer of the ovaries (Platinex). *Adverse effects* include severe nausea and vomiting, damage to the bone marrow producing blood disorders, damage to the kidneys, damage to the nerves of the ear producing tinnitus and deafness, damage to the nerves producing pins and needles in the arms and legs, loss of taste, allergic reactions characterized by swelling of the face, wheezing, rapid beating of the heart and falling blood pressure within a few minutes of drug administration. It may also cause a rise in blood uric acid levels and a fall in magnesium levels. *Precautions:* It should not normally be used in patients with impaired function of their kidneys, bone marrow, nervous system or hearing. It should not be used in patients with a history of allergy to cisplatin or other platinum-containing compounds. It should not be

used in pregnancy or in breastfeeding mothers. It may affect fertility. Since severe allergic reactions may occur in the first few minutes of administration, adrenaline(epinephrine), a corticosteroid and an antihistamine drug should always be at hand. Kidney function, the nervous system and hearing should be monitored throughout the period of treatment.

citalopram (Cipramil) is a 5HT re-uptake blocker used to treat depression. See Chapter 4. *Adverse effects* include nausea, dry mouth, sleepiness, tremor and sweating. *Precautions:* Use with caution in pregnancy, in breastfeeding mothers and in patients with severe impairment of kidney or liver function. *Interactions:* MAOIs, 5HT stimulants, lithium, tryptophan and antipsychotic drugs. Also see adverse effects and precautions listed under fluoxetine (Prozac).

Citanest ➤ prilocaine.

Citramag is an osmotic laxative (see Chapter 21). It is an effervescent powder of magnesium citrate in a sachet. The contents are dissolved in water and taken by mouth to empty the bowel the day before X-ray of, or surgery on, the bowel. It should be used with caution in patients with kidney failure and in the elderly. Patients should drink plenty of fluids and have a low-residue diet the day before the X-ray or surgery.

cladribine (Leustat) is an anti-cancer drug. See Chapter 51. It is used to treat hairy cell leukaemia. *Adverse effects* include damage to the bone marrow producing blood disorders, kidney damage and nerve damage. It may cause fatigue, fever, headache, rash, fluid retention (oedema), rapid beating of the heart, affect breathing and cause muscle pains and cough. *Precautions:* Do not use in pregnancy or in breastfeeding mothers. Use with caution in patients with impaired kidney or liver function or severe bone-marrow damage. Blood counts and kidney and liver function tests must be carried out at regular intervals. Stop the drug at the earliest signs of kidney or nerve damage. *Interaction:*

Other drugs that may damage the bone marrow.

Claforan ➤ cefotaxime.

Clariteyes eye drops ➤ sodium cromoglycate.

clarithromycin (in Heliclear, in Helimet, Klaricid) is a semi-synthetic derivation of the macrolide antibiotic erythromycin (see p. 268). It is better absorbed than erythromycin because it is not affected by the acid in the stomach. *Adverse effects* include nausea, vomiting, diarrhoea, abdominal pains, headache and skin rashes. *Precautions:* It should be used with special caution in patients with impaired kidney or liver function, in pregnancy and in breastfeeding mothers. *Interactions:* Theophylline, oral anticoagulants, digoxin, carbamazepine, terfenadine.

Clarityn ➤ loratadine.

clavulanic acid has little antibacterial action of its own, but enhances the effects of penicillins. By inactivating penicillinase produced by bacteria, the resistance of these bacteria to penicillins is destroyed. It is combined with amoxycillin in *Augmentin* and with ticarcillin in *Timentin*.

clemastine (Tavegil) is a non-sedative antihistamine ➤ antihistamines. *Adverse effects* include drowsiness and rarely bowel and stomach upsets, headache, dizziness, dry mouth, palpitations, excitement, weakness, skin rashes, fatigue and heartburn. *Precautions:* use with utmost caution in pregnancy, in breastfeeding mothers, in patients who suffer from glaucoma, who have difficulty passing urine (e.g. enlarged prostate gland) or any narrowing of the outlet from the stomach (e.g. due to scarring from a duodenal ulcer). *Interactions:* Alcohol, sedatives, sleeping drugs (and any other drug that depresses brain function), MAOIs.

Clexane ➤ enoxaparin.

Climagest preparations contain tablets of oestradiol (an oestrogen) and norethisterone (a progestogen). They are used as HRT ➤ HRT.

Climaval ➤ oestradiol. It is used as hormone replacement treatment in women who have had a hysterectomy ➤ HRT.

Climesse is a bleed-free HRT. It is used to treat women at least twelve months past their last natural period. Each tablet contains oestradiol (an oestrogen) and norethisterone (a progestogen). One tablet is taken *daily* without a break. Irregular bleeding may occur in the first few months of treatment. If taken too soon after the menopause, menstrual bleeding may occur and another form of HRT should be used. *Adverse effects* ➤ HRT.

clindamycin (Dalacin C) is a lincosamide antibiotic (see p. 269). *Adverse effects:* It may cause nausea, vomiting, severe diarrhoea and inflammation of the bowel. It may, rarely, cause blood disorders and jaundice. *Precautions:* Do not use in patients who are allergic to lincomycin. Use with caution in patients with impaired kidney or liver function. Stop if severe diarrhoea develops. *Interactions:* Neuromuscular blocking drugs. Clindamycin is used as cream (Dalacin cream) to treat bacterial vaginal infection. Applied to the vagina it may cause irritation and it may be absorbed into the bloodstream to cause stomach and bowel upsets, severe diarrhoea and inflammation of the bowel (stop immediately). Barrier contraceptives may be less effective. Do not use if the patient is allergic to lincomycin. Clindamycin is also used as a roll-on lotion (Dalacin T) to treat acne. It may cause dry skin or dermatitis.

Clinitar preparations ➤ coal tar.

Clinoril ➤ sulindac.

clioquinol (iodochlorhydroxquinoline) is an antiseptic (see p. 244). It is used in Betnovate C, Locorten-Vioform, Synalar C, Vioform-hydrocortisone. *Adverse effects:* It stains the skin yellow and may cause irritation. *Precautions:* It should not be taken by mouth to treat traveller's diarrhoea because it may damage the nerves of the arms, legs and eyes (myelo-optico-neuropathy).

Clivarine ➤ reviparin.

clobazam (Frisium) is a benzodiazepine used to treat anxiety (see Chapter 2) and epilepsy (see Chapter 15). *Adverse effects and Precautions* ➤ benzodiazepines.

clobetasol (clobetasol propionate, Dermovate, in Dermovate-NN) is a very potent corticosteroid used in skin applications to treat eczema and psoriasis. See corticosteroid skin applications, p. 241.

clobetasone (clobetasone butyrate, Eumovate, in Trimovate) is a moderately potent corticosteroid used in skin applications to treat eczema and psoriasis. See corticosteroid skin applications, p. 241. It is also used in Cloburate eye drops to treat non-infected, inflammatory eye disorders.

Cloburate eye drops ➤ clobetasone.

clodronate sodium ➤ sodium clodronate.

clofazimine (Lamprene) is used in the treatment of leprosy. *Adverse effects:* It may cause stomach and bowel upsets, dry eyes, weight loss, dry skin, itching, and it may colour the urine, skin, hair and secretions red. *Precautions:* Use with caution in pregnancy, breastfeeding mothers, patients with impaired kidney or liver function, and patients with diarrhoea and abdominal pain.

clomethiazole (Heminevrin) is used as a sleeping drug (see Chapter 1), to treat epilepsy (see Chapter 15) and alcohol withdrawal symptoms. *Adverse effects* include headache, nausea, vomiting, nasal congestion and sneezing, sore eyes, dizziness, rashes, stomach and bowel upsets, allergic reactions, drowsiness, excitement and confusion. *Precautions:* Do not use in breastfeeding mothers or in patients with severe chest trouble or in alcoholics who continue to drink. Use with caution in patients with long-term chest complaints, impaired kidney or liver function. It may increase the

effects of alcohol and other depressant drugs. It may trigger off depression in someone who suffers from episodes of severe depressive illness (manic-depressive psychosis). It may interfere with the ability to drive or operate machinery. *Drug dependence* of the barbiturate/alcohol type may develop quickly in certain individuals. Avoid prolonged use and sudden withdrawal. *Interactions:* alcohol, sedatives, sleeping drugs, diazoxide, propranolol, cimetidine.

Clomid ➤ clomifene.

clomifene (clomiphene citrate, Clomid) is used to treat infertility caused by failure to ovulate. It is an anti-oestrogen (see p. 198). *Adverse effects* include hot flushes, nausea, vomiting, dizziness, headache, depression and mood changes, insomnia, breast tenderness, weight gain, abdominal discomfort, ovarian enlargement, skin rashes, hair thinning, visual disturbances (stop immediately), spotting, heavy periods and rarely, convulsions. Over-stimulation (hyperstimulation) of the ovaries may occur (stop treatment if this happens). *Precautions:* It should not be used in patients with liver disease, large ovarian cysts, cancer of the womb or bleeding from the womb, or in pregnancy. Patients should be warned of the possibility of multiple births. Pregnancy should be tested for before and during treatment. Use with caution in polycystic ovary syndrome. Monitor for ovarian hyperstimulation (OHSS), ectopic pregnancy, multiple birth and visual symptoms. Do not use for longer than six menstrual cycles because of the risk of cancer of the ovary if treated for more than six months.

clomiphene ➤ clomifene.

clomipramine (clomipramine hydrochloride, Anafranil) is a tricyclic antidepressant drug. See Chapter 4 and ➤ tricyclic antidepressants.

clonazepam (Rivotril) is a benzodiazepine drug used to treat epilepsy. See Chapter 15 and ➤ benzodiazepines.

clonidine (Catapres, Dixarit) is a central

alpha stimulant used to treat raised blood pressure (see Chapter 25), prevent migraine (see Chapter 34) and relieve menopausal flushing (see p. 201). *Adverse effects* include drowsiness, dry mouth, dizziness, headache and constipation. Occasionally it may cause fluid retention, mood changes, disturbed sleep, vivid dreams and impotence. *Precautions:* Do not use in patients with mental depression. Use with caution in patients with porphyria (a hereditary disorder of metabolism) or disorders of the circulation. Treatment should be stopped gradually over several days in order to avoid a sudden rebound rise in the blood pressure. Use with caution in breastfeeding mothers. *Interactions:* Tricyclic antidepressants, other anti-blood pressure drugs, alpha-blockers, sedatives, sleeping drugs (and other drugs that depress brain function). It may impair ability to drive because it causes drowsiness.

clopamide (in Viskaldix) is a thiazide diuretic ➤ thiazide diuretics.

clopidogrel (Plavix) is an anti-platelet drug used to treat strokes (from day seven until less than six months), heart attack (from a few days until less than thirty-five days), or established peripheral artery disease. See Chapter 28. *Adverse effects* include bleeding, stomach and bowel upsets, skin reactions and nervous system, liver, gall bladder and blood disorders. *Precautions:* Do not use in patients with severe liver damage, active bleeding (e.g. from a peptic ulcer or bleeding from the brain), unstable angina, acute stroke of less than seven days, in pregnancy or while breastfeeding. Use with caution in patients with moderate impairment of liver function, risk of bleeding (e.g. in injury, surgery, acute peptic ulcer or bleeding inside the eyes). Unusual bleeding should be reported.

Clopixol Acuphase oily injection ➤ zuclopenthixol.

Clopixol preparations ➤ zuclopenthixol.

cloral betaine (Welldorm tablets) is a sleeping drug (see Chapter 1) that is broken down in the body to chloral hydrate ➤ chloral hydrate.

clorazepate dipotassium (Tranxene) is a long-acting benzodiazepine used to treat anxiety ➤ benzodiazepines.

Clostet ➤ tetanus vaccine.

Clostridium botulinum type A toxin ➤ Dysport.

Clotam Rapid ➤ tolfenamic acid.

clotrimazole (Canesten, Candiden) is an antifungal drug (see Chapter 47) used in Canesten preparations to treat vaginal infections, outer ear infections and skin infections, in Lotriderm preparations to treat fungal skin infections and in Masnoderm to treat fungal skin infections and vaginal infections. Applied to the skin, ears or vagina it may rarely cause a local burning sensation and irritation and very rarely allergic reactions.

clozapine (Clozaril) is an antipsychotic drug (➤ antipsychotic drugs). It blocks many neurotransmitters in the brain but has less effect than other antipsychotic drugs on blocking dopamine; it therefore produces fewer involuntary movements. *Adverse effects:* Its principal adverse effect is that it may produce a life-threatening fall in the white blood cell count. In addition it may cause drowsiness, fatigue, rapid beating of the heart, stomach and bowel upsets, increased production of saliva, dizziness, headache, urinary retention, incontinence, fall in blood pressure on standing up after sitting or lying down, arrest of the heart and breathing, convulsions, transient parkinsonism, damage to the heart, persistent erection (priapism), disturbances of temperature regulation, raised blood sugar, skin rashes, weight gain and EEG and ECG changes. It may impair judgement and the ability to perform learnt tasks (e.g. driving motor vehicles). *Precautions:* Do not use in patients suffering from psychoses due to alcohol or drugs, who are comatose, or in patients with a history of drug-induced blood disorders, or who have circulatory collapse, severe heart, liver or kidney disease or in breastfeeding mothers. Use with utmost caution in pregnancy and in patients with epilepsy, enlarged prostate gland, glaucoma or an obstruction in the intestine caused by lack of muscle tone (paralytic ileus). Use adequate contraception while on treatment. White blood counts must be carried out before and during treatment. Patients should report any symptoms of infection, for example, sore throat or fever. It should be used cautiously in patients with mild and moderate impairment of liver function, and tests of liver function should be carried out before and at regular intervals during treatment. The drug should be stopped gradually. *Interactions:* Any drug that depresses bone-marrow function, sedatives, sleeping drugs (or any drug that depresses brain function).

Clozaril ➤ clozapine.

coal tar extract (in Alphosyl, in Alphosyl HC, in Clinitar, in Exorex, in Polytar, in Pragmatar) relieves itching of the skin and it has mild antiseptic properties. *Adverse effects* include irritation of the skin, acne-like eruptions and sensitization of the skin to the sun's rays. Rarely, it may produce an allergic rash. *Precautions:* Avoid contact with eyes, or broken or inflamed skin. It may stain the skin, hair and fabrics and it smells of tar. It is used to treat eczema, psoriasis and dandruff.

co-amilofruse (Fru-Co, Frumil, Lasoride) contains the loop diuretic furosemide (frusemide) and the potassium-sparing diuretic amiloride. It is used to treat fluid retention associated with heart failure, liver or kidney disease, particularly when it is important to avoid a fall in blood potassium levels ➤ amiloride, furosemide(frusemide) and see Chapter 29 on diuretics. *Adverse effects* include stomach and bowel upsets, generally feeling unwell, rash and very rarely blood disorders. *Precautions:* Do not use in patients with severe impairment of liver or kidney function or high blood potassium levels. Do not use in pregnancy or in breastfeeding mothers. Use with caution in patients with impairment of kidney or liver function, the elderly, patients with diabetes, prostatic enlargement or difficulty in passing urine, gout or acidosis. *Interactions:* Potassium-sparing diuretics, lithium, digoxin and related drugs.

co-amilozide (Amil-Co, Moduret 25, Moduretic) contains the potassium-sparing diuretic amiloride and the thiazide diuretic hydrochlorthiazide. It is used to treat congestive heart failure, raised blood pressure, and cirrhosis of the liver with ascites, particularly when it is important to avoid a fall in blood potassium levels ➤ amiloride, thiazide diuretics and see Chapter 29 on diuretics. *Adverse effects* include rash, sensitivity of the skin to sunlight, blood disorders, gout. *Precautions:* Do not use in patients with a high blood potassium level or severe kidney failure. Do not use in pregnancy or in breastfeeding mothers. Use with caution in patients with diabetes, acidosis, gout or impaired liver or kidney function. *Interactions:* Potassium supplements, potassium-sparing diuretics, digoxin or a related drug, lithium, anti-blood pressure drugs, ACE inhibitors.

co-amoxiclav (Amiclav, Augmentin) contains the beta-lactamase inhibitor clavulanic acid, and the broad-spectrum penicillin amoxycillin ➤ clavulanic acid, penicillins and see penicillins p. 267. *Warning:* Liver damage, jaundice, severe skin disorders and kidney damage have been reported. Also phlebitis at the site of injection. Do not use for more than fourteen days without careful assessment. Jaundice may occur up to six weeks after co-amoxiclav has been stopped. Clavulanic acid is probably the culprit.

Co-Aprovel is a combination product used in the treatment of hypertension, containing irbesartan and hydrochlorothiazide ➤ irbesartan, hydrochlorothiazide.

Cobalin-H ➤ hydroxocobalamin (vitamin B_{12}).

co-beneldopa (Madopar) contains the

dopa-decarboxylase inhibitor benserazide, and the dopamine precursor levodopa. It is used to treat parkinsonism (see Chapter 16). *Adverse effects and Precautions* ➤ levodopa.

Co-Betaloc preparations contain metoprolol (a selective beta-blocker) and hydrochlorothiazide (a thiazide diuretic). They are used to treat raised blood pressure (see Chapter 25). *Adverse effects and Precautions* ➤ beta-blockers, thiazide diuretics.

COC (combined oral contraceptives), see Chapter 41.

cocaine is the oldest local anaesthetic, but because of adverse effects and risk of drug dependence it is hardly ever used except for local application to the eyes, ears or nose. Unlike all other local anaesthetics it constricts small blood vessels and need not be given with adrenaline(epinephrine). *Adverse effects:* Some people have an idiosyncrasy to cocaine and may become seriously ill, even after a small dose. They develop headaches, faintness and may suddenly collapse and die. In other patients it may cause the general adverse effects of any local anaesthetic – excitation, restlessness, nausea, yawning and vomiting which may be followed by pallor, sweating, fall in blood pressure, twitching, convulsions and unconsciousness. *Precautions:* It should not be given to patients with myasthenia gravis (muscle weakness due to neuromuscular abnormality) and it should be given with caution to patients with disordered heart rhythm or with impaired liver function.

co-careldopa (Sinemet) contains the dopadecarboxylase inhibitor carbidopa, and the dopamine precursor levodopa. It is used to treat parkinsonism (see Chapter 16). *Adverse effects and Precautions* ➤ levodopa.

co-codamol (Parake) contains paracetamol and codeine. It is used to relieve mild to moderate pain. *Adverse effects and Precautions* ➤ paracetamol, codeine.

co-codaprin preparations contain aspirin and codeine. They are used to relieve mild to moderate pain. *Adverse effects and Precautions* ➤ aspirin, codeine.

Cocois scalp ointment contains coal tar, salicylic acid and sulphur in a coconut oil moisturising base. It is used to prevent itching and to remove dead skin in the treatment of chronic eczema and psoriasis of the scalp. *Adverse effects:* It may irritate the skin. *Precautions:* Do not use if scalp is acutely infected or in pustular psoriasis.

co-cyprindiol (Dianette) is a combination of cyproterone acetate and ethinylestradiol used in the treatment of acne in women who also wish to use oral contraception ➤ cyproterone, ethinylestradiol.

coconut oil is used to form absorbable ointment bases for scalp applications. It is used in the manufacture of 'marine' soaps.

Codafen Continus modified release tablets contain ibuprofen (a non-steroidal anti-inflammatory drug) and codeine (a narcotic (opiate) pain-reliever). *Adverse effects and Precautions:* ➤ non-steroidal anti-inflammatory drugs, codeine.

Codalax ➤ co-danthramer.

co-danthramer (Ailax, Codalax) is a laxative (see Chapter 21). It contains a faecal softener (poloxamer 188) and a stimulant laxative (dantron). *Adverse effects and Precautions* ➤ dantron.

co-danthrusate (Capsuvac, Normax) is a laxative (see Chapter 21). It contains the stimulant laxative dantron, and the faecal softener docusate sodium. *Adverse effects and Precautions* ➤ dantron.

codeine (codeine phosphate, codeine sulphate) is an opiate pain-reliever (see Chapter 30). It is a weak cough suppressant (see Chapter 11) and it is also of value in treating diarrhoea (see Chapter 20). *Adverse effects:* The commonest adverse effects are constipation, nausea, vomiting, dry mouth, dizziness and drowsiness. Very rarely, skin rashes may occur in patients who are allergic to codeine. *Precautions:* Codeine should not be given to patients suffering from severe respiratory disorders (e.g. chronic bronchitis). It should be used with caution in patients suffering from an under-active thyroid gland, chronic liver disease, in the elderly and in women in labour. Individuals may become tolerant to effects of codeine. *Drug dependence:* Prolonged use of high doses may rarely produce dependence of the morphine type: see p. xxviii. *Interactions:* Alcohol, MAOIs, sleeping drugs, sedatives and other drugs that depress brain function.

co-dergocrine (co-dergocrine mesylate, Hydergine) is an ergot alkaloid used to stimulate brain cells in elderly patients with mild to moderate dementia (see p. 138). *Adverse effects* include nausea, vomiting, flushing, headache, cramps in the abdomen, blocked nose, dizziness, rash, and fall in blood pressure on standing up after lying or sitting down (may cause faintness and light-headedness). *Precautions:* Use with caution in patients with severe slowing of the heart rate.

Codis tablets contain codeine and aspirin (500 mg). They are used to relieve mild to moderate pain. *Adverse effects and Precautions:* ➤ codeine, aspirin.

cod liver oil is a rich source of vitamins A and D and essential unsaturated fatty acids. It is also included in some soothing ointments, e.g. Morhulin.

co-dydramol preparations contain paracetamol and dihydrocodeine. They are used to relieve mild to moderate pain. *Adverse effects and Precautions* ➤ paracetamol, dihydrocodeine.

co-fluampicil (Magnapen) contains the broad-spectrum penicillin ampicillin, and the penicillinase-resistant penicillin flucloxacillin. *Adverse effects and Precautions* ➤ penicillins.

co-flumactone preparations (e.g. Aldactide) contain the thiazide diuretic hydroflumethiazide, and a potassium-sparing diuretic spironolactone (aldosterone blocker). They are used to treat congestive heart failure ➤ thiazide diuretics,

spironolactone and see Chapter 29 on diuretics. *Adverse effects* include disturbances of salt and water balance in the body, stomach and bowel upsets, loss of control over voluntary movements (ataxia), rash, confusion, sensitivity of the skin to sunlight, enlargement of the breasts (males and females), deepening of the voice, irregularities of the menstrual periods, blood disorders. *Precautions:* Do not use in patients with severe impairment of liver or kidney function, high blood potassium levels, high blood calcium levels, Addison's disease, breastfeeding mothers, or in patients allergic to sulphonamide drugs. Use with caution in patients with mild or moderate impairment of liver or kidney function, cirrhosis of the liver, diabetes, gout, or systemic lupus erythematosis (a disease of unknown cause with symptoms of fever, muscle and joint pain, blood disorders and skin eruptions). Use with utmost caution in pregnancy. Regular monitoring of blood chemistry should be carried out. Be cautious about long-term use in young patients and in the elderly. *Interactions:* Potassium supplements, potassium-sparing diuretics, ACE inhibitors, digoxin and related drugs, carbenoxolone, NSAIDs, lithium and antidiabetic drugs.

Cogentin ➤ benzatropine.

Colazide ➤ balsalazide.

colchicine is used to treat acute gout (see Chapter 33). *Adverse effects:* Large doses quickly produce diarrhoea, nausea, vomiting and abdominal pains. Bone-marrow damage (causing blood disorders), muscle and nerve damage, kidney damage, loss of hair and skin rashes may, rarely, occur with prolonged use. Irritation and thrombophlebitis (inflammation of the vein) may, rarely, occur at the site of injection. *Precautions:* Colchicine should be given with caution to the elderly and debilitated and to patients who suffer from impaired heart, liver or kidney function, or disorders of the stomach or intestine (e.g. colitis). Use with the utmost caution in pregnancy and breastfeeding mothers. *Interactions:* Cyclosporin.

colecalciferol (in Adcal D3, in Cacit D3, in Caleos, in Calcichew D3) is vitamin D3. See Chapter 36.

Colestid preparations ➤ colestipol.

colestipol (colestipol hydrochloride, Colestid) is used to lower blood cholesterol and fat levels (see Chapter 26). *Adverse effects and Precautions* are similar to those described under cholestyramine ➤ cholestyramine. Use with caution in pregnancy and breastfeeding mothers. Supplements of fat-soluble vitamins A, D, E and K may be required. *Interactions:* digitalis, antibiotics, diuretics.

colestyramine (cholestyramine, Questran, Questran Light) breaks down bile salts in the intestine and is used to treat raised cholesterol and blood fat levels (see Chapter 26). It is also used to break down bile salts in patients who suffer from diarrhoea associated with surgical removal of part of the small intestine, Crohn's disease or radiation treatment, and to relieve itching in patients with a partial obstruction of the bile system. *Adverse effects* include constipation, heartburn, wind, nausea, vomiting and diarrhoea. It may rarely cause skin rashes and high doses may cause fats to appear in the stools (steatorrhoea). Long-term use may interfere with the absorption of fat-soluble vitamins (A, D, E and K) – lack of vitamin K may result in a tendency to bleed easily. *Precautions:* Do not use if the bile system is obstructed. Use with caution in pregnancy and in breastfeeding mothers. Patients on long-term treatment should be given supplements of vitamins A, D, E and K. *Interactions:* Digitalis, antibiotics, diuretics, warfarin, thyroxine. Take any other drug one hour before or four–six hours after taking Questran or Questran Light. Questran Light contains the artificial sweetener aspartane, therefore use with caution in patients with phenylketonurea.

colfosceril (Exosurf) is a synthetic surfactant (lubricant) used to treat respiratory distress syndrome (RDS), a hyaline membrane disease in premature babies. In this condition the lungs are immature and because of a lack of natural lubricant (surfactant), the air sacs collapse when the baby breathes out. Colfosceril acts like the natural surfactant; it stops the air sacs from collapsing, improves exchange of gases and reduces the risks of mechanical ventilation. It may cause bleeding in the lungs. The baby must be carefully monitored to avoid too much oxygen entering the blood.

Colifoam aerosol contains hydrocortisone. It is used to treat inflammatory disorders of the bowel and rectum. *Adverse effects* see Chapter 37 on corticosteroids. *Precautions:* Do not use if there is obstruction, perforation or abscess of the bowel and do not use if there is a tuberculous, fungal or viral infection of the bowel. Use with utmost caution in pregnancy and severe ulcerative disease. Avoid prolonged use.

colistimethate sodium (colistin, Colomycin) is a polymyxin antibiotic. *Adverse effects* by mouth and injection include myasthenia gravis (muscle weakness due to neuromuscular abnormality), vertigo, and pins and needles round the mouth and in the hands and feet. Very rarely, it may cause slurred speech, confusion, visual disturbances, kidney damage and the breathing to stop for a moment (apnoea). *Precautions:* Do not use in patients with myasthenia gravis, in pregnancy or in breastfeeding mothers. The dose should be reduced in patients with impaired kidney function. Use with caution in patients with porphyria (a hereditary disorder of metabolism).

colistin ➤ colistimethate sodium.

collodion ➤ pyroxylin.

Colofac preparations ➤ mebeverine.

Colomycin ➤ colistimethate sodium.

colophony is obtained from volatile oils from various species of pine. It is an ingredient of some collodions and plaster-masses and was previously used in ointments for treating boils, etc.

Colpermin ➤ peppermint oil.

co-magaldrox (Maalox, Mucogel) is a mixture of aluminium hydroxide and magnesium hydroxide. It is used as an antacid. (See Chapter 19.) *Adverse effects and Precautions:* ➤ antacids.

combined oral contraceptives (COC), see Chapter 41.

Combivent aerosol inhalation contains ipratropium (antimuscarinic) and salbutamol (selective beta-stimulant). It is used to treat asthma (Chapter 14). *Adverse effects* ➤ ipratropium, salbutamol. It may cause tremor, nervousness, dizziness, headache, rapid beating of the heart, dry mouth, irritation of the throat, retention of urine and a fall in blood potassium levels. *Precautions* ➤ ipratropium, salbutamol. Use with caution in patients with severe disorders of the heart or circulation, disordered heart rhythm, diabetes, over-active thyroid, recent heart attack (myocardial infarction), in pregnancy or in breastfeeding mothers. *Interactions:* Corticosteroids, theophylline, caffeine, diuretics, sympathomimetic drugs, antimuscarinic drugs, beta-blockers.

Combivir is a combination of the two antiviral agents zidovudine and lamivudine ➤ zidovudine, lamivudine.

co-methiamol (Paradote) is a mixture of methionine and paracetamol; methionine has no analgesic activity but it may prevent paracetamol induced liver toxicity which could occur in overdose ➤ paracetamol.

Comixco ➤ co-trimoxazole.

Comtess ➤ entacapone.

Condyline solution ➤ podophyllotoxin.

conjugated oestrogens are natural oestrogens obtained from the urine of pregnant mares. They are used in HRT ➤ oestrogens, HRT.

Conotrane cream contains the water-repellent dimethicone and the antiseptic benzalkonium. It is used to treat nappy rash and pressure sores ➤ dimethicone, benzalkonium.

Contac 400 is a combination product for the treatment of head colds, containing phenylpropanolamine and chlorphenamine ➤ phenylpropanolamine, chlorphenamine.

Contigen is purified collagen from the skin of cattle. It comes in pre-filled syringes and is used to inject into the neck of the bladder to tighten it up in the treatment of patients suffering from incontinence of urine due to ineffective closure of the bladder neck (see p. 283). *Adverse effects* include urinary tract infections, retention of urine and discomfort and bleeding at the site of injection. *Precautions:* Do not use in patients allergic to bovine collagen (skin tests come free with the treatment kits) or to bovine products. Do not use in patients who suffer from severe allergies, a history of autoimmune disease, acute infection of the bladder or urethra or stricture of the bladder neck or urethra Perform skin tests for allergy four weeks before procedure and repeat if results are doubtful. Do not use in pregnancy or breastfeeding mothers. Patients should report immediately if they develop any swelling or discomfort after the procedure has been carried out.

Contimin ➤ oxybutynin.

contraceptives, oral, see Chapter 41.

Convulex ➤ sodium valporate.

Copaxone ➤ glatiramer.

co-phenetrope preparations (e.g. Lomotil) contain the opiate diphenoxylate, and the antimuscarinic drug atropine. They are used to treat diarrhoea. See Chapter 20. *Adverse effects and Precautions* ➤ antimuscarinic drugs, diphenoxylate. Do not use in patients with intestinal obstruction, acute ulcerative colitis (diarrhoeal disorder), pseudomembranous colitis (colitis caused by antibiotics), or jaundice. Use with caution in patients with impaired liver function, in pregnancy and in breastfeeding mothers. Correct fluid and electrolytes before starting treatment. *Warning:* Young children are susceptible to overdose and symptoms may be delayed so keep under observation for forty-eight hours after ingestion.

copper acts as a contraceptive when present in the uterus (IUD). Copper is an essential trace element in the diet. There is no evidence that wearing a copper bracelet for the treatment of rheumatic disorders has any effect.

co-prenozide (Trasidrex) contains the non-selective beta-blocker oxprenolol, and the thiazide diuretic cyclopenthiazide. It is used to treat raised blood pressure See Chapter 25. *Adverse effects and Precautions* ➤ thiazide diuretics, beta-blockers.

co-proxamol preparations (Cosalgesic, Distalgesic) contain paracetamol and the opiate pain-reliever dextropropoxyphene. They are used to treat mild to moderate pain. *Adverse effects and Precautions* ➤ paracetamol, dextropropoxyphene.

Coracten ➤ nifedipine.

Cordarone X ➤ amiodarone.

Cordilox ➤ verapamil.

Cordilox MR ➤ verapamil.

Corgard ➤ nadolol.

Corgaretic tablets contain the non-selective beta-blocker nadolol and the thiazide diuretic bendrofluazide. They are used to treat raised blood pressure. See Chapter 25. *Adverse effects and Precautions* ➤ beta-blockers, thiazide diuretics.

Corlan pellets ➤ hydrocortisone. It is used to treat mouth ulcers. Do not use if mouth is infected. Use with caution in pregnancy.

Coroday MR ➤ nifedipine.

Coro-Nitro pump spray ➤ glyceryl trinitrate.

Corsodyl antiseptic preparations ➤ chlorhexidine. They are used to maintain oral hygiene and to treat mouth ulcers and sore gums.

corticosteroids, see Chapter 37.

corticosteroid skin applications, see p. 241.

corticotrophin ➤ corticotropin.

corticotropin (adrenocorticotrophic hormone, ACTH) stimulates the cortex of the adrenal glands to produce hormones. The effects produced are similar to, but not identical with, those produced by cortisone. See Chapter 37.

cortisol ➤ hydrocortisone.

cortisone (cortisone acetate, Cortisyl) is a corticosteroid. See Chapter 37.

Cortisyl ➤ cortisone.

Cosalgesic ➤ co-proxamol.

co-simalcite preparations (Altacite Plus) contain the anti-wind surfactant drug, activated dimethicone, and the antacid hydrotalcite. They are used to treat wind and indigestion ➤ antacids and see Chapter 19 on drugs used to treat indigestion and peptic ulcers.

Cosmegen-Lyovac ➤ actinomycin D.

Cosmofer is an iron-hydroxide dextran complex given by intravenous injection ➤ iron.

Cosopt is an eye drop containing dorzolamide and timolol ➤ dorzolamide, timolol.

Cosuric ➤ allopurinol.

co-tenidone (Atenix Co, in Katten, Tenchlor, Tenoret 50, Tenoretic, Totaretic) preparations contain the selective beta-blocker atenolol combined with the thiazide diuretic chlorthalidone. They are used to treat raised blood pressure. See Chapter 25. *Adverse effects and Precautions* ➤ beta-blockers, thiazide diuretics.

co-triamterzide (Dyazide, Triam-Co) diuretic preparations contain the potassium-sparing diuretic triamterene and the thiazide diuretic hydrochlorothiazide. They are used to treat raised blood pressure (see Chapter 25) and fluid retention, e.g. in heart failure (see Chapter 23). *Adverse effects and Precautions* ➤ triamterene, thiazide diuretics.

co-trimoxazole preparations (Bactrim, Chemotrim, Comox, Fectrim, Laratrim, Septrin) contain the folic acid inhibitor trimethoprim, and the sulphonamide sulphamethoxazole. They are an antibacterial drug (see p. 273). *Adverse effects* (➤ trimethoprim, sulphonamides) include nausea, vomiting, sore tongue and skin rashes (occasionally very severe). Very rarely, it may cause inflammation of the pancreas, kidney damage, liver damage, inflammation of the bowel, jaundice and blood disorders. *Precautions:* Do not use in pregnancy, in newborn babies (under six weeks of age), in patients with severe impairment of kidney or liver function, with blood disorders, jaundice or porphyria (a hereditary disorder of metabolism). Use with caution in breastfeeding mothers, in the elderly and in patients with moderate impairment of kidney function. Blood counts should be carried out at regular intervals in patients on long-term treatment. Stop if blood disorders or skin rash develop. Drink plenty of fluids. *Warnings on Use:* The use of cotrimoxazole should be limited to treating *Pneumocystitis carinii pneumonia* (PCP) which occurs in patients suffering from AIDS. It may also be used to treat toxoplasmosis and nocardiasis. It should only be used to treat urinary tract infections, chronic bronchitis flare-ups, and middle ear infection in children when there is laboratory evidence that the two drugs it contains will work better than a single antibacterial drug. *Note:* Most severe adverse effects have occurred in elderly patients. *Interactions:* Folate inhibitors, anticoagulants, antidiabetic drugs, digoxin, procainamide and amantadine.

cough and cold preparations, see Chapters 10 and 11.

cough suppressants, see Chapter 11.

coumarins are oral anticoagulants. See Chapter 28.

counter irritants ➤ rubefacients.

Coversyl ➤ perindopril.

Covonia Bronchial Balsam is a cough medicine containing dextromethorphan and menthol; **Covonia Mentholated Cough Mixture** contains liquorice, menthol and squill; **Covonia Nighttime Formula** is a cough medicine containing dextromethorphan and diphenhydramine ➤ individual entry for each drug.

Cozaar ➤ losartan potassium.

Cozaar Comp is a combination of lorsartan potassium and hydrochlorothiazide, used in the treatment of hypertension ➤ lorsartan potassium, hydrochlorothiazide.

Co-Zidocapt (Caposide, Capto-Co) is a combination product for the treatment of mild to moderate hypertension, containing hydrochlorothiazide and captopril ➤ hydrochlorothiazide, captopril.

Cream E45 contains white soft paraffin, light liquid paraffin and wool fat in an emollient base.

Cremalgin balm is a heat rub. It contains methyl nicotinate, oleoresin, capsicum and glycol salicylate ➤ rubefacients.

Creon capsules are used to replace enzymes that are lacking due to a deficiency of the pancreas. Each capsule contains pancreatin, containing the enzymes lipase, amylase and protease. *Adverse effects* include irritation around the anus. Damage to the bowel may occur when high doses are used over a prolonged length of time. *Precautions:* Drink plenty of fluids. Review patients if abdominal symptoms develop.

Crinone Vaginal gel is used in progesterone deficiency ➤ progesterone.

crisantapase (Erwinase) is the enzyme asparginase produced by the plant *Erwinia chrysanthemi*. It is used intramuscularly and subcutaneously to treat acute lymphoblastic anaemia. See Chapter 51 on drugs used to treat cancer. *Adverse effects* include nausea, vomiting, drowsiness, severe allergic reactions and changes in the blood fat level and liver function tests. *Precautions* see Chapter 51. Careful monitoring for early signs of adverse effects is necessary. Facilities for the immediate treatment of severe allergic reactions should be to hand.

Crixivan ➤ indinavir.

Cromogen inhalation ➤ sodium cromoglicate.

cromoglicate ➤ sodium cromoglicate.

cromoglycate ➤ sodium cromoglicate.

crotamiton (Eurax, in Eurax Hydrocortisone) is used as a skin application to relieve itching. See p. 247. *Precautions:* It should be used only on small areas of skin in babies and infants. It should not be used near the eyes or on areas of broken skin. Do not use in patients with acute, weeping eczema.

Crystacide cream contains hydrogen peroxide for the treatment of superficial bacterial skin infections.

crystal violet (gentian violet, methyl violet) is a dye used as an antiseptic. See p. 245. It may rarely cause nausea, vomiting, diarrhoea and ulceration of the lining of the mouth. It may stain clothes. *Precautions:* Keep away from eyes. It may trigger cancer in animals and is not recommended for use on open wounds or in the mouth. It is used to mark out the skin prior to surgery and as an antiseptic on areas of unbroken skin.

Crystapen ➤ benzylphenicillin (penicillin G).

Cuplex gel contains salicylic acid, lactic acid and copper acetate. It is used to treat warts and corns. *Precautions:* Do not use on facial warts or on warts around the anus and/or genitals. Avoid contact with healthy skin and eyes.

Cuprofen ➤ ibuprofen.

Curatoderm ➤ tacalcitol.

Curosurf ➤ poractant alfa.

Cutivate cream and ointment ➤ fluticasone.

CX Powder ➤ chlorhexidine.

cyanocobalamin (Cytacon, Cytamen) is a form of vitamin B_{12}. It is a cobalt-containing substance. It is used to treat anaemias caused by vitamin B_{12} deficiency. See Chapter 36.

Cyclimorph preparations contain morphine and cyclizine (an anti-vomiting drug). *Adverse effects and Precautions* ➤ morphine, cyclizine. In someone who has had a heart attack (myocardial infarction) the cyclizine may make severe heart failure worse and counteract the benefits of the morphine on the circulation.

cyclizine (cyclizine hydrochloride, Valoid) is an antihistamine used to treat motion sickness, and other disorders associated with nausea and vomiting, e.g. in Migril to treat migraine and in Diconal and Cyclimorph to relieve the nausea and vomiting caused by dipipanone and morphine respectively. See Chapter 18. *Adverse effects and Precautions* ➤ antihistamines.

Cyclodox ➤ doxycycline.

Cyclogest suppositories ➤ progesterone.

cyclopenthiazide (Navidrex, in Navidrex K, in Navispare, in Trasidrex) is a thiazide diuretic (➤ thiazide diuretics). It is used to treat heart failure (see Chapter 23) and raised blood pressure (see Chapter 25).

cyclopentolate (Minims cyclopentolate, Mydrilate) is an antimuscarinic drug used to dilate the pupils for eye examinations. *Adverse effects* ➤ antimuscarinic drugs. Local adverse effects on the eyes include stinging, blurred vision and discomfort on looking into the light (photophobia). General effects include dry mouth, rapid beating of the heart, headache and confusion. *Precautions:* Do not use in patients with closed-angle glaucoma or with paralysis of the small intestine. Use with caution if eye is inflamed and in patients with raised pressure in the eyes, enlarged prostate gland, or diseases of the arteries from the heart.

cyclophosphamide (Endoxana) is an anti-cancer drug. See Chapter 51. It is also used as an immunosuppressant to treat rheumatoid arthritis. See p. 166. *Adverse effects:* It may cause nausea, vomiting and diarrhoea, and occasionally inflammation and bleeding of the bowel, bleeding cystitis, bone-marrow damage producing blood disorders, damage to sperm production and loss of periods. Loss of hair is common but it regrows in two or three months even if the drug is continued. *Precautions:* It should not be given in pregnancy, to breastfeeding mothers, to patients with an infection of the urinary tract or bleeding from the bladder, or to patients whose bone-marrow function is reduced. It should be used with caution in elderly and/or debilitated patients, and in diabetes. *Interactions:* Radiotherapy, doxorubicin, sulphonylureas.

Cyclo-Progynova hormone preparations contain oestradiol (an oestrogen) and levonorgestrel (a progestogen) in varying proportions as HRT for the treatment of menopausal symptoms and post-menopausal osteoporosis. See Chapter 40 on female sex hormones. *Adverse effects and Precautions* ➤ HRT.

cycloserine (Cycloserine) is an antibiotic drug used to treat pulmonary tuberculosis. See Chapter 50. It is a second-choice drug and should be given in combination with other anti-tuberculous drugs in order to prevent resistance developing. *Adverse effects* include headache, dizziness, drowsiness, twitching, vertigo, depression, mental disturbances, blood disorders, speech difficulties, convulsions and unconsciousness. Allergic skin rashes occasionally occur, blood sugar levels may be reduced and certain tests for liver function altered. *Precautions:* Cycloserine should not be given to patients with epilepsy, impaired liver function, severely impaired kidney function, porphyria (a hereditary disorder of metabolism), alcohol dependence, severe anxiety or depression or psychotic illness. It should be given with caution to patients with impaired kidney function, in pregnancy, and in breastfeeding mothers. Tests of liver and kidney function should be carried out at regular intervals. Blood levels of the drug should be monitored if kidney function is impaired or the dose greater than 500 mg/day or if signs of toxicity develop. *Interactions:* Isoniazid, phenytoin.

cyclosporin ➤ ciclosporin.

Cyklokapron ➤ tranexamic acid.

Cymalon ➤ sodium citrate.

Cymevene ➤ ganciclovir.

cyproheptadine (cyproheptadine hydrochloride, Periactin) is an antihistamine drug ➤ antihistamines. It also blocks the actions of serotonin and is used to treat migraine (see Chapter 34). It may cause weight gain and has been used for this purpose. It may affect driving skills.

Cyprostat ➤ cyproterone.

cyproterone (cyproterone acetate) is an anti-androgen (see p. 189). It blocks the effects of male sex hormones (androgens) and has some progestogenic effects. The consequence of these effects is to reduce libido (sex drive) and cyproterone is used as Androcur to treat individuals who are considered to have excessive or misdirected male libido. It is also used as Cyprostat to treat cancers of the prostate which are dependent upon male sex hormones for growth. It is included in Dianette to treat acne in females (➤ Dianette). *Adverse effects:* It stops sperm production and causes the testicles to shrink. These changes appear to be reversible but recovery may take up to twenty months after stopping the drug. The consequences of long-term treatment are not known. It may produce swelling of the breasts, milk production and lumps in the breasts. Pain in the testicles may occur and there may be patchy loss of hair on the body with increased growth of hair on the scalp and lightening of hair colour. Increase in weight may occur with female distribution of fat on the breasts and bottom. Stretch marks (striae) may occur on the abdomen and the patient may complain of fatigue, depression, headache, flushing and sweating. It may also cause liver damage, jaundice, osteoporosis and irritability. *Precautions:* It should be used with caution in patients with liver disorders, diabetes or anaemia. Blood tests for these disorders should be carried out at monthly intervals. Tests of adrenal function should also be carried out at regular intervals. Alcohol reduces its effects and it is of no use in chronic alcoholics. A sperm count should be done before starting treatment to establish whether the patient is fertile or not, except for treating cancer of the prostate gland. It should not be used in patients suffering from acute liver disease, severe chronic depression, a malignant or wasting disease, sickle cell anaemia, if there is a history of thrombosis, or in youths under eighteen years of age because bone growth and testicular development could be stopped by the drug. It may affect the ability to drive motor vehicles because of the fatigue produced.

Cystagon ➤ mercaptamine.

cysteine (l-cysteine, in Cicatrin) is an amino acid which is an essential constituent of the diet to form body proteins.

cysteamine ➤ mercaptamine.

Cystemme ➤ sodium citrate.

Cystoleve powder ➤ sodium citrate.

Cystopurin ➤ potassium citrate.

Cystrin ➤ oxybutynin.

Cytacon ➤ cyanocobalamin.

Cytamen ➤ cyanocobalamin.

cytarabine (Cytosar) is an anti-cancer drug (see Chapter 51) used to treat leukaemia. *Adverse effects* include nausea, vomiting, diarrhoea, ulcers in the mouth, damage to the bone marrow producing blood disorders, liver dysfunction, skin rashes, joint pains, inflammation of the nerves, visual disturbances and loss of hair. *Precautions:* It should not be given to patients who are pregnant or to breastfeeding mothers. Frequent blood counts, tests of bone-marrow, liver and kidney function should be carried out. It should not be used in patients with impaired kidney or liver function.

Cytosar ➤ cytarabine.

Cytotec ➤ misoprostol.

cytotoxic drugs, see Chapter 51 on anti-cancer drugs.

dacarbazine (DTIC-Dome) is an anti-cancer drug. See Chapter 51. *Adverse effects* include severe nausea and vomiting, and damage to the bone marrow producing blood disorders. *Precautions:* It is irritant to the skin and mucous membranes and should therefore be handled with great caution. Dacarbazine is combined with doxorubicin (was named Adriamycin), bleomycin and vinblastine in ABVD treatment of Hodgkin's disease.

daclizumab (Zenapax) is used to prevent organ rejection in kidney transplants, in conjunction with treatment to suppress the immune system. *Adverse effects* include allergic reactions. *Precautions:* Do not use in pregnancy or while breastfeeding.

dactinomycin (actinomycin D, Cosmegen-Lyovac) is an anti-cancer drug used principally to treat cancers in childhood. It is given intravenously. *Adverse effects and Precautions* are similar to those listed under doxorubicin except that toxic effects on the heart are not a problem.

Daktacort preparations contain miconazole (an antifungal drug) and hydrocortisone (a corticosteroid). They are used to treat fungal or bacterial infections of inflamed areas of skin. *Adverse effects and Precautions* ➤ miconazole and see corticosteroid skin applications, p. 241.

Daktarin preparations ➤ miconazole.

Dalacin cream contains clindamycin ➤ clindamycin. It is used to treat bacterial infections of the vagina. *Adverse effects* include vaginal irritation, stomach and bowel upsets. Stop the drug if diarrhoea or colitis (inflammation of the bowel) develop. *Precautions:* Do not use in patients allergic to lincomycin. May reduce the effectiveness of barrier contraceptives.

Dalacin C oral preparations ➤ clindamycin.

Dalacin T preparations contain clindamycin ➤ clindamycin. They are used to treat acne. May cause dry skin, dermatitis, infection of hair follicles (folliculitis), diarrhoea or colitis (inflammation of the bowel) (stop immediately). Avoid contact with the eyes and mouth. Do not use in patients allergic to lincomycin.

dalfopristin/quinupristin (Synercid) is used to treat Gram-positive infections, including pneumonia, skin or soft tissue infections, when no other option is appropriate and also to treat infections due to *E.faecium*. See Chapter 46. *Adverse effects* include injection site reactions, rash, stomach and bowel upsets, headache, itching, pain in joints, pain in muscles, excessive bilirubin in the blood and blood disorders. *Precautions:* Do not use in patients with kidney or liver damage, in pregnancy or while breastfeeding.

Dalivit oral drops are a multivitamin preparation containing vitamins A, B group, C and D.

Dalmane ➤ flurazepam.

dalteparin sodium (Fragmin) is a low molecular weight heparin LMWH (see Chapter 28). It is given by subcutaneous injection to treat deep-vein thrombosis (blood clotting) and to prevent blood clots in veins, particularly the risk of clots associated with general and orthopaedic surgery. It is also used to prevent clots in blood circulation systems outside the body which are used during blood dialysis and filtration. It is also used to treat unstable angina. *Adverse effects* include bleeding with high

doses. For other potential harmful effects ➤ heparin. *Precautions:* It should be used with caution in patients at risk of bleeding, with impaired liver function, in pregnancy and in breastfeeding mothers. *Interactions* ➤ heparin.

danaparoid is a heparinoid used to prevent deep-vein thrombosis in patients undergoing general or orthopaedic surgery. It may also be used in patients who develop thrombocytopenia (a low platelet count) while undergoing treatment with heparin ➤ heparinoids.

danazol (Danol) blocks the secretion of gonadotrophins by the pituitary. It is used to treat endometriosis, infertility associated with endometriosis, heavy periods, benign breast disorders, premenstrual syndrome, enlargement of the breasts in males, precocious puberty and other endocrine disorders where control of the release of the pituitary gonadotrophic hormones, luteinizing hormone (LH) and follicle stimulating hormone (FSH), may be beneficial. *Adverse effects:* Masculinization in women, acne, oily skin, mild hirsutism (hairiness), reduction of breast size, menstrual disturbances, flushing, backache, fluid retention, skin rashes, nausea, headache, dizziness, emotional upsets, nervousness, muscle spasms, jaundice, increase in weight and blood, thyroid and circulatory disorders. *Precautions:* Should not be used in pregnancy, in patients with porphyria (a hereditary disorder of metabolism) or in breastfeeding mothers, in patients with severe liver, heart or kidney disease, thrombotic disease, undiagnosed vaginal bleeding or androgenic-dependent tumours. Avoid sexual intercourse or use mechanical contraceptive while on treatment. Use with caution in patients with epilepsy, migraine, raised blood pressure, heart disease, polythaemia (a blood disorder) or any disorders made worse by fluid retention. *Interactions:* Anticoagulants, anti-epileptic drugs, corticosteroids, anabolic steroids, ciclosporin, anti-diabetic drugs, anti-blood pressure drugs, antimigraine drugs, alcohol and alfacalcidol.

Danlax liquid is used to treat constipation ➤ poloxamer 188, dantron.

Danol ➤ danazol.

danthron ➤ dantron.

Dantrium ➤ dantrolene.

dantrolene (Co-danthramer, dantrolene sodium, Dantrium) is a muscle relaxant (see p. 42) used to relieve spasm produced by conditions such as stroke, multiple sclerosis and spinal cord injury. It is also used to treat malignant hypothermia and neuroleptic malignant syndrome (for symptoms ➤ antipsychotic drugs). *Adverse effects:* Transient drowsiness, dizziness, weakness, generally feeling unwell, fatigue, diarrhoea, occasionally urinary or musculoskeletal disturbances and, rarely, jaundice. *Precautions:* Do not use in patients with acute muscle spasm, impaired liver function and use with caution in pregnancy. It should be given with caution to patients with impaired heart or lung function. Tests of liver function should be carried out before starting treatment and at regular intervals during treatment. Desired effects may not develop for a few weeks but if the patient has not improved after about four to six weeks treatment should be stopped. Drowsiness may affect ability to drive or operate machinery. It should not be used in children or when muscle tone serves a purpose, e.g. in walking. *Interactions:* Alcohol, sleeping drugs, sedatives or any drug that depresses brain function.

dantron (in Ailax, in codanthrusate, in Codalax, in Danlax, in Normax) is a stimulant laxative. See Chapter 21. *Adverse effects* include abdominal cramps, nausea, vomiting, malfunctioning of the bowel and a low blood potassium level. The urine may be coloured red and so may the skin around the anus. *Precautions:* Do not use if bowel is obstructed. Use with utmost caution in pregnancy and breastfeeding mothers. Also see p. 108.

Daonil ➤ glibenclamide.

dapsone is used to treat leprosy, dermatitis herpetiformis (an inflammatory skin disease), and combined with pyrimethamine (in Maloprim) in preventative treatment for malaria. *Adverse effects* include nerve damage, loss of appetite, allergic dermatitis, nausea, vomiting, headache, insomnia, rapid heart rate, anaemia, severe mental disturbances (psychoses), weight loss, nerve damage, inflammation of the liver and blood disorders. *Precautions:* Do not use in patients with porphyria (a hereditary disorder of metabolism) or severe anaemia. Use with caution in patients with heart or lung disease and in breastfeeding mothers, in pregnancy, in anaemia and in patients with G6PD deficiency. Give folic acid supplements in pregnancy. *Interactions:* Rifampicin, probenecid, PABA.

Daraprim ➤ pyrimethamine.

darbepoetin (Aranesp) is used for the treatment of anaemia associated with chronic kidney failure. See Chapter 35. *Adverse effects* include headache, high blood pressure, blood clots, pain at injection site. *Precautions:* It should not be administered to breastfeeding mothers, caution should be used in pregnancy, in impaired liver function, sickle cell anaemia or epilepsy.

daunorubicin (Cerubidin, DaunoXome) is used as an intravenous injection to treat acute myelogenous and lymphatic leukaemia. A special emulsion preparation is available which is used to treat HIV-related Kaposi's sarcoma ➤ DaunoXome. *Adverse effects* include ulcers of the mouth, hair loss, fever, nausea, vomiting, diarrhoea, skin rashes, phlebitis (inflammation of the vein) and damage to tissue at the site of injection. The most serious adverse effects are damage to the bone marrow producing a fall in white cell count and damage to the heart causing congestive heart failure. *Precautions:* Do not use in patients who are exposed to chickenpox or shingles. Do not give by intramuscular or subcutaneous injection. Do not use in pregnancy, in breastfeeding mothers or in patients with heart disease. Use with caution in patients with gout or kidney stones. See Chapter 51 on anti-cancer drugs.

DaunoXome ➤ daunorubicin. In Dauno-Xome preparations the daunorubicin is encapsulated in minute fatty capsules (liposomes) to form an emulsion which is given by intravenous infusion. The encapsulation protects the daunorubicin in the bloodstream and decreases its uptake by normal cells but increases its uptake by solid tumour cells. It is used to treat advanced HIV-related Kaposi's sarcoma. *Adverse effects and Precautions* ➤ daunorubicin. It may cause headaches, fatigue, chills, nausea, vomiting, light-headedness. Initial infusion may cause back pain, flushing and chest tightness.

Day Nurse contains paracetamol, dextromethorphan and phenylpropanolamine ➤ individual entry for each drug.

DDAVP nose drops ➤ desmopressin.

DDC ➤ zalcitabine.

DDI ➤ didanosine.

Debrisan preparations contain beads of dextranomer which absorb secretions and tissue debris from wounds and ulcers ➤ dextranomer.

debrisoquine (debrisoquine sulphate) has effects and uses similar to those described under guanethidine. It is used to treat raised blood pressure. See Chapter 25.

Decadron preparations ➤ dexamethasone.

Deca-Durabolin ➤ nandrolone.

De-capeptyl SR ➤ triptorelin.

deferiprone (Ferriprox) is used to treat iron overload in thalassaemia major (a hereditary defect in the ability to produce haemoglobin) where desferrioxamine is unsuitable. *Adverse effects* include a decrease in the number of white cells in the blood (neutropenia or agranulocytosis), discoloration of urine, stomach and bowel upsets, increased appetite, arthritis. *Precautions:* Do not use in patients with a history of recurrent neutropenia or agranulocytosis, in pregnancy or while breastfeeding. Use with caution in patients with kidney or liver damage or scarring of the liver. Signs of infection should be reported immediately.

deflazacort (Calcort) is a corticosteroid used to treat severe asthma, rheumatoid arthritis and other inflammatory reactions. See Chapter 37. *Adverse effects* include suppression of growth in children, high blood pressure, sodium retention, stomach and bowel disorders, water retention, potassium loss, muscle weakness, death of tissue cells at the joints of the thighbone and upper arm-bone, cushingoid changes (after taking corticosteroids the patient may have the appearance of having Cushing's syndrome – a fat face and body), hyperglycaemia, osteoporosis, depression, euphoria, peptic ulcers. *Precautions:* Do not use in patients with infections unless undergoing antibiotic treatment. Use with caution in patients with tuberculosis, infections, amoebic infection, stomach and bowel upsets. Avoid contact with chickenpox or measles.

Delfen is a spermicidal contraceptive foam which contains nonoxinol 9.

Deltacortril ➤ prednisolone.

Deltaprim ➤ mefloquine.

Deltastab ➤ prednisolone.

demeclocycline (demeclocycline hydrochloride, demethylchlortetracycline hydrochloride, in Deteclo, Ledermycin) is a tetracycline antibiotic (see p. 269). It is long-acting. *Adverse effects and Precautions:* These are similar to those described under tetracyclines but there is an increased risk of skin sensitivity to sunlight. Patients should therefore avoid exposure to sunlight when receiving treatment. It is used by mouth to treat severe acne (see p. 250) and general infections.

Demix ➤ doxycycline.

demulcent cough preparations, see Chapter 11.

De-Noltab tablets (tripotassium dicitrato bismuthate) protect the lining of the stomach. They are used to treat peptic ulcers. See Chapter 19. *Adverse effects:* Blackening of the stools usually occurs and darkening of the tongue may occur. *Precautions:* It should not be used in patients with kidney impairment or in pregnancy.

Dentinox Colic Drops contain activated dimethicone which is used to treat gripe, colic or wind pains.

Dentomycin dental gel contains the tetracycline antibiotic minocycline ➤ tetracyclines. It is used to treat pockets of inflammation and infection in the gums. *Adverse effects* include stinging where the gel is applied. *Precautions:* Do not use in patients with complete kidney failure. Use with caution in patients with impaired liver or kidney function, in pregnancy and in breastfeeding mothers. Patients should avoid cleaning their teeth, rinsing their mouth out, drinking or eating for at least two hours after treatment.

Depakote ➤ valproic acid.

Depixol ➤ flupenthixol.

Depo-Medrone depot injection ➤ methylprednisolone.

Depo-Medrone with Lidocaine injection contains methyl prednisolone (a corticosteroid) and lidocaine(lignocaine) (a local anaesthetic). It is used as a local injection to treat inflammatory and rheumatoid conditions. *Adverse effects and Precautions* ➤ lidocaine(lignocaine) and see Chapter 37 on corticosteroids.

Deponit patch is designed to release glyceryl trinitrate from a plaster through the skin and into the bloodstream to prevent attacks of angina. See Chapter 22. *Adverse effects and Precautions* ➤ glyceryl trinitrate. It may cause headache, dizziness and a rash. Treatment should be withdrawn gradually by replacing with increasing doses of a long-acting nitrate by mouth.

Depo-Provera depot injection ➤ medroxyprogesterone.

Dequacaine lozenges contain dequalinium (antiseptic) and benzocaine (local anaesthetic). They are used to treat sore throats. *Adverse effects and Precautions* ➤ dequalinium, benzocaine.

Dequadin lozenges ➤ dequalinium.

dequalinium (dequalinium chloride, Dequadin, Labosept) is an antiseptic (see p. 244) used in throat lozenges and paints. *Precautions:* Its prolonged and repeated use should be avoided. It can cause the skin to become inflamed when applied under dressings and it should not be used around the anus and genitals.

Derbac-M aqueous preparations ➤ malathion.

Dermacort cream ➤ hydrocortisone.

Dermalo is a bath emollient (skin softener) which contains acetylated wool alcohols and liquid paraffin.

Dermamist spray contains white soft paraffin, liquid paraffin and coconut oil. It is used to soften the skin to treat eczema and chronic itching skin rashes ➤ liquid paraffin.

Dermestril patches ➤ estradiol.

Dermidex cream ➤ lidocaine.

Dermol lotion contains benzalkonium chloride, chlorhexidine hydrochloride, liquid paraffin and isopropyl myristate. It is used to soften dry skin.

Dermovate preparations ➤ clobetasol.

Dermovate-N preparations contain clobetasol (a very potent corticosteroid), neomycin (an aminoglycoside antibiotic) and nystatin (an antifungal drug). They are used to treat infected eczema and psoriasis. *Adverse effects and Precautions* see corticosteroid applications p. 241 and ➤ neomycin, nystatin.

Deseril ➤ methysergide.

Desferal ➤ desferrioxamine.

desferrioxamine (Desferal) is used in the treatment of iron poisoning and in patients who store too much iron in their bodies. It joins with the iron, and the combination is excreted in the urine. It is also used to treat aluminium overload in patients receiving kidney dialysis. *Adverse effects* include pain at the site of injection, and a drop in blood pressure, flushing and shock if given too rapidly by IV injection. Fever, stomach and bowel upsets, red urine, allergic skin rashes. Leg cramps and rapid beating of the heart may, rarely, occur. Very rarely, cataract, and disturbances of vision and hearing, slowing of growth, impaired kidney and liver function, blood disorders and nerve damage may occur. *Precautions:* Use with caution in patients with impaired kidney function, in pregnancy and in breastfeeding mothers. Regular eye and hearing tests should be carried out while on treatment. May cause fits in patients with brain malfunction due to overload with aluminium, therefore pre-treat these patients with the anti-epileptic drug clonazepam. Stop treatment if patient develops an infection and do not start again until the infection has cleared up. Monitor heart function in patients taking vitamin C. Measure height and weight in children every three months. *Interactions:* Prochlorperazine, erythropoietin, vitamin C, gallium scintigraphy.

desflurane (Suprane) is a rapidly acting liquid anaesthetic. See Chapter 44. It is not recommended for use in children.

desirudin (Revasc) is used for the prevention of deep-vein thrombosis (blood clots) in elective hip and knee replacement surgery. See Chapter 28. *Adverse effects* include bleeding, nausea, weeping from wounds, fever, injection site reactions, blood clots, anaemia, low blood pressure, urinary retention, thrombophlebitis (inflammation of a vein), high fever, allergic reactions. *Precautions:* Do not use in active bleeding or irreversible blood disorders, severe kidney or liver damage, severe uncontrolled high blood pressure, subacute bacterial endocarditis (inflammation of the lining membrane of the heart), in pregnancy or while breastfeeding. Use with caution in patients with mild liver or kidney damage, damage to the retina due to diabetes which is not being controlled, a history of stroke, a tendency to haemorrhage.

desloratadine (Neoclarityn) is an antihistamine used to treat hayfever. See Chapter 17. *Adverse effects* include headache. *Precautions:* Do not use in patients with an allergy to loratadine or who are breastfeeding. Use with caution in patients with severe kidney damage or in pregnancy.

desloughing applications are used to remove slough, clots and debris from infected wounds and ulcers. Preparations include Aserbine cream (contains propylene glycol and benzoic, malic and salicylic acids), Hioxyl cream (contains hydrogen peroxide) and Varidase (contains the protein-dissolving enzyme streptokinase). Preparations that help to remove secretions also include adsorbent applications.

desmopressin (in DDAVP nasal drops, tablets and injections, Desmotabs tablets, Desmospray nasal spray, Nocutil) is a synthetic relative of the natural anti-diuretic hormone vasopressin (AVP), which is a hormone produced by the posterior pituitary gland. This hormone causes the kidneys to retain water from the urine. Desmopressin is used to treat diabetes insipidus – a condition in which the posterior lobe of the pituitary gland fails to produce the anti-diuretic hormone with the result that the patient drinks excessive amounts of fluids and passes large volumes of weak urine. Desmopressin is also used to treat bedwetting (see p. 283) and to test kidney function. *Adverse effects* include headache, stomach pains, nausea and a low blood sodium level which may trigger convulsions. *Precautions:* It should be used with caution in patients with impaired kidney function, cystic fibrosis, or heart disease and in pregnancy. Avoid fluid overload. Use with caution in asthma, epilepsy, migraine or any disorder that may be made worse by fluid retention. Exclude alcohol abuse or psychological over-drinking of fluids before starting treatment. It should only be used to treat bedwetting in patients who have a normal blood pressure. *Interactions:* Indomethacin, tricyclic antidepressants, chlorpromazine, carbamazepine.

Desmospray ➤ desmopressin. It is a metered dose atomizer for administration up the nose.

Desmotabs ➤ desmopressin.

desogestrel (in Marvelon, in Mercilon) is a progestogen ➤ progestogens.

desoxymetasone (desoxymethasone, in Stiedex preparations) is a topical corticosteroid used to treat skin disorders. *Adverse effects and Precautions* see corticosteroid skin applications p. 241.

desoxymethasone ➤ desoxymetasone.

Destolit ➤ ursodeoxycholic acid.

Deteclo tablets contain the tetracycline antibiotics chlortetracycline, tetracycline and demeclocycline. See tetracyclines, p. 269. They are used to treat severe acne and general infections. *Adverse effects and Precautions* ➤ tetracyclines.

Detrunorm ➤ propiverine.

Detrusitol ➤ tolterodine.

Dettol Antiseptic Pain Relief Spray ➤ lidocaine(lignocaine).

Dettol preparations contain chloroxylenol. See p. 244.

DeWitts analgesic pills contain paracetamol and caffeine ➤ paracetamol, caffeine.

DeWitts antacid powder is an antacid containing calcium, magnesium, sodium bicarbonate, light kaolin and peppermint oil.

DeWitts antacid tablets are antacids containing calcium, magnesium and peppermint oil.

dexamethasone is a corticosteroid. See Chapter 37. It is used orally (Decadron, Dexol) to treat rheumatic, allergic and inflammatory disorders. *Adverse effects and Precautions* see Chapter 37 on corticosteroids. Dexamethasone is included in Dexa-Rhinaspray-Duo used to treat hayfever (see p. 87). It is used in Maxidex, Maxitrol, in Sofradex and in Tobradex eye drops used to treat inflamed eyes. *Adverse effects* of eye drops include a rise in pressure inside the eye, thinning of the cornea, cataract and fungal infections. *Precautions:* Do not use in patients with glaucoma, or a viral, fungal, tuberculous or infection of the eyes. Do not wear soft contact lenses. Dexamethasone is also used to treat eczema of the ear (otitis externa) in Otomize ear spray and in Sofradex ear drops. Ear preparations should not be used if the ear drum is perforated and they should be used with caution in pregnancy. Long-term use in infants should be avoided.

dexamfetamine (Dexadrine) is an amfetamine drug. See Chapter 6. It is used to treat narcolepsy (a periodic uncontrollable tendency to fall asleep) and hyperkinesia (over-activity) in children. *Adverse effects and Precautions* ➤ amfetamine sulphate. It should *not* be used to treat overweight patients, fatigue, depression or weakness.

dexamphetamine ➤ dexamfetamine.

Dexa-Rhinaspray-Duo contains tramazoline (sympathomimetic drug), dexamethasone (corticosteroid) and neomycin (aminoglycoside antibiotic) ➤ tramazoline, dexamethasone, neomycin. It is used as a nasal spray to treat hayfever. It may cause irritation of the nose and prolonged use should be avoided.

Dexedrine ➤ dexamfetamine.

dexketoprofen (Keral) is a non-steroidal anti-inflammatory drug used to treat musculoskeletal pain, difficult or painful menstruation and dental pain. See Chapter 32. *Adverse effects* include stomach and bowel upsets, headache, dizziness, blood disorders. *Precautions:* Do not use in patients with an allergy to aspirin or anti-inflammatory drugs, asthma, severe kidney or liver damage, active or history of recurrent peptic ulcer, chronic indigestion, bleeding disorders, inflammation of the bowel, severe heart failure, in pregnancy or while breastfeeding. Use with caution in patients with a history of bronchial asthma or allergic disease, systemic lupus erythematosis (SLE – a disease of unknown cause with symptoms of fever, muscle and joint pain, blood disorders and skin eruptions), heart disease, mild liver or kidney damage or in the elderly.

Dexomon preparations ➤ diclofenac.

Dexsol ➤ dexamethasone.

dextran infusions are used as plasma substitutes to restore blood volume after accidents or operations ➤ plasma substitutes. *Adverse effects:* Infusions may occasionally cause allergic reactions, e.g. nettle-rash, flushing and wheezing. Rarely, they may cause nausea and vomiting. *Precautions:* They should not be used in patients allergic to dextrans, with severely impaired kidney function, severe congestive heart failure or certain bleeding disorders. Use with caution in patients with mild to moderate congestive heart failure or mild to moderate impairment of kidney function. **Tears Naturale** (artificial tears) contain dextran.

dextranomer (Debrisan powder and paste) cleans wounds and ulcers by absorbing secretions. It is prepared from dextran. It should not be used on deep wounds or cavities (because it may be difficult to remove) and it should not be used on dry wounds or near the eye.

dextromethorphan (dextromethorphan hydrobromide) is a cough suppressant included in several cough medicines. See Chapter 11. *Adverse effects:* It may occasionally cause drowsiness and dizziness.

dextromoramide (dextromoramide tartrate, Palfium) is an opiate pain-reliever. See Chapter 30. It is used to relieve moderate to severe pain. It may be given by mouth, by rectum or by subcutaneous or intramuscular injection. It works for about four hours. *Adverse effects:* Dextromoramide may cause nausea, vomiting, sweating, dizziness, faintness (due to a fall in blood pressure) and insomnia. As with morphine, these are more likely to occur if the patient is up and about. *Precautions:* It should be used with caution in patients with impaired liver function. It is a powerful respiratory depressant and should not be used in women in labour. It should not be used in patients whose breathing is depressed or who have chronic obstructive airways disease. It should be used with caution in pregnancy, in the elderly and in patients with underworking of their thyroid gland. *Interactions:* MAOIs, anaesthetics, sedatives, hypnotics and tranquillizers. After each of the first few doses the patient should lie down for half an hour because of the drug's effects. *Drug dependence:* Regular daily use may lead to tolerance, mood changes and drug dependence of the morphine type.

dextropropoxyphene (in co-proxamol, in Cosalgesic, in Distalgesic, Doloxene, in Doloxene Compound) is an opiate (opioid) pain-reliever. See Chapter 30. *Adverse effects:* Dextropropoxyphene may cause dizziness, headache, dry mouth, blurred vision, drowsiness, excitation, raised mood (euphoria), insomnia, skin rashes, nausea, vomiting, abdominal pains and constipation. *Precautions:* Dextropropoxyphene should be given with caution to patients with severe respiratory disorders, impaired liver or kidney function, and in pregnancy. Regular daily use may lead to tolerance and drug dependence of the morphine type. *Interactions:* MAOIs, alcohol, sedatives, sleeping drugs and other drugs that depress brain function.

dextrose ➤ glucose.

DF 118 and **DF118 Forte** ➤ dihydrocodeine.

DHC Continus tablets contain dihydrocodeine in a controlled release form ➤ dihydrocodeine.

Diabetamide ➤ glibenclamide.

Diagesil ➤ diamorphine.

DIAGLYK ➤ gliclazide.

Dialar ➤ diazepam.

Diamicron ➤ gliclazide.

diamorphine (diamorphine hydrochloride, heroin) has effects and uses similar to those described under morphine. It is more potent than morphine but is shorter-acting – only about two hours. It has less tendency to produce vomiting and constipation. It is also an effective cough suppressant. *Adverse effects and Precautions* ➤ morphine. *Drug dependence:* Diamorphine produces dependence of the morphine type.

Diamox ➤ acetazolamide.

Dianette tablets contain the anti-male sex hormone cyproterone and the female oestrogen sex hormone ethinyloestradiol. They are used to treat severe acne in females, see p. 252. The reason for using it is to try to block the effects of male sex hormones (androgens) which are considered to be a major factor in the development of acne. Dianette is also an effective oral contraceptive and women should *not* take any other oral contraceptive while on this treatment. They are not suitable for treating male acne. It may also be used to treat severe hirsutism (excessive hair growth). *Adverse effects:* Breast enlargement, bloated feeling, fluid retention, cramps, pains in the legs, depression, loss of libido, headaches, nausea, vaginal discharge, superficial ulcers on the neck of the womb, weight gain, breakthrough bleeding and brown patches on the skin of the face (chloasma). *Precautions:* Do not use in pregnancy or in patients who suffer from or who have suffered from angina, coronary heart disease, blood clots, valvular disease of the heart, sickle cell anaemia, jaundice, hepatitis (inflammation of the liver), liver disease or any other disorder in which an oral contraceptive should not be taken. It should be used with caution in patients with hypertension, Raynaud's disease, diabetes, varicose veins, asthma or severe depression, or in patients receiving kidney dialysis. For other precautions see Chapter 41 on oral contraceptives.

Diarphen ➤ co-phenotrope.

Diarrest contains the opiate codeine and the antispasmodic dicycloverine(dicyclomine), combined with electrolytes (potassium chloride, sodium chloride and sodium citrate). It is taken as a liquid with water to treat diarrhoea, see Chapter 20 and ➤ codeine, dicycloverine(dicyclomine). *Adverse effects* include sedation. *Precautions:* Do not use in patients with severe inflammation of the bowel caused by antibiotics or with diverticular disease. Use with caution in patients with overworking of their thyroid gland, heart failure, impaired kidney or liver function, glaucoma or ulcerative colitis (chronic bowel disorder). *Interactions:* MAOIs.

Diasorb ➤ loperamide.

Diazemuls ➤ diazepam.

diazepam (Alupram, Atensine, Diazemuls, Diazepam Rectubes, Rimapam, Solis, Stesolid, Tensium, Valclair, Valium) is a benzodiazepine ➤ benzodiazepines.

diazoxide (Eudemine) is a vasodilator drug used to treat a severe rise in blood pressure (see Chapter 25), particularly if associated with kidney disease. It is also used to treat low blood sugar (hypoglycaemia) (see Chapter 42). *Adverse effects* include rapid beating of the heart, raised blood sugar level, fluid and salt retention, fall in blood pressure on standing up after sitting or lying down (postural hypotension), coma and delayed labour. *Precautions:* Use with caution in patients with severe impairment of kidney, brain or heart function, low blood protein levels, in pregnancy or in labour. Blood sugar levels should be checked at regular intervals. *Interactions:* Diuretics, anti-blood pressure drugs, coumarin anticoagulants.

Dibenyline ➤ phenoxytenzamine.

dibromopropamidine ➤ dibrompropamidine.

dibrompropamidine (isethionate, Brolene, Golden Eye Ointment) is an antibacterial drug used to treat bacterial infections of the eyelids and conjunctiva. It is also used to treat amoebic infections of the cornea (acanthamoeba keratitis).

dichlorobenzyl alcohol is an antiseptic which is used as an ingredient of lozenges in the treatment of minor infections of the mouth and throat.

diclofenac sodium (Acoflam, in Arthrotec, Dexomon, Dicloflex, Diclomax, Diclotard, Diclovol, Diclozip, Digenac XL, Econac, Enzed, Flamrase SR, Flamratak, Flexotard, Lofensaid, Motifene, Pennsaid, Rheumatac, Rhumalgan, Slofenac, Solaraze, Volraman, Volsaid Retard, Voltarol, Voltarol Ophtha) is a non-steroidal anti-inflammatory drug (NSAID) ➤ nonsteroidal anti-inflammatory drugs.

Dicloflex ➤ diclofenac sodium.

Diclomax ➤ diclofenac sodium.

Diclotard ➤ diclofenac sodium.

Diclovol ➤ diclofenac sodium.

Diclozip ➤ diclofenac sodium.

dicobalt edetate (Kelocyanor) is given by intravenous injection to treat acute cyanide poisoning. Because of its toxicity it should only be used if patient has lost or is losing consciousness. *Adverse effects* include fall in blood pressure, rapid heart beat and vomiting.

Diconal tablets contain dipipanone (an opiate pain-reliever) (see Chapter 30), and cyclizine (an antihistamine used as an anti-vomiting drug) (see Chapter 18). *Adverse effects* ➤ morphine, antihistamines. Common adverse effects produced by Diconal include drowsiness, dry mouth and blurred vision. *Precautions:* Do not use in patients whose breathing is depressed or who have obstructive airways disease. Use with caution in patients with severely impaired liver

or kidney function and in pregnancy. *Interactions:* MAOIs, alcohol, sedatives, sleeping drugs and other drugs that depress brain function. *Dependence* ➤ morphine.

dicycloverine(dicyclomine) (dicycloverine hydrochloride, in Diarrest, in Kolanticon, Merbentyl) is an antimuscarinic drug used to treat painful spasms of the stomach and intestine. *Adverse effects and Precautions* ➤ antimuscarinic drugs.

dicyclomine ➤ dicycloverine.

Dicynene ➤ etamsylate.

didanosine (DDI, Videx) is an antiviral drug used to treat patients suffering from HIV infection. See Chapter 48. *Adverse effects* include nausea, vomiting, diarrhoea, confusion, rash, itching, insomnia, weakness, damage to the pancreas, raised blood uric acid levels, convulsions, nerve damage and pneumonia, eye damage, blood disorders and rarely liver damage. *Precautions:* Do not use in patients in whom the drug has previously caused liver damage. Use with utmost caution in patients with a history of inflammation of the pancreas, nerve damage, a raised blood uric acid level, or impaired liver or kidney function. Use with utmost caution in pregnancy and breast-feeding mothers and do not take the drug at the same time as a tetracycline antibiotic because the tablets contain aluminium and magnesium antacids which can interfere with the absorption of tetracyclines. Liver function, blood fats and uric acid blood levels should be monitored at regular intervals. Check for evidence of nerve damage. Monitor serum amylase before and at regular intervals during treatment. Check the eyes in children for retinal changes. Use with caution in patients with phenylketonurea and patients on a low-sodium diet. *Interactions:* Tetracyclines (see above), drugs that affect or are affected by the acid in the stomach, ganciclovir and drugs known to damage nerves or the pancreas.

Didronel ➤ etidronate.

Didronel PMO contains etidronate disodium and calcium carbonate. It is used to treat vertebral osteoporosis ➤ etidronate disodium, calcium carbonate.

diethylstilbestrol (stiboestrol, Tampovagan) is a synthetic oestrogen ➤ oestrogens.

diethyltoluamide is an insect repellent. It can occasionally cause allergic reactions. It should not be applied near the eyes, to mucous membranes, to broken skin or near areas of skin flexion (e.g. elbows) – it can cause irritation and blistering.

Differin ➤ adapalene.

Difflam cream, **Difflam mouthwash** and **Difflam spray** ➤ benzydamine.

Diflucan preparations ➤ fluconazole.

diflucortolone (diflucortolone valerate, Nerisone) is a potent corticosteroid used in skin applications. *Adverse effects and Precautions* see corticosteroid skin applications, p. 241. It is used to treat severe eczema and psoriasis.

diflunisal (Dolobid) is a non-steroidal anti-inflammatory drug, See Chapter 32. It is used to treat rheumatoid arthritis and acute or chronic pain. It is a salicylate (➤ aspirin). *Adverse effects* include stomach pains, nausea, vomiting, indigestion, sleepiness, insomnia, headaches, dizziness, noises in the ears (tinnitus), diarrhoea and skin rashes. *Precautions:* It should not be used in pregnancy or in breastfeeding mothers, or in patients allergic to aspirin or some other NSAIDs. It should not be used in patients with active peptic ulcers. It should be used with utmost caution in patients with a history of peptic ulcers or bleeding from the stomach or intestine, or with impaired kidney or liver function, heart failure or in the elderly. *Interactions:* Anticoagulants, indomethacin, aspirin, codeine, methotrexate, cyclosporin, antacids.

Diftavax is adsorbed diphtheria and tetanus vaccine for adults and adolescents.

Digenac XL ➤ diclofenac.

Digibind infusion contains digoxin-specific antibody fragments. It is used to treat digoxin and digitoxin overdosage. *Adverse effects* include fall in blood potassium levels. *Precautions:* Do not use in patients allergic to ovine protein.

digitoxin. Read Chapter 23 on drugs used to treat heart failure and ➤ digoxin.

digoxin (Lanoxin) is used to treat heart failure and disorders of heart rhythm. See Chapter 23. *Adverse effects* include nausea, loss of appetite, vomiting, diarrhoea, abdominal pain, visual disturbances, fatigue, drowsiness, headache, confusion, delirium, hallucinations, slowing of heart rate and heart block. These adverse effects are usually associated with overdosage. *Precautions:* Do not use in patients with heart block or certain disorders of the heart or heart rhythm. Use with caution in patients who have had a recent heart attack and in patients with an over-active thyroid gland or impaired kidney function. Reduce the dose in the elderly and avoid rapid intravenous infusion because it may cause nausea, vomiting and disorders of heart rhythm. Use with caution in patients with severe lung disease or raised blood calcium levels. Monitor heart rate, ECG and blood chemistry. *Interactions:* Calcium supplements, digoxin-related drugs, any drug that may cause a fall in blood potassium levels, quinidine, lithium, antacids, antibiotics.

digoxin-specific antibody fragments ➤ Digibind.

dihydrocodeine (dihydrocodeine acid tartrate, dihydrocodeine tartrate, in Codydramol, DF 118, DHC Continus, in Paramol, in Remedeine) is a mild to moderate opiate pain-reliever. See Chapter 30. It is also used as a cough suppressant. See Chapter 11. *Adverse effects* include nausea, vomiting, headache, dizziness and constipation. For other potential adverse effects ➤ morphine. *Precautions:* Use with caution in patients with impaired liver or kidney function, allergies, under-active thyroid, in pregnancy and in elderly patients. Do not use in patients with severe respiratory disorders. *Drug dependence:* It may rarely produce dependence of the morphine type. *Interactions:* alcohol, sedatives, sleeping drugs and other drugs that depress brain function.

dihydrotachysterol (AT 10) is related to vitamin D. It is used to treat tetany (spasm or cramps due to disturbed blood chemistry) caused by a low blood calcium level due to underworking of the parathyroid glands. *Adverse effects:* It may cause a rise in blood calcium levels and calcium in the urine, loss of appetite, listlessness, thirst, vertigo, headache, nausea, urgency to pass urine, passing large volumes of urine, paralysis, stupor. *Precautions:* Use with caution in pregnancy, in breastfeeding mothers or if kidney function is impaired. Monitor blood calcium levels. *Interactions:* Thiazide diuretics, digoxin and related drugs, cholestyramine.

dihydroxycholecalciferol is a form of vitamin D. See Chapter 36 on vitamins.

Dijex is an antacid preparation containing aluminium and magnesium.

Dilcardia SR ➤ diltiazem.

diloxanide furoate (Furamide) is used to treat chronic amoebic infections of the intestine. *Adverse effects* include wind, vomiting, itching and nettle-rash. *Precautions:* Use with utmost caution in pregnancy and in breastfeeding mothers.

diltiazem (Adizem, Angitil, Angitil SR, Angiozem, Calcicord CR, Dilcardia SR, Dilzem, Optil SR, Optil XL, Slozem, Tildiem, Viazem XL, Zemtard XL) is a calcium-channel blocker used to treat angina (see Chapter 22) and hypertension (see Chapter 25). *Adverse effects* include slowing of the heart, heart block, fluid retention causing ankle-swelling, headache, nausea, rashes, fall in blood pressure, generally feeling unwell, hot flushes, stomach and bowel upsets. Depression and liver damage have been reported. *Precautions:* Do not use in patients with severe slowing of the heart rate, left ventricular failure, serious heart block, or in pregnancy. Use with caution in patients with impaired liver or kidney function, heart failure, or mild slowing of the heart rate. *Interactions:* Other anti-blood pressure drugs, beta-blockers, digoxin, carbamazepine, cyclosporin, theophylline, cimetidine, lithium.

Dilzem, Dilzem SR and **Dilzem XL** ➤ diltiazem.

dimercaprol (BAL, Dimercaprol) is used to treat poisoning by antimony, arsenic, bismuth, gold, mercury and thallium. It is used with sodium calcium edetate to treat lead poisoning. *Adverse effects* include nausea, vomiting, salivation, runny eyes, sweating, rapid heart beat, raised blood pressure, burning sensation in mouth, throat and eyes, tightness of throat and chest, abdominal pain, headaches, muscle spasms and tingling in the hands and feet. It may cause a fever in children and the injection may cause local pain and abscesses. *Precautions:* Do not use to treat iron, cadmium or selenium poisoning and do not use to treat severe liver involvement unless due to lead. Use with caution in pregnancy, in the elderly and in patients with raised blood pressure and impaired kidney function. Be very cautious if impaired kidney function develops during treatment.

dimethyl sulfoxide (dimethyl sulphoxide, methyl sulphoxide, in Herpid, in Rimso-50) is principally used as a basis for other drugs to be applied to the skin. It increases their effects by aiding their penetration into the skin. It is well absorbed into the bloodstream, broken down in the body to dimethyl sulphide, and excreted in the urine, faeces, breath and skin, which produces a characteristic garlic-like odour in anyone using it. *Adverse effects:* High concentrations applied to the skin may cause a burning sensation, itching, redness and very rarely, blisters. Long-term use may cause nausea, vomiting, abdominal cramps, chest pains, headache, drowsiness and allergic reactions.

dimethyl sulphoxide ➤ dimethyl sulfoxide.

dimeticones (in Conotrane, in Kolanticon, in Siopel, in Sprilon, in Timodine, in Vasogen) are water-repellent silicones used to reduce wind when taken by mouth (they work as anti-foaming agents). They are also used in barrier skin applications as a water-repellent.

dimeticone activated (Altacite Plus, Asilone, Infacol, Maalox) ➤ simethicone.

Dimetriose ➤ gestrinone.

Dimotane preparations ➤ brompheniramine.

Dimotone Co preparations are cough medicines that contain brompheniramine, codeine and pseudoephedrine ➤ brompheniramine, codeine, pseudoephedrine.

Dindevan ➤ phenindione.

Dinnefords Teejel ➤ choline salicylate.

dinoprostone is prostaglandin E2. See Chapter 52. It causes the uterus to contract and the cervix to soften and is used to start off labour or to produce an abortion. Preparations include Prepidil (cervical gel), Propess-RS (vaginal pessaries) and Prostin E2 (tablets, intravenous solution, extra-amniotic solution, vaginal gel and vaginal tablets). *Adverse effects* include nausea, vomiting, diarrhoea, severe contractions of the uterus. Intravenous administration may cause flushing, shivering, dizziness, headache, transient rise in temperature and raised white blood cell count. Intravenous injections may cause pain and redness at site of injection and there is a risk of infection with extra-amniotic injection. *Precautions:* Do not use in women allergic to prostaglandins, who have ruptured membranes, history of Caesarean section or major surgery on the uterus. Do not use if the baby is in the wrong position, in women with untreated pelvic infections, if the baby is distressed, in a multiple pregnancy, in women who have had many babies or a history of difficult childbirth. Do not use extra-amniotic route if patient has an infection of her vagina or cervix. Use with

caution in patients with asthma or glaucoma. Monitor activity of uterus and monitor the baby. *Interactions:* oxytocin.

Diocalm is an anti-diarrhoeal preparation containing attapulgite and morphine.

Diocalm Ultra ➤ loperamide.

Diocaps ➤ loperamide.

Dioctyl ➤ docusate sodium.

dioctyl sodium suphosuccinate ➤ docusate sodium.

Dioderm cream ➤ hydrocortisone.

Dioralyte powders contain sodium chloride, potassium chloride, sodium acid citrate and glucose. They are used to treat fluid and salt loss, especially in babies with diarrhoea and vomiting. See Chapter 20.

Diovan ➤ valsartan.

Dipentum ➤ olsalazine.

diphenhydramine (diphenhydramine hydrochloride) is a sedative antihistamine. See Chapter 17. *Adverse effects and Precautions* ➤ antihistamines. It is present in numerous cold, cough and flu remedies, in Caladryl cream and lotion (➤ Caladryl) and in the pain-relieving compound Propain. Because one of its main adverse effects is drowsiness it is also used in Dreemon, Medinex, Nightcalm, Nytol and in Pandol Night to promote sleep. See Chapter 1.

diphenoxylate (in Lomotil, Tropergen) is an opiate that reduces the movement of the wall of the intestine and is used to treat diarrhoea (see Chapter 20). *Adverse effects* include itching, skin rash, drowsiness, insomnia, dizziness, restlessness, changes in mood, abdominal distension and cramps. *Precautions:* It should not be used to treat diarrhoea after antibiotic use, if the bowel is obstructed, or if the bowel is ulcerated or inflamed after antibiotic use. Use with caution in pregnancy, in breastfeeding mothers, in patients with impaired liver function or inflammatory bowel disease. *Adverse effects* may be exaggerated in infants and children and it should therefore not be used in children under nine. *Drug dependence:* Diphenoxylate may, rarely, produce drug dependence of the morphine type. Diphenoxylate is often combined with atropine ➤ co-phenotrope.

diphenylpyraline (diphenylpyraline hydrochloride) is an antihistamine drug ➤ antihistamines.

diphosphonates ➤ biphosphonates.

dipipanone (piperidyl methadone hydrochloride, in Diconal) is an opiate pain-reliever which produces less sedation than morphine, see Chapter 30. *Adverse effects:* Nausea, vomiting, dizziness, retention of urine and constipation may occur ➤ morphine. *Precautions:* It should not be used in patients with severe respiratory disorders. It should be used with extreme caution in patients with impaired liver or kidney function. *Drug dependence:* Dipipanone may produce drug dependence of the morphine type. It is available combined with cyclizine (an anti-vomiting drug) as Diconal ➤ Diconal.

dipivetrine (Propine) is a sympathomimetic drug used in eye drops to treat chronic open-angle glaucoma, see p. 62. It is a pro-drug of adrenaline which passes rapidly through the cornea to release the adrenaline(epinephrine) inside the front chamber of the eye. *Adverse effects* include transient stinging of the eyes and rebound redness. It may occasionally cause allergic reactions and, very rarely, a raised blood pressure. *Precautions:* Do not use in patients with closed-angle glaucoma. Do not wear soft contact lenses. Use with caution in patients with narrow-angle glaucoma or aphakia (missing a lens in the eye).

dipotassium clorazepate ➤ clorazepate.

Diprivan ➤ propofol.

Diprobase emollient cream and ointment contain liquid paraffin, and white soft paraffin ➤ liquid paraffin.

Diprobath bath emollient contains liquid paraffin and isopropyl myristate. It is used to treat dry skin conditions ➤ liquid paraffin.

Diprosalic ointment and scalp lotion contain betamethasone (a corticosteroid) and salicylic acid (a keratolytic – used for removing dead skin). They are used to treat eczema and psoriasis. *Adverse effects and Precautions* see corticosteroid skin applications, p. 241 and ➤ salicylic acid.

Diprosone preparations ➤ betamethasone.

dipyridamole (in Asasartin Retard, Persantin) is an antiplatelet drug (see p. 143) used with anticoagulants to prevent blood clots around prosthetic heart valves. *Adverse effects:* It may cause headache, dizziness, faintness, rash and stomach and bowel upsets. *Precautions:* It should be used with caution in patients with rapidly worsening angina or narrowing of the main artery from the heart (aortic stenosis). *Interactions:* Antacids.

Dirythmin SA ➤ disopyramide,

disinfectants, see p. 244.

Disipal ➤ orphenadrine.

disodium cromoglycate ➤ sodium cromoglicate.

disodium edetate (in Optiflo G, in Uriflex G, in Uriflex R, in Uro-Tainer) is used in catheter solutions to remove calcium deposits from the bladder. It is used as the trisodium salt (Limclair) to treat raised blood levels of calcium ➤ trisodium edetate.

disodium etidronate ➤ etidronate disodium.

disodium folinate (Sodiofolin) is used to enhance the effects of the anti-cancer drug 5-fluorouracil (5FU) in bowel cancer. See Chapter 51. *Adverse effects* include allergic reactions, fever. *Precautions:* Do not use in pregnancy or while breastfeeding.

disodium pamidronate (Aredia) is used to treat raised blood calcium levels caused by secondary cancer deposits in bone, bone loss and bone pain associated with secondary breast cancer, multiple myeloma and Paget's disease of the bone. *Adverse effects* include nausea, diarrhoea, a mild transient rise in temperature, flu-like symptoms, bone, joint and muscle pains, eye disorders (iritis, uveitis), skin reactions at the site of injection, headache, blood disorders and low blood magnesium and calcium levels. *Precautions:* Do not use in patients known to be allergic to the drug. Use with utmost caution in pregnancy, in breastfeeding mothers, in patients with impaired kidney function, heart disease or previous thyroid surgery. Changes in blood chemistry may possibly trigger convulsions. Monitor blood chemistry and kidney function during long-term use. *Interactions:* Biphosphonates used to lower blood calcium level, plicamycin.

disodium phosphate ➤ sodium phosphate.

disopyramide (disopyramide phosphate, Dirythmin SA, Isomide CR, Rythmodan, Rythmodan Retard) is used to treat disorders of heart rhythm (see Chapter 24). *Adverse effects:* Dry mouth, blurred vision, difficulty in passing water, constipation, stomach and bowel upsets, low blood pressure, low blood sugar levels, low blood potassium levels and disorders of heart rhythm. *Precautions:* Do not use in patients with serious heart block (in absence of a pacemaker), cardiomyopathy (disease of the heart muscles), low blood pressure, or severe collapse due to a heart attack. It should be used with caution in patients with a low blood potassium, with glaucoma, enlarged prostate gland, a tendency to retention of urine, mild heart block, heart failure (should be controlled with digoxin), impaired kidney or liver function, in pregnancy or in patients with myasthenia gravis (muscle weakness due to neuromuscular abnormality). *Interactions:* Other class I anti-arrhythmic drugs, beta-blockers, drugs that lower blood potassium levels, antimuscarinics, erythromycin, rifampicin, phenytoin.

Disprin ➤ aspirin.

Disprin CV ➤ aspirin.

Disprin Direct ➤ aspirin.

Disprin Extra contains aspirin and paracetamol ➤ aspirin, paracetamol.

Disprol suspension ➤ paracetamol. Contains 120 mg paracetamol per 5 ml of sugar-free suspension. It is used to treat fever following vaccination in babies over two months of age. Also used to treat pain and fever in childhood ➤ paracetamol.

Distaclor preparations ➤ cefaclor.

Distalgesic ➤ co-proxamol.

Distamine ➤ penicillamine.

distigmine (distigmine bromide, Ubretid) is an anticholinesterase, see Chapter 9. It is used in the treatment of urinary retention, myasthenia gravis (muscle weakness due to neuromuscular abnormality) and paralysis of the bowel after surgical operations. *Adverse effects and Precautions* ➤ neostigmine.

disulfiram (Antabuse) is used to treat alcoholism. It is not a cure and it is used because it produces unpleasant effects when alcohol is taken. These unpleasant effects are caused by an accumulation in the blood of a breakdown product of alcohol called acetaldehyde. Within fifteen minutes of taking alcohol, disulfiram may produce red eyes, flushed face, throbbing headache, fast-beating heart, dizziness, nausea, sweating and vomiting. An irritation in the throat, deep breathing and a fall in blood pressure, collapse and convulsions may occur. The effects last from a half to one hour in mild cases and up to several hours in severe attacks. The intensity and duration vary greatly between individuals; initial treatment should therefore only be used in hospital. A careful dosage regimen needs to be worked out, starting with a high dose and slowly working down to a maintenance dose. *Adverse effects:* Disulfiram may cause indigestion, bad breath, body odour, nausea, vomiting, drowsiness, fatigue, severe mental symptoms, liver damage, headache, impotence, allergic skin rashes and nerve damage (peripheral neuritis). Even small quantities of alcohol (e.g. in oral medicines) may produce a severe reaction. *Precautions:* Do not take alcohol for at least twelve hours before starting disulfiram. It should not be used in pregnancy, in patients with heart disease, raised blood pressure, history of a stroke, with severe psychological disorders or with drug dependence. It should be used with the utmost caution in patients with impaired liver or kidney function, and in patients with epilepsy, chronic chest disorders or diabetes. *Interactions:* alcohol, barbiturates, warfarin, paraldehyde. Toiletries containing alcohol should be avoided.

dithranol (Dithrocream, Micanol, in Psorin) is used to treat psoriasis. Some patients are sensitive to it and a small area of skin should be tested first. It stains the skin, causes a burning sensation and irritates the eyes. Do not use to treat acute psoriasis. Avoid contact with unaffected skin, eyes and mucous membranes.

Dithrocream preparations ➤ dithranol.

Ditropan ➤ oxybutynin.

Ditropan XL ➤ oxybutynin.

Diumide-K Continus tablets contain furosemide(frusemide) (a loop diuretic) and sustained-release potassium chloride. They are used to treat fluid retention (oedema) in patients suffering from kidney, liver or heart disease where a potassium supplement is required. See Chapter 29. *Adverse effects and Precautions* ➤ furosemide(frusemide), potassium supplements.

diuretics, see Chapter 29.

Diurexan ➤ xipamide.

Dixarit ➤ clonidine.

dobutamine (Dobutrex, Posiject) is a beta-stimulant sympathomimetic drug used to stimulate the heart (see p. 123) in patients whose circulation has collapsed due to sudden heart failure (cardiogenic shock), septic shock or during heart surgery. *Adverse effects* include rapid beating of the heart. A marked rise in systolic blood pressure indicates overdose. *Precautions:* Use with caution in patients with cardiogenic shock whose blood pressure is seriously low.

Dobutrex ➤ dobutamine.

docetaxel (Taxotere) is an anti-cancer drug (see Chapter 51) to treat patients suffering from advanced breast cancer. *Adverse effects* include fall in white blood cell and platelet counts, increased risk of bleeding, anaemia, allergic reactions, fall in blood pressure, wheezing, skin rashes, loss of hair, damage to nails, fluid retention, nerve damage, painful joints and muscles, inflammation of the lining of the mouth and intestine and changes in liver function tests. *Precautions:* Monitor blood counts and liver function. During infusions watch out for allergic reactions and fluid retention. *Interactions:* Cyclosporin, terfenadine, ketoconazole, erythromycin, troleandomycin.

docosahexaenoic acid (DHA) is a constituent of omega-3 marine triglycerides (Maxepa capsules) which also contains eicosapentaenoic acid (EPA). Maxepa is used to lower blood cholesterol and fat levels ➤ Maxepa.

docusate sodium (in co-danthrusate, in Capsuvac, Dioctyl, Docusol, in Fletcher's Enemette, Molcer ear drops, Norgalax micro-enema, in Normax, Waxsol ear drops) is a surface-active agent which lowers surface tension and has detergent properties. It is used as a laxative (see p. 110), to soften wax in the ears (see p. 57), to make tablets disintegrate in the body and as a surface-active agent in industry.

Docusol ➤ docusate sodium.

Do-Do expectorant is a cough mixture containing guaifenesin ➤ guaifenesin.

Do-Do Chesteze is a cough medicine which contains ephedrine and theophylline ➤ ephedrine, theophylline.

Dolmatil ➤ sulpiride.

Dolobid ➤ diflunisal.

Doloxene ➤ dextropropoxyphene.

Dolvan contains paracetamol, diphenhydramine, ephedrine and caffeine ➤ individual entry for each drug.

domiphen (in Bradosol Plus), is an antiseptic with properties similar to those described under cetrimide. It is used in throat lozenges and antiseptic skin applications. In higher concentration it may be used as a disinfectant.

Domperamol contains paracetamol and domperidone ➤ paracetamol, domperidone.

domperidone (in Domperamol, Motilium) is an anti-dopamine drug used to treat acute nausea and vomiting caused by disorders of the stomach or intestine or by anti-cancer drugs, radiotherapy or anti-parkinsonism drugs (levodopa, bromocriptine). See Chapter 18. It may also be used to treat indigestion. *Adverse effects:* It has similar effects to metoclopramide but is less likely to cause sedation and atony (lack of muscle tone). It may send up the level of prolactin in the blood and cause enlargement of the breasts and milk production. It may cause allergic reactions, skin rashes, reduced libido and acute disorders of movement (dystonias). Injections may cause serious disorders of heart rhythm in patients with heart disease or low blood potassium levels. *Precautions:* Do not use regularly every day, or as a routine following surgery. Do not use in pregnancy. Use with caution in patients with impaired kidney function and in breastfeeding mothers.

donepezil (Aricept) is an acetylcholinesterase inhibitor used to treat mild to moderately severe Alzheimer's dementia. See Chapter 9. *Adverse effects* include stomach and bowel upsets, muscle cramps, fatigue, insomnia, dizziness, headache, pain. Rarely, liver damage, psychiatric disturbances, fainting, slow heart beat, seizures, liver dysfunction, loss of appetite, anorexia, stomach and bowel ulcers and haemorrhage, muscle dysfunction. *Precautions:* Do not use in pregnancy or while breastfeeding. Use with caution in patients with altered heart beat, history or risk of stomach or bowel ulcers, asthma, severe difficulty breathing, bladder outflow obstruction, seizures, muscle dysfunction.

Dopacard ➤ dopexamine.

dopa-decarboxylase inhibitors, see p. 79.

dopamine is a sympathomimetic drug (see Chapter 9) used to treat patients whose circulation has collapsed due to sudden heart failure (cardiogenic shock) as a result of a heart attack or during heart surgery, see p. 124. *Adverse effects* include nausea, vomiting, rapid beating of the heart, changes in blood pressure, and coldness and paleness of the skin (vasoconstriction). *Precautions:* Do not use in patients with a tumour of the central nervous system or a rapid heart beat. Any reduction in blood volume must be treated immediately with intravenous blood or fluids. The dose of dopamine must be carefully controlled; low doses may cause dilatation of arteries and increase the flow of blood through the kidneys, whereas high doses may cause constriction of arteries and make the heart failure worse.

dopexamine (Dopacard) is used to treat heart failure (see p. 123) during heart surgery. It is a sympathomimetic drug that stimulates beta$_2$-receptors and dopamine receptors. It also blocks the re-uptake of noradrenaline(norepinephrine) into nerve cells (see Chapter 9). These actions increase the output from the heart by reducing the afterload, by a direct effect on the heart and by reducing pre-load. *Adverse effects* include rapid beating of the heart and extra beats during infusion. Occasionally, high doses may cause nausea, vomiting, tremor and anginal pain. *Precautions:* Do not use in pregnancy or in breastfeeding mothers. Do not use in patients with a tumour of the central nervous system, low platelet count, or obstruction to the outflow of the blood from the heart (e.g. aortic stenosis). Use with caution in patients with acute heart attack, recent anginal attacks, low blood potassium, or high blood sugar.

Dopram ➤ doxapram.

Doralese ➤ indoramin.

Dormonoct ➤ loprazolam.

dornase alfa (Pulmozyme) is a genetically engineered version of a naturally occurring human enzyme that helps to break down and remove the sticky secretions that build up in the lungs in patients suffering from cystic fibrosis. The solution is given by inhalation through a jetnebulizer. *Adverse effects* include sore throat, hoarseness, skin rash and voice changes. *Precautions:* Use with utmost caution in pregnancy or breast-feeding mothers. Do not mix other drugs in the nebulizer.

dorzolamide (in Cosopt, Trusopt) eye drops are used to treat raised pressure in the eyes in open-angle glaucoma. See p. 64. It may be used with beta-blockers or in place of beta-blockers if these are unsuitable. They are a carbonic anhydrase inhibitor diuretic. See Chapter 29. *Adverse effects* include irritation, burning and stinging of the eyes, blurred vision, headache, bitter taste, soreness of the eyelids and conjunctivitis. *Precautions:* Do not use in patients with severe impairment of kidney function, in pregnancy, or in breastfeeding mothers. Do not wear soft contact lenses. Use with caution in patients with impaired liver function, closed-angle glaucoma or allergy to sulphonamide drugs.

Dostinex ➤ cabergoline.

dosulepin(dothiepin) (Dothapax, Prothiaden) is a tricyclic antidepressant drug ➤ tricyclic antidepressants.

Dothapax ➤ dosulepin.

dothiepin ➤ dosulepin.

Doublebase is a skin-softening cream containing isopropyl myristate and liquid paraffin.

Dovonex ➤ calcipotriol.

doxapram (doxapram hydrochloride, Dopram) is given by intravenous infusion to stimulate breathing in patients with respiratory failure. *Adverse effects:* Rise in blood pressure and heart rate, dizziness and perineal warmth. *Precautions:* Do not use in patients with very high blood pressure, uncontrolled short-term severe asthma (status asthmaticus), coronary artery disease, or overworking of the thyroid gland. Use with caution in patients with epilepsy or impaired liver function.

doxazosin (Cardura) is a selective alpha-blocker used to treat raised blood pressure (see Chapter 25). It is also used to improve passing of urine in patients with an enlarged prostate gland, see p. 284. *Adverse effects:* A fall in blood pressure may occur on standing up after sitting or lying down (postural hypotension). This may cause light-headedness and faintness. It may also cause headache, fatigue and weakness, dizziness, runny nose, sleepiness and vertigo. Rarely it may cause incontinence of urine. Fluid retention (oedema) may occur, causing, for example, ankle swelling. *Precautions:* It should not be used by breastfeeding mothers and it should be used with caution in pregnancy. Sleepiness may affect ability to drive.

doxepin (doxepin hydrochloride, Sinequan, Xepin cream) is a tricyclic antidepressant drug ➤ tricyclic antidepressants.

doxorubicin (has replaced adriamycin) (Caelyx, Myocet) is an anti-cancer drug (see Chapter 51). *Adverse effects:* It colours the urine red. Doxorubicin may damage the bone marrow causing blood disorders, and it may cause ulcers of the mouth, loss of hair, nausea, vomiting and diarrhoea and, very rarely, allergic reactions and damage to the heart. It may damage the tissues at the site of injection. *Precautions:* Careful monitoring of the blood and heart should be carried out. It should be used with the utmost caution in patients with impaired heart function and in the elderly.

doxycycline (doxycycline hydrochloride,

Periost, Vibramycin) is a tetracycline anti-biotic, see p. 269. It is well absorbed, even when taken with food, and acts for a long time; its excretion is slow and it is possible to get high blood levels with a single daily dosage. *Adverse effects and Precautions* ➤ tetracyclines.

doxylamine (doxylamine succinate, in Syndol) is an antihistamine drug ➤ antihistamines.

Doxylar ➤ doxycycline.

Dozic ➤ haloperidol.

Dozol contains paracetamol and diphenydramine ➤ paracetamol, diphenydramine.

Drapolene cream contains benzalkonium and cetrimide ➤ benzalkonium, cetrimide.

Dreemon ➤ diphenhydramine hydrochloride.

Driclor antiperspirant ➤ aluminium chloride.

Drogenil ➤ flutamide.

Dromadol XL ➤ tramadol.

Dristan tablets contain aspirin, caffeine, chlorphenamine, phenylephrine ➤ individual entry for each drug.

DTIC-Dome ➤ dacarbazine.

Dubam spray contains glycol salicylate, methyl salicylate, ethyl salicylate and methyl nicotinate. It is used as a rheumatic rub ➤ rubefacients.

Dulco-lax ➤ bisacodyl.

Dumicoat dental lacquer ➤ miconazole. It is used to treat thrush associated with denture infection.

Duofilm liquid contains salicylic acid and lactic acid in a flexible dressing that dries on the skin. It is used to treat plantar and mosaic warts (see p. 262). *Precautions:* Avoid contact with healthy skin. Do not use on facial warts or anogenital warts ➤ salicylic acid.

Duovent aerosol contains fenoterol (a selective beta-stimulant) and ipratropium (an antimuscarinic drug). It is used to treat asthma and chronic obstructive airways disease. See Chapter 14 and ➤ antimuscarinic drugs, fenoterol. *Adverse effects* include dry mouth, headache and increased circulation to the skin (peripheral vasodilatation). *Precautions:* Use with caution in patients with overworking thyroid, coronary artery disease, raised blood pressure, disorders of heart rhythm, glaucoma or enlarged prostate gland. *Interactions:* Sympathomimetic drugs.

Duphalac ➤ lactulose.

Duphaston and **Duphaston HRT** ➤ dydrogesterone. It is a progestogen used in HRT. *Adverse effects* include nausea, headache, bloating, dizziness, breast tenderness, breakthrough bleeding, skin rashes ➤ HRT.

Duragel is a spermicidal gel containing nonoxinol 9.

Durogesic self-adhesive patches ➤ fentanyl.

dusting powders are finely divided powders that contain one or more active ingredients. They are applied to skin folds where friction may occur. They should not be applied to areas that are very moist because they may cake and make the skin sore. *Talc* acts as a lubricant powder but it does not absorb moisture, whereas *starch* is less lubricant but does absorb water. Other inert powders such as zinc oxide and kaolin may also be used.

Dutonin ➤ nefazodone.

Dyazide ➤ co-triamterzide.

dydrogesterone (Duphaston, Duphaston HRT, Fempak, Femoston, Femoston-Conti) is a progestogen, see p. 198. *Adverse effects and Precautions* ➤ progestogens.

Dynamin ➤ isorbide mononitrate.

Dynese antacid ➤ magaldrate.

Dysman preparations ➤ mefenamic acid.

Dyspamet ➤ cimetidine.

Dysport ➤ botulinum toxin.

Dytac ➤ triamterene.

Dytide capsules contain triamterene (a potassium-sparing diuretic) and benz-thiazide (a thiazide diuretic). See Chapter 29. They are used to treat fluid retention (oedema). *Adverse effects and Precautions* ➤ triamterene, thiazide diuretics.

E45 cream contains light liquid paraffin, white soft paraffin and hypoallergenic anhy-drous lanolin. It is used to soften the skin. See p. 236.

ear preparations, see Chapter 13.

EarCalm ➤ acetic acid.

Ebufac ➤ ibuprofen.

Econac ➤ diclofenac.

Econacort cream contains econazole (an antifungal drug) and hydrocortisone (a corticosteroid). It is used to treat fungal infections of the skin that are inflamed. Avoid contact with eyes. *Adverse effects and Precautions* ➤ econazole and see cortico-steroid skin applications p. 241.

Economycin ➤ tetracycline.

econazole (in Econacort, Ecostatin, Gyno-Pevaryl, Pevaryl) is an antifungal drug (see Chapter 47) with some antibacterial activity. It is applied onto the skin to treat fungal infections of the skin, thrush of the vagina and nappy rash infected with thrush. It may occasionally cause irritation at the site of application and, rarely, an allergic reaction.

Ecopace ➤ captopril.

Ecostatin preparations ➤ econazole.

Edronax ➤ reboxetine.

edrophonium (Camsilon) is an anti-cholinesterase drug (see Chapter 9) with a very brief duration of action. It is used to diagnose myasthenia gravis (muscle weak-ness due to neuromuscular abnormality). It is also used to diagnose dual block caused by suxamethonium (a muscle relaxant with a short duration of action). *Adverse effects and Precautions* ➤ neostigmine.

Ednyt ➤ enalapril.

Efalith ointment contains lithium succinate and zinc sulphate. It is used to treat the skin disorder seborrhoeic dermatitis. Lithium has antifungal and anti-inflammatory prop-erties and may also stimulate the immune system. *Adverse effects:* Local irritation. *Pre-cautions:* It should not be used in children. Use with caution in psoriasis. It should not be applied to the eyes or mucous mem-branes (e.g. mouth).

Efamast ➤ gamolenic acid.

efavirenz (Sustiva) is used in combination with other antiretrovirals to treat HIV-1 infection. See Chapter 48. *Adverse effects* include skin rash, nervous system reactions such as dizziness, insomnia, impaired con-centration, psychotic reactions, stomach and bowel upsets, headache, fatigue, raised liver enzymes. *Precautions:* Do not use in patients with severe liver damage, in preg-nancy or while breastfeeding. Use with cau-tion in patients with mild liver or severe kidney damage, hepatitis B or C, a history of mental illness or substance abuse.

Efcortelan skin preparations and injections ➤ hydrocortisone.

Efcortesol injection ➤ hydrocortisone.

Efexor ➤ venlafaxine.

Effercitrate tablets contain citric acid and potassium bicarbonate. They are used to make the urine less acid (i.e. alkaline) in order to reduce the symptoms of cystitis. *Adverse effects* include a rise in blood potass-ium levels, irritation of the stomach and passing more urine than usual. *Precautions:* Do not use in patients with ulceration or obstruction of the bowel. Use with caution in patients with impaired kidney function. *Interactions:* potassium-sparing diuretics.

Effico is a tonic which contains thiamine, nicotinamide, caffeine and compound gen-tian infusion.

eformoterol ➤ formoterol.

Efudix ➤ fluorouracil.

eicosapentaenoic acid (Maxepa) is used to treat high triglyceride levels in patients at risk from heart disease (see Chapter 26) or inflammation of the pancreas. *Adverse effects* include nausea and belching. *Precautions:* Do not use in patients with bleeding disorders or non-insulin dependent diabetes.

Elantan and **Elantan LA** ➤ isosorbide mononitrate.

Elavil ➤ amitriptyline.

Eldepryl ➤ selegiline.

Eldisine ➤ vindesine.

Electrolade sachets contain a powder for dissolving in cool drinking water for the treatment of fluid loss caused by, for example, diarrhoea and vomiting. The powder in each sachet contains sodium chloride, potassium chloride, sodium bicarbonate and glucose. *Precautions:* The made-up solution should not be used in patients with kidney failure and used with caution in patients with severe, acute abdominal pain. Diabetic patients should note the sugar content.

Elleste Duet contains tablets of oestradiol (an oestrogen) and norethisterone (a progestogen). It is used for HRT ➤ HRT.

Elleste Solo ➤ oestradiol. It is used as HRT in women who have had a hysterectomy ➤ HRT.

Elliman's Universal Embrocation is used as a heat rub in muscle pain. It contains acetic acid and turpentine oil.

Elocon preparations ➤ mometasone furoate.

Eloahes 6% intravenous infusion contains hetastarch and sodium chloride ➤ hetastarch

Eloxatin ➤ oxaliplatin.

Eltroxin ➤ levothyroxine.

Eludril spray contains chlorhexidine (an antibacterial drug) and amethocaine (a local anaesthetic). It is used to treat mouth and throat infections. *Adverse effects and Precautions* ➤ chlorhexidine, amethocaine.

Elyzol suppositories ➤ metronidazole.

Emadine ➤ emedastine.

Emblon ➤ tamoxifen.

Emcor ➤ bisoprolol.

emedastine (Emadine) anti-allergy eye drops are used to treat inflammation of the eye caused by hayfever. See Chapter 13. *Adverse effects* include transient stinging in the eye, blurred vision, swelling in the eyes (oedema), headache, inflammation of the lining of the nose and pain. *Precautions:* Do not use in patients with kidney or liver damage, in the elderly, in pregnancy or while breastfeeding. Use with caution in patients with eye damage. Do not insert contact lenses until ten–fifteen minutes after using the eye drops.

Emeside ➤ ethosuximide.

emetics are drugs that cause vomiting. *Ipecacuanha* mixture is occasionally used to empty the stomach after swallowing certain poisons (e.g. salicylates). The chief danger is that some of the vomit from the stomach may be inhaled. There is no evidence that it prevents the absorption of significant amounts of poisons. It must only be used in patients who are fully conscious. It must not be used in patients who have swallowed a corrosive poison or a substance derived from petrol because if these are inhaled they can seriously damage the lungs. It must *not* be used if the poison is known to produce rapid onset of coma or convulsions. Salt solution, copper sulphate and mustard are dangerous and should not be used to produce vomiting.

Emfib ➤ gemfibrozil.

Emflex ➤ acemetacin.

EMLA cream contains the local anaesthetics lidocaine(lignocaine) and prilocaine. It is used as an anaesthetic on the skin and genitals. See Chapter 44. May cause transient reactions at the site of application. Do not apply to wounds or to patients with eczema.

emollients, see p. 236.

Emulsiderm liquid emulsion contains liquid paraffin, isopropylmyristate and benzalkonium. It is used as an antiseptic skin softener to treat dry skin ➤ each constituent drug.

Enacard ➤ enalapril.

enalapril (Edynt, Enacord, Innovace, in Innozide, Pralenel) is an ACE inhibitor used to treat raised blood pressure (see Chapter 25) and heart failure (see Chapter 23). *Adverse effects* include headache, dizziness, fatigue, weakness, nausea, diarrhoea, muscle cramps, altered taste, fall in blood pressure and rarely, skin rashes, allergic swellings of the mouth and throat (angioedema) and a persistent dry irritant cough. Very rarely, it may cause kidney failure. *Precautions:* Do not use in pregnancy or in patients with aortic stenosis or other obstruction to the outflow of blood from the heart. Use with caution in patients with impaired kidney function, raised blood pressure due to kidney disease, severe congestive heart failure, in breastfeeding mothers and during general anaesthesia. Kidney function tests should be carried out before and at regular intervals during treatment. *Interactions:* Other anti-blood pressure drugs, lithium, potassium supplements, potassium-sparing diuretics.

Enbrel ➤ etanercept.

enbucrilate (Histoacryl, Indermil) is used as a tissue adhesive for closure of minor skin wounds and sealing skin wounds that have been stitched. Within twenty seconds the moisture on the wound causes it to bond. It must be applied very thinly. Do not allow it to come into contact with the eyes, blood vessels, internal organs or nerve tissues.

En-De-Kay preparations ➤ fluoride.

Endoxana ➤ cyclophosphamide.

enflurane (Alyrone, Enflurane) is an inhalant anaesthetic similar to halothane but less potent. It is usually given along with a nitrous oxide/oxygen mixture. It depresses breathing which can result in shallow breathing causing the blood level of carbon dioxide to increase. It also depresses the heart and causes a fall in blood pressure. It may interact with dry carbon dioxide adsorbent to form carbon monoxide, therefore do not let carbon dioxide adsorbent dry out.

EnergixB is a vaccine which contains inactivated hepatitis B virus surface antigen. The vaccine is used in individuals who are at high risk of contracting hepatitis B.

Eno preparations are antacids which contain sodium bicarbonate and sodium carbonate.

enoxaparin (in Clexane) is a low-molecular-weight heparin (LMWH) used to prevent thrombosis (blood clotting in veins) particularly during orthopaedic and general surgery. It is also used to prevent the blood clotting during blood dialysis and to treat deep-vein thrombosis. See Chapter 28. *Adverse effects* include a fall in blood platelets (thrombocytopenia) and disorders of liver function. For other potentially harmful effects ➤ heparin. *Precautions:* It should not be used to treat individuals with pericarditis (inflammation of the lining surrounding the heart), serious bleeding disorders, acute peptic ulcers, stroke due to bleeding into the brain, or who have a low blood platelet count. It should not be given by intramuscular injection. It should be used with caution in people with impaired liver function, or a history of peptic or intestinal ulcers, in pregnancy, in breastfeeding mothers and in individuals with uncontrolled high blood pressure. *Interactions:* Oral anticoagulants, anti-platelet drugs, NSAIDs, aspirin, dextran.

enoximone (Perfan) is a selective phosphodiesterase inhibitor which helps to improve the function of heart muscle. It is used to treat congestive heart failure. See

Chapter 23. *Adverse effects* include fall in blood pressure, disorders of heart rhythm, nausea, vomiting, diarrhoea, headache, insomnia and occasionally fever, chills, painful arms and legs and difficulty passing urine. *Precautions:* Use with utmost caution in patients whose heart failure is due to obstruction to the outflow of blood from the heart and in pregnancy and breastfeeding mothers. Reduce the dose in patients with impaired kidney function and carefully monitor the blood pressure, pulse rate, blood chemistry and liver function and carry out repeated electro-cardiography of the heart (ECGs).

entacapone (Comtess) is used in addition to levodopa and a dopa-decarboxylase inhibitor in patients with Parkinson's disease who cannot be stabilized on these combinations alone. See Chapter 16. *Adverse effects* include movement disorders, stomach and bowel upsets, abdominal pain, dry mouth, reduced haemoglobin levels during long-term treatment and discoloration of urine. *Precautions:* Do not use in patients with impaired liver function, phaeochromocytoma (tumour of the sympathetic nervous system), in pregnancy or while breastfeeding.

Enterosan is an anti-diarrhoeal preparation which contains belladona, morphine and kaolin.

Entocort CR slow-release capsules contain enteric coated granules of the corticosteroid, budesonide. They are used to treat Crohn's disease (a chronic diarrhoeal disorder). The formulation reduces the risk of general adverse effects and increases the anti-inflammatory effects on the intestine. **Entacort enema** is used to treat ulcerated bowels affecting the rectum or lower end of the colon. *Adverse effects and Precautions* see Chapter 37 on corticosteroids. *Interactions:* cholestyramine.

Entonox is a mixture of nitrous oxide 50% and oxygen 50% which is used to produce pain relief without loss of consciousness.

Entrotabs is an antacid which contains aluminium, attapulgite and pectin.

Enzed ➤ diclofenac sodium.

enzymes An enzyme is a protein substance that will start a biochemical reaction. Enzymes are produced by living cells and they may act independently of the cells that produce them but they are an essential constituent of these cells. In medicine enzymes are used to break up clots (see fibrolytics, p. 144) and to dissolve dead skin and debris on wounds and ulcers (see Varidase Topical).

Epaderm ointment contains yellow soft paraffin and emulsifying wax. It is used to treat dry skin conditions.

Epanutin preparations ➤ phenytoin.

ephedrine (ephedrine hydrochloride, ephedrine sulphate, in Franol, in Franol Plus, in Haymine) is a sympathomimetic drug, see Chapter 9. It is used as a bronchodilator to treat asthma and chronic obstructive airways disease (see Chapter 14), as a decongestant in nasal preparations (see Chapter 10), to reverse the fall in blood pressure associated with spinal anaesthesia and to treat bedwetting in children (see p. 283). *Adverse effects:* If given to patients sensitive to ephedrine or if given in large doses it may cause nausea, vomiting, giddiness, headache, sweating, thirst, palpitations, anxiety, restlessness, tremor, disorders of heart rhythm, insomnia and muscular weakness. *Precautions:* It should not be used in patients suffering from high blood pressure, blood clots in the heart, overworking of the thyroid gland, enlargement of the prostate gland or closed-angle glaucoma. It should be given with caution to patients suffering from diabetes. *Interactions:* MAOIs, anaesthetics, tricyclic antidepressants.

Ephynal ➤ alpha tocopheryl acetate.

Epiglu is a tissue adhesive which is used for closure of minor skin wounds and for additional suture support. It contains ethylcyanoacrylate and polymethylmeltacrylate.

Epilim ➤ sodium valproate.

Epimaz ➤ carbamazepine.

epinephrine ➤ adrenaline(epinephrine).

Epipen ➤ adrenaline(epinephrine) and see p. 87.

epirubicin (Pharmorubicin preparations) is an anti-cancer drug. See Chapter 51. It is related to doxorubicin and is used to treat severe breast cancer ➤ doxorubicin. Reduce dose in patients with impaired liver function.

Epivir ➤ lamivudine.

epoetin alfa (Eprex) ➤ erythropoietin and see Chapter 35.

epoetin beta (Neorecormon) ➤ erythropoietin and see Chapter 35.

Epogam ➤ gamolenic acid.

epoprostenol (Flolan) is a prostaglandin (see Chapter 52) used to prevent the blood from clotting during kidney dialysis. It stops platelets from sticking together (see Chapter 28) and is given alone or with heparin (➤ heparin). *Adverse effects* include flushing, headache and fall in blood pressure due to its marked effect in dilating blood vessels. High doses may cause pallor, sweating and a drop in heart rate.

Eppy neutral adrenaline(epinephrine) eye drops ➤ adrenaline(epinephrine). It is used to treat open angle glaucoma (see p. 63). *Adverse effects* include headache, discomfort in the eye, redness and discoloration of the eye. General effects are rare. *Precautions:* Do not use to treat closed-angle glaucoma in patients without a crystalline lens in the eye. *Interactions:* MAOIs, tricyclic antidepressants.

Eprex (epoetin alfa) is an erythropoietin used to treat anaemia associated with chronic kidney failure in patients on kidney dialysis ➤ erythropoietin and see Chapter 35.

eprosartan (Teveten) is an angiotensin-II receptor blocker used to treat high blood pressure. See Chapter 25. *Adverse effects* include dizziness, pain in joints, inflammation of the lining of the nose, flatulence, high triglyceride levels. *Precautions:* Do not use in patients with liver or kidney damage, in pregnancy or while breastfeeding. Use with caution in patients with moderate kidney or liver damage.

Epsom salts ➤ magnesium sulphate.

eptacogalfa (Novoseven) is an anti-haemophilic factor VIIa ➤ Novoseven.

eptifibatide (Integrilin) is used in the early stages of a heart attack in patients with unstable angina. It is used in conjunction with aspirin and unfractionated heparin. See Chapter 28. *Adverse effects* include bleeding and heart disorders. *Precautions:* Do not use in patients with stomach, bowel, genitourinary or other abnormal bleeding within past thirty days, who have had a stroke within past thirty days or have a history of stroke; brain disease; major surgery or severe trauma within past six weeks, blood disorders, severe high blood pressure, severe liver or kidney damage, or while breastfeeding. Monitor for signs of bleeding. Use with caution in patients with liver or kidney damage, or in pregnancy.

Equagesic tablets contain aspirin, ethoheptazine (an opiate pain-reliever) and meprobamate (an anti-anxiety drug and muscle relaxant). It is used for the short-term treatment of painful muscles. *Adverse effects* ➤ aspirin, ethoheptazine, meprobamate. Main adverse effects include drowsiness, dizziness, nausea, loss of control over voluntary movements (ataxia), fall in blood pressure, pins and needles, excitation, allergic reactions and bleeding from the stomach and intestine. *Precautions* ➤ aspirin, meprobamate. *Interactions:* alcohol, sleeping drugs, sedatives or any drug that depresses brain function, anti-coagulants, anti-diabetic drugs, phenytoin, griseofulvin, rifampicin, corticosteriods, oral contraceptives, phenothiazines, tricyclic antidepressants.

Equanox is a mixture of nitrous oxide 50% and oxygen 50% which is used to produce pain relief with no loss of consciousness.

Equasym ➤ methylphenidate.

Equilon ➤ mebeverine.

ergocalciferol is vitamin D2.

ergometrine (ergometrine maleate; ergonovine maleate, in Syntometrine) causes contractions of the uterus and is used to prevent bleeding from the uterus after childbirth. *Adverse effects* include nausea, vomiting, headache, dizziness, noises in the ears (tinnitus), breathlessness, chest pain, palpitations, transient rise in blood pressure, very rarely causes a stroke, heart attack or fluid in the lung. *Precautions:* It should not be used during the first or second stages of labour since this may cause death of the foetus and rupture of the uterus. Do not use in patients with severe heart disease, disease of the circulation, poor lung function, severe impairment of liver or kidney function, severe raised blood pressure, infections or eclampsia. Use with caution in patients with mild or moderate heart disease or raised blood pressure, blood disorders, porphyria (a hereditary disorder of metabolism) or multiple pregnancies. *Interactions:* Erythromycin, possibly azithromycin, beta-blockers, sumatriptan.

ergotamine (ergotamine tartrate, in Cafergot, Lingraine, in Migril) is an ergot alkaloid that stimulates and, in large doses, paralyses the endings of the sympathetic nerves. It constricts small arteries and also the uterus. Its main use is in the treatment of migraine. See Chapter 34. *Adverse effects:* The dose used to treat migraine may cause headache, nausea and vomiting, and occasionally myasthenia gravis (muscle weakness due to neuromuscular abnormality) and pain. In large repeated doses it may produce all the symptoms of ergot poisoning – coldness of the skin, severe muscle pains, gangrene of the hands and feet, blood clots, angina, alteration of heart rate and blood pressure, confusion, drowsiness, paralysis and convulsions. Excessive use may cause scarring (fibrosis) in the chest and abdomen. *Precautions:* It should not be used in pregnancy, in breastfeeding mothers, in patients with severe raised blood pressure or over-active thyroid glands, in patients with impaired kidney or liver function, coronary artery disease, arterial disease, Raynaud's syndrome or porphyria (a hereditary disorder of metabolism). It should be used with caution in elderly patients and it should not be used to prevent migraine. Although it relieves headache by contracting small blood vessels it does not relieve visual and other symptoms and it may make vomiting worse. Some patients may become 'addicted' to ergotamine and headache may develop if the drug is stopped suddenly. The drug should not be used more than twice a month. Check dose, frequency of dosage and maximum dose carefully. *Interactions:* Erythromycin and beta-blockers.

Ervenox is a rubella vaccine which is given by deep subcutaneous or intramuscular injection.

Erwinase ➤ crisantaspase.

Eryacne is a gel for the treatment of acne ➤ erythromycin.

Erymax ➤ erythromycin.

Erythrocin ➤ erythromycin.

erythromycin (in Aknemycin Plus, in Benzamycin, Eryacne, Erymax, Erythrocin, Erythroped, Ilosone, in Isotrexin, in Stiemycin, Rommix, Tiloryth, in Zyneryt) is a macrolide antibiotic (see p. 268). Bacteria may quickly become resistant to it. It is partly destroyed by acid in the stomach and has to be taken in specially coated tablets (enteric coated). *Adverse effects* include nausea, vomiting, abdominal discomfort, diarrhoea (pseudomembranous inflammation of the bowel may occur rarely), allergic reactions, skin rashes, large doses may cause reversible loss of hearing and rarely it may cause jaundice (cholestatic jaundice) and heart disorders (chest pain and disorders of heart rhythm). *Precautions:* The estolate should not be used in patients with liver disease. Use all other preparations with caution in patients with liver disease. Use with caution in patients with impaired kidney function, porphyria (a hereditary disorder of metabolism), abnormal ECGs (prolonged QT) because ventricular tachycardia has been reported. Use with caution in pregnancy and in breastfeeding mothers. *Interactions:* Do not use with astemizole or terfenadine; may interact with theophylline, oral anticoagulants, carbamazepine and digoxin.

erythromycin estolate (Ilosone) is an antibiotic which is more rapidly absorbed than erythromycin ➤ erythromycin.

erythromycin stearate (erythromycin stearate, Erythrocin) is an antibiotic. It is more resistant to the acid in the stomach than erythromycin ➤ erythromycin.

Erythroped ➤ erythromycin.

erythropoietin (epoetin alfa: Eprex; epoetin beta: Recormon) is a hormone produced principally by the kidneys that regulates red cell production by the bone marrow through a process known as *erythropoiesis.* Sensors of oxygen levels in the tissues are located in the kidneys; if the oxygen level falls, erythropoietin is produced by the kidneys and travels in the blood to the bone marrow, where it stimulates the production of red blood cells in order to increase the oxygen-carrying capacity of the blood. In kidney disease the ability to produce erythropoietin is impaired and the individual develops a reduction in red cell production (anaemia). Following the isolation of the gene coding for human erythropoietin, it is now possible to manufacture it using DNA technology. It is used to treat anaemia associated with kidney failure and patients receiving dialysis and before they receive dialysis. It is also used to prevent anaemias in premature babies under thirty-four weeks of age. See Chapter 35. *Adverse effects* include raised blood pressure, headache, blood clot at the site of injection, influenza-like symptoms, seizures and skin

rashes. *Precautions:* Do not use in children or in patients suffering from untreated raised blood pressure. It should be used with caution in patients being treated for raised blood pressure, coronary heart disease, disorders of the circulation, a history of epilepsy or liver failure. Other causes of anaemia should be treated and iron supplements may be needed. The haemoglobin level, platelet count, blood pressure and blood chemistry should be checked at regular intervals. Rise in blood pressure will need treatment. Diet and frequency of dialysis may need to be changed. It should be used with special caution in pregnancy and in breastfeeding mothers.

ESBroncial cough medicine contains ammonium bicarbonate, ipecacuanha, senna and squill ➤ individual entry for each drug.

Eskamel contains resorcinol and sulphur which are used to remove dead skin. It is used to treat acne (see p. 250). *Adverse effects and Precautions* ➤ resorcinol, sulphur. It may irritate the skin. Avoid contact with eyes, mouth and nose.

Eskornade sustained-release capsules contain phenylpropanolamine (a sympathomimetic drug) and diphenylpyraline (an antihistamine). They are used as a decongestant to treat colds. See Chapter 10. *Adverse effects and Precautions* ➤ sympathomimetic drugs, antihistamine drugs.

Esmeron ➤ rocuronium.

esmolol (Brevibloc) is a selective beta-blocker used to treat disorders of heart rhythm. See Chapter 24. *Adverse effects and Precautions* ➤ beta-blockers.

esomeprazole (Nexium) is a proton pump blocker used to treat and prevent heartburn. It is used in combination with antibiotics to eradicate and heal *h-pylori*-associated duodenal ulcers and to prevent the relapse of peptic ulcers. See Chapter 19. *Adverse effects* include headache, stomach and/or bowel upsets, skin reactions, dry mouth. *Precautions:* Do not use in patients with an intolerance to fructose, in patients who are unable to absorb glucose and galactose properly, who have disorders of the enzymes sucrose and isomaltese, or who are breast-feeding. Use with caution in patients with severe kidney or liver damage, on long-term therapy or in pregnancy.

essential oils are volatile mixtures of various chemicals that give off particular odours. Taken by mouth volatile oils irritate the mucous membranes of the mouth and stomach and give a feeling of warmth. They increase salivation, and relax the muscles at the entrance to the stomach and the muscles of the intestine. Various essential oils are used to relieve a sore throat, to relieve stomach wind (e.g. gripe water for babies) and to relieve the symptoms of an irritable bowel (e.g. peppermint oil). When applied to the skin essential oils have an irritant effect and some of them are included in rubefacients (rheumatic rubs). They are also used as flavouring agents in some cold and cough remedies. *Adverse effects:* Excessive use by mouth may irritate the stomach and bowel (causing nausea and vomiting and diarrhoea) and the lining of the bladder and urethra (causing symptoms like cystitis). Overdose by mouth may depress breathing and affect the brain producing excitement, convulsions and stupor. They may irritate the skin and cause contact dermatitis.

Estracombi HRT combination pack contains self-adhesive patches that slowly release oestradiol (Estraderm) and oestradiol with norethisterone (Estragest TTS) ➤ HRT.

Estracyt ➤ estramustine.

Estraderm TTS and **Estraderm MX** self-adhesive patches contain oestradiol ➤ HRT.

estradiol (oestradiol benzoate, oestradiol monobenzoate, oestradiol valerate) is the most active of the naturally occurring oestrogens. It is used to treat menopausal symptoms, used in HRT, and to treat primary amenorrhoea. *Adverse effects and Precautions* ➤ oestrogens, HRT.

Estragest TTS self-adhesive patches contain oestradiol and norethisterone ➤ HRT.

estramustine (Estracyt) is used to treat cancer of the prostate gland. It is a combination of an oestrogen and an anti-cancer drug (mustine). It delivers the mustine to the oestrogen receptors in the tumour. *Adverse effects:* Nausea, vomiting, diarrhoea, allergic skin rash and fever, rarely thrombocytopenia (a fall in blood platelets), enlarged breasts (gynaecomastia) and damage to the heart may occur. *Precautions:* It should not be used in patients with peptic ulcers, severe liver disease, severe heart disease or impaired bone-marrow function. *Interactions:* Milk and milk products.

Estrapak contains skin patches which release the oestrogen oestradiol over a twenty-four-hour period, together with tablets of norethisterone (a progestogen) ➤ HRT.

Estring vaginal rings contain a slow-release preparation of oestradiol. It is used as topical HRT for post-menopausal vaginal dryness and shrinkage ➤ HRT. *Adverse effects* in the vagina include irritation, itching, ulcers, urinary infections and abdominal discomfort.

estriol is a naturally occurring oestrogen used to treat post-menopausal vaginal and vulval conditions. *Adverse effects and Precautions* ➤ oestrogens, HRT.

estrogens ➤ oestrogens.

estrone (piperazine oestrone sulphate, Harmogen, in Hormonin) is a naturally occurring oestrogen. It is used to treat menopausal symptoms. *Adverse effects and Precautions* ➤ oestrogens, HRT.

etamsylate (Dicynene) is a haemostatic (it helps to stop bleeding, see p. 145). It is used in the treatment of heavy periods and to prevent bleeding in premature, low birthweight babies. *Adverse effects* include nausea, headache and rashes. *Precautions:*

Do not use in patients suffering from porphyria (a hereditary disorder of metabolism).

etanercept (Enbrel) is an immunosuppressant used to treat active rheumatoid arthritis and active juvenile chronic arthritis which does not respond to methotrexate treatment. *Adverse effects* include injection site reactions, infection, headache, dizziness, weakness, abdominal pain, indigestion, rash, tumours, heart disorders, inflammation of the gall bladder, inflammation of the pancreas, bleeding in the stomach and bowel, inflammation of joints, depression, difficulty breathing, CNS demyelinating disorders (including multiple sclerosis and optic neuritis). *Precautions:* Do not use in patients with infection or at risk of infection, pregnancy (ensure adequate contraception) or while breastfeeding. Use with caution in patients with a history of recurrent infection or a predisposition to infection, immunosuppression, exposure to chickenpox, history of blood disorders, CNS demyelinating disorders (e.g. multiple sclerosis, optic neuritis).

ethambutol (ethambutol hydrochloride) is used to treat tuberculosis. See Chapter 50. *Adverse effects:* Its most serious adverse effect is impaired vision (e.g. colour blindness) which may occur if high doses are used, particularly in patients with impaired kidney function. It is reversible if the drug is stopped early enough. It may also cause nerve damage. *Precautions:* It should be used with caution in pregnancy, in breastfeeding mothers and in patients with impaired kidney function. Blood levels must be checked. The eyes should be examined before treatment and at frequent intervals during treatment. It should not be used in young children or in patients with optic neuritis (inflammation of the optic nerve causing impairment of vision).

ethamsylate ➤ etamsylate.

ethanol ➤ ethyl alcohol.

ethanolamine oleate is used to strengthen the walls of varicose veins. *Adverse effects:* Leakage may lead to damage (necrosis) of the surrounding tissue. It may rarely cause allergic reactions. *Precautions:* It should not be used in patients whose veins are so painful that they cannot walk, who have inflammation of a vein, who are taking oral contraceptive drugs or have obese legs.

ether is occasionally used as a general anaesthetic.

Ethimil MR ➤ verapamil.

ethinylestradiol is an oestrogen ➤ oestrogens.

ethinyloestradiol ➤ ethinylestradiol.

ethoheptazine (in Equagesic) is a mild to moderate opiate pain-reliever. It may produce stomach discomfort, nausea, dizziness, drowsiness and itching. It is structurally related to pethidine.

ethosuximide (Emeside, Zarontin) is an anticonvulsant drug used to treat epilepsy. See Chapter 15. *Adverse effects* include stomach and bowel upsets, headache, fatigue, lethargy, dizziness, hiccups, drowsiness, apathy, mood changes and loss of control over voluntary movements (ataxia). It may, rarely, cause skin rashes, blood disorders, impaired liver and kidney function, systemic lupus erythematosis (SLE – a disease of unknown cause with symptoms of fever, pain, blood disorders and skin eruptions), overgrowth of the gums, swelling of the tongue, irritability, night tremors, sleep disturbances, poor concentration, increased libido, shortsightedness and vaginal bleeding. *Precautions:* Do not use in patients with porphyria (a hereditary disorder of metabolism). It should be given with extreme caution in pregnancy, in breastfeeding mothers and in patients with impaired liver or kidney function. Blood counts and tests of liver and kidney function should be carried out at regular intervals during treatment. The drug should be withdrawn slowly. *Interactions:* Phenothiazines, antihistamines, antidepressants.

ethyl alcohol ➤ alcohol.

ethylene glycol is included in sunscreen lotions and protective creams. It should only be present in a very low concentration and should *not* be applied extensively on the body.

ethyl nicotinate (in Transvasin) is a rubefacient used in rheumatic rubs ➤ rubefacients.

ethynodiol ➤ etynodiol.

Ethyol ➤ amifostine.

etidronate disodium (Didronel) is a diphosphonate that slows down the laying down and dissolving of bone and reduces the increased turnover of bone that occurs in Paget's disease. **Didronel PMO** tablets (etidronate disodium combined with effervescent calcium carbonate) is used to treat osteoporosis of the spine. *Adverse effects* include nausea, diarrhoea and increased bone pain (in Paget's disease). Infusion may cause metallic or altered taste. There is an increased risk of fractures with high doses in Paget's disease. Rare adverse effects include allergic skin reactions (swelling of the face, hands and feet, nettle-rash, itching), abdominal pain, constipation, headache, pins and needles in the hands and feet, nerve damage and blood disorders. Increase in blood calcium and phosphate levels may occur. *Precautions:* Adequate intake of calcium and vitamin D must be maintained. Do not use in patients with moderate or severe impairment of kidney function. Use with caution in patients with mild impairment of kidney function or inflammation of the bowel. Kidney function tests should be carried out before treatment and at regular intervals during treatment. Dose should be reduced if there is mild or moderate impairment of kidney function. Do not use in pregnancy or in breastfeeding mothers. Do not use to treat osteoporosis if blood level of calcium is raised or if there is a high level of calcium in the urine. Do not use to treat adult rickets. Blood phosphate and alkaline phosphatase levels and urinary hydroxyproline levels should be measured before treatment and then every three months.

etodolac (Lodine) is a non-steroidal anti-inflammatory drug (NSAID) ➤ non-steroidal anti-inflammatory drugs.

etomidate (Hypnomidate) is used as an intravenous anaesthetic. It may cause pain at the site of injection. Repeated doses may damp down the adrenal glands causing a fall in the production of corticosteroids (see Chapter 37). It should not be used in patients with porphyria (a hereditary disorder of metabolism).

etonogestrel (Implanon) is an implant used for long-term reversible contraception which lasts for up to three years. The implant is inserted under the skin on the inner side of the upper arm. See Chapter 41. *Adverse effects* include acne, headache, weight gain, breast tenderness, hair loss, depression, changes in libido, emotional swings, abdominal pain and difficult or painful menstruation. *Precautions:* Do not use in patients with thromboembolic disorders (blood clots), progestogen-dependent cancers, history of severe liver disease, undiagnosed vaginal bleeding or in pregnancy. Use with caution in patients with high blood pressure, liver damage, diabetes, chloasma (patchy brown pigmentation on the face), heavier women, history (during pregnancy or previous use of sex steroids) of jaundice, itching due to jaundice, gallstones, porphyria (a hereditary disorder of metabolism), systemic lupus erythematosis (SLE – a disease of unknown cause with symptoms of fever, muscle and joint pain, blood disorders and skin eruptions), haemolytic uraemic syndrome (a blood disorder), Sydenham's chorea (a childhood disorder with symptoms of rapid jerky movements with low muscle tone and reflexes, and mental disturbance), herpes occurring during pregnancy, otosclerosis (the development of an extra bone in the ear causing progressive deafness).

Etopophos ➤ etoposide.

etoposide (Etopophos, Vepesid) is used as an anti-cancer drug. See Chapter 51. *Adverse effects* include nausea, vomiting, loss of hair and damage to the bone marrow causing blood disorders. *Precautions* see Chapter 51.

etynodiol (Femulan) is an oral contraceptive. See Chapter 41.

eucalyptol has the actions and uses of eucalpytus oil but it is less irritating. It is used as a heat rub, and it has some antiseptic properties. It is used in temporary dental fillings.

eucalyptus oil has a pleasant smell and is included in medicines used to treat symptoms of the upper respiratory tract. It is an irritant to the skin, mouth and nose. It is used in some rheumatic liniments and in preparations to treat wind.

Eucardic ➤ carvedilol.

Eucerin preparations are skin softeners ➤ urea.

Eudemine preparations ➤ diazoxide.

Euglucon ➤ glibenclamide.

Eugynon-30 is a combined oral contraceptive. See p. 216.

Eumovate preparations ➤ clobetasone.

Eurax-Hydrocortisone cream contains hydrocortisone (a corticosteroid) and crotamiton. It is used to treat itching skin rashes. *Adverse effects and Precautions* see corticosteroid skin applications p. 241 and ➤ crotamiton.

Eurax lotion and cream ➤ crotamiton.

evening primrose oil ➤ oil of evening primrose.

Evista ➤ raloxifene.

Evorel Patches are self-adhesive patches of estradiol ➤ HRT.

Exelderm cream ➤ sulconazole.

Exelon ➤ rivastigmine.

exemestane (Aromasin) is an anti oestrogen used to treat advanced post-menopausal breast cancer that has progressed following anti-oestrogen therapy. See Chapter 40. *Adverse effects* include hot flushes, nausea, fatigue, sweating, dizziness, headache, insomnia, pain, rash, weight changes, anorexia, abdominal pain, depression, hair loss, swelling of the legs and arms, constipation, indigestion, disorders of the blood. *Precautions:* Do not use in pre-menopausal women, in pregnancy or while breastfeeding. Use with caution in patients with liver or kidney damage.

Ex-lax Senna ➤ sennosides.

Exocin eye solution ➤ oflaxacin.

Exorex is a coal tar preparation used for the treatment of psoriasis ➤ coal tar.

Exosurf Neonatal ➤ colfosceril.

expectorants, see Chapter 11.

Expulin contains chlorphenamine(chlorpheniramine), menthol, pholcodeine and pseudoephedrine; **Expulin Chesty Cough** contains guaifenesin and menthol; **Expulin Decongestant for Babies and Children** contains chlorphenamine(chlorpheniramine) and ephedrine; **Expulin Dry** contains menthol and pholcodeine; **Expulin Paediatric** contains chlorphenamine(chlorpheniramine), menthol and pholcodeine ➤ individual entry for each drug.

Exterol ear drops contain urea hydrogen peroxide in glycerine. It is used to remove ear wax (see p. 57) *Adverse effects:* include irritation. *Precautions:* Do not use if ear drum is perforated.

eye preparations, see Chapter 13.

factor VIIa ➤ NovoSeven.

factor VIII fraction, freeze-dried (human antihaemophilic fraction dried, Alpha VIII, 8SM, 8Y, Haemate P, Helixate, High Potency Factor VIII Concentrate, Monoclate-P, Refacto, Replanate) is dried factor VIII fraction prepared from human plasma. A recombinant human antihaemophilic factor VIII is available as Kogenate and Recombinate. Factor VIII is used to control bleeding in patients suffering from haemophilia A. *Adverse effects* include allergic reactions and chills, fever and a rise in blood fibrinogen level. *Precautions:* Damage to red blood cells (haemolysis) may occur after large and/or frequent doses in patients with blood group A, B, or AB. This is less likely to occur with high potency concentrates. There is a possibility of transmission of viruses that cause hepatitis B and AIDS. Hyate C is a preparation from pigs ➤ Hyate C.

factor VIII inhibitor bypassing fraction is prepared from human plasma. It is used in patients who have developed inhibitors to factor VIII therapy.

factor IX fraction, dried (Alphanine, Benefix, Dried Factor IX Fraction, Human Factor IX Concentrate Heat Treated, Mononine, Replenine-VF) is prepared from human plasma. It also contains clotting factors II, VII and X. It is used to treat haemophilia B due to a deficiency of factor IX and hereditary deficiency of factor IX (Christmas factor). *Adverse effects* include allergic reactions, chills and fever. *Precautions:* Do not use in patients with a generalized clotting disorder (disseminated intravascular coagulation). There is a risk of blood clots with low purity products.

faecal softeners, see Chapter 21.

famciclovir (Famvir) is an antiviral drug (see Chapter 48) used to treat shingles (herpes zoster) and genital herpes (herpes simplex). *Adverse effects* include headache and nausea. *Precautions:* Do not use in pregnancy or breastfeeding mothers. Use with utmost caution in patients with impaired kidney function. It is taken by mouth as tablets.

Famel Expectorant contains guaifenesin; **Famel Original** contains codeine and creosote ➤ individual entry for each drug.

Fam-Lax Senna ➤ sennosides.

famotidine (Pepcid, Pepcid AC) is an H_2 blocker used to treat peptic ulcers and acid reflux (see Chapter 19). *Adverse effects* include headache, dizziness, constipation, diarrhoea. Less frequently, dry mouth, nausea, skin rash, stomach upsets, loss of appetite, fatigue. Rarely it may cause reversible enlargement of the breasts (in men) and a *very serious* skin rash – toxic epidermal necrosis. *Precautions:* Use with caution in patients with impaired kidney function or stomach cancer (may mask symptoms), and use with caution in pregnancy and breastfeeding mothers. See also under cimetidine but famotidine does not affect enzymes in the liver that metabolize certain drugs.

Famvir ➤ famciclovir.

Fanhdi ➤ factor VIII fraction, dried.

Fansidar is used to treat *Plasmodium falciparum* malaria. It contains the sulphonamide sulfadoxine and pyrimethamine. *Adverse effects* ➤ sulphonamides, pyrimethamine. They include skin rashes, stomach and bowel upsets, blood disorders, sore throat and itching and, occasionally, fatigue, headache, fever, and pins and needles in the arms and legs. Very rarely it may cause *serious* skin rashes. *Precautions:* It should not be used in patients known to be allergic to sulphonamides. It should not be used to prevent malaria, or in patients with severe kidney or liver impairment or blood disorders. Treatment should be stopped immediately if itching, skin rashes, sore mouth or sore throat occur. Consider an adverse drug reaction if patient develops a skin rash, jaundice, fever or a general feeling of being unwell during treatment. Because it blocks folic acid in the body it should not be used in pregnancy or in breastfeeding mothers. Excessive exposure to the sun should be avoided and regular blood counts should be carried out during prolonged use (over three months). *Interactions:* Drugs that block use of folic acid – cotrimoxazole, trimethoprim, phenytoin, methotrexate. Also ➤ sulphonamides.

Fareston ➤ toremifene.

Farlutal ➤ medroxyprogesterone.

Fasigyn ➤ tinidazole.

Fasturtec ➤ rasburicase.

Faverin ➤ fluvoxamine.

Fectrim ➤ co-trimoxazole.

Fefol spansules contain ferrous sulphate and folic acid. See Chapters 35 and 36.

felbinac is a non-steroidal anti-inflammatory drug used in Traxam gel to treat sprains and strains (see p. 164). *Adverse effects* include local redness, itching and dermatitis. *Precautions:* Do not use in patients allergic to aspirin or other anti-inflammatory drugs. Use with caution in patients with asthma, in pregnancy and in breastfeeding mothers. Do not use on broken skin and avoid contact with eyes, lips and mouth. Do not put a non-permeable dressing over it ➤ non-steroidal anti-inflammatory drugs.

Feldene ➤ piroxicam.

Feldene Gel contains the NSAID piroxicam. It is used as a rheumatic rub to relieve muscle aches and pains (see p. 164). *Adverse effects and Precautions* ➤ non-steroidal anti-inflammatory drugs. It may cause local irritation, redness, skin rash and itching. Do not use in patients allergic to aspirin or some other NSAID. Use with caution in pregnancy and breastfeeding mothers.

Felicium ➤ fluoxetine.

felodipine (Plendil, Triapin) is used to treat raised blood pressure. See Chapter 25. It is also used to treat angina. See Chapter 22. It is a class II calcium-channel blocker (see p. 116) which has a very selective effect causing arteries to dilate (vasodilation) and less direct effects on the heart than other class I or class II calcium-channel blockers. *Adverse effects* include headache, dizziness, fatigue, flushing, palpitations, fluid retention, itching, skin rash and overgrowth of the gums. *Precautions:* Do not use in pregnancy and in breastfeeding mothers. Use with special caution in patients with severe impairment of liver function, low blood pressure or fast heart rate. *Interactions* ➤ cimetidine, phenytoin, carbamazepine, phenobarbitone.

felypressin (in Citanest with Octapressin) has actions and uses similar to those listed under vasopressin. It is used to constrict blood vessels in local anaesthetic injections for dental use when adrenaline (epinephrine) and related drugs must not be used ➤ vasopressin.

Femapak consists of skin patches containing oestradiol (an oestrogen) and tablets containing dydrogesterone (a progestogen). They are used as HRT ➤ HRT.

Femara ➤ letrozole.

Fematrix self-adhesive patches contain oestradiol (an oestrogen). They are used as HRT ➤ HRT.

Feminax is a pain-relieving preparation which contains paracetamol, caffeine, codeine and hyoscine ➤ individual entry for each drug.

Femodene is a combined oral contraceptive. See p. 216.

Femodette is an oral contraceptive pill containing gestodene and ethinylestradiol. See p. 216.

Femoston preparations contain tablets of oestradiol (an oestrogen) and dydrogesterone (a progestogen). They are used as HRT ➤ HRT.

FemSeven skin patches contain oestradiol (an oestrogen). They are used as HRT. The skin patches need replacing every seven days instead of the usual three to four days. *Adverse effects and Precautions* ➤ HRT.

Femulen is a progestogen-only oral contraceptive containing etynodiol. See p. 217.

Fenbid and **Fenbid Forte Gel** ➤ ibuprofen.

fenbufen (Lederfen) is a non-steroidal anti-inflammatory drug (NSAID) ➤ non-steroidal anti-inflammatory drugs.

fenchone is an essential oil in Rowatinex.
➤ Rowatinex.

Fenning's Children's Cooling Powders
➤ paracetamol.

Fenning's Little Healers is a cough medicine which contains ipecacuanha ➤ ipecacuanha.

fenofibrate (Lipantil, Supralip) is used to lower blood cholesterol and fat levels. See Chapter 26. *Adverse effects* include stomach and bowel upsets, skin rashes, vertigo, headache and fatigue. Rarely, it may cause muscle damage producing weakness and pain, and reduced libido. *Precautions:* Do not use if kidney or liver function is severely impaired. Do not use in patients with gall-bladder disease, in pregnancy or in breastfeeding mothers. Use with caution in patients with mild or moderate impairment of kidney function (➤ fibrates for warnings on muscle damage). *Interactions:* Anticoagulants, phenylbutazone, oral anti-diabetic drugs.

Fenoket ➤ ketoprofen.

fenoprofen (Fenopron) is a non-steroidal anti-inflammatory drug (NSAID) ➤ nonsteroidal anti-inflammatory drugs.

Fenopron ➤ fenoprofen.

fenoterol (fenoterol hydrobromide, in Duovent) is a selective beta$_2$ stimulant. It is used as a bronchodilator to treat asthma. See Chapter 14. *Adverse effects and Precautions* are similar to those described under salbutamol ➤ salbutamol.

Fenox Nasal Drops and Nasal Spray ➤ phenylephrine.

Fentamox ➤ tamoxifen.

fentanyl (Actiz, in Durogesic, Sublimaze) is an opiate pain-reliever (see Chapter 30) used during surgical operations and to depress respiration in patients on ventilators. *Adverse effects* include fall in blood pressure, slowing of pulse rate, depression of respiration, nausea and vomiting. *Precautions:* Use with caution in patients with chronic chest disease, myasthenia gravis (muscle weakness due to neuromuscular abnormality), under-active thyroid, impaired liver function and in elderly patients. Its use in childbirth may depress breathing in the newborn baby.

Fentazin ➤ perphenazine.

fenticonazole (Lomexin) is an antifungal drug (see Chapter 47) used in pessaries to treat thrush infections of the vagina ➤ Lomexin.

Feospan spansules (sustained-release capsules) ➤ ferrous sulphate.

Fepramax ➤ lofepramine.

Ferfolic SV tablets contain folic acid, ferrous gluconate and vitamin C. They are used to treat iron and folic acid deficiency and to prevent neural tube damage (e.g. spina bifida) in women known to be at risk (see p. 179). *Adverse effects* include nausea and constipation. *Precautions:* Do not use to treat megaloblastic anaemia (e.g. pernicious anaemia). *Interactions:* Tetracycline antibiotics.

Fermathron is a sodium hyaluronate preparation which is injected into a knee joint to supplement natural hyaluronic acid in the synovial (joint) fluid. It is used in the treatment of osteoarthritis of the knee.

ferric ammonium citrate (in Lexpec with iron, in Lexpec with iron M) is a form of iron. The mixture should be well diluted with water and sucked through a straw to prevent discoloration of the teeth. See Chapter 35 on iron.

Ferriprox ➤ deferiprone.

Ferrograd ➤ ferrous sulphate.

Ferrograd C timed-release tablets contain ferrous sulphate and ascorbic acid. The vitamin C helps the absorption of the iron. *Precautions:* Do not use in patients with diverticular disease or intestinal obstruction. *Interactions:* Tetracycline antibiotics, levodopa.

Ferrograd Folic timed-release tablets

contain ferrous sulphate and folic acid. They are used to treat anaemia in pregnancy, see p. 179. *Precautions:* Diverticular disease, intestinal obstruction, vitamin B_{12} deficiency. *Interactions:* Tetracycline antibiotics, levodopa.

ferrous fumarate (Fersaday, Fersamal, Galfer, in Pregaday) ➤ iron salts and see Chapter 35.

ferrous gluconate (in Ferfolic SV) ➤ iron salts and see Chapter 35.

ferrous glycine sulphate (Plesmet) ➤ iron salts and see Chapter 35.

ferrous salts ➤ iron salts and see Chapter 35.

ferrous sulphate (Ferrograd, in Ferrograd Folic, Slow-Fe, in Slow-Fe Folic) ➤ iron salts and see Chapter 35.

Fersaday ➤ ferrous fumarate.

Fersamal ➤ ferrous fumarate.

fexofenadine (Telfast) is used to treat seasonal allergic rhinitis (hayfever). See Chapter 17. *Adverse effects* include headache, nausea, dizziness, fatigue. *Precautions:* Do not use in pregnancy. Use with caution in patients who are breastfeeding.

fibrates, see Chapter 26. *Warning:* these drugs can damage muscle tissue causing muscle pains and weakness and a rise in CPK (creatine phosphokinase) in the blood. This enzyme is raised when muscles are damaged and its level gives an indication of the degree of damage. Patients with impaired kidney function or underworking of the thyroid gland are at particular risk. Do not use a fibrate drug with a statin drug or with ciclosporin because this will increase the risks. CPK levels must be measured during treatment and patients should report any muscle pains or weakness.

fibrinogen is a factor in blood which helps it to clot. See Chapter 28.

fibrinolytic drugs, see p. 144.

Fibrablast interferon ➤ interferons, beta.

Fibro-vein ➤ sodium tetradecyl sulphate.

Filair aerosol inhalation ➤ beclometasone.

filgrastim (Neupogen) is used to reduce the incidence and duration of reductions in neutrophil white blood cells (neutropenia) which may occur in individuals being treated with anti-cancer drugs for cancers not affecting the blood-forming tissues. Filgrastim is a bio-engineered human growth factor that stimulates the production of white blood cells. The growth factor is referred to as human granulocyte colony stimulating factor (G-CSF) because it stimulates the growth of colonies of granulocytes (white blood cells) in the bone marrow and elsewhere. Following the injection of a single dose into a vein or under the skin the number of white cells falls during the first hour and then increases over the next four–five hours. The white cell count rapidly returns to normal when the injections are stopped and there is no evidence of a rebound fall in the number of white blood cells. The response to filgrastim is very selective in affecting neutrophils but not other white blood cells. The effect is similar to that seen in healthy individuals during an infection and it therefore helps to reduce the risk of infection which is a problem in anyone whose neutrophil white cell production is knocked out by anti-cancer drugs. *Adverse effects* include pains in joints and muscles, difficulty and/or discomfort on passing urine, raised blood uric acid levels, headache, diarrhoea, nose bleeds, loss of hair, transient fall in blood pressure, disturbances in liver function tests, allergic reactions, proteins and blood in the urine and a transient fall in blood sugar level. Long-term use may be associated with damage to blood vessels in the skin, enlargement of the liver, skin rash and osteoporosis. *Precautions:* Do not use in patients with severe congenital neutropenia (Katsman's syndrome) with abnormal cell genetics. It should not be used within twenty-four hours before or after anti-cancer drug treatment. It should not be used in individuals with cancer of the blood-forming tissues. It should be used with caution in patients with severely impaired kidney and liver function. White blood cell counts must be carried out at frequent intervals because of the risk of over-production of white blood cells. Monitor blood platelet and haemoglobin level and spleen size. Use with utmost caution in pregnancy and breastfeeding mothers. Bone density must be monitored in individuals with osteoporosis on long-term treatment.

finasteride (Proscar) blocks the enzyme that converts the male sex hormone, testosterone, into a more potent form (dihydrotestosterone). This reduces the amount in the body which helps to reduce the size of the prostate gland. This improves passing urine in men with benign enlargement of their prostate gland, see p. 285. *Adverse effects* include impotence, decreased libido, reduced amount of ejaculate, tenderness and enlargement of the breasts and allergic reactions. *Precautions:* Do not use to treat cancer of the prostate. Finasteride is excreted in the semen, therefore a condom should be worn if sexual partner is pregnant or of childbearing potential. Women who are pregnant or of childbearing potential should *not* handle broken or crushed tablets.

Fisonair aerosol inhalation ➤ sodium cromoglicate.

5HT blockers, see p. 41.

5HT stimulants, see p. 41.

5HT noradrenaline re-uptake blockers, see p. 41.

Fixonase Nasule ➤ fluticasone.

Flagyl ➤ metronidazole.

Flamatak MR ➤ diclofenac sodium.

Flamatrol ➤ piroxicam.

Flamazine cream ➤ silver sulphadiazine.

Flamrase SR ➤ diclofenac sodium.

flavoxate (Urispas) is an antimuscarinic drug used as an anti-spasmodic to treat incontinence, frequency, and urgency of passing urine. See Chapter 49. *Adverse effects*

include dry mouth, blurred vision, headache, nausea, diarrhoea and fatigue. *Precautions:* Do not use if there is any blockage to output of urine (e.g. enlargement of prostate gland) or obstruction of the bowel. For other adverse effects and precautions ➤ antimuscarinic drugs.

Flaxedil ➤ gallamine.

Flebogamma ➤ immunoglobulin.

flecainide (flecainide acetate, Tambocor) is used to treat disorders of heart rhythm. See Chapter 24. *Adverse effects* include dizziness, visual disturbances, nausea, vomiting, disturbed liver function, jaundice, nerve damage, pins and needles, unsteadiness of movement (ataxia) and sensitivity of the skin to the sun's rays. *Precautions:* Do not use in patients with heart failure, with a history of a heart attack, with an irregular heartbeat, serious heart valve disease, heart block or sinus node disease in absence of a pacemaker. Use with utmost caution in the elderly and in patients with impaired kidney or liver function, heart disease, in pregnancy, in breastfeeding mothers, or in patients with an irregular heartbeat following heart surgery. *Interactions:* Other class I anti-arrhythmic drugs, digoxin and drugs that depress heart function.

Fleet Enema, Fleet Ready-to-use Enema contain sodium acid phosphate. They are used to treat constipation or bowel evacuation before abdominal procedures such as surgery or endoscopy.

Fleet Phospho-soda is an oral sodium phosphate solution used for clearing the bowel before X-ray, endoscopy or surgery. See Chapter 21. *Precautions:* Do not use if bowel lining is damaged so that its ability to absorb fluid and electrolytes is increased. Do not use in patients suffering from congestive heart failure. Use with caution in patients on a salt (sodium salt) restricted intake.

Fletchers' Arachis Oil Retention Enema contains arachis oil (peanut oil). It lubricates and softens impacted faeces. *Pre-*

caution: The enema should be warmed to body temperature before use. See Chapter 21.

Fletchers' Enemette contains docusate sodium, glycerol, macrogol and sorbic acid. It lubricates and softens impacted faeces. See Chapter 21.

Fletchers' Phosphate Enema contains sodium acid phosphate and sodium phosphate, which act as an osmotic laxative. See Chapter 21.

Flexin Continus ➤ indometacin.

Flixonase aqueous nasal spray ➤ fluticasone.

Flexotard ➤ diclofenac.

Flixotide inhalation preparations ➤ fluticasone.

Flolan ➤ epoprostenol.

Flomax MR ➤ tamsulosin.

Florinef ➤ fludrocortisone.

Floxapen ➤ flucloxacillin.

Flu-Amp ➤ co-fluampicil.

Fluanxol ➤ flupenthixol.

Fluarix is a flu vaccine. See Chapter 53 on vaccines.

Fluclomix ➤ flucloxacillin.

flucloxacillin (flucloxacillin sodium, in co-fluampicil, Floxapen, Fluclomix, Galfloxin, Ladropen, in Magnapen, Zoxin) is a penicillinase-resistant penicillin. *Adverse effects and Precautions* ➤ penicillins.

fluconazole (Diflucan) is an antifungal drug. See Chapter 47. *Adverse effects* include stomach and bowel upsets, and rarely, allergic reactions and *very serious* skin rashes (particularly in patients suffering from AIDS). *Precautions:* It should not be used in pregnancy or in breastfeeding mothers. Use multiple dose treatment with caution in patients suffering from impaired kidney function. *Interactions:* Anticoagulants, theophylline, rifampicin, cyclosporin,

phenytoin, sulphonylurea anti-diabetic drugs, astemizole, terfenadine.

flucytosine (Alcobon, Ancotil) is an antifungal drug. See Chapter 47. *Adverse effects* include nausea, vomiting, diarrhoea, rashes, confusion, hallucinations, convulsions, headache, vertigo, sedation, liver damage and blood disorders. *Precautions:* It should be used with caution in patients with impaired kidney or liver function, in pregnancy, in the elderly, in breastfeeding mothers and in patients with blood disorders.

Fludara injection ➤ fludarabine.

fludarabine (Fludara) is an anti-cancer drug (see Chapter 51) used to treat chronic lymphatic leukaemia. *Adverse effects* include damage to the bone marrow producing blood disorders. It also suppresses the immune system which reduces the individual's resistance to infection. Rarely it may affect the nervous system and lungs. *Precautions:* Reduce dose in patients with impaired kidney function. See Chapter 51.

fludrocortisone (fludrocortisone acetate, Florinef) is a synthetic mineralocorticoid which can regulate the body's water and electrolyte balance. It is used as partial replacement treatment in patients suffering from underworking of the adrenal glands (Addison's disease). *Adverse effects and Precautions* see Chapter 37.

fludroxycortide(flurandrenolone) is a corticosteroid used in Haelan cream to treat inflammatory skin disorders such as eczema. *Adverse effects and Precautions* ➤ corticosteroid skin applications, see p. 241.

flumazenil (Anexate) is a benzodiazepine blocker (antidote). It displaces benzodiazepines from their receptor sites and reverses their sedative and sleep-producing effects within thirty–sixty seconds of an intravenous injection. It is used to reverse the effects of benzodiazepines that have been used during anaesthesia, intensive care or in diagnostic procedures (e.g. endoscopy). *Adverse effects* include nausea, vomiting, flushing, transient rise in blood pressure, increase in heart rate and, rarely, seizures (particularly in epileptics). If awakening is too rapid patient may feel fearful, anxious, and agitated. *Precautions:* Do not use in patients allergic to benzodiazepines. Rapid or excessive amounts of injection may trigger withdrawal symptoms in patients on long-term treatment with benzodiazepines. Do not give to epileptics who are on long-term benzodiazepine treatment. Do not give to a patient under anaesthesia until the effects of any neuro-muscular blocking drug have completely worn off. Flumazenil works for two–three hours, so that any underlying sedation produced by a benzodiazepine may re-emerge. Use with caution in pregnancy and in breastfeeding mothers, in the elderly, in patients with head injury or impaired liver function. It is short-acting and repeated doses may be necessary but note that the effects of benzodiazepines can last for twenty-four hours. Use with caution in patients dependent on benzodiazepines, it may trigger withdrawal symptoms. Do not give injections rapidly in anxious patients and following major surgery.

flumetasone (flumetasone pivalate) is a corticosteroid (see Chapter 37) combined with the antibacterial drug clioquinol in Locorten-Vioform ➤ Locorten-Vioform.

flumethasone ➤ flumetasone.

flunisolide is a corticosteroid used in a nasal spray (Syntaris) to treat hayfever. *Adverse effects* see Chapter 37 on corticosteroids. It may produce irritation of the nose. Do not use in patients with untreated infections of the nose. Use with caution in patients who have recently had ulcers in the nose or injury or surgery to the nose. Use with caution in pregnancy.

flunitrazepam (Rohypnol) is an intermediate acting benzodiazepine drug ➤ benzodiazepines.

fluocinolone (fluocinolone acetonide, Synalar preparations) is a corticosteroid used in skin and scalp applications. *Adverse effects*

and Precautions see corticosteroid skin applications p. 241.

fluocinonide (Metosyn) is a corticosteroid used in skin and scalp applications. *Adverse effects and Precautions* see corticosteroid skin applications p. 241.

fluocortolone (fluocortolone hexanoate, Ultradil plain, Ultralanum plain, in Ultraproct) is a corticosteroid used in skin applications. *Adverse effects and Precautions* see corticosteroid skin applications p. 241.

Fluor-a-day ➤ fluoride.

fluorescein sodium (Minims fluorescein, Minims lignocaine and fluorescein, in Minims proxymetacaine & fluorescein) is used to stain the eye in order to highlight any scar or foreign particle.

Fluoride (En-De-Kay, Fluor-a-Day). It has now been convincingly demonstrated that in those parts of the world where the natural water contains more than one part per million of fluoride, the incidence of dental caries is lower than in comparable areas where the natural water contains less fluoride. Fluoride increases the resistance of the enamel of the teeth to acid, improves the laying down of minerals in teeth and interferes with bacterial growth. It is most effective if it is taken when the enamel is being laid down on the teeth before they erupt – that is, in childhood. If fluoride is deposited at this stage the teeth will be more resistant to dental caries than teeth that have not had fluoride deposited in them. In parts of the world where there is a high concentration of fluoride in the drinking water the teeth may become mottled, with dull and pitted enamel. This is called fluorosis. There is, however, no risk to health and the teeth are resistant to caries. Where the drinking water contains very high amounts of fluoride (over 10 parts per million) the bones may become hardened (sclerosed) and calcium may be laid down in tendons and ligaments. If the natural fluoride content of drinking water is less than one part per million, artificial fluoridation is the most economic method of supplementing fluoride intake. Daily supplements of fluoride should not be used without knowledge of the fluoride content of the local drinking water. They are not necessary if the water contains 0.7 parts or more per million. Infants under six months of age do not require fluoride supplementation. The local effect of fluoride on the enamel and plaque is more effective in stopping caries than systemic fluoride (i.e. fluoride tablets etc. to be swallowed). Local preparations include mouth rinses, gels and varnishes.

fluorometholone (FML) is a corticosteroid used to treat inflammation of the eye. *Adverse effects* include a rise in pressure in the eye, thinning of the cornea, cataract and risk of fungal infections. *Precautions:* Do not use if viral, fungal or tuberculous infection is present. Do not use if infection is causing a yellow discharge (purulent). Do not wear soft contact lenses while on treatment. Use with utmost caution in patients with glaucoma and be cautious about prolonged use in pregnancy and infants.

fluorouracil (Efudix) is an anti-cancer drug, see Chapter 51. *Adverse effects* include nausea, vomiting, loss of appetite, severe diarrhoea, skin rash (dermatitis), loss of hair (alopecia), nail damage, and pigmentation of the skin. It may produce damage to the lining membrane of the mouth, stomach and intestine, fever, bone-marrow damage leading to blood disorders and damage to part of the brain (the cerebellum). *Precautions:* It should not be given to patients whose bone-marrow function may be depressed and it should be given with caution to patients whose liver function is impaired.

fluothane ➤ halothane.

fluoxetine (Felicium, Prozac) is a 5HT reuptake blocker used to treat depression. See Chapter 4. It is also used to treat bulimia and obsessive compulsive disorders. *Adverse effects* include nausea, vomiting, indigestion, abdominal pains, diarrhoea, constipation, loss of appetite, loss of weight, changes in blood sugar levels, dry mouth, anxiety, nervousness, weakness, headache, tremor, palpitations, insomnia, dizziness, drowsiness, sweating, fever, confusion, hypomania, mania, convulsions, sexual dysfunction, movement disorders, neuromalignant syndrome-like events (see under antipsychotic drugs), low blood sodium levels, abnormal liver function tests, rash or allergic reactions (stop if they develop), blood disorders, stroke, bruising, bleeding from the stomach and intestine, inflammation of the pancreas, hair loss, violent behaviour, ideas about violent suicide, and vaginal bleeding when the drug is stopped. *Precautions:* Do not use in patients with severe impairment of kidney function, unstable epilepsy, in breastfeeding mothers or in manic phase of manic depression. Use with caution in patients with heart disease, epilepsy, history of mania, patients recovering from ECT treatment (risk of prolonged convulsions). Use with caution in pregnancy and in patients with diabetes or impaired heart, kidney or liver function. Avoid abrupt withdrawal. *Interactions:* MAOIs, tryptophan, tricyclic antidepressants, lithium, flecainide, tryptophan, vinblastine, carbamazepine, phenytoin.

flupenthixol ➤ flupentixol.

flupentixol (Depixol, Fluanxol) is a thioxanthene antipsychotic drug (see Chapter 3) which also produces antidepressant effects when given in low doses (see Chapter 4). *Adverse effects* include insomnia and restlessness. Occasionally it may cause headache, dizziness, visual disturbances, tremor and movement disorders (e.g. parkinsonism). *Precautions:* Use with caution in patients with heart diseases, impaired kidney or liver function, arteriosclerosis, lung disease, senile confusion, parkinsonism, porphyria (a hereditary disorder of metabolism). Do not use in patients who are over-active and excitable. Do not use in pregnancy or in breastfeeding mothers or in comatose patients. Drowsiness may affect driving ability. *Interactions:* Alcohol, sleeping drugs, sedatives, anti-anxiety drugs or any drug that depresses brain function, opiate pain-relievers, anti-blood pressure drugs, anti-epileptic drugs, levodopa.

fluphenazine (fluphenazine decanoate, fluphenazine enanthate, fluphenazine hydrochloride, Decazate, Modecate, Moditen, in Motipress, in Motival) is a phenothiazine antipsychotic drug ➤ antipsychotic drugs.

flurandrenolone ➤ fludroxycortide.

flurazepam (Dalmane) is a benzodiazepine drug ➤ benzodiazepines.

flurbiprofen (Froben, Strefen) is a non-steroidal anti-inflammatory drug (NSAID) ➤ non-steroidal anti-inflammatory drugs. It is also used in Ocufen eye solution to relieve inflammation after eye surgery and laser treatment on the eye. It also helps to keep the pupil dilated during surgery.

flutamide (Chimax, Drogenil) is a non-steroidal anti-androgen used to treat cancer of the prostate gland. *Adverse effects* include tenderness and enlargement of the breasts with milk production, and occasionally, nausea, vomiting, increased appetite, diarrhoea, tiredness, insomnia, decreased libido, stomach and chest pains, thirst, blurred vision, headache, dizziness, fluid retention, itching, rashes, liver damage, jaundice, blood disorders and harmful effects on the brain (encephalopathy). *Precautions:* Do not use in patients who are allergic to the drug. Tests of liver function should be carried out before and at regular intervals during treatment. It may cause fluid retention in patients which will aggravate heart disease.

fluticasone is a corticosteroid (see Chapter 45) used as a cream (Cutivate) to treat eczema and dermatitis, as a nasal aerosol (Flixonase) to treat hayfever (see p. 87) and as a disk inhaler (Flixotide, in Seretide) to treat and prevent bronchial asthma (see Chapter 14). *Adverse effects and Precautions* see Chapter 37 on corticosteroids. *Inhalations* to treat asthma may cause hoarseness, thrush of the mouth and throat and

may rarely trigger wheezing. They should be used with caution in patients with tuberculosis and in pregnancy. *Nasal sprays* may cause irritation of the nose, disturbances of smell and taste and occasionally nose bleeds. Use with caution in pregnancy and breastfeeding mothers. *Adverse effects and Precautions* see corticosteroid skin applications p. 241.

fluvastatin (Lescol) is a statin drug used to treat raised blood cholesterol levels. See Chapter 26. *Adverse effects and Precautions* are similar to those listed under simvastatin ➤ simvastatin.

Fluvoxamine (fluvoxamine maleate, Faverin) is an antidepressant drug which blocks 5 HT (serotonin) re-uptake. See Chapter 4. *Adverse effects* include sleepiness, agitation, tremor, nausea, loss of appetite, vomiting, diarrhoea, constipation, dry mouth, abdominal pains, indigestion, headache, generally feeling unwell, insomnia, palpitations, sweating, dizziness, anxiety, nervousness, convulsions, liver disorders and decreased heart rate. *Precautions:* It should be used with utmost caution during pregnancy, in breastfeeding mothers, and in patients with epilepsy. Reduced dosage should be used in patients with impaired kidney or liver function. It may increase the effects of alcohol. *Interactions:* Theophylline, aminophylline, clozapine, propranolol, carbamazepine, benzodiazepines, warfarin, MAOIs, tricyclic antidepressants, alcohol, phenytoin, lithium and tryptophan.

FML eye drops ➤ fluorometholone.

folic acid (pteroylglutamic acid, Folicare, Lexpec, Pre-conceive) is necessary for cell division and for the normal production of red blood cells, see Chapter 36 on vitamins. *Adverse effects:* Large and continuous doses of folic acid may lower the blood level of vitamin B_{12} which is essential to the normal production of red blood cells. *Precautions:* Folic acid should not be used to treat pernicious anaemia and other vitamin B_{12} deficiency disorders because it may trigger the onset of spinal cord degeneration. Do not use in cancer patients unless megaloblastic anaemia due to folic acid deficiency is a complication. For use in pregnancy, see p. 179.

Folicare ➤ folic acid.

folinic acid is an active breakdown product (active metabolite) of the B vitamin folic acid. See Chapter 36. Its calcium salt (calcium folinate, Calcium Leucovorin, Refolinon) is used to counter the anti-folate actions of the anti-cancer drugs methotrexate and trimetrexate. It reduces the toxicity of these drugs, a process referred to as 'folinic acid rescue'. Folinic acid is also used to treat folate deficiency megaloblastic anaemias, but it should not be used to treat pernicious anaemia or other megaloblastic anaemias when vitamin B_{12} is deficient. See Chapter 36. Folinic acid (as Lederfolin) also interacts with the anti-cancer drug fluorouracil to benefit patients being treated with fluorouracil for cancer of the bowel that has produced secondaries. *Adverse effects* include occasional allergic reactions and fever following intravenous administration. *Precautions:* Do not give at the same time as methotrexate – give twenty-four hours after the last dose. It must be administered during treatment with trimetrexate and continued for seventy-two hours after the last dose of trimetrexate.

follicle-stimulating hormone (FSH) ➤ gonadotrophin and see Chapter 40.

follitropin alpha (Gonal-F) is a gonadotrophin used to stimulate the ovaries to produce eggs in assisted fertility treatments (e.g. IVF) and to treat women who do not ovulate and have not responded to clomiphene ➤ gonadotrophin. It is produced by genetic engineering rather than extraction from the urine of post-menopausal women. It is given by injection under the skin. *Adverse effects and Precautions* ➤ human menopausal gonadotrophin.

follitropin beta (Puregon) ➤ follitropin alpha.

fomivirsen (Vitravene) is used for second line treatment of cytomegalovirus (CMV) infections of the retina in AIDS patients. See Chapter 48. *Adverse effects* include abnormal vision, swelling at the injection site, inflammation of the eye, cataract, eye pain, bleeding from the eye and detachment of the retina. *Precautions:* Do not use in patients with eye infections. Use with caution in patients who are pregnant or breast-feeding, have CMV infections of the retina in the other eye, CMV infections outside the eye and patients with sight-threatening diseases.

Foradil ➤ formoterol.

forcaltonin ➤ calcitonin (salmon).

formaldehyde solutions (formalin, Veracur) are used in varying strengths as antiseptics, disinfectants, for removing dead skin to treat warts and verrucas and to treat sweaty feet. It may irritate skin. Avoid contact with healthy skin and the eyes and mouth.

formoterol (eformoterol) (Foradil, Oxis, Symbicort) is a selective beta₂ stimulant used as a bronchodilator to treat asthma. See Chapter 14. *Adverse effects and Precautions* are similar to those listed under salbutamol.

Fortagesic tablets contain pentazocine and paracetamol. They are used to treat moderate pain. *Adverse effects and Precautions* ➤ pentazocine, paracetamol.

Fortipine LA ➤ nifedipine.

Fortovase ➤ saquinavir.

Fortral ➤ pentazocine.

Fortum injection ➤ ceftazidime.

Fosamax ➤ alendronate sodium.

foscarnet (Foscavir) is an antiviral drug (see Chapter 48) used to treat cytomegalovirus (CMV) infections of the iris of the eye (iritis) in patients with AIDS in whom ganciclovir (Cymevene) is not suitable (➤ ganciclovir). *Adverse effects* include headache, nausea, vomiting, fatigue, skin rashes, low blood calcium and blood sugar levels, impaired kidney function, genital irritation, epileptic seizures and anaemia (due to a drop in haemoglobin levels). Undiluted solutions may cause inflammation of the vein when injected into a vein. *Precautions:* Do not use in pregnancy or in breastfeeding mothers. Use with caution in patients with impaired kidney function or with low blood calcium levels before treatment. The patient must be given plenty of fluids during treatment. Tests of kidney function should be carried out before treatment and the dose adjusted accordingly. Blood calcium level and kidney function tests (e.g. blood creatinine level) should be carried out every second day during treatment.

Foscavir ➤ foscarnet.

fosfestrol (fosfestrol tetrasodium, Honvan) is broken down in the body to stilboestrol (an oestrogen). It is used in the treatment of cancer of the prostate. *Adverse effects and Precautions:* Burning pain in the perineum, nausea and vomiting, fluid retention, impotence, enlargement of the breasts and thrombosis (blood clots) may occur ➤ stilboestrol.

fosinopril (Staril) is an ACE inhibitor used to treat raised blood pressure (see Chapter 25), and heart failure in combination with a diuretic (see Chapter 23). *Adverse effects* include dizziness, stomach and bowel upsets, cough, chest pain, palpitations, fatigue, skin rash, muscle and joint pains and taste disturbances. Rarely, it may cause allergic swellings of the hands, face and feet (stop the drug immediately) and inflammation of the pancreas. *Precautions:* It should not be used in pregnancy and in breastfeeding mothers. It should be used with caution in individuals with impaired liver or kidney function, congestive heart failure, raised blood pressure associated with impaired kidney function, patients on blood dialysis and patients who are depleted of salt and water. *Interactions:* Potassium-sparing diuretics, potassium supplements, NSAIDs, antacids, lithium, anti-blood pressure drugs.

fosphenytoin (Pro-Epanutin) is given by injection to control epilepsy. It is used to prevent and treat seizures associated with neurosurgery or head trauma. It is used as a substitute for oral phenytoin when oral administration is not possible. See Chapter 15. *Adverse effects* include heart complications, disorders of the blood, nerve disorders, liver and kidney damage, stomach and bowel upset, itching, headache, unusual hair growth, allergic reactions. *Precautions:* Do not use in patients with slow heart beat, heart block, Adams-Stokes syndrome (fainting caused by a problem in the heart), porphyria (a hereditary disorder of metabolism), or while breastfeeding. Use with caution in patients with low blood pressure, impaired heart, kidney or liver function, hypoalbuminaemia (low level of albumin in the blood), diabetes, in the elderly or in pregnancy.

Frador antiseptic tincture contains menthol, chlorbutanol, storax and benzoin (alcoholic extract). It is used to relieve the pain of mouth ulcers. *Adverse effects* ➤ each constituent drug.

Fragmin ➤ dalteparin sodium.

framycetin (framycetin sulphate) is an aminoglycoside antibiotic, see Chapter 46. *Adverse effects and Precautions* ➤ aminoglycoside antibiotics. It is too toxic to be used by mouth or by injection, and is used principally in topical applications. It is included in Sofradex ear and eye drops and ointment, in Soframycin skin ointment and in Sofra-Tulle gauze dressings.

frangula (in Normacol Plus) is a bulk laxative. See Chapter 21.

Franol preparations contain the bronchodilators ephedrine and theophylline. They are used to treat asthma (see Chapter 14). *Adverse effects and Precautions* ➤ ephedrine, theophylline.

fresh frozen plasma is obtained from *one*

donation of whole blood. It is used to replace coagulation factors or other plasma proteins. *Adverse effects* include allergic reactions, chills, fever, wheezing and adult respiratory stress syndrome. *Precautions:* Blood groups must be compatible and overload of the circulation must be avoided.

Frisium ➤ clobazam.

Froben ➤ flurbiprofen.

Froop ➤ furosemide.

Froop-Co ➤ co-amilofruse.

Fru-Co ➤ co-amilofruse.

fructose ➤ laevulose.

Frumil ➤ co-amilofruse.

frusemide ➤ furosemide.

Frusene preparations contain the loop diuretic furosemide(frusemide) and the potassium-sparing diuretic triamterene. They are used to treat congestive heart failure, and fluid retention caused by liver or kidney disease. See Chapter 29 on diuretics. *Adverse effects and Precautions* ➤ thiazide diuretics, furosemide(frusemide).

Frusol ➤ furosemide(frusemide).

FSH ➤ follicle stimulating hormone.

Fucibet cream contains betametasone (a corticosteroid) and fusidic acid (an antibacterial drug). It is used to treat eczema that is bacterially infected. *Adverse effects and Precautions* see corticosteroid skin applications p. 241 and ➤ fusidic acid.

Fucidin ➤ sodium fusidate.

Fucidin H ointment and cream contain hydrocortisone (a corticosteroid) and sodium fusidate (an antibacterial drug). They are used to treat eczema that is bacterially infected. *Adverse effects and Precautions* see corticosteroid skin applications p. 241 and ➤ sodium fusidate.

Fucithalmic eye drops contain fusidic acid. *Adverse effects and Precautions* ➤ fusidic acid. Eye drops may cause transient stinging and allergic reactions.

Fuller's Earth (terra fullonica) consists largely of montmorillonite, an aluminium silicate with chalk (calcite). It is adsorbent and is used in dusting powders, toilet powders and lotions. It is also used to treat paraquat poisoning.

Full Marks ➤ phenothrin.

Fungilin ➤ amphotericin.

Fungizone ➤ amphotericin.

Furadantin ➤ nitrofurantoin.

furosemide(frusemide) (in co-amilofruse, in Diumide-K Continus, Froop, in Fru-Co, in Frumil, in Frusene, Frusol, in Lasical, in Lasilactone, Lasix, in Lasoride, Min-I-Jet furosemide(frusemide), Rusyde) is a loop diuretic (see Chapter 29). *Adverse effects* include a fall in blood sodium, potassium and magnesium and increase in the excretion of calcium. It may cause nausea, vomiting, diarrhoea, blurred vision, yellow vision, headache, dizziness, allergic reactions, skin rashes, sensitivity of the skin to sunlight, fall in blood pressure, raised blood uric acid levels and gout, raised blood glucose, transient increase in blood cholesterol and fats and, very rarely, jaundice and damage to the bone marrow, producing blood disorders. Noises in the ears (tinnitus) and deafness may develop in patients with impaired kidney function, particularly if high doses are given rapidly into a vein. Large doses intravenously may very rarely damage the pancreas (pancreatitis). *Precautions:* Do not use in patients in precomatose states associated with cirrhosis of the liver. It should be used with caution in patients with liver or kidney impairment, diabetes, gout, in pregnancy and in breast-feeding mothers. Because it increases the volume of urine it should be used with caution in anyone who has difficulty in passing urine, for example, men with enlarged prostate glands. It causes a fall in blood potassium and sodium levels and therefore the blood chemistry should be carefully monitored, particularly in elderly patients and in patients with impaired kidney or liver function. *Interactions:* Digoxin and related drugs, lithium, aminoglycoside antibiotics, cephalosporin antibiotics, anti-blood pressure drugs, NSAIDs.

fusafungine (Locabiotal aerosol) is an antibiotic with anti-inflammatory properties used to treat infections of the nose and throat. It works on the surface and is applied by a spray. *Adverse effects* include transient irritation of the nose and throat and allergic reactions. *Precautions:* Do not use in patients allergic to fusafungine or one of the additives in the spray preparation. Avoid spraying into the eyes.

fusidic acid (Fucidin, Fucithalmic) and its salts are antibiotics used to treat penicillin-resistant staphylococcal infections, especially osteomyelitis (inflammation of bone and bone marrow) ➤ sodium fusidate.

Fybogel ➤ ispaghula husk.

Fybogel Mebeverine ➤ ispaghula husk, mebeverine.

Fybozest Orange effervescent granules contain ispaghula husk. They are used to reduce a raised blood cholesterol level. See Chapter 26. *Adverse effects* and *Precautions* ➤ ispaghula husk. Do not use in patients with phenylketonurea and use with caution in patients with diabetes.

gabapentin (Neurotin) is an anti-epileptic drug. See Chapter 15. *Adverse effects* include nausea, vomiting, headache, tremor, fatigue, dizziness, double vision, sleepiness, runny nose, nystagmus (flicking movement of the eyeballs) and loss of control over voluntary movements (ataxia). *Precautions:* Use with caution in patients with impaired kidney function, in pregnancy, in breast-feeding mothers and in the elderly. Avoid sudden withdrawal, taper the dose off slowly over at least one week. *Interactions:* Antacids.

Gabitril ➤ tiagabine.

Galake ➤ co-dydramol.

galantamine (Reminyl) is an acetylcholinesterase inhibitor used to treat mild to moderately severe Alzheimer's dementia. See Chapter 9. *Adverse effects* include stomach and bowel upset, fatigue, dizziness, headache, drowsiness, weight loss, confusion, fall, injury, insomnia, inflammation of the lining of the nose, urinary tract infection. *Precautions:* Do not use in patients with severe liver or kidney damage, intolerance to galactose, disorders of the enzyme lactase, inability to absorb glucose or galactose properly or while breastfeeding. Use with caution in patients with moderate liver damage, heart-beat disturbances, history of peptic ulcer, epilepsy, asthma, severe difficulty breathing, stomach, bowel or urinary outflow obstruction, bladder surgery or pregnancy.

Galcodine and **Galcodine Paediatric** ➤ codeine.

Galenamet ➤ cimetidine.

Galenamox ➤ amoxicillin.

Galenphol and **Galenphol Strong** ➤ pholcodine.

Galfer preparations ➤ ferrous fumarate.

Galfer FA capsules contain ferrous fumarate and folic acid ➤ iron, folic acid. They may cause nausea and constipation. *Interactions:* tetracycline antibiotics.

Galfloxin ➤ flucloxacillin.

gallamine (gallamine triethiodide; Flaxedil) is a non-depolarizing muscle relaxant (see p. 42) which is used along with general anaesthetics in surgical operations. It may produce rapid beating of the heart. It should not be used in patients with severe impairment of kidney function because it is excreted via the kidneys.

Galloways is an expectorant cough medicine ➤ ipecacuanha, squill.

Galpseud contains pseudoephedrine; **Galpseud Plus** contains chlorphenamine (chlorpheniramine) and pseudoephedrine ➤ individual entry for each drug.

Galpamol ➤ paracetamol.

Galprofen ➤ ibuprofen.

Gamanil ➤ lofepramine.

Gammabulin intramuscular injection, see normal immunoglobulin, p. 302.

Gamma Formula capsules contain evening primrose oil ➤ oil of evening primrose.

gamma globulin, see normal immuno-globulins, p. 302.

gamolenic acid (gamma-linolenic acid, GLA) is obtained from oil of evening prim-rose. It is used in **Efamast** to treat painful breasts (mastalgia) which may be cyclical (e.g. with menstrual periods) or non-cyclical. The discomfort appears to be due to sensitivity to female sex hormones which may be caused by an abnormal ratio of saturated to unsaturated fatty acids in the breast tissue. The pain can be relieved by reducing the ratio of these fatty acids by taking gamolenic acid, which provides a high source of unsaturated fatty acids. It may take up to six months to produce any benefit. Gamolenic acid is also available in **Epogam** to provide symptomatic relief of eczema. It increases the levels of essential fatty acids in the skin and may help some individuals. *Adverse effects* include nausea, headache and diarrhoea. *Precautions:* It should be used with caution in individuals with a history of epilepsy. In women who are treated for mastalgia, cancer of the breast should be excluded before treatment. Use with caution in pregnancy.

ganciclovir (Cymevene, Virgon) is an anti-viral drug used to treat life-threatening and sight-threatening cytomegalovirus (CMV) infections in patients suffering from AIDS or other immune deficiency disorders and to prevent cytomegalovirus infections in patients during immunosuppressive treat-ment following organ transplant. *Adverse effects* include blood disorders, itching, fever, rash and abnormal liver function tests. It may also cause nausea, vomiting, diar-rhoea, mouth ulcers, loss of appetite, bleed-ing in the gut, chest and abdominal pains, chills, generally feeling unwell, fluid reten-tion, changes in blood pressure and heart rate, headache, breathlessness, nervousness, confusion, drowsiness, mental disorders, loss of control over voluntary movements (ataxia), nerve damage, tremor, urinary symptoms, fall in blood sugar level, blood in urine, changes to kidney function, eye pain, deafness, hair loss, acne, sweating, itching, pain and swelling at the injection site and detachment of retina in AIDS patients with inflammation of the retina. *Precautions:* Do not use in pregnancy and avoid getting pregnant while on treatment. Men should use a condom during and for ninety days after treatment has stopped. Do not breastfeed until seventy-two hours after the last dose. Do not use in patients allergic to ganciclovir or with a low white blood cell count. Blood counts should be carried out every two weeks and if counts for white cells and/or platelets are low the drug should not be given.

Ganda eye drops contain varying pro-portions of guanethidine and adrenaline-(epinephrine) for the treatment of glau-coma (see p. 64). *Adverse effects* include dis-comfort in the eyes, headache, redness of the eyes and surrounding skin and pigmen-tation of the eye. General effects from guanethidine and adrenaline(epinephrine) are rare. The drops may cause a rise in pressure inside the eye, drooping of the upper eyelids and damage to the cornea. *Precautions:* Do not use in patients with closed-angle glaucoma or who have the lens missing from the eye. Examine the con-junctivae and cornea every six months and stop treatment if there are signs of damage.

ganglion-blocking drugs, see p. 36.

ganirelix (Orgalutran) is used to prevent premature luteinizing hormone (LH) surges in women undergoing controlled ovarian stimulation for assisted reproduction. *Adverse effects* include injection site reac-tions, headache, nausea. *Precautions:* Do not use in patients with moderate or severe kidney or liver damage, severe allergic conditions, in pregnancy or while breastfeeding.

Garamycin ear and eye drops ➤ gentamicin.

Gardenal Sodium injection ➤ phenobarbital.

gargles are liquid preparations for washing out the throat, and are usually not intended for swallowing. They are used to treat sore throats but are of doubtful value.

garlic has been used for its cough expectorant, disinfectant and diuretic properties. There is controversy over claims that garlic helps to lower blood cholesterol and fat levels and reduce the stickiness of blood platelets and may therefore be of benefit in preventing coronary heart disease.

Gastrobid Continus ➤ metoclopramide.

Gastrocote preparations contain alginic acid, or its sodium salt, aluminium hydroxide, magnesium trisilicate and sodium bicarbonate. They are used to treat heartburn and acid reflux (see p. 102). *Adverse effects and Precautions* ➤ antacids.

Gastroflux ➤ metoclopramide.

Gaviscon tablets contain alginic acid, sodium alginate, magnesium trisilicate, dried aluminium hydroxide gel and sodium bicarbonate. **Gaviscon** and **Gaviscon Advance** liquid contains sodium alginate, sodium bicarbonate and calcium carbonate. Both are used to treat heartburn and acid reflux (see p. 102). *Adverse effects and Precautions* ➤ antacids.

G-CSF contains filgrastim and lenograstim ➤ filgrastim, lenograstim.

gelatin is a protein extracted from animal tissues. It is used in the preparation of capsules, suppositories, pastes, pastilles and pessaries, in preparing lubricating eye drops and to make a solution used to restore blood volume after haemorrhage. It is taken by mouth to treat brittle nails. Allergic reactions have occurred after a slow injection of gelatin.

Gelcosal gel contains strong coal-tar solution, pine, tar and salicylic acid. It is used to treat psoriasis and eczema. *Adverse effects and Precautions* ➤ coal tar, salicylic acid.

Gelcotar gel and liquid ➤ coal tar.

Gelofusine is used to increase the volume of the blood. It contains modified gelatin and sodium chloride.

Gel Tears eye gel contains carbomer 940. It is used to treat dry eye conditions.

Gelusil preparations contain the antacids magnesium trisilicate and dried aluminium hydroxide. See Chapter 19. *Adverse effects and Precautions* ➤ antacids.

gemcitabine (Gemzar) is given with cisplatin as a first-line treatment, or alone to relieve the symptoms, of locally advanced or secondary pancreatic cancer; locally advanced or secondary non-small cell lung cancer; cancer of the pancreas not responding to treatment with 5-fluorouracil (5-FU); advanced bladder cancer in combination with cisplatin. See Chapter 51. *Adverse effects* include mild stomach and bowel side-effects and rashes, kidney damage, damage to the lungs and flu-like symptoms.

gemeprost is a prostaglandin used to soften and dilate the cervix to assist surgical operations through the cervix and during abortions in the first twenty-four weeks of pregnancy. *Adverse effects* include pain in the womb, bleeding from the vagina, nausea, vomiting, diarrhoea, flushing, backache, dizziness, myasthenia gravis (muscle weakness due to neuromuscular abnormality), headache, breathlessness, chest pain, mild fever and palpitations. *Precautions:* Do not use in patients allergic to gemeprost or other prostaglandins. Use with caution in patients with obstructive airways disease (e.g. asthma), heart disease, glaucoma or inflammatory conditions of the cervix or vagina, in patients where there is a risk of rupture of the uterus, which is most common in women who have had several babies, a history of surgery on the uterus or if they are also given oxytocic drugs intravenously.

gemfibrozil (Enfib, Lopid) is a fibrate drug used to lower blood cholesterol and fat levels. See Chapter 26. *Adverse effects* include nausea, diarrhoea, vomiting and wind, headache, dizziness, blurred vision, impotence, pains in the hands and feet, skin rashes, jaundice, itching, allergic reactions (e.g. angioedema), disorders of heart rhythm and muscle damage causing pain and weakness. *Precautions:* Before starting treatment patients should have tests for anaemia, liver function and blood cholesterol and fat levels. It should be used with caution in patients with impaired kidney function and patients should have a specialist examination of their eyes every twelve months. Their blood cholesterol and fat levels should be measured at regular intervals. If there is no response or the blood fats go up (a paradoxical response), the drug should be stopped. The latter can happen in alcoholic liver disease. Tests for anaemia should be carried out every two months during the first twelve months of treatment. It should not be used in patients with alcoholic liver disease, gallstones or impaired liver function. It should not be used in pregnancy or in breastfeeding mothers ➤ fibrates for warnings on muscle damage. *Interactions:* Anticoagulants, other statin blood fat lowering drugs, colestipol.

Gemzar ➤ gemcitabine.

Genotropin (somatropin) ➤ growth hormone.

gentamicin (gentamicin sulphate) is an aminoglycoside antibiotic, see p. 270. It is not absorbed by mouth and has to be given by injections (Genticin); it is also used in local applications to treat infections of the eyes (Cidomycin, Garamycin, Minims Gentamycin), ears (Cidomycin, Garamycin, Genticin, in Gentisone HC). *Adverse effects and Precautions:* For general adverse effects and precautions ➤ aminoglycoside antibiotics. *Ear applications* may cause irritation, allergic reactions and superinfections. They should not be used if the ear drum is perforated or in patients allergic to it or other aminoglycoside antibiotics. Use with caution in pregnancy, breastfeeding mothers and avoid prolonged use. *Eye applications:* Do not use in pregnancy or in patients allergic to it or to other aminoglycosides. *Skin applications* may cause irritation, allergic reactions and superinfection. Do not apply to large areas of damaged skin because of the risk of absorption into the blood and damage to hearing. Do not use in patients allergic to it or to other aminoglycosides. Use with utmost caution in pregnancy and breastfeeding mothers, and avoid prolonged use.

gentian mixture, acid is a concentrated mixture of gentian infusion, dilute hydrochloric acid and chloroform water. It is used as a bitter to stimulate the appetite.

gentian mixture, alkaline is a concentrated mixture of gentian infusion, sodium bicarbonate and chloroform water. It is used as a bitter to stimulate the appetite.

gentian violet (crystal violet) is used in antiseptic skin applications (see p. 245) against bacteria, worms and fungi.

Genticin ➤ gentamicin.

Gentisone HC ear drops contain gentamicin (an aminoglycoside antibiotic) and hydrocortisone (a corticosteroid). They are used to treat infected eczema of the outer ear. *Adverse effects and Precautions* ➤ gentamycin and see corticosteroid skin applications p. 241.

Gentran intravenous infusion preparations contain dextran in glucose or in sodium chloride solution ➤ dextran.

Geref injection ➤ sermorelin.

Germoloids is a haemorrhoidal preparation containing the local anaesthetic lidocaine(lignocaine) and the soothing agent zinc oxide.

gestodene (in Femodene ED, in Femodene, in Femodette, in Minulet, in Tri-Minulet, in Triadene) is a progestogen used in oral contraceptives. *Adverse effects and Precautions* ➤ progestogens and see Chapter 41 on oral contraceptives.

Gestone injection ➤ progesterone.

gestonorone (gestronol hexanoate, gestonorone) is a long-acting progestogen. It is given as an intramuscular injection to treat cancer of the womb. It is also used in males to shrink cancer of the prostate gland which helps to reduce difficulty in passing urine. *Adverse effects and Precautions* ➤ progestogens. Temporary breathlessness, coughing and faintness may occur immediately after the injection. In males gestonorone may reduce libido, cause discomfort in the breasts and temporarily reduce the sperm count. Patients with liver disorders on long-term treatment should have tests of their liver function at regular intervals.

gestrinone (Dimetriose) is used to treat endometriosis. It has both anti-oestrogenic and anti-progestogenic properties. It reduces the secretion of luteinizing hormone (LH) and follicle stimulating hormone (FSH) by the pituitary gland and therefore reduces the release of oestrogens and progesterone by the ovaries. It also blocks progesterone receptors in endometrial tissue (i.e. the lining of the womb) and other endometrial deposits, causing them to shrink. It also dries up the menstrual periods. It offers an alternative to danazol and needs to be taken only twice weekly instead of daily. *Adverse effects* include fluid retention, weight gain, acne, stomach and bowel upsets, changes in appetite, hot flushes, spotting, cramps, nervousness, depression, changes in libido, and, very rarely, male-type hair growth and voice changes. *Precautions:* It should not be used in women with severe heart, kidney or liver disorders, or when breastfeeding. It should not be used in women with diabetes or raised blood cholesterol and fat levels. It should not be used in pregnancy or if there is a risk of the woman being pregnant. Women on treatment should avoid sexual intercourse or use a barrier contraceptive (e.g. condom, cap). *Interactions:* Anti-epileptic drugs, oral contraceptives and rifampicin. Refer also to entry on danazol.

gestronol ➤ gestonorone.

GHRH ➤ somatorelin.

Ginseng is a plant, various parts of which are used to make medicines. The leaves are used to make tea and are said to help digestion; the roots are used in tonic remedies. There appears to be as many uses as there are preparations available. The most popular types come from China, Manchuria and Korea. If you think it will do you good it probably will, but we need documented scientific evidence if we are to assess its value. *Adverse effects* include the *ginseng abuse syndrome* – raised blood pressure, nervousness, sleeplessness, skin rashes and diarrhoea in the mornings.

Givitol is a compound iron preparation containing ferrous fumerate and vitamins B group and C ➤ iron.

GLA (gamma-linolenic acid, gamolenic acid) ➤ oil of evening primrose.

Glandosane mouth spray contains carboxymethylcellulose sodium, sorbital, potassium chloride, sodium chloride, magnesium chloride, calcium chloride and dipotassium hydrogen phosphate. It is used to treat dry mouth associated with radiotherapy and the use of antimuscarinic drugs.

glantiramer (Copaxone) is used in relapsing-remitting multiple sclerosis to reduce the frequency of relapses in patients who are able to walk and who have had at least one relapse during the previous two years. *Adverse effects* include immediate post-injection reactions (such as dilation of the blood vessels), chest pain, difficulty breathing, palpitations, rapid heart beat, injection site reactions, weakness, nausea, hypertonia (abnormally high muscle tone), headache, pain in joints, rash, sweating, enlargement of the lymph nodes, tremor, fluid retention, fainting. *Precautions:* Do not use in patients who are allergic to mannitol. Use with caution in the elderly, in patients with kidney damage, a history of cardiovascular disease, in pregnancy or who are breastfeeding.

Glau-opt is an eye drop ➤ timolol.

glibenclamide (Daonil, Diabetamide, Euglucon, Gliken, Semi-Daonil) is a sulphonylurea oral anti-diabetic drug. See Chapter 42 and ➤ sulphonylureas.

Glibenese ➤ glipizide.

gliclazide (DIAGLYK, Diamicron) is a sulphonylurea oral anti-diabetic drug ➤ sulphonylureas.

Gliken ➤ glibenclamide.

glimepiride (Amaryl) is used to treat non-insulin dependent (type II) diabetes. See Chapter 42. *Adverse effects* include low blood glucose level (hypoglycaemia), allergic reactions including skin rash, stomach and bowel upsets, abdominal pain, confusion, dizziness, drowsiness, headache, generally feeling unwell, tremor, visual disturbances, liver disorders, blood disorders, raised liver enzymes. *Precautions:* Do not use in patients with juvenile growth-onset or unstable brittle diabetes, an increase in the level of ketones in the blood, severe kidney or liver damage, endocrine disorders, stress, infections, after surgical procedures, in pregnancy or while breastfeeding. Use with caution in the elderly or in patients with kidney failure.

glipizide (Glibenese, Minodiab) is a sulphonylurea oral anti-diabetic drug ➤ sulphonylureas.

gliquidone (Glurenorm) is a sulphonylurea oral anti-diabetic drug ➤ sulphonylureas.

GlucaGen Kit contains genetically engineered glucagon. It is given by injection to treat low blood sugar levels ➤ glucagon.

glucagon is a hormone produced by the pancreas that stimulates the release of glucose from glucose stores in the liver. It is used in the emergency treatment of hypoglycaemia (low blood sugar) in insulin-dependent diabetic patients. Unlike glucose it can be injected under the skin or into a muscle as well as into a vein. *Adverse effects* include nausea, vomiting, diarrhoea and low blood potassium. Allergic reactions occurred occasionally with glucagon which was obtained from the pancreatic glands of pigs and cows. A genetically engineered glucagon (GlucaGen) has now replaced it. *Precautions:* It should not be used in patients with a phaeochromocytoma (tumour of the sympathetic nervous system), insulin or glucagon producing tumours. It should be used with caution in pregnancy and breastfeeding mothers.

Glucamet ➤ metformin.

Glucobay ➤ acarbose.

glucocorticoids, see Chapter 37.

glucocorticosteroids, see Chapter 37.

Glucophage ➤ metformin.

Glurenorm ➤ gliquidone.

glutaraldehyde (Glutarol) is used as a gel or liquid in the treatment of warts (see p. 262). *Adverse effects:* It may irritate and stain healthy skin brown. *Precautions:* Do not use on facial warts or ano-genital warts. Avoid contact with healthy skin.

Glutarol ➤ glutaraldehyde.

glycerin ➤ glycerol.

glycerine ➤ glycerol.

glycerol (glycerin or glycerine) is used as a sweetening agent in mixtures, linctuses and pastilles. Externally, it is used in creams for its water-retaining and skin softening properties. It is used in Audax ear drops to soften wax, in Micollette and Relaxit micro-enemas. Glycerol (glycerin) suppositories are used to treat constipation. See Chapter 21. Referred to as glycerin in Exterol ear drops and in Massé cream used to treat sore nipples. It is used to sooth the throat in some cough medicines. *Adverse effects and*

Precautions: By mouth glycerol may cause headaches, thirst, nausea, diarrhoea, and a rise in blood sugar levels. Rarely it may cause disorders of heart rhythm and coma. Large doses by injection may damage red blood cells and the kidneys. Use with utmost caution in diabetic patients and patients who are dehydrated.

glyceryl trinitrate (nitroglycerin, trinitrin) is a nitrate vasodilator used to treat angina (see Chapter 22) and heart failure (see Chapter 23). For preparations, see p. 113. It may also be used by injection to relieve pain from kidney stones or gallstones. *Adverse effects* include flushing of the face, rapid beating of the heart, severe throbbing headache, faintness, and dizziness, especially on standing up after sitting or lying down due to a fall in blood pressure (postural hypotension). Overdose may cause restlessness, vomiting, fall in blood pressure and faintness, but these only last for a short time. Rapid intravenous injection can cause a fall in blood pressure, nausea, retching, apprehension, restlessness, muscle twitching, abdominal pains and fainting. *Precautions:* Glyceryl trinitrate should not be used in patients sensitive to nitrates, who have narrowed aortic or mitral valves of the heart (aortic stenosis, mitral stenosis) or certain other heart disorders, in patients with anaemia, head injury, brain haemorrhage or closed-angle glaucoma. It should be used with caution if blood pressure is low (do not use intravenously), in patients with severe impairment of kidney or liver function, underworking of the thyroid gland, malnutrition or recent heart attack. *Tolerance* to its effects can occur. See p. 113.

glycine ➤ aminoacetic acid.

glycol salicylate (in Cremalgin, in Dubam, in Salonair) is related to aspirin and is used in rheumatic rubs ➤ rubefacients.

glycopyrronium (glycopyrronium bromide) is an antimuscarinic (➤ antimuscarinic drugs). It is used as a pre-medication injection (Robinul) before surgery to dry up secretions in the air passages which are increased when a breathing tube is passed down into the lungs and when general anaesthetics are inhaled. It is also combined with neostigmine in Robinul Neostigmine to reverse the effects of nondepolarizing neuromuscular blockers. See Chapter 9.

Glypressin ➤ terlipressin.

Glytrin mouth spray ➤ glyceryl trinitrate.

GM-CSF ➤ molgramostin.

GnRH ➤ gonadorelin.

gold (sodium aurothiomalate, sodium aurothiosuccinate, Myocrisin injections) is a compound of gold used to treat rheumatoid arthritis. See Chapter 32. It is given in a water solution by deep intramuscular injection. It is slowly absorbed, stored in the body and slowly excreted in the urine. It is not known how it works. *Adverse effects:* Severe reactions occur in about 5% of patients. *Adverse effects* include mouth ulcers, liver damage with jaundice, hair loss, skin rashes, itching, blood disorders, kidney damage, lung damage, inflammation of the bowel (colitis), sensitivity of the skin to sunlight and occasionally inflammation of the brain or nerves may occur. An injection may set off an attack of acute rheumatoid arthritis. *Precautions:* Gold should not be given to patients with severely impaired kidney or liver function, to patients with blood disorders, severe lung disorders (pulmonary fibrosis), severe colitis, or to patients with skin disorders. It should not be given in pregnancy or to breastfeeding mothers, to patients who have recently been exposed to radiation or who have porphyria (a hereditary disorder of metabolism). It should be used with caution in the elderly and in patients with colitis, eczema or allergic skin rashes (e.g. nettle-rash). Before each injection patients should be carefully examined, particularly for sore mouths, fever, weakness, bleeding disorders, sore throats and skin rashes. The urine should be examined and repeated blood tests should be carried out. Patients should report any untoward symptoms such as fever, weakness, itching, metallic taste, bruising, heavy periods, sore throat, sore mouth, itching skin rash or diarrhoea as soon as they occur. The injection must be given deep into a muscle and the area gently massaged. *Interactions:* Penicillamine, phenylbutazone. For oral gold ➤ **auranofin.**

Golden Eye drops contain propamidine isethionate ➤ propamidine and **ointment** contains dibromopropamidine isethionate ➤ dibromopropamidine.

gonadorelin (GnRH, LH-RH, HRF) is gonadotrophin-releasing hormone. It stimulates the pituitary gland to secrete LH and FSH (see Chapter 40). When injected intravenously it leads to a rapid rise in plasma-luteinizing hormone (LH) and follicle-stimulating hormone (FSH) concentrations. It is used to treat absence of periods and to treat certain types of infertility, particularly in females. *Adverse effects* include nausea, headaches, abdominal pain and increased menstrual bleeding. Allergic reactions may rarely occur after repeated injections. Pain at the injection site may occur. *Precautions:* Do not use in patients with cysts of the womb or polycystic disease of the ovaries. Do not use to treat loss of periods due to loss of weight (e.g. anorexia nervosa) before weight is put back on (because periods should return without drug treatment). Stop if conception occurs or after six months of treatment. It is also used to assess the function of the pituitary gland.

gonadotrophin is the name of any of several hormones that are produced by the pituitary gland. In women they stimulate the ovaries to produce eggs and female sex hormones (see Chapter 40) and in men they stimulate the testes to produce sperm and male sex hormones (see Chapter 38). The two principal gonadotrophins are FSH (follicle stimulating hormone) and LH (luteinizing hormone). During pregnancy the placenta produces large amounts of chorionic gonadotrophin which has the actions of LH. Its presence in the urine of pregnant women can be used as a test for pregnancy. Post-menopausal women also produce increased amounts of gonadotrophins and they are extracted from their urine. They include human menopausal gonadotrophins (contains FSH and LH) and urofollitrophin (contains FSH). Bioengineered preparations of human FSH (follitropin alpha and follitropin beta) are also available. FSH and LH together (in human menopausal gonadotrophin) or FSH alone (follitropin alpha, follitropin beta, urofollitrophin) are used to treat infertility in women due to underworking of the pituitary gland or who have not responded to clomiphene (➤ clomiphene). They are also used to stimulate egg production in women undergoing IVF treatment for infertility. They may also be used in men (with underworking of their pituitary gland) to stimulate sperm production. Chorionic gonadotrophin has also been used in delayed puberty in the male but it is more beneficial to use the male sex hormone testosterone. Gonadotrophins include *chorionic gonadotrophin* (human chorionic gonadotrophin, HCG, Gonadotrophon LH, Pregnyl, Profasi); *human menopausal gonadotrophins* (Humegon, Normegon, Pergonal); *urofollitrophin* (Metrodin High Purity, Orgafol); and *follitropin alpha* (*Gonal-F*) and *follitropin beta* (Puregon).

gonadotraphin-releasing hormone ➤ gonadorelin.

Gonal-F ➤ follitropin alpha.

Gopten ➤ trandolapril.

goserelin (Zoladex) mimics the action of the gonadotrophin releasing hormone which stimulates the pituitary gland to release luteinizing hormone (LH). *In men* it stimulates the testes to produce the male sex hormone, testosterone. After initial stimulation it leads to a reduction in testosterone production by the testes equivalent to castration. It is used to treat cancers of the prostate gland which are dependent on testosterone for growth. *In women* treatment with goserelin switches off the production of female sex hormones by the ovaries which is of benefit to women suffering from endometriosis or advanced cancer of the breast in pre-menopausal and peri-menopausal women. It is also used to thin the lining of the womb before a scrape. *Adverse effects in women* include breakthrough bleeding, menopausal-type symptoms such as hot flushes, palpitations, increased sweating, vaginal dryness and changes in libido. It may cause headache, nausea, mood changes, breast swelling and tenderness, abdominal pain, fatigue, weight changes, dizziness, drowsiness, nervousness, acne, backache, muscle pains, ovarian cysts, reduced bone density, allergic rashes, itching, white vaginal discharge, blurred vision, changes in body hair and a rise in blood calcium levels in women being treated for breast cancer. *Adverse effects in men* treated for prostate cancer include an increase in bone pain from secondaries (due to the initial rise in testosterone), hot flushes, decreased libido, depression, headache, nausea, vomiting, dizziness, swelling of the breasts and allergic skin rashes. *Precautions in women:* Do not use in breastfeeding mothers or in pregnancy. While on treatment use nonhormonal method of contraception. Do not use in women with undiagnosed vaginal bleeding. Use with caution to treat endometriosis in women at risk of developing osteoporosis. *Precautions in men:* There is a risk of calcium stones blocking the outlet from the kidneys (ureters) and compression of the spinal cord – monitor carefully for the first four weeks whilst testosterone levels are high. May have to use an anti-androgen drug.

gramicidin is an antibiotic used in skin, ear and eye applications. It is too toxic to be given by mouth or injection. It is included in Adcortyl with Graneodin, in Graneodin, Neosporin, Sofradex, Soframycin, Tri-Adcortyl and Tri-Adcortyl-Otic.

Graneodin applications contain the aminoglycosides neomycin and gramicidin. They are used to treat infections of the skin. *Adverse effects* include allergic reactions, damage to the kidneys and to hearing. *Precautions:* Do not use as dressings or apply to large areas of damaged skin and do not use in the ear in patients with a perforated ear drum. Do not use to treat viral or fungal infections of the skin or to treat deep-seated infections.

granisetron (Kytril) is a 5HT blocker used to prevent and treat nausea and vomiting caused by anti-cancer drugs and post-operative nausea and vomiting. See Chapter 18. *Adverse effects* include skin rashes, headache, constipation and changes in liver function tests. *Precautions:* Do not use in breastfeeding mothers. Use with caution in pregnancy and in patients with partial obstruction of the intestine.

Granocyte ➤ lenograstim.

granulocyte-colony stimulating factor (rhG-CSF) stimulates the production of granulocytes (white blood cells) and may reduce the duration of a fall in neutrophil production by the bone marrow, in patients undergoing chemotherapy. Since neutrophils fight infection this is important in reducing the risks from infection in these patients. Preparations include filgrastim and lenograstim. Malgramostim is a recombinant granulocyte macrophage-colony stimulating factor which stimulates production of all granulocytes and monocytes.

granulocyte macrophage-colony stimulating factor ➤ granulocyte-colony stimulating factor.

Gregoderm ointment contains hydrocortisone (a corticosteroid), the aminoglycoside antibiotics neomycin and polymixin B and nystatin (an antifungal drug). It is used to treat infected and inflamed skin disorders. *Adverse effects and Precautions* see corticosteroid skin applications p. 241 and ➤ aminoglycoside antibiotics, nystatin.

griseofulvin (Grisovin) is an antifungal antibiotic (see Chapter 47) used to treat fungus infections of the nails, hair and skin. *Adverse effects* include drowsiness, headaches, allergic reactions, blood disorders, skin sensitivity to sunlight, depression, nausea, vomiting, confusion, dizziness and fatigue. May aggravate or trigger systemic lupus erythematosis (SLE – a disease of unknown cause with symptoms of fever, muscle and joint pain, blood disorders and skin eruptions). *Precautions:* Griseofulvin should not be used in patients suffering from porphyria (a hereditary disorder of metabolism) or severe liver disease. It should not be used in pregnancy. Men should not father a child during and within six months of stopping treatment. It may impair the ability to drive. *Interactions:* Alcohol, coumarin anticoagulants, barbiturates, oral contraceptives.

Grisovin ➤ griseofulvin.

ground nut oil ➤ arachis oil.

growth hormone is a hormone produced by the pituitary gland that stimulates and controls growth of tissues and various metabolic processes in the body. Somatropin is a synthetic human growth hormone produced by DNA bio-technology. It is identical to natural growth hormone. It is used to produce growth in children who are not producing sufficient of their own growth hormone to enable them to grow naturally. It is also used to treat patients with Turner's Syndrome and to treat growth disturbances in pre-pubertal children with chronic impairment of kidney function and as replacement therapy in adults with evidence of growth hormone deficiency. Preparations include Genotropin, Humatrope, Norditropin and Saizen. *Adverse effects:* Injections may cause pain and damage the fat under the skin, causing dents (lipoatrophy). Fluid retention may occur (e.g. swelling of the ankles) and the thyroid gland may become under-active. It may cause headache, raised blood sugar, sugar in the urine, muscle pain and weakness. *Precautions:* Do not use once bone growth has stopped, in patients with an active tumour, in pregnancy or in breast-feeding mothers. Use with caution in patients with diabetes or adrenocorticotropic hormone (ACTH) deficiency. Thy-

roid function tests should be carried out at regular intervals.

GTN 300 mcg aerosol ·spray ➤ glyceryl trinitrate.

guaifenesin reduces the stickiness of sputum and is used as a cough expectorant. See Chapter 11.

guanethidine (guanethidine sulphate, Ismelin) is an adrenergic neurone blocker used to treat raised blood pressure. See Chapter 25. *Adverse effects:* The commonest adverse effects at the start of treatment with guanethidine are diarrhoea and a drop in blood pressure on standing up after sitting or lying down (postural hypotension). This produces dizziness, faintness, weakness and weariness (particularly in the mornings). These decrease in severity as treatment is continued. Other adverse effects include slowing of the heart rate, breathlessness and oedema (often recognized because the ankles swell). Nausea, vomiting, pain in the cheeks (parotid glands), stuffy nose, dry mouth, drowsiness, blurred vision, muscle pains, trembling, dermatitis, failure to ejaculate, frequency in passing urine, depression of mood, blood disorders, parkinsonism and SLE-like effects. *Precautions:* Guanethidine should be used with caution in pregnancy and in patients with defective blood supply to the brain or heart (e.g. arteriosclerosis), impaired kidney function, peptic ulcers or during general anaesthesia. It should not be used in patients with phaeochromocytoma (a tumour of the sympathetic nervous system), kidney or heart failure, porphyria (a hereditary disorder of metabolism), active liver disease or a history of depression. Drowsiness may affect ability to drive. *Interactions:* MAOIs, anti-arrhythmic drugs, digitalis, anti-blood pressure drugs, tricyclic antidepressants, antipsychotic drugs, oral contraceptives, sympathomimetics, anti-diabetic drugs. Guanethidine is used in Ganda eye drops to treat glaucoma, see p. 64 and ➤ Ganda.

Guarem ➤ guar gum.

guar gum (Guarem) is used as a thickening agent in medicines. Also as an additional treatment in patients with diabetes in order to reduce the rise in blood sugar level that occurs after meals. It may slow down the absorption of carbohydrates. It is also used to relieve dumping syndrome (full stomach, nausea, weakness, sweating, palpitations and diarrhoea after a meal) and as a bulking agent to help slimming diets. *Adverse effects* include wind and distension of the abdomen. *Precautions:* Do not use in patients with obstructive disease of the oesophagus, stomach or intestine. Diabetic patients should have their blood sugar levels monitored during initial treatment and their antidiabetic treatment may need to be changed. Guar gum should be taken with a large drink of water and not just before going to bed.

GyneFix is a contraceptive intrauterine device containing copper.

Gyno-Daktarin preparations ➤ miconazole.

Gynol II is a spermicidal contraceptive gel containing nonoxinol 9.

Gyno-Pevaryl preparations ➤ econazole.

H₂ receptor blockers, see Chapter 19.

Haelan preparations ➤ fludroxycortide (flurandrenolone).

Haemaccel infusion contains polygeline (a modified form of gelatin) ➤ gelatin. It is used to restore blood volume after haemorrhage.

haem arginate (Normosang) is used to treat acute liver porphyria (a hereditary disorder of metabolism). *Adverse effects* include thrombophlebitis (inflammation in a vein), fever, allergic reactions. *Precautions:* Use with caution in pregnancy or while breastfeeding.

haemostatics stop bleeding, see p. 145.

HAES-steril intravenous infusion contains hetastarch in sodium chloride solution ➤ hetastarch.

Halciderm preparations ➤ halcinonide.

halcinonide (Halciderm cream) is a very potent corticosteroid used to treat eczema and psoriasis. *Adverse effects and Precautions* see corticosteroid skin applications p. 241. Do not dilute. Monitor patients with psoriasis to ensure cream is effective.

Haldol ➤ haloperidol.

Haldol Decanoate oily injection ➤ haloperidol.

Half Beta-Prograne ➤ propranolol.

Half-Inderal LA capsules ➤ propranolol.

Half-Securon SR ➤ verapamil.

Half-Sinemet CR ➤ co-careldopa.

halibut liver oil is a rich source of fish oils and vitamins A and D.

haloperidol (Dozic, Haldol, Serenace) is used for schizophrenia, psychosis, mania, hypomania, behavioural disorders, dangerously impulsive behaviour, intractable hiccup, agitation in the elderly, severe tics. See Chapter 3. *Adverse effects* include lack of muscle tone, loss of perception of movement, parkinsonism-like syndrome, slowness of movement, dry mouth, nasal stuffiness, difficulty in urination, rapid heart beat, constipation, blurring of vision, low blood pressure, weight gain, impotence, excessive or spontaneous flow of milk, low body temperature, development of breasts in males. *Precautions:* Do not use in patients in comatose states, with depression, Parkinson's disease, lesions of the basal ganglia. Use with caution in patients with liver or kidney failure, epilepsy, disturbed thyroid function, phaeochromocytoma (a tumour of the sympathetic nervous system), severe heart disease, potassium deficiency in the blood, abnormal ECG, in pregnancy or while breastfeeding.

halothane is a general anaesthetic which may cause liver damage.

Harmogen ➤ estrone.

Hartmann's solution is a compound

sodium lactate intravenous infusion ➤ sodium lactate.

Harvix is a hepatitis A vaccine.

Hay-Crom hayfever eye drops ➤ sodium cromoglicate.

Haymine tablets contain chlorphenamine(chlorpheniramine) (an antihistamine) and ephedrine (a sympathomimetic used as a decongestant). They are used to treat hayfever and allergic disorders (see Chapter 17). *Adverse effects* include drowsiness and dizziness. *Precautions:* Do not use in patients with blood clot in the heart, raised blood pressure, overworking of the thyroid gland. *Interactions:* Alcohol, sleeping drugs, sedatives, MAOIs. They may impair ability to drive. *For other Adverse effects and Precautions* ➤ antihistamines, ephedrine.

HB-Vax II is a hepatitis B vaccine.

Hc45 cream ➤ hydrocortisone.

HCG ➤ chorionic gonadotrophin.

Healonid ➤ sodium hyaluronate.

Hedex ➤ paracetamol.

Hedex Extra ➤ paracetamol, caffeine.

Hedex Ibuprofen ➤ ibuprofen.

Heliclear is used to eradicate *helicobacter pylori* in patients with duodenal ulcer. It contains amoxicillin, clarithromycin and lansoprazole ➤ individual entry for each drug.

Helimet is used to eradicate *helicobacter pylori* in patients with duodenal ulcer who are allergic to penicillin. It contains clarithromycin, lansoprazole and metronidazole ➤ individual entry for each drug.

Hemabate ➤ carboprost.

Heminevrin ➤ clomethiazole.

Hemocane is a soothing haemorrhoidal preparation containing benzoic acid, bisthmus oxide, cinnamic acid, lidocaine (lignocaine) and zinc oxide ➤ individual entry for each drug.

Hemofil-M ➤ factor VIII fraction.

Hemohes ➤ pentastarch.

heparin prevents the blood from clotting. See Chapter 28. It is ineffective by mouth and must be given by injection. *Adverse effects:* The main adverse effect is bleeding – from any site. Rarely, fever and allergic reactions may occur. Nosebleeds, red blood cells in the urine and bruising are the signs of overdosage. Temporary loss of hair, damage to the skin (necrosis) and diarrhoea may occur. Osteoporosis may occur after prolonged use. Heparin may cause a fall in blood platelets (thrombocytopenia) producing bleeding into the skin and lining of the mouth, etc. *Precautions:* It should not be used in patients with bleeding disorders (e.g. haemophilia), peptic ulcers, allergy to heparin, recent brain haemorrhage, severely raised blood pressure, severe kidney or liver disease, or after recent surgery on the eye or nervous system. Blood platelet counts should be carried out at regular intervals on patients receiving heparin for longer than five days and treatment should be stopped immediately if there is a fall in blood platelets.

heparinoid is a derivative of heparin. It has anti-inflammatory and anti-clotting actions and reduces the amount of exudate. It is used in Hirudoid and Lasonil applications to relieve bruises, sprains, soft-tissue injuries, and bruising around varicose veins. It should not be used on open wounds or on mucous membranes, e.g. the lining of the mouth or vagina. It is also used in Anacal cream to treat haemorrhoids.

Hepatyrix is a hepatitis A vaccine.

Hep-flush contains heparin. It is used for cleaning out and removing blood clots from injection tubes. It is not for administration to humans.

Heplok contains heparin. It is used for cleaning out and removing blood clots from injection tubes. It is not for administration to humans.

Hepsal contains heparin. It is used for cleaning out and removing blood clots from injection tubes. It is not for administration to humans.

Herceptin ➤ trastuzumab.

heroin ➤ diamorphine.

Herpetad ➤ aciclovir.

Herpid solution is a skin application that contains the antiviral drug idoxuridine in dimethyl sulfoxide. It is used to treat shingles (herpes zoster) and herpes simplex infections (e.g. cold sores), see Chapter 48. *Adverse effects and Precautions* ➤ idoxuridine, dimethyl sulfoxide. Do not use in pregnancy or in breastfeeding mothers.

Hespan ➤ hetastarch.

hetastarch ➤ etherified starch.

Hetrazan ➤ diethylcarbamazine.

Hewletts Cream contains zinc oxide and hydrous wool fat. It is used as a moisturising cream to treat dry, chapped hands ➤ zinc oxide, hydrous wool fat.

hexachlorophane ➤ hexachlorophene.

hexachlorophene (Ster-Zac DC, Ster-Zac Powder) is an antiseptic and disinfectant, see p. 244. *Adverse effects:* Sufficient may be absorbed through damaged skin or burns to cause stimulation of the brain, leading to convulsions. It may also be absorbed through the skin of newborn babies and damage the brain. It may cause allergic reactions on the skin and also sensitize the skin to the sun's rays. *Precautions:* It should not be used on large areas of skin, on damaged or burnt skin, in the mouth, in the vagina, or under non-permeable dressings. It should not be used in pregnancy or in children under two years of age. Blood reduces its effectiveness. Preparations of hexochlorophane may become infected with gram-negative bacteria.

Hexalen ➤ altretamine.

hexamine ➤ methenamine.

Hexastarch ➤ etherified starch.

hexetidine has an antiseptic action and is used in Oraldene solution as a mouthwash and gargle. It may cause stinging.

Hexopal ➤ inositol.

hexyl nicotinate (in Transvasin) is a heat rub ➤ rubefacients.

hexylresorcinol is an antiseptic which is used for the treatment of minor infections of the skin and mucous membranes, in particular the throat.

HFAs ➤ hydrofluoroalkanes.

HGH ➤ somatotrophin.

Hibicet Hospital Concentrate solution contains the antiseptics chlorhexidine and cetrimide ➤ chlorhexidine, cetrimide.

Hibiscrub cleansing solution ➤ chlorhexidine.

Hibisol solution ➤ chlorhexidine.

Hibitane preparations ➤ chlorhexidine.

HibTITER is a haemophilus influenzae type b vaccine.

Hill's Balsam Adult Expectorant is a cough preparation ➤ ipecacuanha, pholcodeine.

Hill's Balsam Cough Suppressant is a cough preparation ➤ pholcodeine.

Hioxyl cream ➤ hydrogen peroxide.

Hiprex ➤ hexamine hippurate.

Hirudoid preparations ➤ heparinoid.

Histalix cough medicine contains diphenhydramine (an antihistamine), ammonium chloride (an expectorant) and menthol ➤ individual entry for each drug and see Chapter 11.

histamine, see Chapter 27.

Histamine H₁-blockers ➤ antihistamines.

Histamine H₂-blockers, see H_2 receptor blockers in Chapter 19.

Histaocryl ➤ enbucrilate.

Hivid ➤ zalcitabine.

HNIG, see normal immunoglobulins p. 302.

homatropine (homatropine hydrobromide, Minims homatropine) is an antimuscarinic drug. See Chapter 9. It is used to dilate the pupils (see p. 61). Its effects last up to twenty-four hours. *Adverse effects and Precautions:* Do not use in patients with closed-angle glaucoma or in patients who are allergic to atropine. For general adverse effects and precautions of antimuscarinic drugs ➤ antimuscarinic drugs.

Hometrophine eye drops ➤ homatropine.

Honvan ➤ fosfestrol.

hormone blockers, see anti-androgens, p. 189, and anti-oestrogens, p. 198.

hormone replacement therapy (HRT) ➤ HRT.

Hormonin tablets contain the natural oestrogens estradiol, estriol and estrone ➤ HRT.

HRF ➤ gonadorelin.

HRT (hormone replacement therapy) is discussed on p. 199. *Adverse effects of combined oestrogen/progestogen HRT* include nausea and vomiting, changes in weight, enlargement and tenderness of the breasts, premenstrual-like syndrome, fluid retention, breakthrough bleeding, depression, headache, rashes, brown patches on the skin of the face, jaundice, impaired liver function and headache on exercise. Skin patches may cause itching and redness. *Precautions:* Do not use in pregnancy or in breastfeeding mothers, or in women with cancer of the breast, genital tract or any other cancer that depends on oestrogens for growth. Do not use in women with endometriosis, undiagnosed vaginal bleeding, blood clots or severe heart, liver or kidney disease. Use with caution in women with a history of blood clots, mild liver disease (monitor liver function every eight to twelve weeks). The following women should be carefully monitored –

those suffering from gallstones, otosclerosis (development of extra bone in the ear causing progressive deafness), migraine, epilepsy, multiple sclerosis, diabetes, raised blood pressure, porphyria (a hereditary disorder of metabolism), fibroids or tetany (spasms or cramps due to disturbed blood chemistry). Check-ups before starting HRT and at regular intervals during treatment should include pelvic examination, blood pressure recording and breast examination. The latter is of particular importance in women with fibrocystic disease of the breasts and/or a family history of breast cancer. There is an increased risk of cancer of the womb from the oestrogen in HRT but this is countered by taking a progestogen as well. See p. 199. There is also a slight possibility that the risk of breast cancer is increased. *Interactions:* See under oestrogens and progestogens. *Adverse effects and Precautions* of oestrogen-only HRT ➤ oestrogens.

HT Defix ➤ factor IX.

Humaject is an insulin preparation. See Chapter 42.

Humaject-M is an insulin preparation. See Chapter 42.

Humalog is an insulin preparation. See Chapter 42.

Human Actrapid is an insulin preparation. See Chapter 42.

human chorionic gonadotrophin (HCG) ➤ chorionic gonadotrophin.

human growth hormone ➤ growth hormone.

Human Insulatard is an insulin preparation. See Chapter 42.

human insulins, see Chapter 42 on insulins.

Human menopausal gonadotrophins (Humegon, Pergonal) are purified extracts from the urine of post-menopausal women. They contain follicle-stimulating hormone (FSH) and luteinizing hormone (LH). They are used to treat women suffering from anovulatory infertility due to underworking of their pituitary gland or who have not responded to clomiphene. They are also used to stimulate the ovaries to produce ova in women undergoing *in vitro* fertilization (IVF). *Adverse effects* include overstimulation of the ovaries (ovarian hyperstimulation), multiple pregnancies, allergic reactions, and pain at the site of injection. *Precautions:* Use with caution in women with ovarian cysts, adrenal or thyroid disorders, high blood levels of prolactin due to a prolactin-producing tumour of the pituitary gland, or women with a tumour of the pituitary gland. For description of ovarian hyperstimulation syndrome ➤ Humegon.

Human Mixtard is an insulin preparation. See Chapter 42.

Human Monotard is an insulin preparation. See Chapter 42.

Human Normal Immunoglobulin is an insulin preparation. See Chapter 42.

Human Ultratard is an insulin preparation. See Chapter 42.

Human Velosulin is an insulin preparation. See Chapter 42.

HumaPen is an insulin preparation. See Chapter 42.

Humatrope is a growth hormone ➤ somatropin.

Humulin I is an insulin preparation. See Chapter 42.

Humulin I Pen is an insulin preparation. See Chapter 42.

Humulin Lente is an insulin preparation. See Chapter 42.

Humulin M is an insulin preparation. See Chapter 42.

Humulin S is an insulin preparation. See Chapter 42.

Humulin Zn is an insulin preparation. See Chapter 42.

Hyalase injection ➤ hyaluronidase.

hyaluronidase (Hyalase) is an enzyme from mammals' semen which makes tissues more permeable. It is used to increase the spread and absorption of drugs from injections, e.g. local anaesthetics and subcutaneous injections. It is also used in Lasonil ointment to help the resorption of fluid and blood under the skin, e.g. a swollen bruise. *Adverse effects:* It may rarely produce a severe allergic reaction. *Precautions:* Do not apply directly to the cornea or to infected cancerous lesions. Do not use to treat insect bites or stings. Do not use intravenously. Use with caution in infants and the elderly – control speed and volume used (especially if patient has impaired kidney function).

Hyate-C is a porcine preparation of anti-haemophilic factor for individuals who develop inhibitors to human factor VIII which is used to control bleeding in patients suffering from haemophilia A.

Hycamtin ➤ topotecan.

Hydergine tablets ➤ co-dergocrine.

hydralazine (hydralazine hydrochloride, Apresoline) is a vasodilator used to treat raised blood pressure, see Chapter 25, and heart failure, see Chapter 23. *Adverse effects* include nausea, vomiting, headache, a fall in blood pressure on standing, rapid beating of the heart, flushing, fluid retention, sweating, breathlessness, skin rashes, difficulty in passing water and depressed mood. These usually occur in the first few weeks of treatment. Very rarely it may cause kidney damage, blood disorders and nerve damage (e.g. pins and needles in the arms and legs). Prolonged use of high doses may, rarely, cause skin disorders. *Precautions:* It should not be used in patients with rapid beating of the heart or narrowing of the aortic or mitral valves, or in the first half of pregnancy. It should be used with caution in patients with diseases of the arteries in the brain or heart, severe kidney failure, impaired liver function, or in breastfeeding mothers. *Interactions:* Tricyclic antidepressants, MAOIs, sleeping drugs, sedatives, anaesthetics, anti-blood pressure drugs, diazoxide.

Hydrea ➤ hydroxycarbonide (hydroxyurea).

Hydrex is an antiseptic ➤ chlorhexidine.

hydrochlorothiazide is a thiazide diuretic ➤ thiazide diuretics.

hydrocortisone is a corticosteroid that is included in many skin preparations. See Chapter 37 on corticosteroids and corticosteroid skin applications, p. 241.

hydrocortisone acetate (cortisol acetate) is used in eye drops, creams and ointments. It may also be injected into painful joints, ligaments and muscles ➤ hydrocortisone.

hydrocortisone-17-butyrate is a potent form of hydrocortisone used in skin preparations (Locoid) to treat severely inflamed skin disorders such as eczemas that have not responded to less potent corticosteroids. See Chapter 37 on corticosteroids and corticosteroid skin applications p. 241.

Hydrocortisone sodium phosphate (Efcortesol) ➤ hydrocortisone.

Hydrocortisone sodium succinate (Efcortelan soluble; Solu-Cortef) is used in hydrocortisone preparations for injection and in lozenges (Corlan) in the treatment of mouth ulcers ➤ hydrocortisone.

Hydrocortistab preparations ➤ hydrocortisone acetate.

Hydrocortone ➤ hydrocortisone.

hydrofluoroalkanes ➤ chlorofluorocarbons (CFCs).

hydrogen peroxide is used as an antiseptic and deodorant, to clean wounds, as a mouthwash and to remove ear wax. Avoid contact with normal skin and use with utmost caution on large or deep wounds. It may bleach fabrics. It is present in Hioxyl cream for cleaning leg ulcers and pressure sores, in Exterol and Otex ear drops to remove wax and in hydrogen peroxide mouthwash (Peroxyl).

Hydromol skin moisturising cream contains arachis (peanut) oil, isopropyl myristate, liquid paraffin, sodium pyrrolidone carboxylate and sodium lactate ➤ arachis oil, isopropyl myristate, liquid paraffin, sodium lactate.

hydromorphine (Palladone) is used for relief of severe pain in cancer. See Chapter 30. *Adverse effects* include constipation, nausea, vomiting, drowsiness. *Precautions:* Do not use in patients with respiratory depression, coma, paralysis of the small intestine, liver damage, raised pressure in the brain or convulsions.

hydrotalcite (Altacite, in Altacite Plus) is a magnesium and aluminium compound used as an antacid. It may very rarely produce diarrhoea and vomiting ➤ antacids.

hydroxocobalamin (vitamin B_{12}, Cobalin-H, Neo-Cytamen) is used to treat pernicious anaemia and other B_{12} deficient anaemias. It may very rarely cause allergic reactions. See Chapter 36.

hydroxyapatite (Ossopan) is used to provide calcium and phosphorous in the treatment of osteoporosis, rickets and during breastfeeding. *Precautions:* It should not be used in patients with a raised level of calcium in their blood or urine. It should be used with caution in patients with a history of kidney stones, impaired kidney function or if the patient is very immobilized.

hydroxycarbamide(hydroxyurea) (Hydrea) is an anti-cancer drug. See Chapter 51. It is used mainly to treat chronic myeloid leukaemia. *Adverse effects:* It may damage the bone marrow, producing blood disorders. Rarely, it may cause nausea, vomiting, skin rashes, loss of hair, abdominal pain, diarrhoea, blood in the motions and kidney damage. *Precautions:* It should not be used in pregnancy or in patients with severe blood disorders.

hydroxychloroquine (hydroxychloroquine sulphate, Plaquenil) is an antimalarial drug. It has effects and uses similar to those described under chloroquine. It is also used in high doses to treat rheumatoid arthritis (see Chapter 32), certain skin disorders and skin disorders made worse by exposure to the sun's rays. *Adverse effects and Precautions:* These are similar to those listed under chloroquine.

hydroxyethylcellulose (in Minims Artificial Tears) has similar properties to methylcellulose ➤ methylcellulose.

hydroxycholecalciferol ➤ alfacalcidol.

hydroxyprogesterone (hydroxyprogesterone caproate) is a progestogen given by intramuscular depot injection (Proluton Depot) to treat recurrent miscarriages. *Adverse effects and Precautions* ➤ progestogens.

hydroxyquinolone (in Quinocort) is used as an antibacterial and antifungal in skin applications. It is also used for removing dead skin and as a deodorant.

hydroxyurea ➤ hydroxycarbamide.

hydroxyzine (hydroxyzine embonate, hydroxyzine hydrochloride, Atarax, Ucerax) is an antihistamine drug (see Chapter 17) used to treat anxiety (see Chapter 2). It is also used to treat generalized itching, see p. 84. *Adverse effects* include drowsiness, headache, dizziness, weakness, confusion and dry mouth. High doses may produce involuntary movements. *Precautions:* Do not use in pregnancy and use with caution if kidney function is impaired. *Interactions:* It increases the effects of alcohol and other depressant drugs. It may affect ability to drive motor vehicles or operate moving machinery.

Hygroton ➤ clorthalidone.

hyoscine is an antimuscarinic drug (see Chapter 9). Hyoscine butyl bromide is used to relieve spasm of the intestine and painful periods (Buscopan preparations). Hyoscine hydrobromide (scopolamine) was used as a pre-medication before surgery to dry up secretions in the airway (in Omnopon scopolamine). It is used to treat nausea, vertigo and travel sickness (Joy-Rides, Kwells, Sco-

poderm TTS), see Chapter 18. *Adverse effects and Precautions:* ➤ antimuscarinic drugs.

hyoscine butylbromide ➤ hyoscine.

hyoscine hydrobromide ➤ hyoscine.

Hypericum, see Chapter 4.

Hypnomidate ➤ etomidate.

hypnotics (sleeping drugs), see Chapter 1.

Hypnovel ➤ midazolam.

Hypolar Retard ➤ nifedipine.

Hypostop gel is a glucose preparation taken orally for the treatment of hypoglycaemia.

Hypotears drops used to treat dry eyes contain macrogalol '8000' and polyvinyl alcohol. Do not use with soft contact lenses ➤ polyvinyl alcohol, macrogalol.

Hypovase ➤ prazosin.

hypromellose has effects and uses similar to those produced by methylcellulose. It is mainly used as eye drops, for artificial tears, e.g. Isopto Alkaline, Isopto Naturale, in Tears Naturale.

Hypurin Isophane is an insulin preparation. See Chapter 42.

Hypurin Lente is an insulin preparation. See Chapter 42.

Hypurin Neutral is an insulin preparation. See Chapter 42.

Hypurin Protamine Zinc is an insulin preparation. See Chapter 42.

Hypurin 30/70 is an insulin preparation. See Chapter 42.

Hytrin ➤ terazosin.

Hytrin BPH ➤ terazosin. It is used to relax smooth muscle in enlarged prostate glands (benign prostate hypertrophy, BPH). This relaxation helps the flow of urine and provides relief from some of the symptoms of obstruction. *Adverse effects and Precautions* ➤ terazosin.

Ibrufhalal ➤ ibuprofen.

IBS relief ➤ mebeverine.

Ibuderm ➤ ibuprofen.

Ibufem ➤ ibuprofen.

Ibugel ➤ ibuprofen.

Ibuleve preparations ➤ ibuprofen.

Ibumousse ➤ ibuprofen.

ibuprofen (Arthrofen, Brufen, Brufen Retard, in Codafen Continus, Deep Relief, Fenbid, Galprofen, Ibrufhalal, Ibumed, Inoven, Lidifen, Motrin, Obifen, Pacifen, Rimafen. OTC preparations include Advil, Anadin Ibuprofen, Anadin Ultra, Cuprofen, Galprofen, Hedex Ibuprofen, Junifen, Librofem, Migrafen, Motrin, Novaprin, Nurofen, PhorPain, Proflex, Relcofen) is a nonsteroidal anti-inflammatory drug (NSAID) ➤ non-steroidal anti-inflammatory drugs. Antirheumatic preparations for use on the skin which contain ibuprofen include Deep Relief, Fenbid gel, Ibuderm, Ibugel, Ibuleve gel and mousse, Ibuleve Sports gel, Ibumousse, Ibuspray, Neurofen Muscular Pain Relief gel and Proflex.

Ibuspray ➤ ibuprofen.

Ibutop ➤ ibuprofen.

ichthammol is a reddish brown to black sticky liquid obtained from the distillation of bituminous shale. It is slightly antibacterial. It may irritate the skin and rarely produce an allergic reaction. It is used in creams, ointments and bandages, often with zinc oxide, to treat skin disorders, e.g. eczema.

idarubicin (Zavedos) is an anti-cancer drug related to daunorubicin. See Chapter 51. It is a cytotoxic antibiotic. *Adverse effects* include damage to the bone marrow (producing blood disorders), nausea, vomiting, diarrhoea, sore mouth and oesophagus, fever, chills and skin rashes. It may affect liver function, cause reversible hair loss and discoloration of the urine. Very rarely, the patient may develop very severe infections and damage to the heart. *Precautions:* It should not be used in individuals with severe impairment of liver or kidney function, or uncontrolled infections, or in women who are breastfeeding. It should be used with caution in people with impaired bone-marrow function, with heart disease or who have received similar drugs in high doses. Patients over fifty-five years of age will need special care during the period when the bone marrow is not working. Uric acid levels should be checked at intervals. Any infection should be treated before treatment starts. Leakage at the site of infection may cause inflammation of the vein. It may irritate the skin and should be handled with caution.

idoxuridine (in Herpid) is an antiviral drug that is used topically to treat herpes zoster infections (shingles) and herpes simplex infections (e.g. cold sores) of the skin. See Chapter 48. *Adverse effects and Precautions:* It should not be used in pregnancy and in breastfeeding mothers. Skin applications may cause stinging and should not be applied near the eyes or mouth. They may stain the clothing.

ifosfamide (Mitoxana) is an anti-cancer drug. See Chapter 51. *Adverse effects and Precautions* ➤ cyclophosphamide. Reduce dose in patients with impaired kidney function.

Ikorel ➤ nicorandil.

Ilube eye drops contain acetylcysteine and hypromellose. They are used to treat dry eyes ➤ acetylcysteine, hypromellose.

Imazin XL contain aspirin and isosorbide mononitrate ➤ aspirin, isosorbide mononitrate.

Imdur ➤ isosorbide mononitrate.

imidapril (Tanatril) is used to treat high blood pressure. See Chapter 25. *Adverse effects* include cough, dizziness, fatigue, stomach and bowel upset, angioedema (allergic swelling of the mouth and throat), severely low blood pressure, kidney failure, allergic reactions. *Precautions:* Do not use in patients with a history of angioedema due to previous ACE inhibitor therapy, heredity or from an unknown cause, high blood pressure, kidney failure with or without blood dialysis, pregnancy or while breastfeeding. Use with caution in patients with a risk of severe low blood pressure (through loss of blood or fluids, sodium deficiency in the blood or heart failure), kidney or liver damage, narrowing of the main artery from the heart (aortic stenosis), hypertrophic cardiomyopathy (enlargement of the muscles of the heart), psoriasis, in surgery, blood dialysis or apheresis (a certain form of blood donation) with high flux membranes.

imidazole antifungal drugs, see Chapter 47.

imiglucerase (Cerezym) is an enzyme administered as replacement therapy in Gaucher's disease which is a hereditary disorder affecting principally the liver, spleen, bone marrow and lymph nodes. *Adverse effects* include itching, pain, swelling or sterile abscesses at injection site, allergic reactions, nausea, vomiting, diarrhoea, abdominal pain, fatigue, headache, dizziness, fever, rash. *Precautions:* Do not use in pregnancy or while breastfeeding.

Imigran ➤ sumatriptan.

imipenem is a broad spectrum antibiotic. See Chapter 46. Because imipenem is partially inactivated by an enzyme in the kidney it is combined in Primaxin with cilastatin, which blocks that enzyme. *Adverse effects* include nausea, vomiting and diarrhoea (colitis may occur rarely), blood disorders and allergic reactions (itching, rash, nettle-rash, fever). Rarely, muscle twitching, convulsions, confusion and mental disturbances may occur with very high doses or in patients with impaired kidney function. It may produce pain, redness and swelling, and inflammation at the site of injection. It may produce changes in biochemical tests of liver and kidney function. It may make the urine red in children. *Precautions:* Do not use in patients who are allergic to imipenem or cilastatin. Use with caution in pregnancy, in breastfeeding mothers, in patients

known to be allergic to penicillins, cephalosporins or other beta-lactam antibiotics, in patients with impaired kidney function, epilepsy, disorders of the central nervous system, or colitis. *Interactions:* Probenecid, ganciclovir.

imipramine (imipramine hydrochloride, Tofranil) is a tricyclic antidepressant drug ➤ tricyclic antidepressants.

imiquimod (Aldara) is used to treat warts on the genitals and around the anus. See Chapter 45. *Adverse effects* include skin reactions where it is applied. *Precautions:* Uncircumcised men with warts under foreskin should wash area daily. Avoid open wounds, do not use non-permeable dressings. Use with caution in the elderly, in pregnancy or while breastfeeding.

Immukin injection ➤ interferon gamma.

Immune interferon, see Chapter 51.

Immunizations, see Chapter 53.

Immunoprin ➤ azathioprine.

immunosuppressants, see Chapter 17.

Imodium ➤ loperamide.

Imodium Plus contains loperamide and simethicone ➤ loperamide, simethicone.

Implanon ➤ etonogestrel.

Imuderm is a skin softening bath additive containing almond oil and light liquid paraffin. It is used to treat dry skin conditions including dermatitis, eczema, pruritis and ichthyosis.

Imunovir ➤ inosine pranobex.

Imuran ➤ azathioprine.

INAH (iso-nicotinic acid hydrazine) ➤ isoniazid.

indapamide (Natrilix, Nindaxa, Opumide, Natramid) is a thiazide-like diuretic (see Chapter 29) used to treat raised blood pressure (see Chapter 25). *Adverse effects* include headaches, dizziness, fatigue, loss of appetite, indigestion, nausea, diarrhoea, constipation, muscle cramps and fall in blood potassium levels. Rarely it may cause rashes (sometimes severe), fall in blood pressure on standing up after sitting or lying down, rise in blood sugar and blood uric acid levels, pins and needles, sensitivity of the skin to the sun's rays, impaired kidney function, impotence and reversible short-sightedness. *Precautions:* Do not use in patients who have had a recent stroke or who have severe impairment of liver function or who are breastfeeding. Use with caution in patients with impaired kidney function (stop if it gets worse), over-active parathyroid glands, gout or in pregnancy. Use with caution in the elderly and monitor blood chemistry. *Interactions:* Diuretics, anti-arrhythmic drugs, digoxin and related drugs, corticosteroids, laxatives, lithium.

Inderal ➤ propranolol.

Inderal-LA ➤ propranolol.

Inderetic capsules contain propranolol (a non-selective beta-blocker) and bendrofluazide (a thiazide diuretic). They are used to treat raised blood pressure (see Chapter 25). *Adverse effects and Precautions* ➤ beta-blockers, thiazide diuretics.

Inderex capsules contain propranolol (a non-selective beta-blocker) and bendrofluazide (a thiazide diuretic). They are used to treat raised blood pressure (see Chapter 25). *Adverse effects and Precautions* ➤ beta-blockers, thiazide diuretics.

Indermil ➤ enbucrilate.

indinavir (Crixivan) is an antiviral drug used to treat patients suffering from HIV infection. See Chapter 48. *Adverse effects* include stomach and bowel upsets, fatigue, dizziness, headache, weakness, insomnia, dry mouth, pins and needles, painful muscles, skin rashes, disturbances of taste, pain on passing urine, kidney stones and changes in blood chemistry. *Precautions:* Do not use in breastfeeding mothers. Use with caution in patients suffering from impaired liver function, haemophilia and in pregnancy. Use with caution in patients with

kidney stones and make sure they drink plenty of fluids. *Interactions:* Alprazolam, astemizole, methadone, phenobarbitone, phenytoin, rifabutin, rifampicin, terfenadine, triazolam.

Indivina is a hormone replacement therapy containing estradiol and medroxyprogesterone ➤ oestrogens.

Indocid ➤ indometacin.

Indocid PDA injection contains the NSAID indometacin. It blocks prostaglandins and is used to treat patent ductus arteriosus (PDA) (a condition in which the duct between the lung and the aorta in the foetus is still there after birth) in premature babies. *Adverse effects* include risk of bleeding (it affects blood platelets), impaired kidney function, disturbances of electrolytes in the blood, fluid retention and flare-up of infections. *Precautions:* Do not use in babies with untreated infections or bleeding into the brain, stomach or intestine. Do not use if baby has low platelet count (thrombocytopenia), blood-clotting defects, significant kidney impairment, necrotizing enterocolitis (inflammation of the bowel causing death of cells) or disorders where it is necessary to keep the ductus open. Risk of kidney failure is increased in babies with congestive heart failure, poisonous infections, impaired liver function or decreased body fluids. Carefully monitor kidney function and blood chemistry and monitor babies for bleeding and dehydration (which can increase risk of kidney failure). *Interactions:* Digoxin, frusemide, aminoglycosides. Also ➤ nonsteroidal anti-inflammatory drugs.

Indocid-R ➤ indometacin.

Indolar SR ➤ indometacin.

Indomax ➤ indometacin.

indometacin (Indocid, Indocid PDA, Indomax, Rimacid. *Modified release preparations:* Flexin Continus, Indocid-R, Indolar SR, Indomax 75 SR, Indomod, Pardelprin, Rheumacin LA Slo Indo) is a non-steroidal anti-inflammatory drug

(NSAID). See Chapter 32 and ➤ non-steroidal anti-inflammatory drugs. *Adverse effects* include loss of appetite, nausea, vomiting, indigestion and diarrhoea. Ulcers of the stomach or intestine with bleeding may occur. Blood disorders, skin rashes, itching, fluid retention, weight gain, raised blood pressure, loss of hair, drowsiness, tinnitus, headache, light-headedness, insomnia, confusion, depression, mental disturbances, nerve damage, allergic reactions (asthma, rashes and angioedema (allergic swellings of the mouth and throat)), hearing disturbances, blurred vision, deposits in the eye and fainting may rarely occur. *Precautions:* It should not be given to patients with active peptic ulcers, bleeding disorders of the stomach or intestine, allergy to aspirin or some other NSAID, in pregnancy or to breastfeeding mothers. It should be used with caution in patients with impaired kidney or liver function, epilepsy, parkinsonism, serious psychotic illness, and elderly people. Regular eye and blood tests should be carried out. It may impair ability to drive and operate moving machinery. Do not use rectal preparations if patient has haemorrhoids or inflammation of the anus or rectum. For *Adverse effects and Precautions of NSAIDs* ➤ nonsteroidal anti-inflammatory drugs. *Interactions:* Salicylates, anticoagulants, lithium, corticosteroids, diuretics, beta-blockers, probenecid, quinolones, other NSAIDs, anti-blood pressure drugs, aminoglycosides, methotrexate, cyclosporin, digoxin, phenylpropanolamine.

indomethacin ➤ indometacin.

Indomod ➤ indometacin.

indoramin is a selective alpha$_1$-blocker used as Baratol to treat raised blood pressure. See Chapter 25. It is also used as Doralese to relax smooth muscles in benign enlargement of the prostate gland in order to improve the passing of urine (see p. 284). *Adverse effects* include sedation, weakness, drowsiness, headache, palpitations, fall in blood pressure (especially on standing), rapid heart beat, dry mouth, nasal congestion, weight gain, dizziness, depression and failure to ejaculate. *Precautions:* Do not use in patients with heart failure. Drowsiness may occur in the first few days of treatment and patients should be warned not to drive motor vehicles or operate moving machinery. It should be used with caution in patients with impaired kidney or liver function or in patients with epilepsy, depression or parkinsonism. Impaired heart function should be treated with digoxin and a diuretic. *Interactions:* MAOIs, other anti-blood pressure drugs.

Infacol liquid ➤ activated dimethicone.

Infadrops is sugar-free concentrated solution of paracetamol (100 mg/ml) ➤ paracetamol.

Infanrix is a triple vaccine containing diptheria, tetanus and pertussis vaccine.

Infanrix-Hib is Infanrix vaccine, see above, with haemophilus influenzae vaccine added.

infliximab (Remicade) is used to treat severe active Crohn's disease (chronic diarrhoeal disorder) or fistulizing Crohn's disease in patients unresponsive to corticosteroid and/or immunosuppressant therapy. See Chapter 17. *Adverse effects* include viral infection, fever, headache, vertigo, dizziness, high blood pressure, flushing, urinary tract infections, upper or lower respiratory tract infection, difficulty breathing, sinusitis, stomach and bowel upset, skin reactions, fatigue, chest pain. *Precautions:* Do not use in patients with infections or abscesses, allergy to murine proteins, in pregnancy (ensure adequate contraception) or while breastfeeding within six months of dose. Use with caution in patients with liver or kidney damage, or in the elderly.

Influvac is influenza vaccine.

inhalations of warm, moist air may help to relieve cold and cough symptoms. They are usually made by adding menthol or eucalyptus oil to near-boiling water and inhaling the steam with a towel over the head. Boiling water should not be used because of the risk of scalding. An alternative is to squeeze the oil(s) on to a handkerchief and inhale the vapour (➤Karvol capsules). *Do not use vapour inhalations in children under three months of age.* Inhalation, using special devices, is a very effective way of treating asthma (see Chapter 14).

Innohep ➤ tinzaparin.

Innovace ➤ enalapril.

Innozide tablets contain the ACE inhibitor, enalapril, and the thiazide diuretic, hydrochlorothiazide. They are used to treat raised blood pressure. See Chapter 25. *Adverse effects and Precautions* ➤ enalapril, thiazide diuretics.

inosine pranobex (Imunovir) is used as an antiviral drug by mouth to treat herpes simplex infections and genital herpes. It is also used to treat a viral brain infection (subacute sclerosing panecephalitis). *Adverse effects:* It may cause a rise in uric acid levels in the blood and urine. *Precautions:* It should be used with caution in patients with impaired kidney function, gout or raised blood uric acid level. See Chapter 48.

inositol nicotinate (Hexopal) is a nicotinic acid derivative used to improve the circulation. See Chapter 27. *Adverse effects and Precautions* ➤ nicotinic acid.

inotropic drugs have a positive action in strengthening the muscular contractions of the heart, e.g. digoxin.

Inoven ➤ ibuprofen.

Instillagel (gel in a disposable syringe) contains the anaesthetic lidocaine(lignocaine) with the antiseptic chlorhexidine. Instillagel acts as a local anaesthetic and disinfectant lubricant and is used when passing a catheter or instrument through the urethra into the bladder. *Adverse effects and Precautions* ➤ lidocaine(lignocaine), chlorhexidine. Use with utmost caution if there is local bleeding.

insulins, see Chapter 42.

Insuman Basal is an insulin preparation, see Chapter 42.

Insuman Comb is an insulin preparation, see Chapter 42.

Insuman Rapid is an insulin preparation, see Chapter 42.

Intal preparations ➤ sodium cromoglicate.

Integrilin ➤ eptifibatide.

Integrin ➤ oxypertine.

Interferon alfa (Intron A, Roferon-A, Viraferon, Peginteron, ViraferonPeg) see Chapter 51.

Interferon beta (Avonex, Betaferon, Rebif), see Chapter 51.

interferon gamma-1b (immune interferon, Immukin) is an interferon, see p. 292. It is used with antibiotics to reduce the frequency of serious infections occurring in patients with chronic granulomatous disease which is an inherited disease that weakens the ability of white blood cells to kill invading bacteria. *Adverse effects* include nausea, vomiting, headache, fever, chills, muscle and joint pains, fatigue and rashes. *Precautions:* Use with utmost caution in patients with severe impairment of liver or kidney function or heart disease. Blood counts, urine tests, blood chemistry tests and liver and kidney function tests should be carried out at regular intervals. It may impair ability to drive or operate machinery. Adverse effects may be increased by alcohol.

Interferons, see Chapter 51.

interleukin-2 ➤ aldesleukin.

Intralgin preparations contain salicylamide (a rubefacient) and benzocaine (a local anaesthetic). They are used to relieve muscle aches and pains. *Adverse effects and Precautions* ➤ salicylamide, benzocaine.

Intron A ➤ interferon alpha-2b.

Invirase ➤ saquinavir.

Iocare eye irrigation solution contains salts

of sodium, calcium and potassium. It is used during eye surgery.

iodine and its salts (**iodides**) in various forms are used as disinfectants and antiseptics (see p. 244). They are also used to treat overworking of the thyroid gland (see Chapter 43) and in some cough medicines (see Chapter 11). *Adverse effects:* Iodine and iodides may cause the thyroid gland to underwork, producing goitre. This may also occur in infants born to mothers who took iodine or iodides during pregnancy. Iodine preparations can cause allergic reactions whether taken by mouth or applied to the skin. These reactions include nettle-rash (urticaria), angioedema (allergic swelling of the mouth and throat), fever, painful joints, swollen glands and a rise in white blood cells (oesinophils). Prolonged use can cause *iodism* – metallic taste in the mouth, increased salivation, burning sensation in the mouth, running nose, a swollen, sore throat and swelling and irritation of the eyes. An acne-like rash, fluid on the lungs (pulmonary oedema) and stomach and bowel upset may occur. *Precautions:* Do not use in patients with a history of allergy to iodine or iodides. Do not take regularly during pregnancy or when breastfeeding. Do not cover iodine or iodide skin applications with a non-permeable dressing. Iodine preparations may interfere with laboratory tests of thyroid function. The use of cough medicines that contain iodine or iodides should be limited, they should not be used in pregnancy and preferably not when breast feeding. They should not be used in adolescents because of the risk of acne and their effects on the thyroid gland and they should not be used in patients with goitre. Do not apply iodine or iodide-containing preparations to severe burns or large areas of the skin, they may cause iodine adverse effects (see above) and interfere with thyroid function.

iodine, radioactive, is used to treat overactive thyroids. See Chapter 43.

Iodoflex gauze dressing contains cadex-omer iodine. It is used to treat chronic leg ulcers ➤ cadexomer iodine.

Iodosorb powder ➤ cadexomer-iodine. It is used to treat chronic leg ulcers and bedsores.

Ionax Scrub is an abrasive gel that contains the antibacterial drug benzalkonium and abrasive polyethylene granules. It is used to treat acne (see p. 251) ➤ benzalkonium.

Ionil T shampoo application contains salicylic acid, benzalkonium and tar solution in an alcoholic base. It is used to treat psoriasis and excessive oily secretions on the scalp. Avoid contact with eyes. *Adverse effects and Precautions* ➤ coal tar, benzalkonium, salicylic acid.

Iopidine eye drops ➤ apraclonidine.

ipecacuanha (the dried roots of *Cephaelis ipecacuanha*) in very small doses is used as a cough expectorant. See Chapter 11. It is also used to produce vomiting after swallowing certain poisons. *Adverse effects:* Ipecacuanha has an irritant effect upon the stomach and intestine. Large doses produce vomiting and diarrhoea, and sometimes bleeding from the stomach or intestine. Regular misuse (e.g. to lose weight) may damage the heart muscle and kidneys and may cause death.

ipratropium (ipratropium bromide, Atrovent, Ipratropium Steri-Neb, in Combivent, in Duovent, Respartin) is an antimuscarinic drug used to treat bronchial asthma (see Chapter 14) and as Rinatec nose spray to treat perennial hayfever (see p. 88). *Adverse effects and Precautions* ➤ antimuscarinic drugs. To treat asthma, it is used by inhalation, which may cause dry mouth, difficulty in passing urine and constipation. It may rarely produce increased wheezing. To treat perennial hayfever it is used by nasal spray. It may cause dryness and irritation of the nose. It should be used with caution in patients with glaucoma or enlarged prostate glands.

irbesartan (Aprovel, in Co-Approvel) is used to treat high blood pressure. See

Chapter 25. *Adverse effects* include dizziness, musculoskeletal pain, flushing, allergic reactions. *Precautions:* Do not use in pregnancy or while breastfeeding. Use with caution in patients with high blood pressure, kidney or liver damage, heart failure, narrowing of the mitral valve or of the main artery (aorta) from the heart, obstructive hypertropic cardiomyopathy (enlargement of the heart due to muscle damage), blood dialysis.

irinotecan (Campto) is used in combination with 5-fluorouracil (5-FU) and folinic acid for the first-line treatment of advanced bowel cancer and treatment of secondary bowel cancer that has failed to respond to a therapy containing 5-fluorouracil (5-FU). See Chapter 51. *Adverse effects* include delayed diarrhoea, decrease in certain kinds of white blood cells, anaemia, decrease in number of platelets in the blood, liver damage, nausea, vomiting, acute cholinergic syndrome, weakness, hair loss, difficulty breathing, cramps, abnormal sensations such as tingling, burning or tightness. *Precautions:* Do not use in patients with chronic inflammatory bowel disease, bowel obstruction, liver or kidney damage, suppression of blood cell production, in pregnancy or while breastfeeding.

iron is an essential element in the body. It is discussed in Chapter 35. Iron preparations are used to treat and prevent iron deficiency anaemia, see Chapter 35. Preparations of iron salts are taken by mouth, usually as ferrous salts. Iron may also be given by intramuscular or intravenous injection. *Adverse effects:* Iron salts are astringent and they may irritate the stomach lining, producing nausea and pains in the stomach. They may also cause constipation and diarrhoea. These symptoms are related to the amount of elemental iron in the preparation. Iron salts may colour the stools black. Oral iron, particularly modified release preparations, may make diarrhoea worse in patients suffering from chronic inflammatory diarrhoeal disorders such as ulcerative colitis or Crohn's disease. *Precautions:* Iron preparations by mouth should not be used in patients with diverticulitis or obstruction of the bowel. Use with caution in patients with a delayed intestinal transit time due to some intestinal disorder. Because of the risk of constipation elderly patients should use them with caution – there is a risk of faecal blockage (impaction) of the bowel. The body can become overloaded with iron (haemosiderosis) if iron preparations are taken when they are not needed, particularly in patients who have disorders of iron storage or absorption from the intestine. Iron preparations should not be given to patients receiving repeated blood transfusions or to treat anaemias that are not due to iron deficiency. Do not use oral iron together with injections of iron. Liquid mixtures containing iron salts should be taken well diluted with water and through a straw to prevent blackening of the teeth. *Interactions:* Iron reduces the absorption of tetracyclines, ciprofloxacin, norfloxacin, ofloxacin, levodopa, penicillamine and zinc.

iron-hydroxide dextran complex (Cosmofer injection) is an iron preparation ➤ iron.

iron sodium edetate (Sytron elixir) is an iron preparation ➤ iron.

iron sorbitol citric acid complex ➤ Jectofer.

Irriclens aerosol contains sodium chloride. It is used to irrigate wounds.

Isib 60XL ➤ isosorbide mononitrate.

Ismelin ➤ guanethidine.

Ismo and **Ismo Retard** ➤ isosorbide mononitrate.

isocarboxazid (Marplan) is an MAO inhibitor antidepressant drug. See Chapter 4. *Adverse effects and Precautions* are similar to those under phenelzine.

Isocard spray ➤ isosorbide dinitrate.

Isodur ➤ isosorbide mononitrate.

isoflurane (Aerrane) is a volatile general anaesthetic with actions similar to halothane.

Isogel ➤ ispaghula.

Isoket and **Isoket Retard** ➤ isosorbide dinitrate.

isometheptene is a sympathomimetic drug. See Chapter 9. It is combined with paracetamol in Midrid capsules used to treat migraine. See Chapter 34. *Adverse effects and Precautions* ➤ sympathomimetic drugs.

Isomide and **Isomide CR** ➤ disopyramide.

isoniazid (isionicotinic acid hydrazine, INAH, in Rifater, in Rifinah, in Rimactazid) an antibacterial drug used to treat tuberculosis. See Chapter 50. *Adverse effects:* Isoniazid may cause nausea and vomiting. High daily doses may cause inflammation of nerves (peripheral neuritis), producing numbness, pins and needles and weakness. This may be prevented by giving vitamin B6 (pyridoxine) 10 mg daily. Isoniazid usually lifts the mood but it may also cause mental disturbances which are usually reversed on withdrawal of the drug; it may very rarely cause damage to the nerve of the eye (optic neuritis), convulsions and systemic lupus erythematosis (SLE – a disease of unknown cause with symptoms of fever, muscle and joint pain, blood disorders and skin eruptions). Allergic reactions include fever, skin rashes, swollen glands (lymphadenopathy) and, rarely, blood disorders, liver damage and jaundice (stop immediately if jaundice develops or if signs of liver damage appear – persistent nausea, vomiting and generally feeling unwell). Raised blood sugar and swollen breasts in men (gynaecomastia) have been associated with isoniazid treatment. Withdrawal symptoms may occur on stopping the drug; these include headache, irritability, nervousness, insomnia and excessive dreaming. *Precautions:* It should not be used in patients with porphyria (a hereditary disorder of metabolism) or a history of liver damage caused by drugs. Do not use in patients suffering from manic or hypomanic psychosis. It should be given with caution to patients suffering from epilepsy, history of serious mental illness, chronic alcoholism or with impaired kidney or liver function. It should be used with caution in pregnancy and breastfeeding mothers. Some patients inactivate it slowly and therefore they may develop adverse effects on smaller doses. Tuberculosis bacteria rapidly become resistant to isoniazid and therefore it should not be used alone. *Interactions:* Phenytoin, primidone, carbamazepine.

Isophane insulin, see Chapter 42.

isoprenaline (isoprenaline hydrochloride, isoprenaline sulphate) is a non-selective beta-stimulant used to treat asthma (see Chapter 14). It is also used (as Saventrine IV) to treat disorders of the heart, see Chapter 24. *Adverse effects* include rapid beating of the heart, chest pain, dry mouth, faintness, dizziness, headache, nervousness, tremor, diarrhoea and weakness. Irregularities of heart rate may occur. *Precautions:* Isoprenaline should not be used in patients with heart disease, asthma due to heart disease, disorders of heart rhythm or overactive thyroid. It should be used with caution in patients with raised blood pressure or diabetes and in pregnancy. Tolerance may develop to isoprenaline taken in an aerosol; in such cases the dose should not be increased but the drug should be stopped and an alternative drug used. *Interactions:* MAOIs, sympathomimetic drugs, tricyclic antidepressants.

isopropyl myristate (in Dermol, in Diprobath, in Emulsiderm, in Hydromol) is resistant to oxidation and water and does not become rancid. It is used in skin applications to make them relatively free from greasiness. It is used as a solvent and is absorbed readily by the skin. It is also used as a food additive.

Isopto Alkaline eye drops contain hypromellose, as a lubricant. Do not wear soft contact lenses.

Isopto Atropine eye drops contain atropine with the lubricant hypromellose. They are used to dilate the pupil. See p. 61. *Adverse effects* include transient stinging, dry mouth, blurred vision, photophobia (discomfort in the light), rapid beating of the heart, headache, mental upsets and behavioural disturbances. *Precautions:* Do not use in patients with closed-angle glaucoma. Do not wear soft contact lenses ➤ antimuscarinic drugs.

Isopto Carbachol eye drops contain carbachol with the lubricant hypromellose. They are used to treat glaucoma. See p. 63. *Adverse effects and Precautions:* Do not use if the cornea is damaged or in patients with inflammation of the iris in the eye. Do not wear soft contact lenses.

Isopto Carbine eye drops contain pilocarpine with the lubricant hypromellose ➤ pilocarpine.

Isopto Frin eye drops contain phenylephrine with the lubricant hypromellose. They are used to relieve minor irritation of the eye causing redness. *Adverse effects and Precautions:* Do not wear soft contact lenses. Use with caution in patients with closed-angle glaucoma ➤ phenylephrine.

Isopto Plain eye drops contain the lubricant hypromellose.

Isordil preparations ➤ isosorbide dinitrate.

isosorbide dinitrate (sorbide dinitrate, for preparations, see p. 113) is a nitrate vasodilator used to treat and prevent angina (see Chapter 22) and heart failure (see Chapter 23). *Adverse effects and Precautions:* ➤ glyceryl trinitrate.

isosorbide mononitrate (Dynamin, Elantan preparations, Imazin XL, Imdur, Ismo, Isotard XL, Isotrate, MCR 50, Monit, Mono Cedocard, Monomax) is a nitrate vasodilator. It has very similar effects to isosorbide dinitrate, but has a longer action and is more reliably absorbed. It is used to treat and prevent angina (see Chapter 22) and treat heart failure (see Chapter 23). *Adverse effects and Precautions:* ➤ glyceryl trinitrate.

Isotard preparations ➤ isosorbide mononitrate.

Isotrate ➤ isosorbide mononitrate.

isotretinoin (Roaccutane) is a vitamin A derivative used to treat severe acne, see p. 252. Its use is restricted to hospitals. *Adverse effects* are mainly related to the dose and include itching, drying, scaling, thinning, fragility and redness of the skin, dryness of the lining of the nose with nosebleeds, dryness of the lips and mouth, dryness of the eyes, visual disturbances (optic neuritis, photophobia, corneal opacities, cataracts), thinning of the hair, headache, nausea, vomiting, sweating, pigmentation of the face, hoarseness, increased hair growth (hirsutism), drowsiness, lethargy, mood changes, painful joints and muscles, changes in liver function tests, raised blood fat levels, seizures, irregularities of the menstrual periods, hearing loss, allergic reactions affecting the blood vessels, bone changes, kidney damage and swollen glands. The skin may become fragile and blister. *Precautions:* Prescriptions for isotretinoin must be written by a named skin specialist. Do not use in pregnancy or in breastfeeding mothers. Do not use in patients with impaired kidney or liver function. Pregnancy must be excluded before starting treatment and sexual intercourse must be avoided, or effective contraception used, one month before, during and for at least one month after treatment. Tests of liver function and blood fat levels must be carried out before starting and every four weeks during treatment. Do not donate blood while on treatment, or for one month after it. *Interactions:* Avoid tetracycline antibiotics and high doses of vitamin A. Isotretinoin is also available for topical application as Isotrex gel and Isotrexin gel.

Isotrex gel ➤ isotretinoin. It may irritate the skin. Do not use if there is a family history of skin cancer (epithelioma), in pregnancy or in breastfeeding mothers.

Avoid contact with eyes, mouth and mucous membranes, damaged or sunburnt skin. *Interactions:* Keratolytics (products for removing dead skin). Avoid UV light.

Isotrexin gel ➤ isotretinoin. It may irritate the skin. Do not use if there is a family history of skin cancer (epithelioma), in pregnancy or in breastfeeding mothers. Avoid contact with eyes, mouth and mucous membranes, damaged or sunburnt skin. *Interactions:* Keratolytics (products for removing dead skin). Avoid UV light.

Isovorin ➤ calcium levofolinate.

ispaghula husk (Fybogel, in Fybogel mebervine, Fybozest, Isogel, Konsyl, in Manevac, Regulan) is the dried ripe seeds of *Plantago ovata*. It is used as a bulk laxative (see Chapter 21) because the seeds take up a large amount of water in the intestine to form a gummy mass. It is also used to treat diarrhoea (see Chapter 20) and irritable bowel syndrome and to lower raised blood cholestorol levels (see Chapter 26). *Adverse effects* include wind, distension of the abdomen, impaction of bowel contents causing obstruction, and allergic reactions. *Precautions:* Do not use in patients who have difficulty in swallowing or any obstructive disorder of the bowel.

isradipine (Prescal) is a calcium-channel blocker used to treat raised blood pressure. See Chapter 25. *Adverse effects* include rapid beating of the heart, palpitations, flushing, headache, dizziness, swelling of the ankles, abdominal discomfort, weight gain, fatigue and skin rashes. *Precautions:* Use with caution in pregnancy and in patients with heart disorders. In elderly patients, and those with impaired kidney or liver function, start with half the recommended daily dose. *Interactions:* Anti-epileptic drugs.

Istin ➤ amlodipine.

itraconazole (Sporanox) is an antifungal drug. See Chapter 47. *Adverse effects* include headache, dizziness, indigestion, abdominal pains, constipation, menstrual disorders, allergic reactions (e.g. itching, skin rashes, nettle-rash, angioedema (allergic swelling of the mouth and throat)), liver damage and jaundice (especially if treatment exceeds one month), nerve damage (stop treatment immediately) and severe skin lesions. Long-term treatment may rarely cause a fall in blood potassium level and hair loss. *Precautions:* Do not use in pregnancy. Sexual intercourse should be avoided or contraceptives used during and for one month after treatment. Do not use when breastfeeding. Use with caution in patients with impaired liver function and in those who have had liver damage produced by some other drug. Tests of liver function should be carried out before treatment starts and after one month if patient on long-term treatment. Check liver function if patient develops loss of appetite, nausea, vomiting, fatigue, abdominal pain or dark urine. Stop treatment if the tests are abnormal. Use with caution in patients with impaired kidney function, AIDS or reduced white cell count because effectiveness of the drug may be reduced. Blood levels of itraconazole should be monitored. *Interactions:* Avoid astemizole, terfenadine and cisapride. Other interactions include rifampicin, cyclosporin, H_2-blockers and antacids.

Jectofer is an iron sorbitol/citric acid complex given by injection to treat iron deficiency anaemia (see Chapter 35). *Adverse effects* include nausea, vomiting, dizziness, flushing and occasionally severe disorders of heart rhythm. *Precautions:* Do not use in patients with seriously impaired function of their liver or kidneys, acute leukaemia, untreated infection of the urinary tract, early pregnancy. Use with utmost caution in patients with heart disorders such as angina or disorders of heart rhythm. Oral iron treatment should be stopped twenty-four hours before starting treatment with Jectofer. It is effective only in iron-deficiency anaemia and will not work in other anaemias.

Jomethid XL ➤ ketoprofen.

Joy-rides tablets ➤ hyoscine.

juniper tar ➤ cade oil.

Juno Junipah salts is a stimulant laxative which contains juniper berry oil, sodium bicarbonate, sodium phosphate, sodium sulphate.

Kabiglobulin, see normal immunoglobulin (human), p. 302.

Kabikinase ➤ streptokinase.

Kabivial ➤ somatrophin.

Kaletra ➤ lopinavir.

Kalspare preparations contain clorthalidone (a thiazide diuretic) and triamterene (a potassium-sparing diuretic). See Chapter 29. They are used to treat a mild to moderate rise in blood pressure (see Chapter 25) and fluid retention. See Chapter 23 on drugs used to treat heart failure. *Adverse effects and Precautions* ➤ thiazide diuretics, triamterene.

Kalten capsules contain atenolol (a selective beta-blocker) amiloride (a potassium-sparing diuretic) and hydrochlorothiazide (a thiazide diuretic). They are used to treat raised blood pressure (see Chapter 25). *Adverse effects and Precautions* ➤ beta-blockers, thiazide diuretics, amiloride.

Kamillosan preparations ➤ chamomile.

Kaodene contains codeine and kaolin. It is used to treat diarrhoea (see Chapter 20). *Adverse effects and Precautions* ➤ codeine, kaolin.

kaolin is a hydrated aluminium silicate. Kaolin preparations are used as dusting powders, as poultices and in suspensions to treat diarrhoea.

Kapake ➤ co-codamol.

Kaplon ➤ captopril.

Karvol inhalant capsules contain menthol, chlorbutol, cinnamon oil, pine oil, terpineol and chlorothymol ➤ inhalations.

Kay-Cee-L syrup contains potassium chloride ➤ potassium supplements.

Kefadim ➤ cefazidime.

Kefadol ➤ cephamandole.

Keflex preparations ➤ cefalexin.

Kefzol ➤ cephazolin.

Kelfizine W ➤ sulfametopyrazine.

Kemadrin ➤ procyclidine.

Kemicetine ➤ chloramphenicol.

Kenalog ➤ triamcinolone.

keratolytics, see p. 247.

Kentene ➤ piroxicam.

Keppra ➤ levetiracetam.

Keral ➤ dexketoprofen.

Keri Lotion ➤ liquid paraffin.

Kerlone ➤ betaxolol.

Ketalar injection ➤ ketamine.

ketamine (Ketalar) is an injectable anaesthetic, mainly used for children. *Adverse effects* include increased pressure in the arteries, rapid beating of the heart and hallucinations.

Ketil CR ➤ ketoprofen.

Ketocid ➤ ketoprofen.

ketoconazole (Nizoral) is a broad-spectrum antifungal drug. See Chapter 47. *Adverse effects* include stomach and bowel upsets, headache, itching and, very rarely, enlargement of the breasts (in males), blood disorders and serious liver damage (if given for more than two weeks). *Precautions:* Do not use in patients with porphyria (a hereditary disorder of metabolism), active liver disease or impaired liver function, or in pregnancy. For treatment longer than fourteen days liver function tests must be carried out before and during treatment. *Interactions:* Anticoagulants, phenytoin, rifampicin, cyclosporin. Its absorption from the stomach depends upon the presence of acid; it is therefore better absorbed when taken with a meal and poorly absorbed if taken with any drug that reduces acid production, e.g. antimuscarinics, H_2 blockers, antacids. Such drugs should be taken not less than two hours after a dose of ketoconazole. Do not use with astemizole, terfanadine, or cisapride. *Nizoral cream* is used to treat seborrhoeic dermatitis. It may cause irritation where it is applied. *Nizoral Shampoo* is used to treat seborrhoeic dermatitis of the scalp and dandruff. It may irritate the scalp.

ketoprofen (Fenoket, Jomethid XL, Ketil CR, Ketocid, Ketpron, Ketpron XL, Ketotard, Ketovail, Ketozip XL, Larafen CR, Orudis, Oruvail) is a non-steroidal anti-inflammatory drug (NSAID) ➤ nonsteroidal anti-inflammatory drugs. Also available in a gel (Oruvail gel, Powergel) to relieve muscle aches and pains. These preparations may cause irritation where it is applied and should not be used in patients allergic to aspirin or an NSAID or in patients with asthma. They should be used with caution in patients with impaired kidney function, in pregnancy and in breastfeeding mothers.

ketorolac trometamol (Toradol) is a nonsteroidal anti-inflammatory drug used to relieve moderate to severe pain following surgery. It can be given by mouth or by injection. *Adverse effects and Precautions* ➤ non-steroidal anti-inflammatory drugs. Do not use in pregnancy or in breastfeeding mothers. It is also available as eye drops (Acular).

Ketotard ➤ ketoprofen.

ketotifen (Zaditen) has antihistamine properties and is used by mouth to prevent asthma (see Chapter 14) and hayfever. See Chapter 17. *Adverse effects* include drowsiness, dry mouth, agitation, weight gain and dizziness. *Precautions:* Do not use in pregnancy or in breastfeeding mothers. *Interactions:* Sleeping drugs, sedatives or any drug that depresses brain function, oral anti-diabetic drugs, antihistamines. Withdraw the drug slowly over two–four weeks. It may increase the effects of alcohol and because it produces drowsiness it may impair the ability to drive motor vehicles or operate moving machinery.

Ketovail ➤ ketoprofen.

Ketovite is a multivitamin preparation used in the prevention of deficiency in disorders of carbohydrate or amino acid metabolism.

Ketozip XL ➤ ketoprofen.

Ketpron and **Ketpron XL** ➤ ketoprofen.

Kiflone ➤ cefalexin.

Kinidin Durules ➤ quinidine.

Klaricid ➤ clarithromycin.

Klean-Prep contains polyethylene glycol, sodium sulphate, sodium bicarbonate, sodium chloride and potassium chloride. It is an osmotic laxative (see Chapter 21) used to clear the bowels before surgery. *Adverse effects* include nausea, bloated feeling, distension of the abdomen and, occasionally, abdominal cramps, vomiting and irritation of the anus. Very rarely, it may cause allergic reactions. *Precautions:* Do not use in children. Do not use if there is a blockage or ulcers in the stomach or intestine. Use with caution in patients with oesophageal disorders, impaired gag-reflex or ulcerated bowel, in pregnancy or in breastfeeding mothers. *Interactions:* Give any oral medicine at least one hour before giving Klean-Prep.

Kliofem preparations contain tablets of oestradiol (an oestrogen) and tablets of norethisterone (a progestogen). They are used as HRT ➤ HRT.

Kliovance is a hormone replacement therapy ➤ estradiol, norethisterone.

Kloref preparations contain betaine hydrochloride and potassium salts. They are used as a potassium supplement ➤ betaine, potassium supplements.

Kogenate ➤ factor VIII fraction, dried.

Kolanticon gel contains dicyloverine (dicyclomine) (an antimuscarinic drug), the antacids aluminium hydroxide and magnesium oxide and the anti-foaming drug, dimethicone. It is used as an antacid ➤ antacids, dicyloverine(dicyclomine), dimethicone.

Konakion ➤ phytomenadione.

Konakion MM Paediatric is a preparation of the vitamin K derivative phytomenadione which can be given by mouth to healthy newborn babies to prevent vitamin K deficiency bleeding disorders. An intramuscular or intravenous preparation of vitamin K should be used in premature babies or newborn babies born at term who are at special risk. *Adverse effects and Precautions:* ➤ phytomenadione.

Konsyl preparations ➤ ispaghula husks.

Kwells preparations ➤ hyoscine.

Kytril preparations ➤ granisetron.

labetalol (labetalol hydrochloride, Trandate) is an alpha- and beta-blocker. It is used to treat raised blood pressure and raised blood pressure in pregnancy, see Chapter 25, and angina associated with a raised blood pressure. See Chapter 22. *Adverse effects:* Fall in blood pressure on standing up after sitting or lying down, headache, tiredness, weakness, nausea, vomiting, rashes, tingling of the scalp, difficulty in passing water, pains in the stomach, liver damage and skin rash. For other potential *adverse effects* ➤ beta-blockers. *Precautions* ➤ beta-blockers. It should be used with utmost caution in patients suffering from heart block, heart failure and asthma; and particularly in late pregnancy and breastfeeding mothers. The dose should be reduced in liver disease and abrupt withdrawal of the drug should be avoided. It can interfere with laboratory tests for adrenaline(epinephrine)-like substances. At first sign of liver damage (e.g. changes in liver function tests, jaundice) the drug should be stopped. *Interactions* ➤ beta-blockers.

Labiton liquid tonic contains thiamine, kola nut dried extract, alcohol and caffeine ➤ caffeine, kola. Do not use in patients suffering from inflammation of the liver. *Interactions:* Sleeping drugs, sedatives and other drugs that depress brain function.

Labosept pastilles ➤ dequalinium.

lacidipine (Motens) is a class II calcium-channel blocker used to treat raised blood pressure. See Chapter 25. *Adverse effects* include dizziness, headache, palpitations, weakness, flushing, ankle-swelling, rash, itching, stomach and bowel upsets, passing large volumes of urine, swelling of the gums, chest pains. *Precautions:* Do not use in children, in pregnancy or in breastfeeding mothers. Use with utmost caution in patients with conduction defects of their hearts or poor heart function or impaired liver function. Stop the drug immediately if chest pains develop after starting treatment. *Interactions:* cimetidine.

Lacri-Lube lubricant eye ointment contains soft paraffin, liquid paraffin and lanolin ➤ liquid paraffin.

lactic acid is used to prepare compound sodium lactate injections which are given for acidosis (when the blood acid/base balance becomes disturbed). It may be used in vaginal douches for the treatment of vaginal discharge, in skin preparations to treat chronic dry skin and as a paint to treat warts.

Lacticare moisturising lotion contains lactic acid and sodium pyrrolidonecarboxylate in an emulsion base. It is used to treat chronic dry skin, see emollients p. 236.

Lactitol (lactitol monohydrate) is an osmotic laxative used to treat constipation. See Chapter 21. *Adverse effects* include wind, bloatedness, itchy anus and stomach discomfort. *Precautions:* Do not use in patients with intestinal obstruction or galactosaemia (inability to convert galactose to glucose). Use with caution in pregnancy. Drink plenty of fluids.

Lactugal solution ➤ lactulose.

lactulose (Duphalac, Lactugal, Osmolax, Regulose) is an osmotic laxative used to treat constipation (see Chapter 21). *Adverse effects* include wind, cramps and abdominal discomfort. *Precautions:* Do not use in patients with intestinal obstruction or galactosaemia (inability to convert galactose to glucose). Use with caution in patients with lactose intolerance.

Ladropen ➤ flucloxacillin.

laevulose (fructose) is a sugar, used medicinally in the same way as glucose.

Lamictal ➤ lamotrigine.

Lamisil ➤ terbinafine.

lamivudine (in Combivir, Epivir, in Trizivir, Zeffix) is an antiviral drug used to treat patients suffering from HIV infection. See Chapter 48. *Adverse effects* include blood disorders, headache, generally feeling unwell, nausea, fatigue, diarrhoea, abdominal pain, vomiting, insomnia, cough, blocked nose, muscle and joint pains, nerve damage, inflammation of the pancreas and changes in liver function tests. *Precautions:* Use with caution in patients with impaired kidney function, advanced liver disease due to hepatitis B, in pregnancy, in breastfeeding mothers and in patients with diabetes or signs of inflammation of the pancreas. *Interactions:* Ganciclovir, foscarnet, cotrimoxazole.

lamotrigine (Lamictal) is an anti-epileptic drug. See Chapter 15. *Adverse effects* include flu-like symptoms, skin rash, fever, tiredness, drowsiness, headache, stomach and bowel upsets, dizziness, blurred vision, irritability, agitation, confusion, aggression, double vision and unsteadiness of movement (ataxia). Very rarely it may cause serious skin disorders, blood disorders, liver damage and sensitivity of the skin to the rays of the sun. *Precautions:* Do not use in patients with severe impairment of liver function. Patients must be closely monitored for adverse effects and seizure control especially in first month of treatment and especially if lamotrigine is given with other anti-epileptic drugs when serious worsening of the patient's condition may occasionally occur. Use with caution in pregnancy and breastfeeding mothers. *Interactions:* Antidepressants, cimetidine, cholestyramine, other anti-epileptic drugs (see above).

Lamprene ➤ clofazimine.

Lanacane cream is a soothing haemorrhoidal preparation containing benzocaine and chlorothymol ➤ benzocaine, chlorothymol.

Lanacort preparations ➤ hydrocortisone.

lanolin ➤ wool fat.

Lanoxin ➤ digoxin.

lanreotide (Somatuline LA) is used for the relief of symptoms associated with overproduction of growth hormone due to a pituitary tumour (acromegaly) and when levels of growth hormone remain elevated after surgery or radiotherapy. *Adverse effects* include pain at injection site, stomach and bowel upset, gallstones. *Precautions:* Do not use in pregnancy or while breastfeeding. Use with caution in patients with diabetes, risk of gallstones, kidney or liver damage.

Lanvis ➤ thioguanine.

lansoprazole (in Heliclear, in Helimet, Zoton) is a proton pump blocker used to treat acid indigestion. See Chapter 19. *Adverse effects* include stomach and bowel upsets, headache, irritation of the skin and changes in liver function tests. Rarely it may cause painful joints, ankle swelling, blood disorders and depression. *Precautions:* Use with caution in pregnancy and breastfeeding mothers. It may mask symptoms of cancer of the stomach: monitor patients with stomach ulcers carefully to exclude the possibility of cancer. *Interactions:* Oral contraceptives, phenytoin, theophylline, warfarin, antacids, sucralfate.

Lanvis ➤ tioguaine.

Larafen CR ➤ ketoprofen.

Largactil ➤ chlorpromazine.

Lariam ➤ mefloquine.

Laryng-O-Jet is a disposable kit for laryngo-tracheal anaesthesia. It contains a jet spray of lidocaine(lignocaine) (local anaesthetic) ➤ lidocaine(lignocaine).

Lasikal tablets contain furosemide(frusemide) (a loop diuretic) and slow-release potassium chloride (a potassium supplement). They are used to treat fluid retention when a potassium supplement is required (see Chapter 29). *Adverse effects and Precautions* ➤ furosemide(frusemide), potassium supplements.

Lasilactone capsules contain furosemide (frusemide) (a loop diuretic) and spironolactone (a potassium-sparing diuretic). They are used to treat fluid retention not responding to other diuretic therapies (see Chapter 29). *Adverse effects and Precautions* ➤ furosemide(frusemide), spironolactone.

Lasix ➤ furosemide(frusemide).

Lasonil ointment contains heparinoid and hyaluronidase. It is used to reduce swelling in bruises and sprains ➤ heparinoid, hyaluronidase. Do not use on open or infected wounds.

Lasoride tablets contain furosemide (frusemide) (a loop diuretic) and amiloride (a potassium-sparing diuretic). They are used to treat fluid retention when a quick response is needed and when it is important not to let the blood potassium level fall (see Chapter 29). *Adverse effects and Precautions* ➤ furosemide(frusemide), amiloride.

Lassar's paste contains zinc oxide and salicylic acid. It is used to treat dry, thickened skin (e.g. in eczema). *Adverse effects and Precautions* ➤ salicylic acid, zinc oxide.

latanoprost (Xalatan) is a prostaglandin used for open-angle glaucoma and high blood pressure in the eye where other treatments have failed or are not tolerated. See Chapters 13 and 52. *Adverse effects* include blurred vision, red eye, a feeling that something is in the eye and changes in the colour of the eyes. The iris becomes increasingly

brown due to the deposit of the brown pigment melanin. This occurs predominantly in patients with mixed coloured eyes and rarely in patients with eyes of one colour whether blue, grey, brown or green. *Precautions:* Do not use while wearing contact lenses, in pregnancy or while breastfeeding. Use with caution in patients with congenital glaucoma, disorders of the lens and severe asthma.

lauromacrogols are used as lubricants, surfactants and as spermicidal agents in some contraceptive preparations.

laxatives (purgatives or cathartics) are used to treat constipation (see Chapter 21).

Laxoberal ➤ sodium picosulfate.

lecithins consist of groups of fatty acids obtained from animal and vegetable sources, e.g. egg lecithins, vegetable lecithins, soya lecithins. Vegetable lecithin differs from egg lecithin in so far as it does not contain cholesterol and contains a lower percentage of phosphorus. Lecithins are used as emulsifiers and stabilizers in the preparation of creams and ointments and in the food industry.

Ledclair ➤ sodium calcium edetate.

Lederfen ➤ fenbufen.

Lederfolin preparations contain the calcium salt of folinic acid ➤ folinic acid.

Ledermycin ➤ demeclocycline.

leflunomide (Arava) is used for active rheumatoid arthritis. See Chapter 32. *Adverse effects* include increased blood pressure, stomach and bowel upset, disorders in the mouth, abdominal pain, altered liver function, decrease in white blood cells, headache, dizziness, weakness, abnormal sensations such as tingling, burning or tightness, weight loss, allergy. Rarely severe liver toxicity and Stevens-Johnson syndrome. *Precautions:* Do not use in patients with severe immunodeficiency, bone-marrow dysfunction, disorders of the blood, serious infections, liver damage, severe kidney impairment, severe protein deficiency in the blood, mouth ulcers, pregnancy – contraception is required for both males and females during treatment and for two years after use or while breastfeeding.

lemon oil (juice) is used as a flavouring agent and to break up wind in e.g. flatulence and colic.

Lemsip Blackcurrant, **Lemsip Lemon**, **Lemsip Cold and Flu Breathe Easy**, **Lemsip Cold and Flu Max Strength** and **Lemsip Max Strength** contain paracetamol and phenylephrine; **Lemsip Cold and Flu Combined Relief** contains paracetamol, caffeine and phenylephrine; **Lemsip Power and Paracetamol** contains paracetamol and pseudoephedrine; **Lemsip Power Plus** contains ibuprofen and pseudoephedrine ➤ individual entry for each drug.

lenograstim (Granocyte) is genetically engineered human granulocyte stimulating factor (G-CSF). It is used to stimulate the production of white blood cells in patients when white cell production by the bone marrow has been knocked out by anticancer drugs. It is also used to stimulate white cell production in patients who have undergone bone-marrow transplantation. *Adverse effects and Precautions* are similar to those listed under filgrastim ➤ filgrastim.

Lentaron ➤ formestone.

Lentizol ➤ amitriptyline.

lepirudin (Refludan) is used for anticoagulation (preventing or slowing the formation of blood clots) in patients with thrombocytopenia type II (where heparin is unsuitable) and thromboembolic disease, requiring anti-blood-clot therapy by injection. See Chapter 28. *Adverse effects* include bleeding, anaemia, fever, kidney failure, allergic reactions, injection site reactions. *Precautions:* Do not use in conditions likely to cause bleeding, in pregnancy or while breastfeeding. Use with caution in patients with kidney or liver damage.

lercanidipine (Zanidip) is used to treat high blood pressure. See Chapter 22. *Adverse effects* include flushing, swelling of the arms and legs, rapid heart beat, headache, dizziness and weakness. *Precautions:* Do not use in patients with heart disorders.

Lescol ➤ fluvastin.

letrozole (Femara) is used to treat advanced post-menopausal breast cancer in patients in whom tamoxifen or other antioestrogens (see p. 198) have failed to help. About one-third to one-half of breast cancers depend on oestrogens to stimulate their continued growth. In post-menopausal women whose ovaries have stopped working, their main oestrogen supply comes from converting male sex hormones into oestrogens. These male sex hormones are produced naturally by the adrenal glands and are converted in the tissues to oestrogens by an enzyme (aromatase). Letrozole blocks this action – it is an aromatase inhibitor. *Adverse effects* include headache, nausea, vomiting, constipation or diarrhoea, fatigue, muscle and joint pains, cough, breathlessness, chest pain, hot flushes, abdominal pains and risk of viral infections. *Precautions:* Do not use in premenopausal women, in pregnancy, in breastfeeding mothers or in patients suffering from severe impairment of liver function. Use with caution in women with very severe impairment of kidney function.

Leucomax ➤ molgramostim.

leucovorin ➤ folinic acid.

Leukeran ➤ chlorambucil.

leuprorelin (leuprorelin acetate, Prostap SR) is used to treat serious cancer of the prostate gland. It is a gonadotrophin-releasing hormone analogue which stimulates the pituitary gland to release LH and FSH; this initially stimulates the testes to produce testosterone, but subsequently it causes the pituitary to switch off the production of LH and FSH, causing the blood level of testosterone to fall, so that within about three weeks an effect similar to castration is achieved (chemical castration). *Adverse* *effects:* include decreased libido, impotence, hot flushes, sweating, ankle-swelling, fatigue and nausea. It may cause pain at the injection site and initially, when blood testosterone levels are up, it may cause bone pain and difficulty in passing urine. *Precautions:* To reduce the flare-up of symptoms at the start of treatment an anti-male sex hormone drug (anti-androgen) should be given three days before starting treatment and continued for two–three weeks. Leuprorelin (Prostap SR) is also used to treat *endometriosis* in women. It causes the production of female sex hormones by the ovaries to be switched off. *Adverse effects* in women include hot flushes, emotional upsets, headaches and dry vagina. *Precautions:* Do not use in pregnancy and avoid risk of getting pregnant, but do not use an oral contraceptive. Do not use in breastfeeding mothers or in women with undiagnosed vaginal bleeding. Because it stops oestrogen production, use with utmost caution in women at risk of developing osteoporosis.

Leustat ➤ cladribine.

levamisole is used to treat *Ascaris lumbricoides,* a parasitic worm infection of the intestine producing general ill-health and weakness. It is also used, in some countries, to stimulate the immune system in disorders such as rheumatoid arthritis. *Adverse effects:* When used as a single dose to kill worms it may cause nausea, vomiting, headache, dizziness and abdominal pains. When used over a period of time (e.g. as an immunostimulant) it may cause flu-like symptoms, painful joints, muscle pains, skin rash, fatigue, headache, confusion, insomnia, dizziness, excitation, convulsions, blood disorders, stomach and bowel upsets and an abnormal taste in the mouth. *Precautions:* Do not use in patients with severe kidney or liver disease or with pre-existing blood disorders.

levetiracetam (Keppra) is used as additional therapy in epilepsy and seizures. See Chapter 15. *Adverse effects* include accidental injury, headache, anorexia, stomach and bowel upset, weakness, drowsiness, amnesia, unsteadiness of movement (ataxia), convulsions, dizziness, depression, emotional swings, hostility, insomnia, nervousness, tremor, vertigo, skin rash, double vision. *Precautions:* Do not use while breastfeeding. Use with caution in patients with kidney or severe liver damage, in the elderly or in pregnancy.

levobunolol is a beta-blocker used in Betagan eye drops to treat glaucoma. See p. 64. *Adverse effects* include irritation of the eyes, dizziness and headache. For general effects of beta-blockers ➤ beta-blockers. *Precautions:* Use the eye drops with caution in patients with diabetes or asthma, and in breastfeeding mothers.

levobupivacaine (Chirocaine) is a form of bupivacaine (➤ bupivacaine). It is used for surgical anaesthesia (e.g. epidural, intrathecal, peripheral nerve block, local infiltration, peribulbar block in ophthalmic surgery) and pain management (e.g. postoperative pain, pain relief during labour and general pain relief). *Adverse effects and Precautions:* ➤ bupivacaine.

levocabastine (Livostin) is an antihistamine (see Chapter 17) that can be applied locally up the nose as a spray and in the eyes as eye drops to treat the symptoms of hayfever. It is rapid acting and produces prolonged effects. *Adverse effects* include headache, fatigue, sleepiness, local irritation, wheezing, nettle-rash, blurred vision and swelling (oedema) where it is applied. *Precautions:* Do not use in patients with severe impairment of kidney function. Use with caution in pregnancy. Use eye drops with caution if patient wears soft contact lenses.

levocetirizine (Xyzal) is a non-sedative antihistamine (see Chapter 17). *Adverse effects* include drowsiness, headache, dry mouth, stomach and bowel upsets, agitation and dizziness. *Precautions:* Do not use if breastfeeding. Use with caution in pregnancy and in patients with impaired kidney function. Increases effects of alcohol.

Although it produces less drowsiness than sedative antihistamines it may still affect driving skills. For other adverse effects and precautions of antihistamines ➤ antihistamines.

levodopa (in Madopar, in Sinemet) is used to treat parkinsonism. See Chapter 16. *Adverse effects* include loss of appetite, nausea, vomiting, dizziness and faintness (due to a fall in blood pressure on standing), insomnia, agitation, rapid beating of the heart, reddish coloration of the urine and other body fluids, allergic reactions and irregularities of heart rhythm. It may also produce involuntary movements, e.g. of the tongue, jaw and neck. These are dose-related. It may produce mental disturbances, depression, psychosis, mania, drowsiness, headache, flushing, sweating, bleeding from the stomach and intestine, nerve damage and changes in tests for liver function. *Precautions:* It should not be used in patients with severe mental illness, closed-angle glaucoma or a history of malignant melanoma. It should be used with caution in patients with kidney, liver or heart disease, disorders of the circulation, peptic ulcers, adult rickets, chronic chest disease, diabetes, open-angle glaucoma, in breastfeeding mothers or in pregnancy. The patient's heart, liver and kidney function should be checked at regular intervals. Blood tests should be carried out regularly, as well as assessments of the patient's mental state. It should be stopped eight weeks before surgery because of the risk of producing disorders of heart rhythm. The drug should be withdrawn slowly. It should be used with utmost caution in pregnancy and breastfeeding mothers. *Interactions:* MAOIs, pyridoxine (vitamin B_6), antiblood pressure drugs, sympathomimetics, ferrous sulphate.

levofloxacin (Tavanic) is a quinoline antibiotic. It is used for mild to moderate infection including acute sinusitis, acute exacerbation of chronic bronchitis, community-acquired pneumonia, complicated urinary tract infection, inflammation of the kidney and soft tissue infections. See Chapter 46. *Adverse effects* include stomach and bowel upset, raised liver enzymes, tendon disorders. *Precautions:* Do not use in patients with epilepsy, fluoroquinolone related tendon disorders, in pregnancy or while breastfeeding. Use with caution in patients with kidney damage, G-6-phosphate dehydrogenase deficiency, porphyria (a hereditary disorder of metabolism), severe persistent diarrhoea (discontinue). Avoid strong UV light.

levomepromazine(methotrimeprazine) (methotrimeprazine hydrochloride, methotrimeprazine maleate, Nozinan) is a phenothiazine antipsychotic drug ➤ antipsychotic drugs.

Levonelle-2 is an emergency contraceptive containing levonorgestrel ➤ levonorgestrel. It is used for post-coital contraception. It should not be administered if menstrual bleeding is overdue or if unprotected intercourse occurred more than seventy-two hours previously.

levonorgestrel is a progestogen used in combined oral contraceptives (see Chapter 41), in HRT (➤ HRT) and in the morning-after pill (see p. 207). *Adverse effects and Precautions* ➤ progestogens.

levothyroxine sodium(thyroxine sodium) (Eltroxin) is a preparation of the thyroid hormone thyroxine used to treat patients with under-active thyroid glands. See Chapter 43. *Adverse effects* include sweating, rapid beating of the heart, diarrhoea, flushing, muscle cramps, excessive weight loss, headaches, restlessness, excitability, irregularities of heart rhythm and angina. *Precautions:* It should be used with caution in breastfeeding mothers, in pregnancy, in the elderly, in patients with adrenal deficiency and in patients with coronary artery disease. It has a delayed and cumulative effect and may take up to two weeks to be effective; the dose must therefore be controlled carefully. *Interactions:* Anticoagulants, anti-diabetic drugs, antiepileptic drugs, tricyclic antidepressants, cholestyramine, digoxin and related drugs, sympathomimetic drugs.

Lexotan ➤ bromazepam.

Lexpec preparations ➤ folic acid.

Lexpec syrup with iron contains ferric ammonium citrate and folic acid ➤ iron, folic acid.

Lexpec syrup with iron-M contains ferric ammonium citrate and folic acid ➤ iron, folic acid.

LH ➤ luteinizing hormone.

LH-RH ➤ gonadorelin.

Liberate ➤ factor VIII.

Librium ➤ chlordiazepoxide.

Librofem ➤ ibuprofen.

Lidifen ➤ ibuprofen.

lidocaine(lignocaine) is a local anaesthetic. See Chapter 44. Preparations for injection include lidocaine, Min-I-Jet Lignocaine hydrochloride, Xylocaine Preparations for dental use include Lignospan, Lignostab A, Xylocaine, Xylotox. Preparation for surface anaesthesia include Emla cream, Instillagel gel, Laryng-O-Jet spray, Xylocaine gel, lidocaine ointment and spray. Preparations to apply to the eye as drops include Minims Lignocaine and Fluorescein. It is also present in the following topical applications: Betnovate Rectal, Bradosol Plus, Calgel, Perinal, Xyloproct. It is also used as Xylocard to treat irregular heartbeat associated with a heart attack. See Chapter 24. *Adverse effects* of injections include confusion, depressed breathing, convulsions, fall in blood pressure, slowing of the heart rate (may cause the heart to stop), and allergic reactions. *Precautions:* Do not use in patients with a complete heart block, low blood volume, or with adrenaline(epinephrine) to anaesthetize a finger, toe or penis. Use with caution in patients suffering from epilepsy, impaired liver or respiratory function, conduction defects of the heart, slow heart rate or porphyria (a hereditary disorder of metab-

olism). Reduce the dose in the elderly or debilitated and always have resuscitative equipment immediately to hand.

lignocaine ➤ lidocaine.

Lignospan ➤ lidocaine. It is used for local anaesthesia in dentistry.

Lignostab A injection ➤ lidocaine.

Li-Liquid oral solution ➤ lithium.

Limclair ➤ trisodium edetate.

linezolid (Zyvox) is an antibiotic used for the treatment of pneumonia, skin and soft tissue infections.

Lingraine ➤ ergotamine.

Lioresal ➤ baclofen.

liothyronine (liothyronine sodium, l-triiodothyronine sodium, Tetroxin) is a thyroid hormone used to treat severe thyroid deficiency and as a test for hyperthyroidism. See Chapter 43. *Adverse effects* include rapid beating of the heart, disorders of heart rhythm, pain from angina, excitability, restlessness, headache, flushing, sweating, diarrhoea, muscle cramps and excessive loss of weight. *Precautions:* Use with caution in patients with angina or heart disease, in breastfeeding mothers, the elderly and in patients with adrenal insufficiency. *Interactions:* Anticoagulants, anti-diabetic drugs, anti-epileptic drugs, tricyclic antidepressants, digoxin and related drugs, sympathomimetics.

Lipantil ➤ fenofibrate.

Liparol XL ➤ bezafibrate.

lipid lowering drugs, see Chapter 26.

Lipitor ➤ atorvastatin.

Lipobase emollient cream contains cetostearyl alcohol, cetomacrogol, liquid paraffin and white soft paraffin ➤ liquid paraffin and see emollients p. 236.

Lipobay ➤ cerivastatin.

Lipostat ➤ pravastatin.

Liqui-Char ➤ activated charcaol.

liquid paraffin (mineral oil) is a mixture of liquid saturated hydrocarbons obtained from petroleum. It is used as a moisturizer in skin preparations (see p. 236) and as a lubricant to treat dry eyes (e.g. Lacri-Lube, Lubri-Tears). It is also used as a lubricant laxative (see Chapter 21). *Adverse effects:* Taken by mouth it may leak from the anus and cause irritation. Inhalation of drops of oil may cause pneumonia (lipoid pneumonia). There is slight absorption of emulsified forms of liquid paraffin from the intestine and this may cause patches of irritation leading to scarring in the wall of the intestine (granulomatous reactions). *Precautions:* Avoid prolonged use by mouth and do not use in children under three years of age. By mouth it may interfere with the absorption of fat soluble vitamins A, D, E and K.

Liquifilm Tears ➤ polyvinyl alcohol. It is used to lubricate the eyes and as a tear substitute. Do not wear soft contact lenses.

Liqufruita is a cough preparation ➤ guaifenesin.

lisinopril (Carace, in Carace Plus, Zestril in Zestoretic) is an ACE inhibitor used to treat congestive heart failure (see Chapter 23) and raised blood pressure (see Chapter 25). It may also be used to prevent heart failure in patients who have had a heart attack (myocardiac infarction) provided they are not in shock and their systolic blood pressure is above 100. *Adverse effects and Precautions* are similar to those listed under captopril ➤ captopril.

Liskonum ➤ lithium.

lisuride (lysuride maleate) stimulates dopamine receptors and is used to treat Parkinson's disease. See Chapter 16. *Adverse effects* include nausea, vomiting, headaches, dizziness, drowsiness, lethargy, generally feeling unwell, fall in blood pressure, constipation, skin rashes, abdominal pain, mental disturbances including hallucinations, and, very rarely, coldness of the fingers and toes (Raynaud's phenomenon). *Precautions:* Do not use in patients with severe disorders of the circulation or with coronary artery disease. Use with caution in patients with pituitary tumours, psychotic illness, porphyria (a hereditary disorder of metabolism) and in pregnancy. Fall in blood pressure can cause dizziness, faintness and light-headedness in the first few days of treatment, therefore care must be exercised when driving or operating moving machinery. *Interactions:* Antipsychotic drugs, dopamine blockers.

lithium salts (lithium carbonate (Camcolit, Liskonum, Lithonate, Priadel); lithium citrate (Li-liquid, Priadel Liquid)) are used to treat mania and hypomania and prevent recurrent manic-depressive illness. See Chapter 4. *Adverse effects:* These develop slowly as the drug accumulates in the body; they are related to dosage. They include loss of appetite, nausea, vomiting, myasthenia gravis (muscle weakness due to neuromuscular abnormality), weight gain, fluid retention, excessive thirst and passing a lot of urine. Higher dosage results in higher blood levels which produce more serious adverse effects – confusion, slurred speech, diarrhoea, drowsiness, exaggerated jerky movements, blurred vision, increased nausea, vomiting and loss of appetite, myasthenia gravis, giddiness, serious mental disturbances, and unsteadiness of movement (ataxia). If these symptoms occur treatment should be stopped. Severe overdosage can cause convulsions, psychosis, fainting and coma. It may cause a drop in blood potassium levels, under-activity of the thyroid, goitre, kidney damage, and flare-up of psoriasis. Changes on electrocardiograms have been reported. *Precautions:* Lithium should not be given to patients with impaired heart or kidney function, Addison's disease, under-active thyroid or disturbance of sodium levels in the body. It should not be used in breastfeeding mothers. Use with caution in pregnancy, in elderly people, and ensure adequate intake of salt (sodium chloride) and water. Thyroid function should be checked at regular intervals. Blood levels of lithium should be monitored regularly. Patients should have their kidney, heart and thyroid function thoroughly checked before starting treatment with lithium. *Interactions:* Diuretics, NSAIDs, carbamazepine, phenytoin, haloperidol, metoclopramide, tricyclic and tetracyclic antidepressants, tetracycline antibiotics. *Note:* Lithium Succinate is used in Efalith ointment to treat seborrhoeic dermatitis ➤ Efalith.

lithium carbonate is a lithium salt.

lithium citrate is a lithium salt.

lithium succinate is a lithium salt.

Lithonate ➤ lithium salts.

Livial ➤ tibolone.

Livostin nasal spray and eye drops ➤ levocabastine.

Lloyd's cream is a heat rub ➤ diethyl salicylate.

Locabiotal ➤ fusafungine.

local anaesthetics, see Chapter 44.

local anaesthetic skin applications, see p. 247.

Loceryl ➤ amorolfine.

Locoid preparations ➤ hydrocortisone 17-butyrate.

Locoid C cream contains hydrocortisone butyrate (a potent corticosteroid) and chlorquinalol (an anti-infective drug). It is used to treat severe eczema when there is an added infection. *Adverse effects and Precautions* see corticosteroid skin applications p. 241.

Locoid Crelo emulsion ➤ hydrocortisone butyrate.

Locorten-Vioform ear drops contain clioquinol (an anti-infective drug) and flumethasone (a corticosteroid). They are used to treat infected, inflammatory conditions of the external ear (otitis externa). *Adverse*

effects: It may cause irritation and discolour the hair. *Precautions:* Do not use in patients with a perforated ear drum or primary infection of the external ear. Use with caution in breastfeeding mothers. See also corticosteroid skin applications, p. 241 and clioquinol.

Lodiar ➤ loperamide.

Lodine SR ➤ etodolac.

Iodoxamide (Alomide) eye drops are used to treat allergic conjunctivitis. *Adverse effects* include itching, stinging, mild transient burning sensation and watering of the eyes. *Precaution:* Do not wear soft contact lenses. Use with caution in pregnancy and in breastfeeding mothers.

Loestrin 20 and **Loestrin 30** are combined oral contraceptives. See p. 216.

Lofensaid ➤ diclofenac.

lofepramine (lofepramine hydrochlorine, Feprapax, Gamanil, Lomont) is a tricyclic antidepressant drug ➤ tricyclic antidepressants.

lofexidine (BritLofex) is used to relieve the symptoms of patients undergoing withdrawal of heroin or other opioids. It is a central-acting alpha stimulant, see p. 130. *Adverse effects* include dry mouth, throat and nose, drowsiness, fall in blood pressure and slowing of the heart rate. On stopping treatment the blood pressure may shoot up (rebound hypertension). *Precautions:* Use with caution in patients with diseases of the arteries from the heart, recent heart attack, or other heart disorders, low heart rate, impaired kidney function, history of depression, in pregnancy and in breastfeeding mothers. Monitor pulse rate and blood pressure frequently. Withdraw lofexidine slowly over several days in order to prevent a rebound rise in blood pressure. *Interactions:* Alcohol, any drug that depresses brain function.

Logynon is a triphasic oral contraceptive. See p. 217.

Logynon ED is a combined oral contraceptive. See p. 217.

lomefloxacin (Okacyn) is a quinolone antibiotic eye drop that is used to treat infection of the eye. See Chapter 13. *Adverse effects* include mild transient burning sensation. *Precautions:* Do not use while wearing contact lenses, in pregnancy or while breastfeeding.

Lomexin (fenticonazole) pessaries are used to treat thrush infections of the vagina. *Adverse effects:* It may produce mild irritation. *Precautions:* Use with caution in pregnancy and in breastfeeding mothers. *Interactions:* Damages latex condoms and diaphragms.

Lomont ➤ loperamine.

Lomotil preparations contain diphenoxylate (an opiate) and atropine (an antimuscarinic drug). They are used to treat diarrhoea (see Chapter 20). *Adverse effects* include allergic skin reactions, abdominal cramps and bloating. For adverse effects of opiates ➤ morphine, and for atropine ➤ antimuscarinic drugs. *Precautions:* Do not use in patients with intestinal obstruction, ulcers or inflammation of the bowel, or jaundice. Use with caution in pregnancy, breastfeeding mothers and patients with impaired liver function. Correct fluid and electrolyte loss before taking Lomotil. *Interactions:* MAOIs, sleeping drugs, sedatives and any drug that depresses brain function.

lomustine is an anti-cancer drug. See Chapter 51. *Adverse effects* include loss of appetite, nausea and vomiting, bone-marrow damage causing blood disorders (may be delayed for four–six weeks), mouth ulcers, loss of hair and liver damage. *Precautions:* See Chapter 51.

Loniten ➤ minoxidil.

loop diuretics, see Chapter 29.

LoperaGen ➤ loperamide.

loperamide (loperamide hydrochloride, Diasorb, Diocaps, Imodium, Lodiar, Loper-aGen, Norimode, Normaloe. OTCs:– Arret, Boots Diareze capsules, Diasorb, Diocalm Ultra) is an opiate which acts on the muscles of the intestinal wall and slows down its movements. It is used to treat diarrhoea (see Chapter 20). *Adverse effects* include bloating, abdominal cramps, paralysis of the small intestine (paralytic ileus), and skin rashes. *Precautions:* Do not use in patients whose abdomens are distended, who have paralytic ileus, or inflammation or ulcers of the bowel.

Lopid ➤ gemfibrozil.

lopinavir (Kaletra) is used for the treatment of HIV-1 infected adults and children in combination with other anti-retroviral agents. See Chapter 48. *Adverse effects* include stomach and bowel upset, weakness, headache, abdominal pain, rash. *Precautions:* Do not use tablets or solution in patients with severe kidney failure. Do not use solution in patients with severe kidney failure or liver failure. Use with caution in patients with severe kidney or moderate liver damage, hepatitis B or C, haemophilia, lipid disorders, inflammation of the pancreas, diabetes or in pregnancy.

Lopranol LA ➤ propranolol.

loprazolam (Dormonoct) is a benzodiazepine drug ➤ benzodiazepines.

Lopresor preparations ➤ metoprolol.

loratadine (Clarityn) is a non-sedative antihistamine. See Chapter 17 and ➤ antihistamines. *Adverse effects* include headache, nausea, fatigue, hair loss, severe allergic reactions, abnormal liver function tests and serious disorders of heart rhythm (supraventricular tachyarrhythmias). *Precautions:* Do not use in pregnancy or if breastfeeding.

lorazepam (Ativan) is a benzodiazepine drug ➤ benzodiazepines.

lormetazepam is a benzodiazepine drug ➤ benzodiazepines.

lornoxicam (Xefo) is a non-steroidal anti-inflammatory drug (NSAID) used to relieve pain and inflammation in arthritis or to treat post-operative pain ➤ non-steroidal anti-inflammatory drugs.

Loron ➤ sodium clodronate.

losartan potassium (Cozaar, in Cozaar Comp) is used to treat raised blood pressure. See Chapter 25. It is a specific angiotensin II receptor blocker. *Adverse effects* include dizziness, fall in blood pressure on standing after sitting or lying down, raised blood potassium levels and, rarely, skin rashes and changes in liver function tests. *Precautions:* Do not use in pregnancy or breastfeeding mothers. Use with caution in patients with impaired kidney or liver function or narrowing of the arteries to the kidneys (renal stenosis). Monitor blood potassium levels particularly in the elderly and patients with impaired kidney function. *Interactions:* Potassium-sparing diuretics.

Losec ➤ omeprazole.

Lotriderm cream contains betamethasone (a corticosteroid) and clotrimazole (an antifungal drug). It is used for the *short-term* treatment of inflamed fungal infections of the skin, *Adverse effects and Precautions:* See corticosteroid skin applications p. 241 and ➤ clotrimazole. The cream may cause mild burning, irritation and allergic reactions on the skin.

Loxapac ➤ loxapine.

loxapine (Loxapac) is an antipsychotic drug. See Chapter 3. *Adverse effects* include weakness, faintness, drowsiness, dizziness, muscle twitching, confusion, changes in blood pressure, rapid beating of the heart, dry mouth, blurred vision, constipation, nausea, vomiting, headache, breathlessness, parkinsonism and other disorders of involuntary movement, and very rarely transient impairment of vision and neuroleptic malignant syndrome (for symptoms ➤ antipsychotic drugs). *Precautions:* Do not use in patients who are comatose or semi-comatose. Use with caution in patients with disorders of the heart or circulation, with glaucoma, or with difficulty in passing urine

(e.g. from enlarged prostate gland), in pregnancy, in breastfeeding mothers and in patients with epilepsy. It may impair mental alertness and coordination, and impair the ability to drive motor vehicles or operate moving machinery. *Interactions:* Sedatives, sleeping drugs or any drug that depresses brain function, antimuscarinic drugs.

Luborant (artificial saliva) contains calcium, magnesium and potassium chlorides, potassium and magnesium acid phosphates, sodium fluoride and sodium carboxymethyl cellulose. It is used to treat dry mouth caused by radiotherapy or sicca (dry) syndrome.

Lubri-Tears ➤ liquid paraffin.

Ludiomil ➤ maprotiline.

Lugol's solution ➤ aqueous iodine solution.

Lustral ➤ sertraline.

luteinizing hormone (LH), see Chapter 40.

Lutropin alfa (Luveris) is used to treat infertility by stimulating the development of follicles in women with severe deficiencies in luteinizing hormone (LH) and follicle stimulating hormone (FSH). *Adverse effects* include pain, redness and swelling at the injection site, headache, sleepiness, nausea, abdominal pain, pelvic pain, over-stimulation of the ovaries, ovarian cyst and breast pain. *Precautions:* Do not use in patients with tumours of the hypothalamus, pituitary gland, ovary, uterus or breast, undiagnosed vaginal bleeding or any deficiency of the ovaries which would preclude pregnancy. Any endocrine disorders should be treated first.

Luveris ➤ lutropin alfa.

Lyclear creme-rinse conditioner ➤ permethrin.

lymecycline (Tetralysal) is a tetracycline antibiotic ➤ tetracyclines.

lysuride ➤ lisuride.

Lysovir ➤ amantadine.

Maalox and **Maalox TC** preparations contain aluminium hydroxide and magnesium hydroxide in varying proportions. **Maalox plus** preparations also contain dimethicone. They are used to treat indigestion and heartburn. See Chapter 19. *Adverse effects and Precautions* ➤ antacids. *Interactions:* tetracyclines antibiotics.

MabCampath ➤ alemtuzumab.

MabThera ➤ rituximat.

Maclean is an antacid preparation containing aluminium, calcium and magnesium ➤ antacids and individual entry for each drug.

Macrobid ➤ nitrofurantoin.

Macrodantin ➤ nitrofurantoin.

macrogols (polyethylene glycols) are polymers that can combine with water and are used to make water-based ointments and creams.

Madopar preparations ➤ co-careldopa.

magaldrate is an aluminium and magnesium hydroxide combination used as an antacid ➤ antacids.

Magnapen preparations contain ampicillin (a broad spectrum penicillin) and flucloxacillin (a penicillinase-resistant penicillin). *Adverse effects and Precautions* ➤ penicillins.

Magnatol is an antacid preparation containing alexitol, magnesium, potassium bicarbonate, xanthan gum.

Magnesia, cream of ➤ magnesium hydroxide mixture.

magnesium alginate (in Algicon, in Gaviscon Infant) is a magnesium salt of alginic acid ➤ alginic acid.

magnesium carbonate: Heavy magnesium carbonate and light magnesium carbonate are used as antacids and osmotic laxatives ➤ antacids and see Chapter 21 on drugs used to treat constipation.

magnesium chloride is used as a source of magnesium and chloride in kidney dialysis solutions. It is used to provide a source of magnesium in tube feeds and is a constituent of some mouth and skin preparations.

magnesium citrate (Citramag, in Picolax) is used as an osmotic laxative before X-ray of, or surgery on, the bowel. See Chapter 21.

magnesium hydroxide is used as an antacid (➤ antacids) and as an osmotic laxative. See Chapter 21.

magnesium oxide is used as an antacid (➤ antacids) and as an osmotic laxative. See Chapter 21.

magnesium sulphate (Epsom salts, in Andrews Liver Salts, in Kest) is used as an osmotic laxative. See Chapter 21. Also given intravenously or intramuscularly to correct magnesium deficiency and in the treatment of serious disorders of heart rhythm (particularly if blood potassium is low). Its value in patients suffering from a suspected heart attack requires further research. *Adverse effects:* Injections may cause a raised blood magnesium level causing nausea, vomiting, thirst, flushing, drowsiness, confusion, fall in blood pressure, depressed breathing and myasthenia gravis (muscle weakness due to a neuromuscular abnormality). By mouth it may cause colic and diarrhoea. *Precautions:* Use with caution in patients with impaired kidney or liver function. If given by injection monitor blood level of magnesium and other electrolytes very closely.

magnesium trisilicate is used as an antacid ➤ antacids.

Malarone is an antimalarial product containing proguanil and atovaquone ➤ proguanil, atovaquone.

malathion (Derbac-M, Prioderm, Quellada M, Soleo-M) is an organophosphorus insecticide used to treat head and pubic lice (see p. 256), scabies (see p. 261) and in mosquito control. *Adverse effects* include skin irritation and allergic reactions. *Precautions:* Do not use on broken or secondarily infected skin. Contact with the eyes should be avoided. Alcoholic preparations

(Prioderm lotion and Suleo-M lotion) should not be used in young children, in patients suffering from asthma, or to treat crabs or scabies. Use water-based solutions instead. Do not use more than once a week for three weeks at a time.

malgramostim (Leucomax) is used to reduce the severity of neutropenia (a decrease in certain kinds of white blood cells) brought on by anti-cancer drugs or ganciclovir and to speed up recovery following bone-marrow transplant. *Adverse effects* include pains in joints and muscles, difficulty or discomfort on passing urine, raised blood uric acid levels, headache, diarrhoea, nosebleeds, loss of hair, transient fall in blood pressure, disturbances of liver function, allergic reactions, proteins and blood in the urine and a transient fall in blood sugar level. Long-term use may be associated with damage to blood vessels in the skin, enlargement of the liver, skin rash and osteoporosis. *Precautions:* Do not use in patients with severe congenital neutropenia (Katsman's syndrome) with abnormal cell genetics. It should not be used within twenty-four hours before or after anti-cancer drug treatment. It should not be used in individuals with cancer of the blood-forming tissues. It should be used with caution in patients with severely impaired kidney and liver function. White blood cell counts must be carried out at frequent intervals because of the risk of over-production of white blood cells. Monitor blood platelet and haemoglobin level and spleen size. Use with utmost caution in pregnancy and breastfeeding mothers. Bone density must be monitored in individuals with osteoporosis on long-term treatment.

malic acid (in Aserbine) is a mild acid present in apples, pears and many other fruits. It is used as a food additive, and to give acidity to some skin applications.

Maloprim is used to prevent malaria. It contains dapsone and pyrimethamine. *Adverse effects and Precautions* ➤ dapsone, pyrimethamine. It may cause blood disorders, anaemia and allergic skin reactions. It should be used with caution in patients with impaired liver or kidney function, in breastfeeding mothers and in pregnancy (extra folic acid should be given daily). *Interactions:* Folate-blockers.

Mandanol ➤ paracetamol.

mandelic acid (Uro-Tainer, Mandelic Acid) is an antibacterial drug which is used to prevent infections of the urinary tract from catheters, usually as an ammonium or a calcium salt. See Chapter 49. *Adverse effects* include dizziness, noises in the ears (tinnitus), stomach upsets, pain on passing urine, blood in the urine and, rarely, nettle-rash. *Precautions:* It should not be used in patients with impaired kidney function.

Manerix ➤ moclobemide.

Manevac laxative contains ispaghula and sennosides. See Chapter 21 and ➤ ispaghula, sennosides.

mannitol is an osmotic diuretic See Chapter 29. It is used intravenously to reduce fluid retention in the brain and to reduce the pressure of fluid in the eye in glaucoma. See p. 62. *Adverse effects:* It may produce diarrhoea when given by mouth. Rapid injection into a vein may cause headache, chills, fever, chest pains and depress the respiration. *Precautions:* Do not use in patients with congestive heart failure or fluid on the lungs. Leakage from a vein may cause inflammation of the vein.

Manusept ➤ triclosan.

MAOIs ➤ monoamine-oxidase inhibitors.

maprotiline (maprotiline hydrochloride, Ludiomil) is a tetracyclic antidepressant drug. See Chapter 4. *Adverse effects:* It may cause antimuscarinic effects (e.g. dry mouth, blurred vision, constipation, rapid beating of the heart, difficulty passing urine). Occasionally it may cause convulsions and, very rarely, skin rashes, severe blood disorders and severe mental symptoms may occur. Other occasional adverse effects reported with tetracyclic antidepressants include drowsiness, dizziness, sweating, fall in blood pressure on standing up after sitting or lying down (they may produce faintness and light-headedness), tremor, pins and needles in the hands and feet, vivid dreams and impotence. *Precautions:* Do not use in patients with mania, severe impairment of liver or kidney function, a history of epilepsy, closed-angle glaucoma, difficulty passing urine (e.g. from enlarged prostate gland), or in patients who have had a recent heart attack or have a conduction defect of the heart. It should be used with caution in patients with heart disease, in the elderly, in pregnancy, in breastfeeding mothers and in patients with schizophrenia, cyclical depression, suicidal tendencies, fall in blood pressure on standing or sitting up after lying down (postural hypotension), raised pressure inside the eyes, chronic constipation or overworking of their thyroid gland. *Interactions:* MAOIs, anti-blood pressure drugs, sympathomimetics, barbiturates, antipsychotic drugs, alcohol, anaesthetics, phenytoin, benzodiazepines, cimetidine, SSRIs, anti-blood clotting drugs (coumarins), antimuscarinic drugs, quinidine, methylphenidate, anti-diabetic drugs.

Marcain local anaesthetic ➤ bupivacaine.

Marevan ➤ warfarin.

Marvelon is a combined oral contraceptive. See p. 216.

Masnoderm preparations ➤ clotrimazole.

Maxalt ➤ rizatriptan.

Maxepa concentrated fish oil capsules (Omega-3 marine triglycerides) contain eicosapentaenoic acid and docosahexaenoic acid, used to lower raised blood cholesterol and fat levels. See Chapter 26. *Adverse effects* include nausea and belching. *Precautions:* Patients with bleeding disorders and patients taking anti-blood-clotting drugs should be carefully monitored.

Maxidex eye drops contain dexamethasone (a corticosteroid) and hypromellose (a lubricant). They are used to treat inflammation of the eye. *Adverse effects* include rise in pressure inside the eye, thinning of the cornea, cataract, fungal infections. *Precautions:* Do not use if patient has a viral, fungal or tubercular infection of the eyes or in patients with glaucoma. Do not wear soft contact lenses. Be cautious about prolonged use in pregnancy or in infants. See Chapter 37 on corticosteroids.

Maxitrol eye ointment and drops contain dexamethasone (a corticosteroid) and the aminoglycoside antibiotics neomycin and polymixin B. They are used to treat infected eye disorders. *Adverse effects* include a rise in pressure inside the eyes, thinning of the cornea, cataract and fungal infections. *Precautions:* Do not use to treat viral, fungal, tuberculous or pus-filled infections. Do not wear soft contact lenses. Use with caution in infants and avoid prolonged use in pregnancy.

Maxivent aerosol inhalation ➤ salbutamol.

Maxolon ➤ metoclopramide.

Maxtrex ➤ methotrexate.

MCR-50 ➤ isosorbide mononitrate.

mebendazole (Boots Threadworm Treatment, Ovex, Pripsen Mebendazole, Vermox) is used to treat infestation with threadworms, hookworms, whipworms and roundworms. It may cause stomach and bowel upsets. It should not be used in pregnancy.

mebeverine (mebeverine hydrochloride, Colofac, Equilon, in Fybogel Mebeverine, IBS Relief) is an antispasmodic used to relieve painful spasm of the stomach and intestine, and irritable bowel syndrome. *Adverse effects and Precautions:* It should not be used in patients with porphyria (a hereditary disorder of metabolism) or paralysis of the small intestine. Use with caution in pregnancy and in breastfeeding mothers.

meclozine (meclozine hydrochloride, Sealegs) is an antihistamine drug (➤ antihistamines). It is used mainly to treat motion sickness, nausea, vomiting and vertigo. See Chapter 18. *Adverse effects and Precautions* ➤ antihistamines. Main adverse effects include drowsiness, dry mouth and blurred vision. Drowsiness may affect ability to drive. Increases the effects of alcohol.

Mectizan ➤ ivermectin.

mecysteine (methyl cysteine hydrochloride, Visclair) is a mucolytic used to liquefy sputum in patients with chronic bronchitis. See Chapter 11. It may cause stomach and bowel upsets.

Medicoal effervescent granules ➤ activated charcoal.

Medijel ➤ aminoacridine, lidocaine.

Medinex ➤ diphenhydramine.

Medinol paediatric preparations ➤ paracetamol.

Medised pain-relieving preparations contain paracetamol and promethazine (an antihistamine). They are used to relieve pain ➤ paracetamol, antihistamines.

Medocodene is an analgesic combination product ➤ codeine, paracetamol.

Medrone ➤ methylprednisolone.

medroxyprogesterone is a progestogen. See Chapter 40. It is used as a deep intramuscular depot injection (Depo-Provera) to provide contraception which lasts about twelve weeks. It can be given within five days of childbirth if not breastfeeding or after six weeks if breastfeeding. It is also used (Farlutal tablets and injection and Provera tablets) to treat cancer of the breast, womb, prostate and kidney. Medroxyprogesterone (Adgyn Medro, Provera) is also used by mouth to treat mild to moderate endometriosis, heavy periods and secondary loss of periods (secondary amenorrhoea). Improvera HRT contains tablets of piperazine oestrone (an oestrogen) and tablets of medroxyprogesterone and Tridestra HRT contains tablets of oestradiol (an oestrogen) and tablets of medroxyprogesterone ➤ HRT. *Adverse effects* produced by medroxypro-

gesterone include fluid retention, weight gain, stomach and bowel upsets, acne, nettle-rash, changes in libido, premenstrual symptoms, discomfort in the breasts, irregular periods, depression, insomnia, sleepiness, hair loss, allergic reactions, excessive hair growth, and rarely jaundice. *Precautions:* Do not use in pregnancy, in women with undiagnosed vaginal bleeding, impaired liver function, active liver disease, porphyria (a hereditary disorder of metabolism), blood clots, cancer of the breast or genital tract. Use with caution in patients with diabetes, raised blood pressure or kidney or liver disease ➤ progestogens. *Note:* When used as depot injections for contraception it may cause temporary infertility on stopping treatment. It may also cause prolonged and heavy vaginal bleeding during the first two–three cycles as well as headache, dizziness, weakness and abdominal pains. For contraception it should not be used in women with hormone-dependent cancer. In the high doses used to treat cancer it may cause adverse effects similar to those produced by corticosteroids (e.g. moonface). See Chapter 37. *Interactions:* Cyclosporin, rifampicin.

mefenamic acid (Dysman, Meflam, Ponstan, Ponstan Forte) is a non-steroidal anti-inflammatory drug (NSAID) (➤ non-steroidal anti-inflammatory drugs). It is used to relieve mild to moderate pain, headache, painful periods, and to treat rheumatoid arthritis. See Chapter 32. *Adverse effects* include indigestion, diarrhoea, and irritation of the stomach with bleeding. It may rarely cause drowsiness, dizziness, skin rashes, kidney damage and blood disorders. *Precautions:* Do not use in patients with peptic ulcers, ulcerative colitis, with a history of allergy to aspirin or an NSAID, impaired kidney or liver function. Use with caution in the elderly, in patients with asthma or allergic disorders, in breastfeeding mothers, in patients with heart failure or epilepsy or in pregnancy. *Interactions:* Anticoagulants, quinolones, sulphonylurea anti-diabetic drugs, hydantoins.

Meflam ➤ mefenamic acid.

mefloquine (Lariam) is an antimalarial drug. It is a derivative of quinine. *Adverse effects* include dizziness, loss of balance, nausea, vomiting, loss of appetite and bowel upsets. It may rarely cause slowing of the heart rate, headache, visual disturbances, conduction defects of the heart, weakness, nerve damage, itching, disturbances of liver function tests, painful muscles, loss of appetite, weakness, noises in the ears (tinnitus), dizziness, loss of balance, sleepiness, bad dreams, sleep disturbances, painful joints, hair loss, fall in blood pressure, nettle-rash, blood disorders and a severe skin disorder (Stevens-Johnson syndrome). Mefloquine may cause mild to very serious psychotic disturbances (e.g. anxiety, depression, sleep disturbances, nightmares, hallucinations, psychotic illness) and convulsions. If any of these occur stop the drug immediately. *Warning:* Patients receiving mefloquine to prevent malaria should take medical advice *before* taking the next weekly dose if they develop any kind of nerve, mood or mental symptoms. Start mefloquine at least one week before departure to give time for assessing whether the drug is going to be tolerated. *Precautions:* When used to prevent malaria it should not be given to patients who have impaired kidney or liver function, a history of psychiatric illness, or convulsions (or a family history of convulsions). Do not use in first three months of pregnancy or in breastfeeding mothers or in patients allergic to quinine. Women of childbearing potential should avoid sexual intercourse or use contraceptives during and for three months after treatment. Do not use to prevent malaria in patients with epilepsy or conduction defects of the heart. *Interactions:* Sodium valproate, oral live typhoid vaccination, halofantrine (danger of fatal irregularities of heart rhythm). Delay use until twelve hours after taking quinine or a related compound. May affect ability to drive for up to three weeks.

Mefoxin ➤ cefoxitin.

Megace ➤ megestrol.

megestrol (Megace) is a progestogen ➤ progestogens.

Meggezones lozenges ➤ menthol.

Melleril ➤ thioridazine.

meloxicam (Mobic) is a non-steroidal anti-inflammatory drug (NSAID) which has less risk of damaging the lining of the stomach or causing kidney damage (see Chapter 32). *Adverse effects and Precautions* ➤ non-steroidal anti-inflammatory drugs (NSAIDs).

melphalan (Alkeran) is an anti-cancer drug. See Chapter 51. *Adverse effects* include nausea, vomiting, diarrhoea, mouth ulcers, bleeding from the intestine, and loss of hair. It damages the bone marrow, producing blood disorders (this may become apparent for four–six weeks). *Precautions* see Chapter 51 on anti-cancer drugs.

Meltus Dry Cough (Junior) contains dextromethorphan and pseudoephedrine; **Meltus Expectorant (Junior)** contains guaifenesin; **Meltus Expectorant with Decongestant (Adult)** contains guaifenesin, pseudoephedrine and menthol ➤ individual entry for each drug.

menadiol (menadiol sodium diphosphate) is a water-soluble preparation of vitamin K used to treat or prevent bleeding in patients with obstructive jaundice and to prevent vitamin K deficiencies in malabsorption syndromes. *Adverse effects:* It may cause haemolytic anaemia. In newborn babies (especially if they are premature) it may cause kernicterus. *Precautions:* It should not be used in newborn babies, infants or in late pregnancy.

Mengivac (A+C) is a meningococcal vaccine given by deep subcutaneous injection or by intramuscular injection.

Meningitec is a meningoccal vaccine given by intramuscular injection.

Menjugate is a meningoccal vaccine given by intramuscular injection.

Menogon ➤ menotrophin.

Menopur ➤ menotrophin.

Menorest skin patches contain oestradiol (an oestrogen) used for HRT ➤ HRT.

menotrophin (Menogon, Menopur) is a gonadotrophic hormone (➤ gonadotrophins). It is used to treat anovulatory infertility and to stimulate ovulation in IVF treatment. It is also used to treat males with underdeveloped testicles due to a deficient production of gonadotrophic hormones by the pituitary gland. In males it may cause allergic reactions. *Adverse effects* in females include over-stimulation of the ovaries (➤ Humegon), multiple births and allergic reactions. It may cause discomfort at the site of injection and, rarely, fever and joint pains. Very rarely the ovaries may enlarge and rupture. *Precautions:* It should not be used in pregnancy. In both males and females any endocrine disorders or related brain disorders should be treated before therapy starts.

menthol is a colourless, crystalline substance with a strong odour and aromatic taste. By mouth it gives a warm feeling followed by a cold sensation in the mouth and throat. Inhalations have the same effect on the nose. It may be obtained from volatile oils of *Mentha* or manufactured from thymol. It is included in preparations to treat muscular rheumatism (➤ rubefacients), to be inhaled (in hot water) to relieve a blocked nose and catarrh, sucked as pastilles or applied to the chest as a vapour rub.

Mentholatum contains amylmetacresol and menthol ➤ amylmetacresol, menthol.

mepacrine (mepacrine hydrochloride) is used to treat giardiasis (a bowel infection). It is also occasionally used to treat discoid lupus erythematosus (a skin disorder). *Adverse effects* include headache, stomach and bowel upsets and dizziness. Large doses may cause nausea and vomiting and occasionally acute toxic psychosis and stimulation of the nervous system. Prolonged treatment may colour the skin and urine yellow. It may rarely cause severe skin peeling, liver damage, damage to red cell production (causing aplastic anaemia), a blue/black discoloration of the palate and nails and deposits in the cornea of the eyes causing visual disturbances. *Precautions:* Do not use in patients with psoriasis. Use with caution in patients with a history of psychosis, impaired liver function and in the elderly.

mepivacaine (mepivacaine hydrochloride, in Estradurin, Scandonest) is a local anaesthetic. See Chapter 44.

Mepranix ➤ metoprolol.

meprobamate (in Equagesic) is an anti-anxiety drug. See Chapter 2. *Adverse effects* include drowsiness, loss of appetite, nausea, vomiting, diarrhoea, weakness, headache, dizziness, loss of control over voluntary movements (ataxia) and disturbance of vision. Rarely, it may cause rapid beating of the heart, a drop in blood pressure, skin rashes, allergic reactions and blood disorders. Some patients become excited instead of calm. *Precautions:* Do not use in patients with porphyria (a hereditary disorder of metabolism), severe lung disorders, alcoholism or in breastfeeding mothers. Use with caution in patients with impaired kidney or liver function, epilepsy, depression, in pregnancy, in patients with a history of alcohol or drug abuse, severe personality disorders, in the elderly or debilitated or in patients with chronic breathing disorders. It may produce dependence, increase the effects of alcohol and impair ability to drive motor vehicles or operate moving machinery. The drug should be withdrawn very gradually. *Interactions:* Alcohol, sleeping drugs and any other drugs that depress brain function.

meptazinol (meptazinol hydrochloride, Meptid) is an opiate (opioid) pain-reliever with similar properties to morphine (see Chapter 30), but it is less likely to depress breathing. *Adverse effects and Precautions* ➤ morphine.

Meptid ➤ meptazinol.

mepyramine (Anthisan cream) is an antihistamine cream used in the treatment of insect bites, stings and nettle-rash.

Merbentyl ➤ dicycloverine.

mercaptamine (cysteamine) (Cystagon) is used to treat nephropathic cystinosis (an anomaly of kidney tubular function in which there is impaired re-absorption of cystine leading to nerve damage). *Adverse effects* include breath and body odour, nausea, vomiting, diarrhoea, anorexia, lethargy, fever, rash, dehydration, high blood pressure, abdominal discomfort, gastroenteritis, drowsiness, disorder of the brain (encephalopathy), headache, nervousness, depression, anaemia, decrease in white blood cells. *Precautions:* Do not use while pregnant or breastfeeding or in patients with an allergy to mercaptamine or penicillamine.

mercaptopurine (Puri-Nethol) is an anticancer drug. See Chapter 51. *Adverse effects* include nausea, vomiting, diarrhoea, ulcers in the lining of the intestine and liver damage. It causes bone-marrow damage, which produces blood disorders. *Precautions:* See Chapter 51 on anti-cancer drugs.

Mercilon is a combined oral contraceptive. See p. 216.

Merocaine antiseptic lozenges contain cetylpyridinium (an antiseptic) and benzocaine (a local anaesthetic). They are used to treat sore mouths and throats. *Adverse effects and Precautions:* ➤ cetylpyridinium, benzocaine.

Merocet preparations ➤ cetylpyridinium.

Meronem ➤ meropenem.

meropenem (Meronem) is a beta-lactam antibiotic (see p. 266). *Adverse effects* include nausea, vomiting, diarrhoea, abdominal pain, headache, itching, rashes, pins and needles, convulsions, blood disorders and disturbances of liver function. Rarely it may cause thrush infections and colitis. It may cause pain and inflammation at the site of injection. *Precautions:* Use with caution in patients allergic to penicillins, cephalosporins or other beta-lactam antibiotics, in patients with impaired liver or kidney function, history of colitis, in pregnancy or in breastfeeding mothers. Do not use in patients allergic to meropenem.

mesalazine (Asacol, Pentasa, Salofalk) is 5-aminosalicylic acid (a salicylate) used to treat ulcerative colitis and Crohn's disease (chronic diarrhoeal disorders). *Adverse effects* include headache, nausea, diarrhoea, abdominal pain, flare-up of colitis, liver or kidney damage, blood disorders, heart and lung damage and, rarely, reversible damage to the pancreas. *Precautions:* Do not use in patients allergic to aspirin or other salicylates, or in patients with severe impairment of kidney function. Use with caution in patients with mild or moderate impairment of kidney function, if the blood urea is raised, or if there is protein in the urine. Use with caution in pregnancy and breastfeeding mothers. *Interactions:* Do not use with lactulose.

mesna (Uromitexan) is used in patients who are receiving ifosfamide or cyclophosphamide anti-cancer therapy, to prevent these drugs from damaging the bladder. *Adverse effects* include stomach upset, headaches and fatigue if given above maximum recommended dose. Limb and joint pains, depression, irritability, rash, low blood pressure, increase in heart rate and allergic reactions may occur. *Precautions:* Do not use in patients allergic to thiol-containing drugs. See Chapter 51.

mesterolone (Pro-Viron) is a male sex hormone. *Adverse effects and Precautions* are similar to those listed under testosterone ➤ testosterone.

Mestinon ➤ pyridostigmine.

mestranol (Norinyl 1) is a synthetic oestrogen ➤ oestrogens.

Metalyse ➤ tenecteplase.

Metanium ointment contains titanium salts in a silicone base ➤ titanium, silicone. It is used to treat and prevent nappy rash.

metaraminol (Aramine) is a vasoconstrictor sympathomimetic drug which has been used to treat an acute fall in blood pressure. See p. 124. *Adverse effects and Precautions* ➤ noradrenaline(norepinephrine). It is longer-acting than noradrenaline(norepinephrine) and may cause rapid beating of the heart or a prolonged rise in blood pressure.

Metatone tonic mixture contains calcium, potassium, sodium and manganese glycerophosphates, and vitamin B ➤ glycerophosphates.

Meted shampoo contains salicylic acid and sulphur. It is used to treat psoriasis of the scalp, dandruff and seborrhoeic dermatitis ➤ salicylic acid, sulphur.

Metenix ➤ metolazone.

metformin (metformin hydrochloride, Glucamet, Glucophage) is an oral antidiabetic drug. See Chapter 42. *Adverse effects* include loss of appetite, nausea, diarrhoea and vomiting, which are usually related to the dose. Skin rashes, loss of weight and weakness may occasionally occur. It may, rarely, cause lactic acidosis (a metabolic disorder) especially in patients with kidney failure. *Precautions:* Do not use in patients with impaired liver or kidney function, heart failure or dehydration, during pregnancy, in breastfeeding mothers or in patients with alcohol dependence. It may decrease the absorption of vitamin B_{12}. It should not be used by diabetic patients with infections, after surgery or injury – such patients will require insulin. Use with caution in elderly patients. *Interactions:* Beta-blockers, MAOIs, corticosteroids, corticotrophin, diuretics, oral contraceptives, alcohol, bezafibrate, clofibrate, oral anticoagulants, aspirin, phenylbutazone, cyclophosphamide, rifampicin, sulphonamides, chloramphenicol, glucagon.

methadone (amiodarone hydrochloride, Methadose, Methex, Methorose, Physeptone) is an opiate pain-reliever. See Chapter 30. It is used to relieve severe pain, as a cough suppressant and also in treating heroin addicts. Methadone produces less sedation than morphine. *Adverse effects:* Minor adverse effects, particularly in ambulant patients, include nausea, vomiting, dizziness, euphoria, sedation, faintness, dry mouth and constriction of the pupils. Methadone may cause a fall in blood pressure and depress respiration. Children tolerate only very small doses. *Precautions:* Methadone depresses respiration; it is therefore undesirable as a pain-reliever in childbirth. It should not be used in doses to relieve pain in patients with severe chest disorders or in patients who are up and about. It should be used with caution in patients with chronic liver disease. *Drug dependence:* Methadone produces drug tolerance and dependence of the morphine type. See p. xxviii.

Methadose ➤ methadone.

Metharose ➤ methadone

methenamine (hexamine, Hiprex) is used to treat infections of the urinary system, see Chapter 49. It forms formaldehyde in the urine and only works if the urine is made acid. *Adverse effects:* It may cause stomach and bowel upsets. If taken in large doses it may cause painful and frequent urination, cystitis and blood in the urine. Skin rashes may occasionally occur. *Precautions:* It should not be given to patients who are severely dehydrated, or who have severe impaired kidney function or acidity of the blood (metabolic acidosis). *Interactions:* Sulphonamides, alkalizing drugs.

Methex ➤ methadone.

methionine (in Paradote) is an essential amino acid in the diet. It is used as an antidote to treat paracetamol overdosage, see p. 160.

methocarbamol (Robaxin) is a skeletal muscle relaxant. See p. 42. *Adverse effects* include light-headedness, dizziness, drowsiness, nausea, allergic reactions, weariness, restlessness, anxiety, confusion, and convulsions. *Precautions:* Do not use in patients allergic to it or in patients in a coma, with brain damage, epilepsy or myasthenia gravis (muscle weakness due to a neuromuscular abnormality). Do not use injections in patients with impaired kidney function. Use with caution in pregnancy, in breastfeeding mothers and in patients with impaired kidney or liver function. May increase effects of alcohol and impair ability to drive motor vehicles or operate moving machinery. *Interactions:* Alcohol, sedatives, sleeping drugs or any drug that depresses brain function, stimulants, antimuscarinic drugs.

methotrexate (Maxtrex) is an anti-cancer drug (see Chapter 51) which is also used to treat psoriasis (see p. 260) and severe rheumatoid arthritis (see p. 261). *Adverse effects* include nausea, vomiting, diarrhoea, abdominal pain, skin rashes and loss of hair. Ulcers in the mouth and intestine may occur with high doses. It may cause severe allergic reactions, sensitivity of the skin to sunlight, liver damage and bone-marrow damage leading to serious blood disorders. *Precautions:* Do not use in patients with severe impairment of liver or kidney function, serious anaemia or depressed white cell count, in pregnancy or in breastfeeding mothers. Use with caution in patients with evidence of impaired kidney or liver function, depressed bone-marrow function, disorders of the stomach or intestine or psychiatric disorders. Use with utmost caution in the elderly and in children. Regular tests of liver, kidney and bone-marrow function should be carried out. *Interactions:* alcohol, live vaccines, folic acid, etretinate, anti-epileptic drugs and NSAIDs.

methotrimeprazine ➤ levomepromazine.

methoxamine (Vasoxine) is a vasoconstrictor sympathomimetic drug used to treat an acute fall in blood pressure which can occur under general anaesthesia. See p. 124. *Adverse effects and Precautions* ➤ nor-

adrenaline(norepinephrine). It is longer-acting than noradrenaline(norepinephrine) and therefore it may cause a prolonged rise in blood pressure.

methylcellulose (Celevac) is a bulking agent which swells in water and is used to treat constipation (see Chapter 21) and diarrhoea (see Chapter 20). It also absorbs water in the stomach and is said to relieve hunger because it swells and makes the stomach feel full. It is used as a slimming drug. See Chapter 8. *Adverse effects* include wind, abdominal distension, intestinal obstruction. *Precautions:* Do not use in patients with a bowel obstruction. Drink plenty of fluids.

methyl cysteine ➤ mecysteine.

methyldopa (Aldomet) is a central alpha stimulant used to treat raised blood pressure. See Chapter 25. *Adverse effects:* Drowsiness may occur in the first few days of treatment; this usually disappears on its own or on reduction of the dose. Other adverse effects include diarrhoea, dryness of the mouth, nausea, depression, mental disturbances, nightmares, fluid retention, stuffiness of the nose, fever, dizziness and failure to ejaculate. Rarely, joint and muscle pains, impotence, skin rashes, parkinsonism, jaundice, and weakness may occur. Blood disorders (haemolytic anaemia) have been reported and liver function may be impaired in the first few weeks of treatment. Methyldopa may occasionally make the urine dark. *Precautions:* Do not use in patients with depression, active liver disease, porphyria (an error of metabolism) or phaeochromocytoma (a tumour of the sympathetic nervous system). Methyldopa should be used with caution by patients with anaemia, impaired kidney or liver function, or with a history of liver disease. A severe fall in blood pressure may occur during anaesthesia in patients on methyldopa. A positive direct Coombs' test may occur in 20% of patients. This may affect the cross-matching of blood for a blood transfusion. Liver function tests and blood counts should be carried out at regular intervals during treatment. *Interactions:* Tricyclic antidepressants, phenothiazine antipsychotic drugs, lithium, MAOIs, sympathomimetic drugs. Injections of methyldopa contain methyldopate hydrochloride.

methyl hydroxybenzoate (in Instillagel) is used as a preservative in creams and ointments and also in foods.

methylphenidate (methylphenidate hydrochlorate, Ritalin) is a stimulant (see Chapter 5) used to treat hyperactive children (attention deficit disorder). *Adverse effects* ➤ amfetamine. They include stomach and bowel upsets, headache, insomnia, decreased appetite, rash, fever, nettle-rash, painful joints, hair loss, skin peeling and blood disorders. *Precautions:* Do not use in children with marked anxiety, agitation or tension, tics, a family history of Tourette's syndrome, disordered heart rhythm, glaucoma, or over-active thyroid gland. Use with caution in children with psychoses, raised blood pressure, emotional instability or epilepsy. Monitor height, weight, blood pressure and blood count at regular intervals. *Interactions:* Anticoagulants, anti-epileptic drugs, tricyclic antidepressants, MAOIs, guanethidine, alcohol.

methylphenobarbital (methylphenobarbitone, Prominal) is a long-acting barbiturate used in the treatment of epilepsy. See Chapter 15. *Adverse effects and Precautions* ➤ phenobarbital.

methylphenobarbitone ➤ methylphenobarbital.

methylprednisolone is a corticosteroid (see Chapter 37). It is present in Depo-Medrone and Depo-Medrone with Lidocaine injections, Medrone tablets, and in Solu-Medrone injections. *Adverse effects and Precautions:* See Chapter 37.

methylrosanilium chloride ➤ crystal violet.

methyl salicylate (oil of wintergreen, in Balmosa, in Radian-B) is used in rheumatic rubs and liniments ➤ rubefacients. It is also present in Monphytol and Phytex preparations used to treat fungal infections of the skin (e.g. athlete's foot).

methyl undecenoate (in Monphytol) is an antifungal drug, see p. 244.

methysergide (methysergide maleate, Deseril) is used to prevent migraine. See Chapter 34. *Adverse effects* include nausea, drowsiness, dizziness, restlessness, cramps in the legs, mood changes, vomiting, heartburn, stomach upsets, angina, diarrhoea or constipation, loss of control over voluntary movements (ataxia), weakness, weight gain, disorders of circulation in the arms and legs, confusion, insomnia, skin rashes, loss of hair, painful joints and muscles, pains in the chest, breathlessness, heart murmurs, discomfort on passing urine, fall in blood pressure on standing, rapid beating of the heart, and blood disorders. Prolonged use may produce fibrosis (scarring) of tissues at the back of the abdomen (retroperitoneal). *Precautions:* It should not be taken during pregnancy or when breastfeeding and should not be taken by patients with heart or circulatory disorders, with high blood pressure, impaired kidney or liver function, chest disease, urinary tract disorders, severe wasting, or collagen diseases. It should be used with caution in patients with peptic ulcers. Maximum duration of treatment should be six months. Leave one month between courses of treatment. To stop treatment, reduce daily dose slowly over two–three weeks. Patients should have a full medical examination at regular intervals. *Interactions:* Ergot drugs and drugs that constrict the blood vessels.

metipranolol (Minims metipranolol eye drops) is a beta-blocker used to treat glaucoma (see p. 62) in patients who are allergic to the preservatives used in eye drops or who are wearing soft contact lenses. *Adverse effects* include slight stinging of the eyes and transient headache. For general effects ➤ beta-blockers. *Precautions:* It should not be used in patients with asthma or chronic obstructive airways disease, slow disordered heart rhythms, or heart failure. It should be used with caution in pregnancy and in patients with a slow heart rate due to heart block. *Interactions:* Verapamil, other beta-blockers.

metoclopramide (Gastrobid Continus, Gastroflux, Maxolon, in Migramax, Primperan) is an anti-dopaminergic drug used to treat nausea and vomiting. See Chapter 18. It is also used to treat indigestion and acid reflux. See Chapter 19. Metoclopramide is also used in Migravess and Paramax to treat migraine. See Chapter 34. *Adverse effects:* It may cause restlessness, drowsiness, dizziness, and bowel upsets (e.g. diarrhoea, constipation). Prolonged treatment, especially in children and adolescents may cause involuntary movement of the arms, legs and body and, rarely, parkinsonism and tardive dyskinesia (➤ antimuscarinic drugs). It stimulates secretion of the milk-producing hormone prolactin, and may cause breast enlargement in men and milk production. It may also cause depression, neuroleptic malignant syndrome (for symptoms ➤ antipsychotic drugs) and disorders of conduction in the heart (following intravenous use). *Precautions:* Do not use in patients who have had recent surgery on the stomach or intestine, who have a prolactin-dependent breast cancer, or a phaeochromocytoma (tumour of the sympathetic nervous system). Use with caution in pregnancy, in breastfeeding mothers, in patients with impaired kidney or liver function, in patients with porphyria (a hereditary disorder of metabolism), epilepsy or in the elderly, young adults and children. *Interactions:* Antimuscarinic drugs, phenothiazines and butyrophenone antipsychotic drugs. See Chapter 3.

metolazone (Metenix) is a thiazide-like diuretic drug. See Chapter 29. *Adverse effects and Precautions* ➤ thiazide diuretics.

Metopirone ➤ metyrapone.

metoprolol (Betaloc, in Co-Betaloc, Lopresor, Mepranix) is a selective beta-receptor blocker used to treat angina and raised blood pressure ➤ beta-blockers.

Metosyn cream contains fluocinonide.

Metrodin High Purity ➤ urofollitrophin.

Metrogel ➤ metronidazole. It is used on the skin to treat acute flare-ups of acne rosacea. It may cause irritation and it should not be used in pregnancy.

Metrolyl ➤ metronidazole.

metronidazole (Anaback gel, Flagyl, in Flagyl Compak, in Helimet, Metrogel, Metrolyl, Metrotop, Neutratop, Noritate, Rozex, Vaginyl, Zidoval, Zyomet) is a nitroimidazole antibacterial drug. See p. 272. *Adverse effects* include loss of appetite, nausea, vomiting, stomach and bowel upsets, drowsiness, headache, dizziness, loss of control over voluntary movements (ataxia), generally feeling unwell, unpleasant taste, coated tongue, dryness of the mouth, skin rashes, and allergic reactions. Prolonged treatment may cause nerve damage and a reduced white blood cell count and high doses may, very rarely, cause seizures. It may cause the urine to be stained brown. *Precautions:* When taken with alcohol the patient may experience flushing of the face, headache, dizziness and nausea. It should be used with caution in pregnancy and in breastfeeding mothers, in patients with impaired liver function or nerve or brain disorders. *Interactions:* Alcohol, oral anticoagulants, phenobarbitone, lithium. Patients should be carefully monitored for adverse effects if treatment goes on for more than ten days.

Metrotop gel contains metronidazole. It is used to deodorize certain tumours by killing anaerobic bacteria that break down tissue to release an offensive smell. It may cause irritation where it is applied and it should not be used in pregnancy or in breastfeeding mothers ➤ metronidazole.

metyrapone (Metopirone) is an aldosterone-blocker used to treat Cushing's syndrome and fluid retention due to increased aldosterone secretion (see p. 148). *Adverse effects* include nausea and vomiting, dizziness, headache, allergic reactions and a drop in blood pressure. *Precautions:* Do not use in pregnancy or in breastfeeding mothers. Do not use in patients with underactivity of the adrenal glands. Use with caution in patients with underworking of the pituitary gland.

mexiletine (mexiletine hydrochloride, Mexitil) is used to treat disorders of heart rhythm. See Chapter 24. *Adverse effects* include nausea, vomiting, dizziness, drowsiness, constipation, confusion, pins and needles, double vision, alterations of heart rate, fall in blood pressure, and very rarely tremor, difficulty in speaking, confusion, mental disturbances, jaundice, liver damage and blood disorders. *Precautions:* Do not use in patients with slow heart rate (bradycardia) or severe heart block. Use with caution in patients with impaired liver function. Monitor blood pressure and ECG closely.

Mexitil and **Mexitil PL** ➤ mexiletine.

Miacalcic ➤ calcitonin (salmon).

mianserin (mianserin hydrochloride) is a tetracyclic antidepressant. See Chapter 4. *Adverse effects* include drowsiness and occasionally damage to the bone marrow, producing serious blood disorders (particularly in the elderly). Other adverse effects include tremor, sweating, faintness and light-headedness on standing up after lying or sitting down, disorders of liver function and jaundice, convulsions, swelling of the breasts with milk production and soreness of the nipples, fluid retention (e.g. ankleswelling), joint pains, arthritis, flu-like symptoms, skin rashes and increased heart rate. *Precautions:* Do not use in patients with mania, severe liver disease or in breastfeeding mothers. Use with caution in pregnancy, in the elderly, and in patients with an enlarged prostate gland or who have had a heart attack (myocardial infarction).

Because of the risk of blood disorders, patients should have a blood test before treatment starts and every four weeks during the first three months of treatment. The drug should be stopped if the patient develops a fever, sore throat, sore mouth or other signs of infection. It should also be stopped if patient develops jaundice, hypomania or convulsions. *Interactions:* MAOIs, alcohol, anticoagulants.

Micanol cream is used in the treatment of psoriasis ➤ dithranol.

Micardis ➤ telmisartan.

Micolette micro-enema contains sodium citrate, sodium laurylsulphoacetate and glycerol. It is used to treat constipation and to clear the bowel before and after surgery and before a rectal examination. Do not use in patients suffering from inflammatory or ulcerative disorders of the bowel or acute stomach or bowel disorders. See Chapter 21.

miconazole (miconazole nitrate, in Daktacort, Daktarin, Dumi-coat, in Gyno-Daktarin) is an antifungal drug. See Chapter 47.

Micralax micro-enema contains sodium citrate, sodium alkylsulphoacetate and sorbic acid ➤ sodium citrate. It is used to treat constipation and to clear the bowel before endoscopy or X-ray examination. See Chapter 21. Do not use in patients with inflammatory bowel disease.

Microgynon-30 is an oral contraceptive, see p. 216.

Micronor is a progestogen-only contraceptive, see p. 217.

Micronor HRT tablets ➤ norethisterone.

Microval is a progestogen-only oral contraceptive, see p. 217.

Mictral effervescent granules contain nalidixic acid, sodium citrate, citric acid and sodium bicarbonate ➤ nalidixic acid. They are used to treat cystitis, see p. 281.

midazolam (Hypnovel) is a benzodiazepine drug used before surgical procedures to produce sedation with amnesia. *Adverse effects and Precautions* ➤ benzodiazepines.

Midrid capsules contain paracetamol and isometheptene. They are used to treat migraine and throbbing headaches. See Chapter 34 and ➤ paracetamol, isometheptene.

Mifegyne ➤ mifepristone.

mifepristone (Mifegyne) is a progesterone blocker used to produce an abortion up to sixty-three days of pregnancy. Progesterone (see Chapter 40) plays a central role in the establishment and maintenance of pregnancy. It stimulates the lining of the womb (which has become thickened by oestrogens in the first two weeks of the menstrual cycle) to become secretory in order to provide nutrition in case a fertilized egg embeds on its surface. If this occurs, the lining, under the influence of progesterone, develops further in order to provide more nutrition. The increased production of progesterone also causes the neck of the womb to close off, and blocks the effects of other chemicals (prostaglandins) which, if fertilization does not occur, cause the shedding of the lining of the womb (a menstrual period). It also blocks the effects of a hormone (oxytocin) that causes the womb to contract to produce a menstrual period. In addition, progesterone prevents the growth of other follicles in the ovaries (see p. 197). These effects produced by progesterone are aimed at protecting the embryo and providing its nutrition. Progesterone produces its effects by stimulating progesterone receptors in the womb, ovaries and elsewhere. Mifepristone competes with progesterone at these progesterone receptors and blocks its effects. This results in the death of the embryo because its nutrition is cut off and its attachment to the lining of the womb is loosened. The blocking of progesterone receptors also causes a profound fall in chorionic gonadotrophin produced in the womb by the developing embryo (see Chapter 40). This causes the corpus luteum in the ovary to shrink and cut off the supply of progesterone, thus adding to the direct anti-progesterone effects of mifepristone. The changes triggered in the lining of the womb (endometrium) result in the release of prostaglandins which further add to the effects of mifepristone, resulting in the expulsion of the embryo through its loosening from the endometrium, increased contractions of the womb and softening and opening of the neck of the womb (cervix). In other words, it causes an abortion. Mifepristone produces an abortion in about 88% of cases, but when it is combined with a prostaglandin (prostaglandin E, an analogue of gemeprost) it produces a complete evacuation of the womb in 95% of women up to sixty-three days from the first day of their last period. *Adverse effects* include generally feeling unwell, fainting, nausea, vomiting and rashes, and gemeprost may cause flushing, dizziness, chills, headache and, very rarely, heart and circulatory disorders. The combined treatment with mifepristone by mouth and gemeprost by vaginal pessary thirty-one–forty-eight hours later may cause two major problems: excessive vaginal bleeding and pain. The blood loss may be so severe that the woman has to be given a blood transfusion and the womb scraped (curettage). The pain is often so severe that about one in three women will need a morphine-like drug to relieve the pain. *Precautions:* The abortion treatment should not be given if there is the slightest suspicion of an ectopic pregnancy or if the woman has adrenal failure (mifepristone produces some anti-glucocorticosteroid effects because of the similarity between progesterone receptors and glucocorticosteroid receptors). It should not be given to any woman who has had long-term treatment with a glucocorticosteroid, has a bleeding disorder or who is receiving anticoagulant drugs. It should not be used in women over thirty-five years of age who are moderate or heavy smokers, or who have impaired kidney or liver function. The abortion treatment should be used with the utmost caution in women who suffer from asthma or chronic airways disease, heart disease or raised blood pressure. Women with artificial heart valves or a past history of infective endocarditis (infection and inflammation of the lining of the heart) should be given full antibiotic cover. For two days before, during the day of treatment and for one day after treatment with gemeprost, women should not smoke or consume alcohol. *Interactions:* Do not take aspirin or an NSAID for at least eight–twelve days after treatment with mifepristone.

Migrafen ➤ ibuprofen.

Migraleve pink tablets contain buclizine, paracetamol and codeine; yellow tablets contain paracetamol and codeine. They are used to treat migraine. See Chapter 34. *Adverse effects and Precautions* ➤ buclizine, paracetamol, codeine.

MigraMax is a powder for the treatment of migraine. It contains aspirin and metoclopramide ➤ aspirin, metoclopramide.

Migril tablets contain ergotamine, cyclizine and caffeine. They are used to treat migraine. See Chapter 34, *Adverse effects and Precautions* ➤ ergotamine, cyclizine.

Mildison Lipocream contains hydrocortisone in a cream base with 70% oil. It is used to treat eczema and dermatitis ➤ hydrocortisone.

Milpar contains liquid paraffin and magnesium hydroxide. It is used as a laxative. See Chapter 21 and ➤ liquid paraffin, magnesium hydroxide.

milrinone (Primacor) is a phosphodiesterase-blocker used in the short-term treatment of severe congestive heart failure. See Chapter 23. *Adverse effects* include fall in blood pressure, angina, headache, disorders of heart rhythm, and tremor. *Precautions:* It should be used with caution in pregnancy and in breastfeeding mothers. Tests of blood chemistry and kidney function should be carried out at regular intervals. Also ➤ enoximone.

mineralocorticoids, see Chapter 37.

Minihep ➤ heparin.

Min-I-Jet Adrenaline ➤ adrenaline(epinephrine).

Min-I-Jet Atropine Sulphate ➤ atropine.

Min-I-Jet Bretylium Tosylate ➤ bretylium.

Min-I-Jet Calcium Chloride ➤ calcium chloride.

Min-I-Jet Frusemide ➤ furosemide.

Min-I-Jet Glucose ➤ glucose.

Min-I-Jet Isoprenaline ➤ isoprenaline.

Min-I-Jet Lignocaine ➤ lidocaine.

Min-I-Jet Morphine Sulphate ➤ morphine.

Min-I-Jet Naloxone ➤ naloxone.

Min-I-Jet Sodium Bicarbonate ➤ sodium bicarbonate.

Minims* Amethocaine single-dose eye drops ➤ amethocaine. May cause transient burning sensation and dermatitis. *Interactions:* sulphonamides.

Minims* Artificial Tears are single-dose eye drops containing hydroxyethylcellulose and sodium chloride.

Minims* Atropine single-dose eye drops ➤ atropine. Do not use in patients with closed-angle glaucoma.

Minims* Benoxinate single-dose eye drops ➤ oxybuprocaine.

Minims* Chloramphenicol eye drops contain chloramphenicol. They are used to treat bacterial infections of the eye. *Adverse effects:* May produce allergic reactions in the eye (stop the drug immediately) and blood disorders (aplastic anaemia) ➤ chloramphenicol. *Precautions:* Remove contact lenses. *Interactions:* Chymotrypsin.

Minims* Cyclopentolate single-dose eye

---

* All Minims eyedrop preparations are preservative free.

drops ➤ cyclopentolate. Do not use in patients with closed-angle glaucoma.

Minims* Dexamethasone single-dose eye drops ➤ dexamethasone.

Minims* Fluorescein single-dose eye drops ➤ fluorescein. Do not wear soft contact lenses.

Minims* Gentamicin single-dose eye drops ➤ gentamicin.

Minims* Homatropine single-dose eye drops ➤ homatropine. Do not use in closed-angle glaucoma.

Minims* Lidocaine and Fluorescein single-dose eye drops ➤ lidocaine and fluorescein.

Minims* Metipranolol single-dose eye drops ➤ metipranolol.

Minims* Neomycin single-dose eye drops ➤ neomycin.

Minims* Phenylephrine single-dose eye drops ➤ phenylephrine.

Minims* Pilocarpine single-dose eye drops ➤ pilocarpine. Do not use in patients with closed-angle glaucoma, raised blood pressure, coronary artery disease, overactive thyroid or diabetes. *Interactions:* Beta-blockers, MAOIs, tricyclic antidepressants.

Minims* Prednisolone single-dose eye drops ➤ prednisolone. May cause rise in pressure in the eye, thinning of the cornea, cataract, fungal infections. Do not use in pregnancy, glaucoma, or viral, tuberculous or bacterial infections.

Minims* Proxymetacaine single-dose eye drops are used as a local anaesthetic in surgical procedures on the eye. *Adverse effects* include irritation of the eye and rarely severe allergic reactions. *Precautions:* Use with caution in patients with a history of allergy, heart disease or overactive thyroid gland,

* All Minims eyedrop preparations are preservative free.

in pregnancy or in breastfeeding mothers. Avoid prolonged use.

Minims* Proxymetacaine and Fluorescein see individual entries above.

Minims* Rose Bengal single-dose eye drops ➤ rose bengal.

Minims* Sodium Chloride single-dose eye drops ➤ sodium chloride.

Minims* Tropicamide single-dose eye drops ➤ tropicamide.

Minitran self-adhesive patches ➤ glyceryl trinitrate.

Minocin preparations ➤ minocycline.

minocycline (Aknemin, Dentomycin, Minocin) is a tetracycline antibiotic. *Adverse effects* include dizziness and vertigo (more common in women), severe peeling skin rashes (exfoliative dermatitis), pigmentation of the skin (sometimes doesn't clear up when drug is stopped), liver damage, blood disorders and raised blood pressure in the brain (benign intracranial hypertension). For other adverse effects ➤ tetracyclines. *Precautions:* Do not use in patients with systemic lupus erythematosis (SLE – a disease of unknown cause with symptoms of fever, muscle and joint pain, blood disorders and skin eruptions), kidney failure, in pregnancy or in breastfeeding mothers. Use with caution in patients with impaired kidney or liver function. For other precautions and interactions ➤ tetracyclines.

Minodiab tablets ➤ glipizide.

minoxidil (Loniten) is a vasodilator drug used to treat raised blood pressure. See Chapter 25. *Adverse effects* include sodium and water retention, ankle-swelling and rapid beating of the heart. Increased growth of hair, which is reversible; skin rashes, weight gain, stomach and bowel upsets, breast tenderness and changes in kidney function tests may occur. *Precautions:* Do not use in patients with a phaeochromocytoma (tumour of the sympathetic nervous system) or porphyria (a hereditary disorder of metabolism). It should not be given to patients with fluid retention and it should always be given with a diuretic and a beta-blocker. It may aggravate heart failure and angina. Lower doses are needed in patients on renal dialysis. Use with caution in patients with angina or who have had a heart attack. Minoxidil is also available as a scalp application to treat male-type baldness ➤ Regaine.

Mintec capsules ➤ peppermint oil.

Minulet is an oral contraceptive. See p. 216.

Miochol solution contains acetylcholine and mannitol. They are used to constrict the pupil during surgery on the front chamber of the eye or removal of a cataract. Do not use in pregnancy or in breast feeding mothers. *Interactions:* Topical non-steroidal anti-inflammatory drugs (NSAIDs) ➤ acetylcholine, mannitol.

Mirapexin ➤ pramipexole.

Mirena is an intrauterine progestogen-only contraceptive. It is inserted into the uterine cavity within seven days of onset of menstruation and is effective for five years.

mirtazapine (Zispin) is used for the treatment of depressive illness. See Chapter 4. *Adverse effects* include weight gain, drowsiness, raised liver enzymes, fluid retention, low blood pressure on standing, skin eruptions, mania, decrease in the number of white blood cells. Signs of infection should be reported. *Precautions:* Do not use in pregnancy or while breastfeeding. Use with caution in patients with kidney or liver damage, epilepsy, brain damage, angina, heart disorders, recent heart attack, low blood pressure, increase in the size of the prostate, glaucoma or diabetes.

misoprostol (in Arthrotec, Cytotec, in Napratec) has a similar structure to a prostaglandin. See Chapter 52. It blocks acid production in the stomach and helps to protect its lining. See Chapter 19. It is used to treat peptic ulcers and to treat and prevent peptic ulcers caused by non-steroidal anti-inflammatory drugs (NSAIDs). *Adverse effects* include diarrhoea (occasionally severe) which may be reduced by taking a smaller dose and avoiding antacid mixtures that contain magnesium. It may occasionally cause nausea, indigestion, rash, dizziness, abdominal pain and wind. It may cause abnormal vaginal bleeding (bleeding between periods, heavy periods and periods in post-menopausal women). *Precautions:* Do not use in pregnancy. Women of childbearing potential should avoid sexual intercourse or use contraception while on treatment because it causes the muscles of the womb to contract. It may cause a fall in blood pressure and should therefore be used with caution in patients with diseases of the heart and circulation. Do not use in breastfeeding mothers.

mistamine ➤ mizolastine.

mitobronitol (Myelobromol) is an anti-cancer drug. See Chapter 51. *Adverse effects* include nausea, vomiting and diarrhoea, loss of hair, skin rashes, irregular periods and bone-marrow damage leading to severe blood disorders. *Precautions* see Chapter 51 on anti-cancer drugs.

mitomycin (Mitomycin C Kyowa) is an anti-cancer antibiotic. See Chapter 51. *Adverse effects* include delayed bone-marrow damage causing blood disorders, loss of hair, impairment of kidney and liver function, fever, nausea and vomiting, and lung damage. *Precautions:* See Chapter 51 on anti-cancer drugs.

Mitomycin C Kyowa ➤ mitomycin.

Mitoxana ➤ ifosfamide.

mitoxantrone (Novantrone, Onkotrone) is an anti-cancer drug. See Chapter 51. *Adverse effects* include loss of hair, bone-marrow damage causing blood disorders, loss of appetite, diarrhoea, fatigue, weakness, fever, bleeding from the intestine, changes in liver function and heart failure. *Precautions:* See Chapter 51 on anti-cancer drugs.

mitozantrone ➤ mitoxantrone.

Mivacron ➤ mivacurium chloride.

mivacurium (Mivacron) is a muscle relaxant used in surgical operations and in patients receiving long-term ventilation in intensive care units, see muscle relaxants p. 42.

mizolastine (Mistamine, Mizollen) is used to treat hayfever and nettle-rash. See Chapter 17. *Adverse effects* include drowsiness, weakness, increased appetite, dry mouth, diarrhoea, indigestion, headache. *Precautions:* Do not use in patients with severe liver damage, heart diseases including arrhythmias, QT prolongation, hypokalaemia (low potassium levels in the blood), slow heart beat; in pregnancy or while breastfeeding. Use with caution in the elderly or in patients with diabetes.

Mizollen ➤ mizolastine.

Mobic ➤ meloxicam.

Mobiflex ➤ tenoxicam.

moclobemide (Manerix) is a *reversible* monoamine oxidase A inhibitor antidepressant drug. See Chapter 4. It is used to treat major depression. *Adverse effects* include nausea, headache, dizziness, agitation, sleep disturbances, restlessness, confusion and changes in liver function tests. *Precautions:* Do not use in patients suffering from acute confusional states or phaeochromocytoma (a tumour of the sympathetic nervous system). Use with caution in agitated and excited patients, in patients with overworking of their thyroid gland or severe impairment of liver function, in pregnancy or in breastfeeding mothers. It may trigger manic episodes in patients suffering from manic depressive illness. *Interactions:* 5HT reuptake blockers, tricyclic and tetracyclic antidepressants, trazodone, cimetidine, some sympathomimetic drugs, pethidine, codeine, morphine, fentanyl. Avoid excessive amounts of tyramine-rich foods. See p. 20.

modafilil (Provigil) is used to treat narcolepsy (a rare sleeping disorder in which the patient keeps falling asleep during the daytime). See Chapter 6. *Adverse effects* include nervousness, excitation, aggression, insomnia, personality disorders, anorexia, headache, euphoria, abdominal pain, stomach and bowel upset, dry mouth, palpitations, rapid heart beat, high blood pressure, tremor and itching. *Precautions:* Do not use in patients with heart disorders, severe liver or kidney failure, pregnancy (use adequate contraception), or while breastfeeding. Use with caution in patients with severe liver or kidney failure.

Modalim ➤ ciprofibrate.

Modecate ➤ fluphenazine.

Modisol XL ➤ isosorbide mononitrate.

Moditen ➤ fluphenazine.

Modrasone cream and ointment ➤ alclometasone.

Modrenal ➤ trilostane.

Moducren tablets contain timolol (a nonselective beta-blocker), amiloride (a potassium-sparing diuretic) and hydrochlorothiazide (a thiazide diuretic). They are used to treat raised blood pressure. See Chapter 25. *Adverse effects and Precautions* ➤ beta-blockers, thiazide diuretics, amiloride.

Moduret-25 ➤ co-amilozide.

Moduretic ➤ co-amilozide.

moexipril (Perdix) is an ACE inhibitor. It is used to treat raised blood pressure (see Chapter 25). *Adverse effects* include headache, dizziness, fatigue, flushing, cough and skin rashes. *Precautions:* Do not use in patients with a history of angioedema (allergic swelling of the mouth and throat) – stop at the earliest signs. Do not use in pregnancy or in breastfeeding mothers. Use with caution in patients with impaired kidney or liver function, or obstruction to the flow of blood from the heart into the main artery (aortic stenosis) or into the artery to a kidney (renal stenosis). *Interactions:* Diuretics, calcium-channel blockers, lithium and drugs that affect blood potassium levels.

Mogadon ➤ nitrazepam.

Molcer ear drops ➤ docusate sodium.

molgramostim (Leucomax) is a bioengineered human growth factor that stimulates the production of white blood cells. It is used to reduce the incidence and duration of reductions in white blood cells (neutrophils) in individuals being treated with anti-cancer drugs for cancer not affecting blood-forming tissues. It is also used to stimulate white cell production in patients who have had a bone-marrow transplant and in patients whose white cell production has been reduced by ganciclovir which is used to treat AIDS-related cytomegalovirus infections of the eyes. *Adverse effects* include loss of appetite, nausea, diarrhoea, vomiting, weakness, fatigue, breathlessness, flushing, chills, fever, muscle and joint pains, headache, sweating, abdominal pain, itching and dizziness. Rarely, severe complications may develop such as severe allergic reactions, heart failure, disorders of heart rhythm, confusion and convulsions. *Precautions:* Do not use in patients under eighteen years of age. Use with caution in pregnancy and breastfeeding mothers. Monitor blood cells and proteins at regular intervals. Carefully monitor patients with chest disorders and immune deficiency disorders (e.g. AIDS).

Molipaxin ➤ trazodone.

mometasone (mometasone furoate, Elocon) is a potent corticosteroid used in skin applications to treat dermatitis, psoriasis and eczema. *Adverse effects and Precautions:* See corticosteroid skin applications p. 241. It is also used as a nasal spray (Nasonex) to prevent and treat hayfever.

Monit, **Monit SR** and **Monit XL** ➤ isosorbide mononitrate.

monoamine-oxidase inhibitors (MAOIs), see Chapter 4.

Mono Cedocard Retard ➤ MCR-50.

Monoclate-P ➤ factor VIII fraction, dried (human anti-haemophilic fraction, dried).

Monocor ➤ bisoprolol.

monoethanolamine oleate ➤ ethanolamine oleate.

Monomax SR ➤ isosorbide mononitrate.

Mononine ➤ factor IX fraction (dried).

Monoparin and **Monoparin Calcium** contain heparin calcium ➤ heparin.

Monosorb XL ➤ isosorbide mononitrate.

Monotrim preparations ➤ trimethoprim.

Monovent preparations ➤ terbutaline.

Monozide 10 tablets contain bisoprolol (a selective beta-blocker) and hydrochlorothiazide (a thiazide diuretic). They are used to treat raised blood pressure. See Chapter 25. *Adverse effects and Precautions* ➤ beta-blockers, thiazide diuretics.

Monphytol paint contains chlorbutanol, methyl undecenoate, salicylic acid, methyl salicylate, propyl undecenoate. It is used to treat athlete's foot. It may occasionally sting when applied to an inflamed area of skin. *Precautions:* Do not apply to extensive areas of skin. Do not use in pregnancy.

montelukast (Singulair) is used as supplementary therapy in mild to moderate asthma, inadequately controlled by inhaled corticosteroids and short-acting β_2-stimulants. It is also used to treat exercise-induced bronchoconstriction. See Chapter 14. *Adverse effects* include abdominal pain, stomach and bowel upset, headache, rash, insomnia, dizziness, fatigue, drowsiness, pain in joints or muscles, generally feeling unwell, nightmares, irritability, restlessness, allergic reactions. *Precautions:* Do not substitute for inhaled or oral steroid therapy. Do not use to relieve an asthma attack. Use with caution in pregnancy or while breastfeeding.

Moorland is an antacid containing aluminium, bismuth, calcium, magnesium, light kaolin ➤ individual entry for each drug.

MOPP contains three anti-cancer drugs: mustine, vincristine (Oncovin) and procarbazine and prednisolone (a corticosteroid). See Chapter 51 on anti-cancer drugs and Chapter 37 on corticosteroids.

Moraxen are rectal tampons (i.e. non-dissolving suppositories) containing morphine ➤ morphine.

Morcap SR capsules contain sustained-release pellets of morphine ➤ morphine.

Morhulin ointment contains cod liver oil and zinc oxide. It is a skin softener used to treat disorders such as nappy rash, eczema and pressure sores.

moroctocog alfa (Refacto) is a recombinant human factor VIII used to prevent and treat bleeding in haemophilia A.

morphine (morphine hydrochloride and morphine sulphate, in Cyclimorph, Min-I-Jet Morphine Sulphate, Moraxen, Morcap SR, MST Continus, MXL, Oramorph solution, Sevredol, Zomorph) is an opiate pain-reliever; see Chapter 30. *Adverse effects* include nausea, loss of appetite, constipation, vomiting, dry mouth, blurred vision, drowsiness and confusion, difficulty in passing urine, vertigo, palpitations, flushing of the face, slowing of the heart rate, fall in body temperature (hypothermia), hallucinations, small pupils, itching, fall in blood pressure on standing up after lying down, restlessness, change in mood and euphoria. These effects occur more often if the patient is up and about rather than in bed. Sneezing and skin rashes may occur. Rarely, large doses may cause depression of breathing, fall in blood pressure, collapse and coma. Convulsions may occur in children. *Precautions:* Babies and young children are very sensitive to the effects of morphine and it should not be given to children under one year of age. Alarming and unusual reactions may occur in the elderly and the debilitated. It should not be used in patients with severe respiratory disorders or after operations on the gallbladder. Do not use in patients who have had a head injury or raised pressure in the brain because it affects the pupils and may interfere with the neurological diagnosis. It should not be used in acute alcoholism and convulsive disorders. It should be used with caution in patients with under-active thyroids or chronic liver disease, low blood pressure, impaired liver function, asthma (do not use during an attack), poor lung function, breastfeeding mothers or in elderly and/or debilitated patients. *Interactions:* Its effects may be increased by MAO inhibitor antidepressant drugs and depressant drugs such as anaesthetics, sleeping drugs, sedatives, anti-anxiety drugs, phenothiazines and other antipsychotic drugs. Alcohol increases the sedative and blood pressure lowering effects of morphine. *Drug dependence:* Drug dependence of the morphine type is a state arising from repeated use of morphine or a morphine-like drug. It is characterized by an overwhelming desire to go on taking the drug, by a tendency to increase the dose, and by psychological and physical dependence. Withdrawal symptoms include running eyes and nose, sneezing, trembling, headache, weakness, sweating, anxiety, insomnia, restlessness, nausea, loss of appetite, vomiting, diarrhoea, muscle cramps and a rise in temperature. See p. xxix.

Motens ➤ lacidipine.

Motifene ➤ diclofenac sodium.

Motilium preparations ➤ domperidone.

Motipress is an antidepressant containing fluphenazine (an antipsychotic drug) and nortriptyline (an antidepressant drug) ➤ fluphenazine, nortriptyline.

Motival ➤ fluphenazine.

Motrin ➤ ibuprofen.

Movelat is a topical heat cream ➤ salicylic acid, thymol.

Movical contains polyethylene glycol and the salts sodium bicarbonate, sodium chloride and potassium chloride. It is used to treat constipation, see Chapter 21. *Adverse effects* include nausea and abdominal distention. *Precautions:* Do not use in patients suffering from an obstructed bowel, ulcers, inflammation or distension of the bowel.

moxisylyte(thymoxamine) (thymoxamine hydrochloride, Opilon) is a selective alpha₁ blocker used as a vasodilator to treat Raynaud's disease. See Chapter 27. *Adverse effects* include nausea, headache, diarrhoea, flushing, dizziness and liver damage. *Precautions:* Do not use in patients allergic to it, in pregnancy, in breastfeeding mothers or in patients with acute liver disease. Use with caution in patients with diabetes, angina or recent heart attack.

moxonidine (Physiotens) is used to treat raised blood pressure (see Chapter 25). It acts on blood pressure controlling centres in the brain by stimulating certain receptors. This reduces the activity of the sympathetic nerves supplying blood vessels in the body, which causes them to dilate. As a consequence peripheral resistance is reduced and the blood pressure falls. *Adverse effects* include headache, dry mouth, dizziness, weakness, nausea, disturbed sleep and flushing. *Precautions:* Do not use in patients with allergic swelling of the face, hands and feet, certain disorders of heart rhythm or heart block, heart failure, coronary heart disease, impaired liver or kidney function or severe slowing of the heart rate. Use with caution in patients with moderate impairment of kidney function, Raynaud's disease, Parkinson's disease, epilepsy, depression or glaucoma. Use with caution in pregnancy and breastfeeding mothers. Withdraw the drug gradually. If stopping treatment with moxonidine and a beta-blocker, withdraw the beta-blocker gradually and stop a few days before withdrawing moxonidine gradually. *Interactions:* Alcohol, sleeping drugs, sedatives, anti-anxiety drugs, tricyclic antidepressants, other anti-blood pressure drugs.

Mrs Cullen's Powders ➤ aspirin.

MST Continus ➤ morphine.

Mucaine suspension contains oxetazaine (local anaesthetic) and the antacids aluminium hydroxide and magnesium hydroxide. It is used to treat inflammation of the oesophagus. *Adverse effects and Precautions* ➤ oxetazaine, antacids.

mucin (in Saliva Orthana artificial saliva) contains glycoproteins. It is present in mucus and in the salivary glands, skin, tendons and cartilage.

Mucodyne preparations ➤ carbocisteine.

Mucogel contains the antacids aluminium hydroxide and magnesium hydroxide ➤ antacids.

mucolytics are used to reduce the stickiness of the sputum (see Chapter 11) and to treat impaired mucus production and tear deficiency in the eyes ➤ Ilube eye drops which contain the mucolytic acetylcysteine.

Mu-Cron tablets contain paracetamol and phenylpropanolamin ➤ paracetamol, phenylpropanolamin

Multiparin ➤ heparin.

mupirocin (Bactroban skin ointment, Bactroban Nasal ointment) is a broad spectrum antibiotic used to treat bacterial skin infections such as impetigo and boils. It is applied up the nose to knock out the source of infection in individuals who carry staphylococci (including methicillin-resistant staphylococci) up their nose. Avoid contact with the eyes. Use with caution in patients with impaired kidney function because the ointment contains macrogol. It may sting the skin.

muscle relaxants, see p. 42.

MUSE ➤ alprostadil.

mustine ➤ chlormethine.

MVPP treatment consists of using three anti-cancer drugs: mustine, vinblastine, procarbazine and the corticosteroid prednisolone ➤ entry on each individual drug and see Chapter 51 on anti-cancer drugs.

MXL sustained-release capsules ➤ morphine.

Mycil ➤ undeconoates.

Mycobutin ➤ rifabutin.

mycophenolate mofetil (Cellcept) is an immunosuppressant drug (see Chapter 17) used to prevent kidney transplant rejection. It is used in combination with cyclosporin and corticosteroids. *Adverse effects* include stomach and bowel upsets, blood disorders, raised blood pressure, chest pains, breathlessness, fluid retention, cough, headache, risk of infections, raised blood sugar levels, raised blood cholesterol levels, kidney damage, acne, blood in the urine, mouth ulcers, allergic reactions, sore gums, rapid heart rate, weight gain, and disorders of the metabolism. *Precautions:* Do not use in pregnancy or in breastfeeding mothers. Use with caution in the elderly and patients with ulcers of the stomach or intestine. Full blood counts should be carried out during therapy. *Interactions:* Aciclovir, antacids, azathioprine, cholestyramine, probenecid.

Mycota cream and powder contains the antifungal drugs zinc undecenoate and undecenoic acid. The spray contains undecenoic acid and dichlorophen. They are used to treat athlete's foot. *Adverse effects and Precautions* ➤ undecenoic acid.

Mydriacyl eye drops ➤ tropicamide.

Mydrilate eye drops ➤ cyclopentolate.

Myleran ➤ busulfan.

Myocet ➤ doxorubicin.

Myocrisin ➤ gold.

myoneural blocking drugs, see p. 42.

Myotonine preparations ➤ bethanecol.

Mysoline ➤ primidone.

myometrial relaxants ➤ uterine relaxants.

nabilone is chemically related to one of the constituents of cannabis. It is used to control nausea and vomiting in patients taking anti-cancer drugs (see Chapter 18). *Adverse effects* include drowsiness, confusion, depression, tremors, vertigo, euphoria, loss of control over voluntary movements (ataxia), difficulty concentrating, sleep disturbances, difficulty with speech, headache, nausea, disorientation, hallucinations, psychosis, dry mouth, decreased appetite, cramps in the abdomen, rapid heart rate, fall in blood pressure on standing up after lying down, and blurred vision. *Precautions:* Use with caution in patients with severe liver disease, a history of serious mental illness, in the elderly and in patients with raised blood pressure or heart disease. Do not use in pregnancy or in breastfeeding mothers. It may impair ability to drive. *Interactions:* It may increase the effects of alcohol, opiate pain-relievers, sedatives and sleeping drugs.

nabumetone (Relifex) is a non-steroidal anti-inflammatory drug (NSAID) ➤ non-steroidal anti-inflammatory drugs.

nadolol (Corgard, in Corgaretic) is a nonselective beta-receptor blocker ➤ beta-blockers.

nafarelin (Synarel) is used to treat endometriosis. It is a synthetic analogue of gonadotrophin-releasing hormone (GnRH). It is given by metered dose nasal spray twice daily between days two and four of the menstrual cycle for a maximum period of six months. It stimulates the release of pituitary gonadotrophins luteinizing hormone (LH) and follicle stimulating hormone (FSH), subsequently causing a desensitization of GnRH receptors in the pituitary. This results in a *decreased* production of LH and FSH, thus preventing growth of an ovarian follicle, ovulation and the effects of LH causing a decline in the production of oestrogens and progesterone, producing a relief of symptoms from endometriosis. *Adverse effects* include allergic reactions, changes in bone density, hot flushes, changes in libido, dryness of the vagina, headaches, emotional upsets, painful muscles, decreased breast size, depression, nerve damage (pins and needles), acne, hair loss, migraine, palpitations, blurred vision and ovarian cysts.

The nasal spray may cause irritation of the lining of the nose. *Precautions:* It should not be used in pregnancy, in breastfeeding mothers or in undiagnosed vaginal bleeding. Sexual intercourse should be avoided or a mechanical form of contraception (not the pill) should be used throughout the period of treatment. It should be used with caution in women with cysts of the ovaries or whose ovarian hormonal control is already suppressed. It should be used with caution in women at risk of developing osteoporosis. *Interactions:* Nasal decongestants.

naftidrofuryl (naftidrofuryl oxalate, Praxilene, Stimlor) activates cells and is used to treat disorders of circulation to the brain and limbs. See Chapter 27. *Adverse effects:* Nausea, stomach pain, rash and liver damage.

nalbuphine (Nubain) is an opiate pain-reliever. See Chapter 30. *Adverse effects and Precautions* ➤ morphine.

nalcrom is an oral preparation of sodium cromoglycate used to treat food allergies. It may cause nausea, joint pains and rashes ➤ sodium cromoglycate.

nalidixic acid (in Mictral, Negram, Uriben) is a quinolone antibacterial drug. See p. 272. It is used in the treatment of infections of the bladder, kidneys and intestine. *Adverse effects* include nausea, vomiting, diarrhoea, dizziness and drowsiness. Myasthenia gravis (muscle weakness due to neuromuscular abnormality) and pains, allergic reactions (e.g. rashes, fever), painful joints (stop drug immediately) and sunlight sensitivity of the skin may occur occasionally. Rarely, headache, blurred vision, weakness, nerve damage, toxic psychosis (depression, confusion, hallucinations and excitement) may occur. Blood disorders, jaundice, haemolysis (in patients with G6PD deficiency) and convulsions have occurred very rarely. *Precautions:* Nalidixic acid should be given with caution to patients with impaired liver function or with disorders of the nervous system, to breastfeeding mothers or in pregnancy. It should not be given to patients subject to convulsions, people with brain disorders, impaired kidney function or porphyria (a hereditary disorder of metabolism), or to babies, children or growing adolescents because of the risk of joint damage. Exposure to strong sunlight should be avoided during treatment. *Interactions:* anticoagulants, antibacterial drugs, melphalan, probenecid.

Nalorex ➤ naltrexone.

naloxone (naloxone hydrochloride, Narcan) is an opiate blocker which is used to reverse the effects of opiate pain-relievers. See Chapter 30. It is also used to treat depressed breathing in newborn babies resulting from the use of opiate pain-relievers during the mother's labour. It may also be used to diagnose acute opiate overdosage. *Adverse effects* include nausea, vomiting and disorders of heart rhythm and rate. In patients dependent upon narcotic drugs naloxone will produce typical withdrawal symptoms. *Precautions:* It should be used with caution in pregnancy (except in labour), in patients with heart disease and in patients physically dependent on opiates. Keep patient under close observation because repeat doses may be needed.

naltrexone (Nalorex) is an opiate blocker used as maintenance treatment in detoxified individuals who were formerly addicted to an opiate (e.g. heroin). *Adverse effects* include abdominal cramps, nausea, vomiting, nervousness, sleep difficulties, headache, reduced energy, dizziness, drowsiness, and muscle and joint pains. It may occasionally cause loss of appetite, constipation, thirst, chest pain, sweating, runny eyes, mood changes, irritability, chills, delayed ejaculation, blood disorders, skin rashes and abnormalities of liver function. *Precautions:* Do not use to treat individuals who are addicted to opiates or who suffer from acute inflammation of the liver or liver failure. Use with caution in patients with impaired liver and kidney function. Tests of liver function should be carried out before and at regular intervals during treatment. Naloxone should be used to test for dependence to opiates.

nandrolone (Deca-Durabolin) is an anabolic steroid. See Chapter 39. It is used in the treatment of aplastic anaemia and post-menopausal osteoporosis. *Adverse effects* include acne, sodium retention producing fluid retention, masculinization and loss of periods in females, loss of sperm in males, stunted growth in young people and, very rarely, liver tumours. *Precautions:* Do not use in pregnancy or in patients with porphyria (a hereditary disorder of metabolism), severe impairment of liver function, prostate cancer or male breast cancer. Use with caution in patients with impaired kidney, heart or liver function, raised blood pressure, diabetes, epilepsy or migraine. Monitor bone growth in young patients. There is a risk of a rise in blood calcium levels in patients with secondary cancer of the bone. *Interactions:* Anti-diabetic drugs.

Napratec combination pack contains tablets of naproxen (an NSAID) and misoprostol (a prostaglandin). The misoprostol protects the stomach lining (see Chapter 19) from damage by naproxen and the combination is used to treat rheumatoid arthritis (see Chapter 32). *Adverse effects and Precautions* ➤ non-steroidal anti-inflammatory drugs (NSAIDs), misoprostol.

Naprosyn ➤ naproxen.

naproxen (Laraflex, in Napratec, Naprosyn, Nycopren, Synflex) is a non-steroidal anti-inflammatory drug (NSAID) ➤ non-steroidal anti-inflammatory drugs.

naratriptan (Naramig) is used to treat acute migraine with or without aura. See Chapter 34. *Adverse effects* include generally feeling unwell, fatigue, dizziness, nausea, pain or sensation of warmth, heaviness or pressure in any part of the body including throat or chest, slow heart beat, rapid heart beat, visual disturbance. *Precautions:* Do not use in patients with heart disorders, severe kidney or liver damage. Use with caution

in patients with moderate liver or kidney damage, an allergy to sulphonamides, those at risk of coronary artery or heart disease, in pregnancy or while breastfeeding.

Naramig ➤ naratriptan.

Narcan ➤ naloxone.

Narcan Neonatal injection ➤ naloxone.

narcotic analgesics ➤ narcotic pain-relievers.

narcotic blockers ➤ opiate blockers and see Chapter 30. For use of the terms narcotic, opiate and opioid see p. 153.

narcotic pain-relievers ➤ opiate pain relievers and see Chapter 30. For use of the terms narcotic, opiate and opioid see p. 153.

Nardil ➤ phenelzine.

Naropin ➤ ropivacaine

Nasacort ➤ triamcinoline.

nasal decongestants, see Chapter 10.

Nasciodine is a heat rub for muscles containing camphor, iodine, menthol, methyl salicylate and turpentine oil.

Naseptin cream contains the antibacterial drugs chlorhexidine and neomycin. It is applied to the inside of the nostrils to eradicate staphylococcal bacteria ➤ chlorhexidine, neomycin.

Nasobec aqueous nasal spray ➤ beclometasone. It is used to treat hayfever. See p. 87. *Adverse effects* include irritation of the nose, disturbances of taste and smell and nosebleeds. *Precautions:* Use with caution in pregnancy and breastfeeding mothers and in patients with untreated infections of the nose. Use with caution when transferring patients from corticosteroids by mouth.

Nasonex ➤ mometasone furoate.

nateglinide (Starlix) is used in combination with metformin in Type II diabetes inadequately controlled by a maximum tolerated dose of metformin alone. See Chapter 42. *Adverse effects* include symptoms of low blood glucose level (hypoglycaemia). Rarely, allergic reactions, raised liver enzymes. *Precautions:* Do not use in patients with Type I diabetes, increase in ketones in diabetes, severe liver damage, in pregnancy or while breastfeeding. Use with caution in patients with a risk of hypoglycaemia, particularly in elderly, in malnourished patients and those with adrenal or pituitary insufficiency.

Natramid ➤ indapamide.

Natrilix and **Natrilix SR** ➤ indapamide.

Navelbine ➤ vinorelbine.

Navidrex ➤ cyclopenthiazide.

Navispare tablets contain cyclopenthiazide (a thiazide diuretic) and amiloride (a potassium-sparing diuretic). They are used to treat raised blood pressure. See Chapter 25. *Adverse effects and Precautions* ➤ thiazide diuretics, amiloride.

Navoban ➤ tropisetron.

Nebcin ➤ tobramycin.

Nebilet ➤ nebivolol.

nebivolol (Nebilet) is a beta-blocker used to treat hypertension. See Chapter 22 and Chapter 25. *Adverse effects* include cold extremities, sleep disturbances, slow heart beat, tiredness on exertion, bronchospasm, heart failure, low blood pressure, stomach and bowel upset, hair loss, decrease in number of platelets in the blood (thrombocytopenia). Unexplained dry eyes or skin rash should be reported. *Precautions:* Do not use in patients with heart disorders, diseases of the arteries, low blood pressure, tumour of the sympathetic nervous system (phaeochromocytoma), acidity of the blood. Use with caution in patients with obstructive airway disease, diabetes, weakness, inadequate blood flow to the brain, atopy (a hereditary disorder giving a predisposition to allergic conditions), liver or kidney damage, hyperthyroidism, in pregnancy or while breastfeeding.

nedocromil sodium (Tilade aerosol) is used to prevent attacks of asthma. See Chapter 14. *Adverse effects* include a bitter taste in the mouth, nausea, stomach and bowel upsets, cough, headache and, rarely, wheezing. *Precautions:* It should be used with caution during pregnancy and in breastfeeding mothers. Nedocromil sodium (Rapitil eye drops) is used to treat allergic conjunctivitis. *Adverse effects* include transient irritation of the eyes and bitter taste in the mouth. *Precautions:* Do not wear contact lenses. Use with caution in pregnancy. See Chapter 17.

nefazodone (Dutonin) is a 5HT re-uptake blocker used to treat depression. See Chapter 4. *Adverse effects* include dry mouth, nausea, weakness, dizziness, sleepiness, fever, chills, fall in blood pressure on standing up after lying or sitting down (postural hypotension), constipation, pins and needles, light-headedness, confusion, ataxia (loss of control over voluntary movements), visual disturbances and, rarely, fainting. *Precautions:* Do not use in breastfeeding mothers. Use with caution in patients with epilepsy, a history of mania or hypomania, in the elderly (especially females), in pregnancy and in patients with impaired kidney or liver function. *Interactions:* Benzodiazepines, lithium, haloperidol, MAOIs, anti-blood pressure drugs, general anaesthetics, alcohol.

nefopam (Acupan) is a non-opiate pain-reliever, See p. 156. *Adverse effects:* Nausea, vomiting, dry mouth, light-headedness, blurred vision, drowsiness, insomnia, sweating, headache and rapid beating of the heart. *Precautions:* It should not be used to relieve the pain of a heart attack. It should be used with caution in patients with impaired kidney or liver function, who suffer from retention of urine, or in pregnancy. It should not be used in patients with a history of convulsions. *Interactions:* MAOIs, antimuscarinic drugs, sympathomimetic drugs, tricyclic antidepressants.

Negram ➤ nalidixic acid.

NeisVac-C is a meningococcal vaccine which is given by intramuscular injection.

nelfinavir (Viracept) is used in combination with antiretroviral nucleoside analogues to treat HIV-1 infected patients with advanced or progressive immunodeficiency. See Chapter 48. *Adverse effects* include stomach and bowel upset, rash, increased creatinine kinase, decreased neutrophils, inflammation of the liver, lipodystrophy (a disturbance of fat metabolism in which the subcutaneous fat disappears over some parts of the body), high cholesterol levels, insulin resistance, diabetes. *Precautions:* Do not use while breastfeeding. Use with caution in patients with kidney or liver damage, haemophilia, diabetes or in pregnancy.

Neo-Bendromax ➤ bendroflumethiazide.

Neoclarityn ➤ desloratadine.

Neo-Cortef ointment and ear drops contain neomycin (an antibiotic) and hydrocortisone (a corticosteroid). They are used as ear drops to treat otitis externa and as eye drops to treat inflammation of the eyes when a secondary bacterial infection is suspected. *Adverse effects and Precautions* ➤ neomycin, hydrocortisone. *Adverse effects* of Neo-Cortef eye applications include rise in pressure inside the eye, thinning of the cornea, cataract and allergic reactions. *Precautions:* Do not use to treat viral, fungal, tubercular or infections of the eye or in glaucoma. Prolonged use in pregnancy and infants should be given with utmost caution. *Adverse effects* of Neo-Cortef ear drops include allergic reactions and superinfections. *Precautions:* Do not use if the ear drum is perforated or in the presence of a viral, fungal, tubercular or pus-filled bacterial infection.

Neo-Cytamen ➤ hydroxocobalamin.

Neogest is a progestogen-only oral contraceptive. See p. 218.

Neo-Mercazole ➤ carbimazole.

neomycin (neomycin sulphate, Neosporin, Nivemycin) is an aminoglycoside antibiotic (➤ aminoglycoside antibiotics). It is used to treat infections of the skin, ears and eyes, and to prepare the bowel before surgery. *Adverse effects:* Neomycin should not be given by injection because it may cause kidney damage, deafness and disorders of balance after a few days of treatment. The deafness is permanent. *Adverse effects* by mouth ➤ aminoglycoside antibiotics. Allergy may occur, producing skin rashes and itching after application to the eyes, ears or skin. *Precautions:* Skin preparations should not be applied to raw areas or wounds. Prolonged use in creams, ointments and drops should be avoided as it may cause allergy which may be obscured but not prevented by the use of preparations of neomycin containing corticosteroids. Do not use ear preparations containing neomycin in patients with a perforated ear drum.

Neo-NaClex ➤ bendrofluazide.

Neo-NaClex-K tablets contain bendrofluazide, a thiazide diuretic (see Chapter 29) and potassium chloride. *Adverse effects and Precautions* ➤ thiazide diuretics, potassium supplements. They are used to treat raised blood pressure (see Chapter 25) and fluid retention (see Chapter 29).

Neoral ➤ ciclosporin.

NeoRecormon ➤ epoetin beta.

Neosporin eye drops contain polymyxin B, neomycin and gramicidin. They are used to treat bacterial infections of the eye. *Adverse effects* include allergic reactions to the neomycin. *Precautions:* If absorbed into the blood-stream neomycin can cause damage to hearing and to the kidneys. Polymyxin B and gramicidin can cause kidney damage ➤ aminoglycosides. However, these effects are unlikely with eye applications unless they enter the fluid in the eye during surgery. They should not be used if there is this risk.

neostigmine (neostigmine bromide, neostigmine methylsulphate, in Robinul neostigmine) acts upon the parasympathetic division of the autonomic nervous system. It is an anticholinesterase drug which prevents the destruction of acetylcholine by cholinesterase, thus allowing the concentration of acetylcholine to build up. See Chapter 9. It is used in the treatment and diagnosis of myesthenia gravis, to relieve retention of urine and paralysis of the bowel (paralytic ileus), and to reverse the effects of nondepolarizing neuromuscular blocking drugs (see p. 42). *Adverse effects:* Nausea, vomiting, increased salivation, diarrhoea and abdominal cramps. Signs of overdose are increased stomach and bowel discomfort, bronchial secretions, sweating, involuntary opening of the bowel and emptying of the bladder, visual disturbances, slowing of the pulse rate, fall in blood pressure, agitation, excessive dreaming, and weakness eventually leading to paralysis. *Precautions:* It should not be used in patients with intestinal or urinary obstruction. It should be used with caution in patients suffering from asthma, slow heart rate, recent heart attack, epilepsy, low blood pressure, parkinsonism, and in pregnancy. Atropine or another antidote may be necessary (particularly when neostigmine is given by injection) but it should not be given routinely as it may mask signs of overdosage. *Interactions:* Depolarizing muscle relaxants, cyclopropane, halothane.

Neotigason ➤ acitretin.

Nephril ➤ polythiazide.

Nerisone preparations ➤ diflucortolone.

Netillin ➤ netilmicin.

netilmicin (netilmicin sulphate, Netillin) is an aminoglycoside antibiotic ➤ aminoglycoside antibiotics.

Neulactil preparations ➤ pericyazine.

Neupogen ➤ filgrastim.

Neuro Bloc ➤ botulumin toxin B.

neuroleptics ➤ antipsychotic drugs.

neuromuscular blocking drugs, see p. 37.

Neurontin ➤ gabapentin.

Neutratop ➤ metronidazole.

Neutrexin ➤ trimetrexate.

nevirapine (Viramune) is used in combination therapy for HIV infections in patients with advanced or progressive immunodeficiency. See Chapter 48. *Adverse effects* include rash, nausea, fatigue, fever, headache, drowsiness, stomach and bowel upset, abdominal pain, pain in muscles, abnormal liver function, jaundice, inflammation of the liver. *Precautions:* Do not use in patients with kidney or liver failure, in pregnancy or while breastfeeding. Use with caution in patients with liver or kidney damage. Discontinue if there are signs of severe rash or rash with fever, blistering, oral lesions, conjunctivitis, muscle or joint pain or generally feeling unwell.

Nexium ➤ esomeprazole.

nicardipine (nicardipine hydrochloride, Cardene) is a calcium-channel blocker used to treat angina (see Chapter 22) and raised blood pressure (see Chapter 25). *Adverse effects* include dizziness, headaches, nausea, swelling of the ankles and palpitations, abdominal pain, diarrhoea, constipation, vomiting, loss of appetite, heartburn, weariness, feelings of warmth, flushing, noises in the ears (tinnitus), salivation, drowsiness, itching, skin rash, backache, frequency of passing urine and insomnia. It may make angina worse, cause disorders of heart rhythm and impair the functioning of the kidneys and liver. Infrequently, it can cause a fall in blood pressure upon standing up from a sitting or lying position (postural hypotension). *Precautions:* A change from a beta blocker to nicardipine should be carried out with caution. The dose of betablocker should be reduced slowly over ten days. Some patients can get angina within half an hour of starting the drug or on increasing the dose; if this happens the treatment should be stopped. It should be used with caution in patients with impaired kidney or liver function, congestive heart failure and in the elderly. It should not be used in pregnancy and breastfeeding mothers, or in patients with advanced aortic stenosis (obstruction to the flow of blood from the heart into the main artery). *Interactions:* Digoxin, cimetidine.

Nicep ➤ cefradine.

niclosamide (Yomesan) is used to treat tapeworm infections. It is not effective against larval worms. *Adverse effects* include nausea, retching, itching, abdominal pains and light-headedness.

nicorandil (Ikorel) is a potassium channel activator used to treat angina. See Chapter 22. *Adverse effects* include transient headache at the start of treatment, flushing, weakness, nausea and vomiting. High doses may cause the blood pressure to fall and/or increase the heart rate. *Precautions:* Do not use to treat patients with sudden heart failure, left-sided heart failure, low blood pressure or fluid on the lungs, in pregnancy or in breastfeeding mothers.

Nicorette preparations ➤ nicotine.

nicotinamide (niacinamide) is a member of the vitamin B group. See Chapter 36.

nicotine is the principal alkaloid in tobacco. It is very rapidly absorbed into the bloodstream by inhalation from tobacco smoke, through the lining of the nose from snuff, through the mouth from chewing tobacco and through the skin. Nicotine causes a rise in blood pressure, an increase in heart rate, a reduced blood supply to the skin and stimulation of the brain and central nervous system. Psychological dependence to nicotine is common, tolerance occurs so that bigger and bigger doses are needed to produce the same effect and withdrawal symptoms occur if the drug is stopped suddenly. Nicotine is a 'drug of addiction' and various nicotine preparations are available to help individuals to give up smoking. To stop smoking is important not only because of the nicotine addiction but also because tobacco smoking is associated with cancer of the lungs, chronic bronchitis and emphysema, coronary artery disease, arterial disease, peptic ulcers, raised blood pressure and harmful effects on the unborn baby.

Nicotine preparations are available in the form of skin patches (Niconil, Nicorette, Niquitin CQ, TTS), chewing-gum (Nicorette, Nicotinell) and nasal sprays (Niconette). *Adverse effects* of nicotine products for stopping smoking include nausea, headache, dizziness, cold and flu-like symptoms, indigestion, vivid dreams, insomnia, painful muscles, palpitations, chest pain, anxiety, irritability, sleepiness, difficulty in concentrating, painful periods, changes in blood pressure, hiccups, stomach and bowel upsets, allergic reactions and dependence. *Skin patches* may irritate the skin (stop if severe); *nose sprays* may cause nosebleeds, watery eyes, snoring and irritation of the throat; *chewing gum* may cause mouth ulcers, increased salivation, swelling of the tongue and sore throat. *Precautions:* Do not use nicotine preparations if you have severe heart disease, severe disorders of heart rhythm, if you have recently had a heart attack (myocardial infarction) or a stroke, if you have severe blood pressure or if you are pregnant or breastfeeding. Do not use skin patches if you have had a serious generalized skin disorder such as eczema, do not apply to broken skin and because skin patches provide a continuous release of nicotine do not use them if you are an occasional smoker. Use nicotine preparations with caution if you have any disorder of the heart or circulation, over-active thyroid gland, diabetes, phaeochromocytoma (a tumour of the sympathetic nervous system), impaired kidney or liver function or a history of peptic ulcers or inflammation of the stomach. Do not use nicotine preparations in combination with smoking.

Nicotinell preparations ➤ nicotine.

nicotinic acid (niacin) is a member of the vitamin B group. It is used to treat disorders of the circulation since it causes dilation of the blood vessels. See Chapter 27. It is also used to lower blood cholesterol and fat levels. See Chapter 26. *Adverse effects* include flushing, dry skin, itching, skin rashes, nausea, vomiting, diarrhoea, headache, weakness, loss of appetite, flare-up of peptic ulcers, jaundice, and increased blood sugar and uric acid levels. Symptoms can be reduced by starting with small doses taken with meals or by taking an aspirin tablet half an hour before the dose. *Precautions:* Do not use in pregnancy or in breastfeeding mothers. Use with caution in patients with diabetes, gout, liver disease or peptic ulcers.

nicomualone ➤ acenocoumarol.

Nifedepress ➤ nifedipine.

Nifedotard ➤ nifedepine.

nifedipine (Adalat preparations, Adipine MR, Angiopine MR, in Beta-adalat, Calanif, Cardilate MR, Coracten, Coroday MR, Fortipine LA, Hypolar Retard 20, Nifedepress MR, Nifedotard MR, Nifopress Retard, Slofedipine, Slofedipine XL, in Tenif, Tensipine MR) is a calcium-channel blocker used to treat angina (see Chapter 22), hypertension (see Chapter 25) and Raynaud's disease (see Chapter 27). *Adverse effects* include headache, flushing, lethargy, dizziness, anginal pains, swelling of the fingers and ankles (peripheral oedema), rapid beating of the heart, palpitations, increased frequency of passing urine, depression, telangiectasia, overgrowth of the gums, eye pain, stomach and bowel upsets, fall in blood pressure, pins and needles, skin rashes, muscle pains, tremor, visual disturbances, impotence and swelling of the breasts in men (gynaecomastia). Stop the drug if anginal pains occur. *Precautions:* Do not use in patients with sudden heart failure, in pregnancy, in patients with porphyria (a hereditary disorder of metabolism) or aortic stenosis (obstruction to the flow of blood from the heart into the main artery). Use with caution in patients with impaired heart function, low blood pressure, impaired liver function (reduce dose), diabetes or in breastfeeding mothers. It may stop labour. Stop the drug if angina occurs or gets worse shortly after starting treatment. *Interactions:* Other anti-blood pressure drugs, cimetidine, quinidine, digoxin.

Niferex Elixir and **Niferex Paediatric** con-

tain polysaccharide-iron complex. They are used to prevent and treat iron deficiency in infants born prematurely. They are also used in children. *Niferex capsules* are used by mouth to treat adults. *Interactions:* Tetracyclines by mouth ➤ iron and see Chapter 35.

Nifopress Retard ➤ nifedipine.

Nightcalm ➤ diphenydramine.

Night Nurse contains paracetamol, dextromethophen and promethazine ➤ individual entry for each drug.

Nimbex ➤ cisatracurium.

nimodipine (Nimotop) is a calcium-channel blocker used to relieve spasm of brain arteries which may occur following bleeding between the membranes of the brain (subarachnoid haemorrhage). *Adverse effects* include fall in blood pressure, flushing, headache, nausea, stomach and bowel upsets, warm feeling, increased or decreased heart rate, and thrombocytopenia (a fall in the number of blood platelets). Temporary abnormal tests of liver function after intravenous injection may occur. *Precautions:* Use with caution if there is swelling of the brain (cerebral oedema), if the pressure inside the brain is increased, in patients with impaired kidney function, cirrhosis of the liver or in pregnancy. Check blood pressure at very regular intervals. Nimodipine is incompatible with PVC; avoid contact during treatment. *Interactions:* Other calcium-channel blockers, beta-blockers, anti epileptic drugs, cimetidine, drugs that may damage the kidneys. Avoid using tablets and infusions of nimodipine together.

Nimodrel MR ➤ nifedipine.

Nimotop intravenous infusion ➤ nimodipine.

Nindaxa ➤ indapamide.

Nipent ➤ pentostatin.

Niquitin CQ preparations ➤ nicotine.

niridazole is used to kill and remove guinea worms from body tissues.

Nirolex Day Cold Comfort contains paracetamol, pholcodine and pseudoephedrine; **Nirolex Night Cold Comfort** contains paracetamol, pholcodine, pseudoephedrine and diphenhydrate; **Nirolex For Night Time Coughs** containes diphenhydramine and pholcodine ➤ individual entry for each drug.

nisoldipine (Syscor MR) is a calcium-channel blocker used to treat angina (see Chapter 22) and raised blood pressure (see Chapter 25). *Adverse effects* include fluid retention, flushing, headache, dizziness, rapid beating of the heart and stomach and bowel upsets. *Precautions:* Do not use in patients in shock from heart failure, with aortic stenosis (obstruction to the flow of blood from the heart into the main artery), impaired liver function, unstable angina, malignant hypertension, in pregnancy or in breastfeeding mothers. Use with caution in patients with a low blood pressure.

nitrates used to treat angina (see Chapter 22) and to treat heart failure (see Chapter 23). For tolerance to, see p. 113.

nitrazepam (Mogadon, Remnos, Somnite) is a benzodiazepine sleeping drug ➤ benzodiazepines.

Nitrocine ➤ glyceryl trinitrate.

Nitro-Dur self-adhesive patches ➤ glyceryl trinitrate.

nitrofurantoin (Furadantin, Macrobid, Macrodantin) is an antibacterial drug used to treat infections of the urinary tract. See Chapter 49. *Adverse effects* include loss of appetite, nausea, diarrhoea, vomiting, abdominal discomfort and drowsiness. Skin rashes, nerve damage (peripheral neuritis) and lung damage (asthma) have been reported. These are commonest in patients with impaired kidney function and patients on prolonged treatment with large doses. Blood disorders, allergic reactions, jaundice, inflammation of the pancreas, painful joints, temporary hair loss, serious skin rashes and liver damage may occur. *Precautions:* Nitrofurantoin should not be taken by patients with impaired kidney function or by patients with a deficiency of glucose-6-phosphate-dehydrogenase (G6PD) since they may develop anaemia. It should not be used in patients who have previously developed allergy or asthma while on nitrofurantoin, who are not producing urine or who are at the end of pregnancy. It should be used with caution in patients with anaemia, diabetes, disturbed blood chemistry, impaired liver function, chest disorders, vitamin B deficiency, weakness, in pregnancy, in breastfeeding mothers and in the elderly. Lung and liver function should be checked before and at regular intervals during prolonged therapy and in the elderly. It may colour the urine yellow or brown and cause false positive tests for glucose in the urine. Stop treatment if signs of lung, liver, nerve or blood damage appear. *Interactions:* Magnesium trisilicate, probenecid, sulphinpyrazone, quinolones.

nitroglycerin ➤ glyceryl trinitrate.

Nitrolingual preparations ➤ glyceryl trinitrate.

Nitromin pump spray ➤ glyceryl trinitrate.

Nitronal injection ➤ glyceryl trinitrate.

nitroprusside ➤ sodium nitroprusside.

nitrous oxide is used for induction and maintenance of anaesthesia and, in sub-anaesthesia concentrations, for pain relief in a variety of situations. It is also known as laughing gas.

Nivaquine ➤ chloroquine.

Nivemycin ➤ neomycin.

Nizatidine (Axid, Zinga) is an H_2 receptor blocker used to heal and prevent stomach and duodenal ulcers. See Chapter 19. *Adverse effects* include bad dreams, sleepiness, sweating, abnormal tests for liver function, anaemia, nettle-rash, jaundice, liver damage and enlargement of the breasts (in men).

Precautions: Use with caution in patients with impaired kidney or liver function, in pregnancy and in breastfeeding mothers. *Interactions* ➤ salicylates.

Nizoral preparations ➤ ketoconazole.

Nocutil ➤ desmopressin.

Nolvadex preparations ➤ tamoxifen.

nonacog alfa (Benefix) is used to control and prevent haemorrhage in patients with haemophilia B previously treated with other drugs. *Adverse effects* include allergic reactions, development of resistance to nonacog alfa, pain at injection site, altered taste, burning sensation in jaw, dizziness, headache, cough, fever, inflammation of a vein. *Precautions:* Allergic reactions should be reported.

non-depolarizing muscle relaxants, see p. 42.

nonoxinol (Delfen, Double Check, Durex Duragel, Gynol II, Ortho Crème, Ortho Forms) is a spermicidal contraceptive but it does not give sufficient protection if used alone. It can be used with barrier methods.

non-sedative antihistamines (See Chapter 17 and ➤ antihistamines). *Adverse effects:* Astemizole and terfenadine are non-sedative antihistamines that affect the electrochemistry of cells in heart muscle, prolonging the QT interval on tracings of the heart (ECG). They can trigger disorders of heart rhythm if the blood levels are high. This usually occurs at doses in excess of those recommended, especially in patients with impaired liver function. To avoid the risk of serious disorders of heart rhythm, astemizole and terfenadine should not be used together and they should not be taken in doses above those recommended. They should not be used in patients with severe impairment of liver function, and they should not be taken at the same time as drugs that block their breakdown in the liver such as ketoconazole, itraconazole and related imidazole antifungal drugs (see Chapter 47) or with macrolide anti-biotics (erythromycin, clarithromycin). They should not be used in patients with a low blood potassium level or prolonged QT on ECG and they should not be used with drugs known to produce disorders of heart rhythm such as anti-arrhythmic drugs, antipsychotics, tricyclic antidepressants, quinine or drugs likely to cause disturbances of the blood chemistry, particularly a fall in blood potassium levels (e.g. thiazide and loop diuretics).

Fexofenadine (Telfast) is an active breakdown product of terfenadine that undergoes negligible breakdown in the liver. It can therefore be given to patients with impaired liver function and the dose need not be reduced when given with drugs that block the breakdown of terfenadine (see above). Because it does not produce the electrochemical changes in the cells of heart muscle that terfenadine produces it is unlikely to produce toxic effects on the heart leading to a prolonged QT on ECG and the risk of disorders of heart rhythm. No reduction in dosage is needed in the elderly or in patients with impaired kidney or liver function.

non-steroidal anti-inflammatory drugs (NSAIDs) are discussed in Chapter 32. *Adverse effects* of NSAIDs differ in the various drugs and in the individual patient. They vary in frequency, severity and type. Most harmful effects produced by NSAIDs are mild and are usually related to the dose used. They can easily be controlled by reducing the dose. More serious harmful effects are rare and are usually caused by high doses and/or how a particular individual reacts. Not all of the following adverse effects have been reported with every NSAID, but they have been reported with one or more of them and should be borne in mind whenever a NSAID is used. They include nausea, vomiting, loss of appetite, indigestion, constipation, diarrhoea, ulcers and bleeding from the stomach and intestine. Very rarely, they may cause kidney damage, liver damage with jaundice, blood disorders, blood in the urine, allergic reactions (itching skin rashes), allergic swelling of the face, hands and feet, wheezing, headache, sleepiness, dizziness, tremor, confusion, insomnia, ringing in the ears (tinnitus), reduced hearing and vision, palpitations, sweating, nervousness, fluid retention (may trigger heart failure in elderly patients), aseptic meningitis, sensitivity of the skin to the sun's rays, reversible kidney failure, lung damage and inflammation of the pancreas. *Precautions:* They should not be used in people allergic to aspirin or any one of the NSAIDs; they may trigger an asthma attack in a patient with a history of asthma or allergic disorders. They should not be used in anyone with an active peptic ulcer or bleeding from the stomach or intestine. They should be used with caution in people with a history of peptic ulcers or inflamed bowel disorders. Because of the risk of fluid retention they should be used with caution in people with heart failure or raised blood pressure, and they should be used with great caution in anyone with impaired kidney or liver function, in pregnancy, in breastfeeding mothers and in the elderly. Because they may cause a deterioration in kidney function the dose should be kept as low as possible and tests of kidney function should be carried out before and at regular intervals during treatment. If a patient who really needs treatment with an NSAID develops stomach or bowel ulcers, treatment should be stopped until symptoms clear up and then an NSAID should be given with an H₂ blocker (see p. 97) or a proton-pump blocker (see p. 97). This may reduce the risks. Risks of stomach and bowel upsets from NSAIDs are greatest with azopropazone and lowest with ibuprofen and meloxicam. Diclofenac, indomethacin, ketoprofen, piroxicam and naproxen carry intermediate risk. To reduce the risk of stomach problems NSAIDs should be taken with food or milk and never on an empty stomach. *Interactions:* ACE inhibitors, other NSAIDs, 4-quinolone antibiotics, anticoagulants, anti-diabetic drugs, anti-blood pressure drugs, beta-blockers, cyclosporins, anti-cancer drugs, diuretics, lithium. *Warning:* If a patient's asthma gets worse it could be due to their taking an NSAID either prescribed or bought over the counter. Also, NSAIDs applied topically to relieve muscle aches and pains may make a patient's asthma worse.

Nootropil ➤ piracetam.

noradrenaline(norepinephrine) (noradrenaline tartate, norepinephrine) is the chemical transmitter released by adrenergic nerves. See Chapter 9. It is a sympathomimetic drug used to treat a sudden fall in blood pressure and/or sudden stoppage of the heart. *Adverse effects* include palpitations, headache, slowing of the heart rate, raised blood pressure, disorders of heart rhythm and reduced blood supply to the hands and feet. Also ➤ adrenaline(epinephrine). *Precautions:* Use with caution in patients with coronary thrombosis, or other thromboses, following a heart attack, overworking of the thyroid gland, diabetes, or in the elderly. Do not use in pregnancy or in patients with raised blood pressure. Blood pressure and rate of flow must be measured frequently. Leakage at the site of injection may seriously damage the surrounding tissue.

Norcuron ➤ vecuronium bromide.

Nordiject (somatrophin) ➤ growth hormone.

Norditropin (somatropin) ➤ growth hormone.

norepinephrine ➤ noradrenaline.

norethisterone enantate (norethisterone acetate, norethindrone, Micronor, Noriday, Noristerat, Primolut N, SH 420, Utovlan) is a progestogen. See Chapter 40. It is used to treat menstrual irregularities, to delay menstruation and to treat painful periods. It is included in several combined oral contraceptives and progestogen-only contraceptives and HRTs. *Adverse effects and Precautions* ➤ progestogens.

norfloxacin (Utinor) is a 4-quinolone antibiotic used to treat infections of the urinary tract. See Chapter 49. *Adverse effects* include nausea, heartburn, abdominal cramps, diarrhoea, loss of appetite, depression, anxiety, ringing in the ears (tinnitus), headache, dizziness, anxiety, irritability, sleep disturbances, convulsions, allergic reactions, confusion, liver, blood and pancreatic disorders, sensitivity of the skin to the sun's rays and serious skin rashes. Inflamed tendons (tendonitis) may develop (stop treatment and rest the limb if this occurs). Rarely a tendon may rupture. *Precautions:* It should not be used in pregnancy, in breastfeeding mothers, in pre-pubertal children and growing adolescents. It should be used with caution in individuals who have suffered from epilepsy, or who have impaired kidney function or G6PD deficiency. *Interactions:* Nitrofurantoin, theophylline, cyclosporin, oral anticoagulants, sucralfate, iron, zinc, antacids, probenecid and other quinolones.

norgestimate (in Cilest) is a synthetic progestogen that produces minimal androgenic (male hormone) effects ➤ progestogens.

Norgeston is a progestogen-only oral contraceptive. See p. 218.

norgestrel (Cyclo-Progynova, Neogest, Schering PC4) ➤ levonorgestrel.

Norgolax micro-enema contains docusate sodium and glycerol. It is used to treat constipation. See Chapter 21. *Adverse effects and Precautions* ➤ docusate sodium, glycerol.

Noriday is a progestogen-only oral contraceptive. See p. 218.

Norimin is a combined oral contraceptive. See p. 216.

Norimode ➤ loperamide.

Norinyl-1 is a combined oral contraceptive. See p. 216.

Noristerat injection ➤ norethisterone.

Noritate is a metronidazole cream used in the treatment of acne rosacea ➤ metronidazole.

Normacol and **Normacol Plus** granules contain the bulk laxatives sterculia and frangula. They are used to treat constipation.

See Chapter 21. *Adverse effects* ➤ sterculia, frangula. *Precautions:* Do not use if there is an obstruction of the bowel. Use with caution in pregnancy. Avoid taking at bedtime. Drink plenty of fluids.

Normaloe ➤ loperamide.

Normasol powder makes a sterile solution of sodium chloride. It is used to irrigate the eyes and also wounds and burns.

Normax capsules contain docusate sodium and dantron.

Normosang ➤ haem arginate.

Norphyllin SR ➤ aminophylline.

Norprolac ➤ quinagolide.

nortriptyline (nortriptyline hydrochloride, Allegron in Motipress, in Motival) is a tricyclic antidepressant drug ➤ tricyclic antidepressants.

Norvir ➤ ritonavir.

Novantrone ➤ mitoxantrone.

Novaprin ➤ ibuprofen.

Nova-T is an intra-uterine contraceptive device which contains copper.

Novonorm ➤ repaglinide.

NovoRapid ➤ insulin.

NovoSeven dried powder contains recombinant antihaemophilic factor VIIa. It is used to treat haemophiliac patients who develop serious bleeding or undergo surgery when they have developed resistance to factor VIII or IX. Because it is bioengineered it does not carry the risk of viral contamination (e.g. HIV, inflammation of the liver). *Adverse effects* include irritation of the skin, nausea, generally feeling unwell, fever, changes in blood pressure, disorders of the circulation, angina, disorders of heart rhythm and shock. *Precautions:* Do not use in patients allergic to mouse, hamster or bovine protein. Use with caution in pregnancy and breastfeeding mothers. Should be used only at special haemophiliac centres.

Interactions: Prothrombin coagulation factor concentrates.

Noxyflex S ➤ noxythiolin.

noxythiolin (Noxyflex S) is an antifungal, antibacterial drug used to inject into the abdomen in patients suffering from life-threatening peritonitis due to bile or faeces in the peritoneal cavity. Must be specially prepared and used within seven days.

Nozinan ➤ levomepromazine.

NSAID ➤ non-steroidal anti-inflammatory drugs.

Nubain injections (nalbuphine hydrochloride) ➤ nalbuphine.

Nuelin and **Nuelin SA** ➤ theophylline.

Nulacin is an antacid containing calcium, magnesium, peppermint oil ➤ individual entry for each drug.

Numark Cold Relief powders ➤ paracetamol.

Nupercainal ointment ➤ cinchocaine.

Nurofen, **Nurofen Children** and **Nurofen Muscular Pain Relief gel** contain ibuprofen; **Nurofen Cold and Flu** contains ibuprofen and pseudoephedrine. **Nurofen Plus** contains ibuprofen and codeine ➤ individual entry for each drug.

Nurse Sykes' balsam ➤ guaifenesin.

Nurse Sykes' powders contains aspirin, paracetamol and caffeine ➤ individual entry for each drug.

Nu-Seals Aspirin ➤ aspirin.

Nutraplus cream ➤ urea.

Nutrizym preparations ➤ pancreatin.

Nuvelle tablets contain the natural oestrogen oestradiol and the progestogen levonorgestrel. They are used in hormone replacement therapy ➤ HRT.

Nuvelle TS sequential HRT skin patches deliver oestradiol (a natural oestrogen) in the first set of patches and oestradiol plus levonorgestrel (a progestogen) in the second set of patches ➤ HRT.

Nycopren ➤ naproxen.

Nylax with senna ➤ senna.

Nystaform cream and ointment contains nystatin (an antifungal drug) and chlorhexidine (an antibacterial drug). They are used to treat skin infections. *Adverse effects and Precautions* ➤ nystatin, chlorhexidine.

Nystaform-HC contains chlorhexidine (an antibacterial drug) and hydrocortisone (a corticosteroid). It is used to treat eczema and dermatitis that is infected. *Adverse effects and Precautions:* See corticosteroid skin applications p. 241 and ➤ chlorhexidine.

Nystamont ➤ nystatin.

Nystan preparations ➤ nystatin.

nystatin (Nystamont, Nystan) is an antifungal drug (see Chapter 47) which is active against a wide range of fungi and yeasts. When given by mouth, little is absorbed. It is mainly used to treat *Candida* infections (e.g. thrush) of the skin, mouth, genitals and intestine. *Adverse effects:* High doses may cause nausea, vomiting and diarrhoea. Treatment by mouth may irritate the mouth and rarely cause an allergic reaction. Very rarely it may cause urticaria (nettle-rash) and Stevens-Johnson syndrome (a severe form of inflammatory skin disease).

Nytol ➤ diphenhydramine.

Obifen ➤ ibuprofen.

Occlusal application contains salicylic acid in polyacrylic solution ➤ salicylic acid. It is used to treat warts (see p. 262).

Octaplus is a preparation of treated human plasma (frozen).

octocog alfa (Helixate, Kogenate/Recombinate/Refacto) is used to prevent and treat haemophilia A. *Adverse effects* include allergic reactions, injection site reactions, chest tightness, dizziness, mild low blood pressure, nausea. *Precautions:* Do not use in patients who are mouse or hamster protein sensitive. It does not contain von Willebrand Factor, therefore do not use for von Willebrand's disease (a bleeding disorder associated with increased bleeding time and low Factor VIII activity). Use with caution in pregnancy or in breastfeeding mothers.

Octogam ➤ immunoglobulin.

octreotide (Sandostatin) is related to somatostatin, which blocks the release of growth hormone by the pituitary gland. It is used as short-term treatment for acromegaly (due to overworking of the pituitary gland) prior to surgery on the pituitary gland; as long-term treatment for patients not improved by surgery, dopamine blockers or radiotherapy to the pituitary gland; to relieve symptoms of tumours of the pancreas and other tumours that may affect the bowel (e.g. carcinoid tumour). *Adverse effects* include loss of appetite, nausea, bloating, vomiting, abdominal pain, diarrhoea and fat in the stools (steatorrhoea). Rarely, it may cause a persistent rise in blood glucose levels, gallstones, gall-bladder colic and an impairment of liver function. It may produce pain, stinging and redness at the injection site. *Precautions:* Do not use in pregnancy or in breastfeeding mothers. Patients should be monitored for gallstones (by ultrasound scan every twelve months) and for disorders of thyroid function. *Interactions:* Cyclosporin, cimetidine. It may reduce the response to anti-diabetic drugs in patients being treated for diabetes.

Ocufen eye drops contain flurbiprofen (a non-steroidal anti-inflammatory drug in polyvinyl alcohol) (Liquifilm Tears). They are used as an anti-inflammatory following eye surgery, also to prevent contraction of the pupil during eye surgery.

Oculotect ➤ povidone.

Odrik ➤ trandolapril.

oestradiol ➤ estradiol.

oestrial ➤ estriol.

Oestrogel (gel in pressurized dispenser) contains estradiol (an oestrogen). It is used as HRT and applied to arms, shoulders and inner thighs ➤ HRT.

oestrogens are discussed in Chapter 40. *Adverse effects* include salt and water retention producing oedema, weight gain, nausea, vomiting, headache, dizziness, migraine, depression, enlargement and tenderness of the breasts, breakthrough bleeding, spotting, changes in menstrual periods, premenstrual-like syndrome, loss of periods during or after treatment, thrush of the vagina, jaundice, changes in liver function, skin rashes, chloasma (brown patches on the face), and headache on vigorous exercise. There is a risk of cancer of the womb, which can be prevented if oestrogens are given cyclically (three weeks on and one week off) with an added progestogen (see Chapter 40). For risks of blood clots, see Chapter 41 on oral contraceptives. Skin patches may cause local redness and itching. *Precautions:* Oestrogens should not be used in women who suffer from oestrogen-dependent cancer of the breast, undiagnosed bleeding from the vagina, blood clots or a history of blood clots, a history of itching during pregnancy, worsening otosclerosis (the development of extra bone in the ear causing progressive deafness), sickle-cell anaemia, acute or chronic liver disease, jaundice, porphyria (a hereditary disorder of metabolism), disorders of fat metabolism, or endometriosis. They should not be used if there is known or suspected pregnancy, or in breastfeeding mothers. They should be used with caution in women suffering from raised blood pressure, coronary or cerebral artery disease, asthma, varicose veins, hyperthyroidism, or diabetes. Oestrogens may cause fluid retention and aggravate epilepsy, migraine, heart disease and kidney disease. Patients with these disorders should be kept under close medical supervision. Also see Chapter 41 on oral contraceptives.

oestrone ➤ estrone.

ofloxacin (Tarivid) is a synthetic quinolone

antibacterial drug (see p. 272) structurally related to nalidixic acid. It is used to treat infections of the urinary tract, lower respiratory tract and genital tract (gonorrhoea and non-gonococcal infections). *Adverse effects* include stomach and bowel upsets, skin rashes, allergic reactions, dizziness, sleep disorders, itching, fever, changes in tests of liver and kidney function, joint and muscle pains, damage to the bone marrow producing blood disorders, inflammation and rupture of tendons (stop drug at first signs of pain or inflammation in tendons), damage to blood vessels (vasculitis), anxiety, ataxia (loss of control over voluntary movements), tremor, pins and needles, nerve damage, restlessness, depression, hallucinations, confusion, disturbances of taste, vision and smell, psychotic reactions, rapid beating of the heart and fall in blood pressure. *Precautions:* Do not use in pregnancy, in breastfeeding mothers, in growing adolescents or in people with a history of epilepsy. Use with caution in patients with mental illness or impaired kidney function (reduce dose accordingly), G6PD deficiency or in patients receiving blood dialysis or peritoneal dialysis. Avoid exposure to strong sunlight or UV rays. Dizziness and visual disturbances may affect the ability to drive a motor vehicle or operate moving machinery. *Interactions:* Magnesium and aluminium antacids, sucralfate, glibenclamide, iron, NSAIDs, anticoagulants, barbiturates, intravenous anaesthetics, anti-blood pressure drugs. It is used in **Exocin** eye drops to treat bacterial infections of the eyes. *Adverse effects:* The eye drops may cause transient irritation and rarely nausea, dizziness, numbness and headache. *Precautions:* Use with caution in pregnancy and breastfeeding mothers. Do not wear soft contact lenses.

Oilatum cream ➤ arachis oil.

Oilatum emollient and gel ➤ light liquid paraffin.

Oilatum Plus contains liquid paraffin, and the antiseptics benzalkonium and triclosan

➤ benzalkonium, triclosan. It is used to treat eczema where there is a risk of infection of the affected area of skin.

oily cream ➤ hydrous ointment.

Okacyn ➤ lomefloxacin.

Olbetam ➤ acipimox.

olive oil is used for soothing and to soften ear wax.

olanzapine (Zyprexa) is an antipsychotic drug used to treat schizophrenia. See Chapter 3. *Adverse effects* include dizziness, gain in weight, sleepiness, increased appetite, swelling of the ankles, fall in blood pressure on standing up after sitting or lying down (postural hypotension), temporary antimuscarinic effects (➤ antimuscarinic drugs). *Precautions:* Do not use in breastfeeding mothers or in patients with closed-angle glaucoma. Use with caution in patients with impaired liver or kidney function, enlarged prostate gland, blood disorders, seizures, tardive dyskinesia (➤ antipsychotic drugs), and in pregnancy. Monitor blood pressure in elderly patients. A lower dose is normally used in elderly female patients, particularly if they smoke. See risks of *neuroleptic malignant syndrome* under entry on antipsychotic drugs – patient should report early symptoms such as fever and muscle rigidity. *Interactions:* Drugs known to affect heart tracings (increased QT), activated charcoal, smoking and drugs that damage the liver. Also see under antipsychotic drugs.

olsalazine (olsalazine sodium, Dipentum) is a salicylate used to treat ulcerative colitis. *Adverse effects* include watery diarrhoea, abdominal cramps, nausea, indigestion, headache, painful joints, skin rashes, blood disorders and very rarely reversible inflammation of the pancreas. *Precautions:* Do not use in patients allergic to aspirin or other salicylates. Do not use in pregnancy or in patients with a severe impairment of kidney function. Patients should report any unexplained bruising, sore throat or if generally feeling unwell and a blood test should be carried out to check whether the drug is causing blood disorders.

omega-3 triglycerides (omega-3 marine triglycerides, Maxepa) are obtained from fish oils. They contain two essential unsaturated fatty acids – eicosapentaenoic acid and docosahexaenoic acid. They reduce the blood level of cholesterol and fats (triglycerides). See Chapter 26. Eicosapentaenoic acid (EPA) is also involved in the manufacture of a prostaglandin that makes platelets in the blood less sticky. *Adverse effects* include nausea and belching. *Precautions:* Use with caution in patients with bleeding disorders. *Interactions:* Anticoagulants.

omeprazole (Losec) is a proton pump-blocker used to treat peptic ulcers, acid reflux and ulcers caused by non-steroidal anti-inflammatory drugs (NSAIDs) (see Chapter 19). *Adverse effects* include headache, nausea, diarrhoea, constipation, wind, abdominal pain, dizziness, vertigo, generally feeling unwell, insomnia, sleepiness, faintness, muscle and joint pains, blurred vision, ankle-swelling, sweating, enlargement of the breasts in men, impotence, loss of taste, fever, wheezing, itching, skin rashes, hair loss, sensitivity of the skin to the sun's rays, blood disorders, kidney damage, liver damage, confusion, agitation, depression and hallucinations in severely ill patients. *Precautions:* Do not use in pregnancy or in breastfeeding mothers. It may mask symptoms of cancer of the stomach; therefore monitor patients with stomach ulcers carefully to exclude the possibility of cancer. *Interactions:* Diazepam, phenytoin, warfarin, digoxin.

Omnopon ➤ papaveretum.

OncoTice ➤ Bacillus Calmette-Guérin.

Oncovin ➤ vincristine.

ondansetron (Zofran) is a 5HT blocker used to treat nausea and vomiting caused by anti-cancer drugs and radiotherapy and to treat post-operative nausea and vomiting (see Chapter 18). *Adverse effects* include constipation, headaches, flushing of the face

and abdomen. Very rarely, it may cause allergic reactions and changes in liver function tests. Intravenous use may cause transient visual disturbances. *Precautions:* Do not use in breastfeeding mothers and use with caution during pregnancy.

One-Alpha preparations contain alfacalcidol. They are related to vitamin D and are used to treat patients suffering from bone disease caused by kidney failure, parathyroid disorders and rickets. *Precautions:* Use with caution in patients with kidney failure, in pregnancy and in breastfeeding mothers. Check blood calcium at regular intervals. *Interactions:* Barbiturates, anti-epileptic drugs, danazol, digitalis, thiazide diuretics, antacids, mineral oils, cholestyramine, colestipol, sucralfate.

Onkotrone ➤ mitoxantrone.

Opas is an antacid containing calcium, magnesium and sodium bicarbonate ➤ individual entry for each drug.

Opazimes is an anti-diarrhoeal preparation containing belladona, morphine, aluminium and kaolin ➤ individual entry for each drug.

Opthalin and **Opthalin Plus** ➤ sodium hyaluronate.

opiate analgesics ➤ opiate pain-relievers.

opiate blockers see Chapter 30. For use of the terms narcotic, opiate and opioid, see p. 153.

opiate pain-relievers see Chapter 30. For use of the terms narcotic, opiate and opioid, see p. 153.

Opilon ➤ moxisylite.

opioid analgesics ➤ opiate pain-relievers.

opioid blockers ➤ opiate blockers.

opioid pain-relievers ➤ opiate pain-relievers.

opium (raw opium, powdered opium) has effects and uses similar to those described under morphine, which is its main constituent. It is more constipating than morphine alone. See Chapter 30.

Oprisine ➤ azathioprine.

Opticrom preparations ➤ sodium cromoglicate.

Optil, Optil SR and Optil XL ➤ diltiazem.

Optilast ➤ azelastine.

Optimax ➤ tryptophan.

Optimine preparations ➤ azatadine.

Optrex Allergy eyedrops ➤ sodium cromoglicate.

Opumide ➤ indapamide.

Oralbalance gel is used as artificial saliva to treat dry mouth due to radiotherapy or sicca syndrome. It contains xylitol and peroxidase and oxidase enzymes.

Orabase ointment contains carmellose, sodium, pectin and gelatin in equal parts. It is used to protect lesions in the mouth and moist body surfaces.

Oragard ➤ cetylpyridirium, lidocaine(lignocaine).

Orahesive powder contains the same ingredients as Orabase and is used on moist body surfaces to protect them.

oral contraceptives, see Chapter 41.

oral hypoglycaemic drugs ➤ antidiabetic drugs (oral) and see Chapter 42.

Oraldene mouthwash and gargle ➤ hexetidine.

Oramorph oral preparations ➤ morphine.

Orap ➤ pimozide.

orciprenaline (orciprenaline sulphate, Alupent) is a partially selective beta-stimulant used to treat asthma. See Chapter 14. Its effects are similar to those described under salbutamol. *Adverse effects* include rapid beating of the heart, headache, dizziness, nausea, tremor, nervous tension, flushing and disorders of heart rhythm. Difficulty in passing urine may also occur.

Precautions: Do not use in patients with acute coronary artery disease, overworking of the thyroid gland and asthma caused by heart disease. Use with caution in patients with raised blood pressure or diabetes. *Interactions:* MAOIs, tricyclic antidepressants, sympathomimetic drugs.

Orelox ➤ cefpodoxime.

Orgalutran ➤ ganirelix.

Orgaran injection ➤ danaparoid sodium.

Orimeten ➤ aminoglutethimide.

Orlept ➤ sodium valproate.

orlistat (Xenical) is a supplement to diet in a weight reduction programme in obese patients. See Chapter 8. *Adverse effects* include faecal incontinence, oily stools, stomach and bowel upset, respiratory infection, influenza, headache, menstrual irregularity, anxiety, fatigue, urinary tract infection. *Precautions:* Do not use in patients who cannot absorb the nutrients from food properly, with cholestatis (stoppage or slowing of flow in biliary channels), in pregnancy or while breastfeeding. Eat diet rich in fruit and vegetables, containing approx 30% calories from fat.

Orovite Complement B6 ➤ pyridoxine.

orphenadrine (orphenadrine citrate, orphenadrine hydrochloride, Biorphen, Disipal, Norflex) is an antimuscarinic drug used to treat parkinsonism (see Chapter 16) and also muscle spasm due to injury (often combined with a pain-reliever). *Adverse effects and Precautions* ➤ benzhexol, antimuscarinic drugs. It may cause euphoria, confusion, agitation, insomnia, rash in high doses and antimuscarinic effects. Do not use in patients with closed-angle glaucoma, enlargement of the prostate gland, porphyria (a hereditary disorder of metabolism), or tardive dyskinesia (➤ antipsychotic drugs). Use with caution in patients with obstruction of the stomach or intestine, or heart disorders. Withdraw slowly. *Interactions:* Phenothiazines and other antipsychotic drugs, antihistamines and antidepressants.

Ortho-Creme ➤ nonoxynol.

Orthoforms ➤ nonoxinol.

Ortho-Gynest is an intravaginal cream containing oestriol (an oestrogen) ➤ HRT. It may damage latex condoms and diaphragms.

Ortho-Gynest pessaries ➤ oestriol.

Orudis ➤ ketoprofen.

Oruvail gel ➤ ketoprofen.

Osmolax solution ➤ lactulose.

Ossopan preparations ➤ hydroxyapatite.

Ostram ➤ calcium supplements.

Otex ear drops ➤ urea hydrogen peroxide.

Otomize spray suspension contains neomycin (an antibiotic), acetic acid and dexamethasone (a corticosteroid). It is used to treat inflammation of the outer ear (otitis externa). *Adverse effects* include transient stinging and burning. *Precautions:* Use with caution in patients with a perforated ear drum and in pregnancy ➤ neomycin, dexamethasone.

Otosporin ear drops contain the antibiotics neomycin and polymyxin B and hydrocortisone (a corticosteroid). They are used to treat bacterial infections and inflammation of the outer ear (otitis externa). *Adverse effects* include superinfection. *Precautions:* Do not use in patients with a perforated eardrum or untreated viral, fungal or tubercular infection. Avoid long-term use in infants.

Otradrops ➤ xylometazoline.

Otraspray ➤ xylometazoline.

Otrivine-Antistin eye drops contain xylometazole (a sympathomimetic drug) and antazoline (an antihistamine). They are used to treat allergic conjunctivitis. *Adverse effects* include transient stinging, headache, drowsiness, blurred vision and rebound congestion when drops are stopped. *Precautions:* Do not use in patients with closed-angle glaucoma. Do not wear contact lenses.

Use with caution in patients with raised blood pressure, overworking of the thyroid gland, diabetes, coronary artery disease or dry eyes. *Interactions:* clonidine. For *general adverse effects and precautions* ➤ sympathomimetic drugs, antihistamines.

Otrivine nasal preparations ➤ xylometazoline.

Ovestin preparations ➤ oestriol.

Ovex ➤ mebendazole.

Ovitrelle ➤ choriogonadotropin.

Ovran 30 is a combined oral contraceptive, see p. 216.

Ovranette is a combined oral contraceptive, see p. 216.

Ovysmen is a combined oral contraceptive, see p. 216.

oxaliplatin (Eloxatin) is used in combination with 5-fluorouracil (5-FU) and folinic acid to treat secondary cancer of the bowel. See Chapter 51. *Adverse effects* include damage to the nerves affecting the senses, absence of feeling in the pharynx or larynx, anaemia, decrease in certain kinds of white blood cells (neutropenia), decrease in number of platelets in the blood (thrombocytopenia), diarrhoea, inflammation of mucous membranes, hair loss, raised liver enzymes, allergic reactions, damage to the ears, kidney function disturbance, transient loss of visual sharpness. *Precautions:* Do not use in patients with severe kidney damage, neutropenia, thrombocytopenia, damage to the nerves affecting the senses, in pregnancy or while breastfeeding. Use with caution in patients with moderate kidney damage, diarrhoea or a history of sensitivity to platinum compounds.

oxazepam is a benzodiazepine drug ➤ benzodiazepines.

oxcarbazepine (Trileptal) is used to treat epilepsy – partial seizures with or without secondary generalized tonic-clonic seizures. See Chapter 15. *Adverse effects* include fatigue, weakness, stomach, bowel and visual disturbances, low blood sodium level, skin reactions, Stevens-Johnson syndrome (disease causing severe inflammation of the skin and mucous membranes), decrease in number of platelets in the blood. *Precautions:* Do not use while breastfeeding. Use with caution in patients with kidney damage, a history of allergy to carbamazepine, heart disease, in the elderly or in pregnancy.

oxerutins (Paroven) are bioflavonoids used to treat varicose veins and haemorrhoids. They strengthen small blood vessels (capillaries) and reduce their permeability. *Adverse effects* include flushing, headache and stomach upsets.

oxetacaine is a local anaesthetic. It is an ingredient of Mucaine ➤ Mucaine.

oxethazaine ➤ oxetacaine.

Oxiprenix SR ➤ oxprenolol.

Oxis ➤ formoterol.

oxitropium (Oxivent) is an antimuscarinic drug administered by inhaler to treat asthma. See Chapter 14. *Adverse effects* include local irritation of the throat, dry mouth and nausea. Rarely, it may produce general antimuscarinic effects such as blurred vision, constipation and difficulty in passing urine ➤ antimuscarinic drugs. *Precautions:* It should not be used in individuals allergic to atropine or ipratropium and it should be used with caution in people with glaucoma or enlarged prostate gland. Contact with the eyes should be avoided. It should not be used in pregnancy or in breastfeeding mothers. It should be stopped if wheezing, coughing or tightness in the chest develop.

Oxivent ➤ oxitropium.

oxpentifylline ➤ pentoxifylline.

oxprenolol (oxprenolol hydrochloride, Slow-Trasicor, Trasicor, in Trasidrex) is a non-selective beta-blocker ➤ beta-blockers.

oxybenzone is used as a sunscreen agent.

oxybuprocaine (Minims Benoxinate) is a local anaesthetic used in eye drops.

oxybutynin (Contimin, Cystrin, Ditropan, Promictuline) is used to treat frequency and urgency of passing urine associated with incontinence, and to treat bedwetting. See Chapter 49. It is an antispasmodic/antimuscarinic drug that relaxes the bladder muscle and delays the initial desire to pass urine, allowing the bladder to hold more urine. *Adverse effects* include facial flushing and antimuscarinic effects (➤ antimuscarinic drugs). *Precautions:* It should not be used in patients with obstruction of the bladder, obstruction of the bowel, severe ulcerative colitis, myasthenia gravis (muscle weakness due to neuromuscular abnormality), glaucoma, or in breastfeeding mothers. It should be used with caution in patients with impaired kidney or liver function, over-active thyroid gland, coronary artery disease, congestive heart failure, rapid heart beat, disorders of heart rhythm, enlarged prostate gland, porphyria (a hereditary disorder of metabolism), hiatus hernia, or in pregnancy. *Interactions:* Phenothiazines, butyrophenone antipsychotic drugs (see p. 12), amantadine, digoxin, levodopa, tricyclic antidepressants, other antimuscarinic drugs.

oxycodone (Oxynorm, Oxycontin) is an opiate pain-reliever. See Chapter 30. *Adverse effects and Precautions* ➤ morphine.

OxyContin ➤ oxycodone.

oxymel is a preparation of purified honey in acetic acid and water.

oxymetazoline (oxymetazoline hydrochloride, Afrazine, Sudafed Nasal Spray) is a sympathomimetic drug (➤ sympathomimetic drugs). It narrows blood vessels to relieve nasal congestion. See Chapter 10. *Adverse effects:* It may occasionally cause stinging or burning where it is applied, sneezing, headache, insomnia, rapid beating of the heart and dryness of the mouth and throat. *Precautions:* Prolonged use should be avoided because it may cause rebound congestion of the nose and a continually blocked nose. It should be used with caution in patients with raised blood pressure, coronary artery disease, over-active thyroid or diabetes.

Oxymycin ➤ oxytetracycline.

Oxynorm ➤ oxycodone.

oxypertine is an antipsychotic drug that is related to the phenothiazines ➤ antipsychotic drugs.

oxytetracycline (Berkmycen, Oxytetramix, Oxymycin, in Terra-Cortril, in Terra-Cortril Nystatin, in Trimovate) is a tetracycline antibiotic ➤ tetracyclines.

Oxytetramix ➤ oxytetracycline.

oxytocin (Syntocinon injection, Syntometrine) is a natural hormone produced and secreted by the pituitary gland. It increases the contractions of the uterus during normal labour and it stimulates milk production. It is used to assist labour or abortion. It is given after delivery of the baby's shoulder to speed up the expulsion of the afterbirth (placenta). It is also used with ergometrine to stop bleeding after childbirth and abortion. *Adverse effects:* At low doses it may make the uterus go into spasm and at high doses it may make the uterus contract violently producing distress in the baby and occasionally rupture of the uterus. It may cause nausea, vomiting, disturbed heart rhythm and allergic reactions in the mother. The large volume of water in the infusion may cause water intoxication and a fall in blood sodium levels in the mother. *Precautions:* Do not use in women who have a mechanical obstruction to vaginal delivery, if the baby is distressed, if the baby or the placenta are in the wrong position, if the umbilical cord is prolapsed, in women who have had many babies, if the uterus is scarred due to surgery or a Caesarean section, or if the mother has severe heart disease or raised blood pressure. Use with caution if pelvis is small compared with the baby's head (avoid if significant), if the mother has raised blood pressure or

heart disease triggered by the pregnancy, in women over thirty-five years of age with a history of lower segment Caesarean section, if the baby is dead, if there is meconium in the amniotic fluid, if the mother has water intoxication and low blood sodium levels (avoid large volumes at infusion and restrict fluids by mouth). *Interactions:* Careful monitoring is needed if used with prostaglandins. Anaesthetics may possibly reduce the effects of oxytocin and increase risk of a fall in blood pressure and disorders of heart rhythm.

Pabrinex is a multivitamin preparation which is given by intravenous or intramuscular injection. It contains vitamins B and C.

Pacifene preparations ➤ ibuprofen.

paclitaxel (Taxol) is an anti-cancer drug. See Chapter 51. It is used to treat ovarian cancer with secondaries when standard platinum treatment has failed. It is given by intravenous infusion. *Adverse effects:* It may produce severe allergic reactions and therefore a corticosteroid, an antihistamine and an H_2 blocker should be given routinely before treatment is started. Resuscitation equipment must be immediately to hand. It may cause a fall in blood pressure and heart rate, nausea, vomiting, hair loss, muscle pains, nerve damage, disorders of heart rhythm and damage to the bone marrow producing blood disorders. *Precautions:* see Chapter 51.

Paldesic ➤ paracetamol.

Palfium ➤ dextromoramide.

palivizumab (Synagis) is used to prevent respiratory syncytial virus (RSV) infection in children born at thirty-five weeks gestation or less and under six months old at onset of RSV season, or in children over two years old who have had treatment for bronchopulmonary dysplasia (overinflated lungs) within last six months. *Adverse effects* include fever, injection site reactions, nervousness. *Precautions:* Use with caution in patients with congenital heart disease, severe infection, feverish illness, allergic reactions, decrease in number of platelets in the blood, coagulation disorders.

Palladone ➤ hydromorphone.

Paludrine ➤ proguanil.

Paludrine/Avloclor is a travel pack of two antimalarial preparations. Avloclor ➤ chloroquine and Paludrine ➤ proguanil.

Pamergan P100 contains pethidine (an opiate pain-reliever) and promethazine (a sedative antihistamine). It is used by intramuscular injection to relieve pain in childbirth. It is also used as a pre-medication before surgery. *Adverse effects and Precautions* ➤ morphine, antihistamines.

pamidronate disodium (Aredia) ➤ disodium pamidronate.

Panadeine preparations contain paracetamol and codeine ➤ paracetamol, codeine.

Panadol preparations contain paracetamol; **Panadol Extra** contains paracetamol and caffeine; **Panadol Night** contains diphenhydramine and paracetamol; **Panadol Ultra** contains paracetamol and codeine ➤ individual entry for each drug.

Panaleve Elixir, **Panaleve Junior** and **Panaleve 6+** ➤ paracetamol.

Pancrease ➤ pancreatin.

pancreatin supplements contain extracts of pancreatic glands from pigs. They contain pancreatic enzymes which help to digest starch, fats and protein. They are given by mouth to treat patients who have impaired function of their pancreas (e.g. cystic fibrosis) or who have had their pancreas removed. The acid in the stomach inactivates the enzymes so they should be taken with or after food, with drugs that block acid production (see Chapter 19) or they should be taken as capsules that have a special acid-resistant coating (enteric coated). Enteric-coated preparations include Creon, Nutrizym GR, Pancrease and Pancrex V. They should be swallowed whole without chewing. *Adverse effects* include

irritation of the skin around the mouth and anus, nausea, vomiting and abdominal discomfort. Very high doses may cause an increase in the uric level in the blood and urine. They may occasionally cause allergic reactions which may affect those who handle it. Very rarely pancreatin may cause scarring in the bowel. *Precautions:* Pancreatin is inactivated by heat so avoid excessive heat if pancreatin is mixed with foods or drinks; these mixtures should not be kept for more than one hour. Drink plenty of fluids. Report any unusual abdominal symptoms if taking high doses.

Pancrex V preparations ➤ pancreatin.

pancuronium (pancuronium bromide, Pavulon) is a non-depolarizing muscle-relaxant drug (see p. 42) used with general anaesthetics in surgical operations.

Panoxyl preparations ➤ benzoyl peroxide.

pantoprazole (Protium) is a protein pump blocker that reduces stomach acid production. It is used to treat duodenal ulcer, stomach ulcer and moderate or severe oesophagitis (inflammation of the gullet). See Chapter 19. *Adverse effects* include headache, dizziness, diarrhoea, itching and skin rash. *Precautions:* Use with caution in patients with cirrhosis of the liver and impaired liver function, in pregnancy and in breastfeeding mothers.

Papaveretum (previously called Omnopon) injection contains morphine, papaverine and codeine. It is used to relieve post-operative pain and as a pre-medication before surgery. *Adverse effects and Precautions* ➤ morphine.

papaverine is a smooth muscle relaxant injected directly into the penis (intracavernosal) to produce an erection in men suffering from inability to attain an erection. *Adverse effects* include persistence of erection which, if it lasts for more than four hours, will need emergency treatment (aspiration of blood from the erect penis). If this fails metaraminol injections into the penis may be needed. Local side-effects include burning pain at the site of the injection, bruising and scarring (which may cause a distortion of the penis).

Papulex Gel ➤ nicotinamide.

paracetamol (acetaminophen) is a mild pain-reliever; it also reduces fever. Unlike aspirin, it has no anti-inflammatory properties. There are a large number of preparations which contain paracetamol, both on prescription and over-the-counter. See Chapter 31. *Adverse effects:* Skin rashes and blood disorders may occur very rarely. Prolonged daily use may occasionally cause inflammation of the pancreas. Overdose may cause liver damage and, less frequently, kidney damage. See p. 159. *Precautions:* Paracetamol should be taken with caution by patients with impaired kidney or liver function, or dependence on alcohol which damages the liver.

Paracets ➤ paracetamol.

Paracets Plus contains paracetamol, caffeine and phenylephrine ➤ individual entry for each drug.

Paraclear ➤ paracetamol.

Paracodol contains paracetamol and codeine ➤ paracetamol, codeine.

Paradote tablets contain paracetamol and an antidote (methionine). See p. 160. *Precautions:* Do not use in patients with active liver disease. Use with caution if kidney or liver function is severely impaired. Use with caution in pregnancy and in breastfeeding mothers. *Interactions:* Levodopa, MAOIs.

paraffin (hard paraffin) is obtained from petroleum and is used to form a base for ointments.

Parake tablets contain paracetamol and codeine ➤ paracetamol, codeine.

paraldehyde is a quick-acting sleeping drug and anticonvulsant. Because of its nasty smell, taste and part-excretion in the breath it is seldom used except in hospitals to treat epilepsy. See Chapter 15. *Adverse effects:* Because it irritates the stomach it is

usually given by injection, which may be painful and cause a sterile abscess. It may also be given as an enema which may cause irritation of the rectum. *Adverse effects* include skin rashes and, rarely, liver and kidney disorders. Nerve damage may occur if injected close to a main nerve. *Precautions:* If given by mouth or by rectum it should be well diluted. Intramuscular injections should be given with caution to patients with impaired liver function. *Drug dependence:* Paraldehyde may produce dependence of the barbiturate/alcohol type. See p. xxvii.

Paramax preparations contain paracetamol and metoclopramide (an anti-nauseant, anti-vomiting drug, see Chapter 18). It is used to treat migraine. See Chapter 34. *Adverse effects and Precautions* ➤ paracetamol, metoclopramide.

Paramol tablets contain paracetamol and dihydrocodeine, an opiate pain-reliever. *Adverse effects and Precautions* ➤ paracetamol, dihydrocodeine.

Paraplatin ➤ carboplatin.

parasiticidal preparations are used to treat scabies (p. 261) and head and body lice (p. 256).

Pardelprin ➤ indometacin.

Pariet ➤ rabeprazole.

Parlodel ➤ bromocriptine.

Parnate ➤ tranylcypromine.

Paroven ➤ oxerutins.

paroxetine (Seroxat) is used to treat depression. See Chapter 4. It is a selective 5-HT re-uptake blocker. *Adverse effects* include dry mouth, nausea, sleepiness, sweating, weakness, tremor, insomnia and impaired sexual function. It may produce movement disorders and spasm of facial muscles. *Precautions:* It should be used with caution in pregnancy, in breastfeeding mothers, in patients with severe impairment of kidney or liver function, with disorders of the heart or circulation, with epilepsy or a history of mania. Avoid abrupt withdrawal because of the risk of withdrawal symptoms. Reduce daily dose slowly over a few weeks. May impair ability to drive. Do not use in patients during manic phase of manic depressive illness. *Interactions:* MAOIs, tryptophan, lithium, phenytoin, and anti-epileptic drugs.

Parvolex ➤ acetylcysteine.

Pavacol D is a cough mixture containing pholcodeine ➤ pholcodeine.

Pavulon ➤ pancuronium.

peanut oil ➤ arachis oil.

PegIntron is a peginterferon alfa ➤ Interferon.

Penbritin ➤ ampicillin.

penciclovir is an antiviral drug used as a cream (Vectavir) to treat cold sores (herpes simplex virus). *Adverse effects* include temporary burning and stinging. *Precautions:* Use with caution in patients with immuno-deficiency disorders due to disease (e.g. AIDS) or drugs (e.g. chemotherapy). Avoid contact with eyes and use with caution in pregnancy and breastfeeding mothers.

penicillamine (Distamine) is a derivative of penicillin that is very effective at binding (chelating) various metal ions in the body and helping their excretion. It can be used as an antidote to treat copper and lead poisoning and to treat Wilson's disease where there is an accumulation of copper in the liver and eyes. It is also used to treat rheumatoid arthritis (see Chapter 32), chronic active inflammation of the liver and cystinuria (a hereditary kidney disorder). *Adverse effects* vary in incidence and severity according to the dose that is used and the disorder being treated. Reported harmful effects include allergic reactions, nettle-rash, redness of the skin if temperature goes above 41°C, nausea, vomiting, loss of appetite, loss of taste (for about six weeks), mouth ulcers, bleeding into the skin, protein in the urine, kidney damage, blood disorders which may be serious, myasthenia gravis (muscle weakness due to neuro-muscular abnormality), fever and systemic lupus erythematosis (SLE – a disease of unknown cause with symptoms of fever, muscle and joint pain, blood disorders and skin eruptions). *Precautions:* Do not use in patients allergic to penicillamine or who suffer from impaired kidney function, depressed bone-marrow function, or lupus erythematosus. Do not use in patients receiving gold treatment, chloroquine, hydrochloroquine or immunosuppressive drugs. Use with caution in patients with impaired kidney function or allergy to penicillin. Regular tests of kidney function, urine tests and blood counts should be carried out in patients on long-term treatment. In rheumatoid arthritis, no improvement will occur for six to twelve weeks. If improvement continues after this period the dose should be slowly reduced at intervals of twelve weeks. Nausea may be prevented by taking the drug with food or on going to bed, and by starting with small doses which are gradually increased. Rashes are common. Those that occur in the first few months usually clear up if the drug is stopped, then started at a lower dose which is increased gradually. Rashes occurring late in treatment are more difficult to clear up and usually require the drug to be stopped. Patients should report to their doctor immediately if they develop a sore throat, mouth ulcers, bruising, fever, skin rash or generally feeling unwell. *Interactions:* Gold salts, antimalarial drugs, anti-cancer drugs, phenylbutazone, antacids, zinc salts, iron salts.

penicillin G (benzylpenicillin) ➤ penicillins.

penicillin V ➤ phenoxymethyl penicillin.

penicillins are discussed in Chapter 46. *Adverse effects:* Allergic reactions to penicillins occur occasionally (e.g. skin rash, joint pains, fever, swellings of the skin, mouth and throat), and very rarely they may be severe (anaphylactic shock). Allergic reactions are more common after injections and in people who have previously had an allergic reaction to a penicillin or a cephalosporin. Cross-allergy occurs between penicillins. All penicillins given by mouth may cause diarrhoea, heartburn and itching of the anus. Diarrhoea is commonest with ampicillin, which may (rarely) cause colitis (inflammation of the bowel) and occasionally a very serious form of bowel inflammation known as pseudomembranous colitis. Very rarely, extremely high doses of penicillins given by injection, or standard doses given to people with impaired kidney function, may cause irritation of the brain (encephalopathy). Injections of penicillin into the spinal cord may cause convulsions and death and should not be used. Some preparations are high in sodium and potassium salts and should be used with caution in patients with kidney disease. Penicillins given by mouth may occasionally cause a black tongue due to a fungal infection. Very rarely, penicillins may cause blood disorders and superinfection. Ampicillin and amoxicillin may cause a measles-like rash (which is not an allergic rash) in patients with glandular fever or chronic lymphatic leukaemia and possibly AIDS. *Precautions:* Penicillins should not be used in patients known to be allergic to one of the penicillins. Those who suffer from nettle-rash, asthma or hayfever, or who are allergic to a cephalosporin, are more prone to allergic reactions from penicillin than other people. The dosage of amoxicillin, ampicillin, azlocillin, mezlocillin and piperacillin should be reduced in patients with impaired kidney function. Bacampicillin and pivampicillin should not be used in patients who suffer from severe impairment of kidney or liver function.

Ampicillin and *amoxicillin* should be used with caution in patients suffering from glandular fever.

Flucloxacillin may rarely cause liver damage and jaundice. This may occur several weeks after stopping the drug. The risk is increased with advancing age and treatments that go on for more than two weeks. Use with caution in patients with porphyria (a hereditary disorder of metabolism).

Co-amoxiclav (amoxicillin plus clavulanic acid) should be used with utmost caution in patients with impaired liver function (carry out regular tests of liver function) and in pregnancy. It may rarely cause liver damage and jaundice (may occur up to six weeks after stopping the drug, and is due to the clavulanic acid). Severe skin disorders, kidney damage and inflammation of the vein at site of injection may occur.

Pivampicillin: Do not use in patients with porphyria (a hereditary disorder of metabolism) and carry out kidney and liver function tests at regular intervals.

Carbenicillin may cause a fall in blood potassium levels and changes in platelet function affecting blood clotting.

Timentin (ticarcillin plus clavulanic acid) may cause liver damage with jaundice due to the clavulanic acid.

Pentacarinat ➤ pentamidine.

Pennsaid ➤ diclofenac.

pentamidine (pentamidine isoethinate, Pentacarinat powder in vial) is an antiprotozoal drug used to treat the early stages of African trypanosomiasis ('sleeping sickness'), other diseases transmitted by tsetse flies and some forms of Leishmaniasis. It is also available as a nebulizer solution for inhalation (Pentacarinat Nebulizer Solution) to treat *Pneumocystis carinii* pneumonia (PCP) in patients infected with HIV. *Adverse effects:* Pentamidine by injection is a toxic drug and adverse effects are frequent and sometimes severe. They include kidney and liver damage, blood disorders, a fall in blood glucose levels (hypoglycaemia) and also a rise in blood glucose level triggering diabetes. Rarely, it may damage the pancreas. Rapid intravenous injection of pentamidine may produce a sudden fall in blood pressure, headache, dizziness, vomiting, rapid heart beat, breathlessness and fainting. Slow intravenous injections or intramuscular injections may also cause a fall in blood pressure. Intramuscular injections may cause pain, swelling and skin abscesses at the sites of injection. Intravenous injections may cause inflammation of the vein. Rarely, it may cause a fall in blood calcium levels, a rise in blood potassium levels, fever, flushing, nausea, vomiting, taste disturbances, confusion, hallucinations, disorders of heart rhythm, skin rashes and Stevens-Johnson syndrome (a disease causing severe inflammation of the skin and mucous membranes). *Precautions:* Patients receiving injection treatment with pentamidine should be under close supervision in hospital; they should remain lying in bed (supine) and their blood pressure should be checked at regular intervals. Heart tests (ECG) and tests of kidney and liver function, blood glucose levels, blood cell counts and blood potassium and calcium levels should be carried out at regular intervals. The dose should be reduced in patients with impaired kidney function, and other drugs that may damage the kidneys should be avoided. *Pentacarinat* ready-to-use Nebulizer Solution of pentamidine is used to prevent and treat PCP. The nebulizer solution is given once daily for three weeks in treatment and once a month in prevention. The risks of adverse effects are reduced by using a nebulizer which produces a tenfold higher concentration of the drug in the lungs than if the drug is given by injection.

Pentasa enema ➤ mesalazine.

Pentaspan intravenous infusion contains pentastarch in sodium chloride ➤ etherified starch.

pentastarch ➤ etherified starch.

pentazocine (in Fortagesic, Fortral) is a partial opiate blocker used as a pain-reliever (see Chapter 30). *Adverse effects* include nausea, vomiting, dizziness, light-headedness, changes in mood and sweating. It may occasionally cause headache, dry mouth, constipation, flushing, rapid heart rate, blood pressure changes, nightmares, pins and needles, insomnia, itching, retention of urine, visual disturbances, chills, allergic reactions, disorientation, hallucinations and, very rarely, convulsions. These adverse effects are more likely to occur if the patient is up and about rather than in bed. *Precautions* ➤ morphine. Do not use in patients who are dependent on opiates, who have depressed breathing, raised pressure in the brain, head injury or serious brain disorders, alcoholism, acute asthma or heart failure. Use with caution in patients with porphyria (a hereditary disorder of metabolism), impaired kidney, lung or liver function or in pregnancy. *Interactions:* MAOIs, opiate pain-relievers, alcohol. Prolonged use of high doses may lead to drug dependence.

Pentostam ➤ sodium stibogluconate.

pentostatin (Nipent) is an anti-cancer drug (see Chapter 51) effective against hairy cell leukaemia. *Adverse effects* include damage to the blood-forming tissues in the bone marrow and damage to the immune system. *Precautions:* See Chapter 51.

pentoxifylline(oxpentifylline) (Trental) is a xanthine used to treat disorders of the circulation. See Chapter 27. *Adverse effects* include nausea, stomach and bowel upsets, dizziness and flushing. *Precautions:* It should be given with caution to patients with low blood pressure, severe coronary artery disease, recent heart attack or impaired kidney function. *Interactions:* Anti-blood pressure drugs.

Pentrax shampoo ➤ coal tar.

Pepcid preparations ➤ famotidine.

peppermint oil (in Carbellon, Colpermin, Mintec) is obtained from the dried leaves and flowering tops of *Mentha piperita*. There are two varieties, known as black peppermint and white peppermint. Peppermint oil is used to relieve wind. Enteric-coated capsules of peppermint oil (Colpermin, Mintec) are used to treat colic and distension of the abdomen, irritable bowel syndrome and spastic colon. *Adverse effects* of peppermint oil used in this way include heartburn and, very rarely, allergic reactions, rash, headache, slowing of the heart rate, muscle tremor and loss of control over voluntary movements (ataxia). *Precautions:* Should be used with caution in patients with active ulceration of the bowel (e.g. ulcerative colitis) and paralysis of the small intestine. Capsules should not be chewed or broken because the released peppermint may cause irritation of the mouth and oesophagus.

Peptac liquid is an antacid containing sodium bicarbonate, sodium alginate and calcium carbonate ➤ individual entry for each drug.

Peptimax ➤ cimetidine.

Pepto-Bismol suspension ➤ bismuth salicylate.

Percutol ointment ➤ glyceryl trinitrate.

Percuvac is a vaccine used for immunization against tuberculosis. See Chapters 50 and 53.

Perdix ➤ moexipril.

Perfan ➤ enoximone.

pergolide (pergolyde mesylate, Celance) is used to treat Parkinson's disease. See Chapter 16. It is derived from ergot and mimics the actions of dopamine by stimulating dopamine receptors in the brain. This produces a reduction in tremor, improves movement and reduces rigidity. It has a long duration of action and helps to reduce the wearing-off effects (end-of-dose effects) associated with the use of levodopa preparations, and allows the daily dosage of levodopa to be reduced. *Adverse effects* include sleepiness, confusion, abnormal movements (dyskinesia), hallucinations, fall in blood pressure, rapid heart beat, indigestion, nausea, abdominal pains, insomnia, constipation or diarrhoea, runny nose, breathlessness, double vision and, very rarely, neuroleptic malignant syndrome (for symptoms see p. 331). *Precautions:* It should be used with caution in patients with heart disease, disorders of heart rhythm, a history of hallucinations or confusion. It should be used with caution in pregnancy, in breastfeeding mothers and in patients with porphyria (a hereditary disorder of metabolism). Treatment should be tapered off, not stopped suddenly. It should be used with

caution in patients who have suffered pleurisy or pericarditis (inflammation of the lining of the lungs or heart) from taking ergot drugs used to treat migraine. See Chapter 34. *Interactions:* Dopamine blockers, anti-blood pressure drugs, anticoagulants.

Periactin ➤ cyproheptadine.

pericyazine (Neulactil) is a phenothiazine antipsychotic drug ➤ antipsychotic drugs.

perindopril (Coversyl) is an ACE inhibitor used to treat raised blood pressure (see Chapter 25) and heart failure (see Chapter 23). *Adverse effects* include fall in blood pressure, nausea, abdominal pain, impaired taste, headache, cough, fatigue, weakness, generally feeling unwell, itching, flushing, localized skin rashes, angioedema (allergic swelling of the mouth and throat), blood disorders and impaired kidney function. *Precautions:* Do not use in preg- nancy or in breastfeeding mothers. Use additional treatment with diuretics with caution, particularly potassium-sparing diuretics; use potassium supplements with caution. Use perindopril with caution in patients with impaired kidney function, raised blood pressure due to kidney disease, and in patients with low blood pressure. Use with caution in elderly people because their kidney function may be impaired. Tests of kidney function should be carried out before and at regular intervals during treatment. *Interactions:* Other anti-blood pressure drugs, potassium supplements, potassium-sparing diuretics, lithium, antidepressants.

Periostat ➤ doxycycline.

permethrin (Lyclear) is a synthetic derivation of the naturally occurring insecticide pyrethrin. It is used as a hair preparation (Lyclear Cream Rinse) to treat head lice (see p. 256) and as a skin cream (Lyclear Dermal Cream) to treat scabies (see p. 261). *Precautions:* It should be used with caution in children under two years, in pregnancy and in breastfeeding mothers. Contact with the eyes should be avoided. Do not use on broken or secondarily infected skin. The use of skin cream for scabies and cream rinse for head lice in children aged two months to two years should be under the supervision of a doctor or nurse.

Permitabs solution tablets ➤ potassium permanganate.

Peroxyl ➤ hydrogen peroxide.

perphenazine (Fentazin, in Triptafen) is a phenothiazine antipsychotic drug ➤ antipsychotic drugs.

Persantin ➤ dipyridamole.

Peru balsam (in Anugesic HC, in Anusol, in Anusol HC) is a balsam exuded from the trunk of *myroxylon balsamum*. It has a mild antiseptic action by virtue of its content of cinnamic and benzoic acids. It is used in ointments for the treatment of eczema and itching of the skin, and in suppositories for the relief of haemorrhoids. It may cause allergic reactions.

pethidine (pethidine hydrochloride, meperidine hydrochloride, in Pamergan P100) is a synthetic opiate pain-reliever (see Chapter 30). It has actions and uses similar to those described under morphine but it is not as powerful and its effects are less prolonged. It is less likely to cause constipation and it produces less depression of breathing in newborn babies when used to relieve pain in labour. It has little effect upon coughs. *Adverse effects:* It may cause a lift in mood, dizziness, sweating, dry mouth, nausea, vomiting, constipation and retention of urine. These are all much less frequent than with morphine. Injection into a vein may cause a fall in blood pressure. Its use during childbirth may depress the respiration of the baby at birth (but see above). *For other potential adverse effects* ➤ morphine. *Precautions:* Pethidine should not be given to patients with severe liver or kidney disease or to relieve gall-bladder pains. *For other precautions* ➤ morphine. *Drug dependence:* Pethidine may cause drug dependence of the morphine type. Tolerance is not always complete and addicts may develop twitching, tremor, mental confusion and hallucinations. Sometimes convulsions and death may occur from pethidine dependence. Withdrawal symptoms come on more quickly than with morphine. *Interactions* ➤ morphine.

petroleum jelly ➤ paraffin, white soft and yellow soft.

Pevaryl preparations ➤ econazole.

Pharmalgen are preparations of bee venom extract (*Apis mellifera*) and wasp venom extract (*Vespula*). They are used to desensitize patients who are allergic to bee or wasp venom. *Adverse effects:* Allergic reactions, especially in small children. *Precautions:* Do not use in pregnancy or in patients suffering from acute asthma or who have a fever. Facilities for full cardiopulmonary resuscitation must be immediately to hand (see p. 87). Monitor patient closely for one hour after each injection.

Pharmorubicin injection ➤ epirubicin.

phenazocine (Narphen), see p. 154.

phenelzine (phenelzine sulphate, Nardil) is a monoamine oxidase inhibitor antidepressant drug. See Chapter 4 on antidepressants. *Adverse effects and Precautions* ➤ MAOIs.

Phenergan preparations ➤ promethazine.

phenindione (phenylindanedione, Dindevan) is an oral anticoagulant used to treat deep-vein blood clots (see Chapter 28). *Adverse effects:* Early signs of overdose are bleeding from the gums, nose or elsewhere, and red blood cells in the urine. It may cause vomiting, diarrhoea, skin rashes and fever. Sore throat may be an early sign of allergy which may lead to blood disorders, liver damage and kidney damage. Phenindione may cause a brownish pigmentation of the fingernails, fingers and palms of the hands of the person handling it. It sometimes colours the urine pink. *Precautions:* It should be given with caution to patients with impaired liver or kidney function, raised blood pressure, acute illness, vitamin

K deficiency, or to elderly patients. It should not be used in pregnancy or within twenty-four hours of childbirth or surgery. It should not be used in patients with severe liver or kidney disease, or bleeding disorders. Mothers who are taking phenindione should not breastfeed their babies. *Interactions:* NSAIDs, oral anti-diabetic drugs, sulphonamides, quinidine, antibiotics, phenformin, cimetidine, corticosteroids.

phenobarbital sodium (phenobarbitone sodium, Gardenal Sodium) is a long-acting barbiturate used to treat epilepsies. See Chapter 15. *Adverse effects* of barbiturates include hangover, dizziness, lethargy, drowsiness, mental depression, allergic skin rashes and depression of breathing. High doses may cause incoordination of movements (ataxia). Elderly people may become restless and confused, and children may become over-excitable. Some people may get a paradoxical effect and become excited instead of calm. Folic acid deficiency anaemia may develop after prolonged use (responds to folic acid by mouth) and, very rarely, liver damage may occur. *Precautions:* Barbiturates should not be used in patients with uncontrolled pain, in young adults, the elderly and debilitated, in pregnancy, in breastfeeding mothers, in patients with a history of alcohol or drug abuse or with porphyria (a hereditary disorder of metabolism). They should be used with caution in children and people with impaired kidney or liver function, or impaired breathing. They cause drowsiness and can affect the ability to drive motor vehicles and operate moving machinery. *Interactions:* Alcohol, sleeping drugs, sedatives, anti-anxiety drugs and other drugs that depress brain function, coumarin-type anticoagulants, oestrogens, progestogens, oral contraceptives, corticosteroids, griseofulvin, rifampicin, phenytoin, metronidazole, chloramphenicol. *Drug dependence:* Barbiturates may cause drug dependence of the barbiturate/alcohol type (see p. xxvii). Avoid sudden withdrawal.

phenobarbitone ➤ phenobarbital.

phenol is used as a disinfectant and antiseptic.

phenothiazines, see p. 12.

phenothrin (Full Marks shampoo) is used to treat head lice. See p. 256. Contact with the eyes should be avoided. Use with caution in children under six months of age. It may irritate the skin. Do not use on broken or secondarily infected skin. It may cause wheezing in asthmatic patients.

phenoxybenzamine (Dibenyline) is a non-selective alpha-blocker used to treat episodes of raised blood pressure in a patient suffering from a phaeochromocytoma (tumour of the sympathetic nervous system) (see Chapter 25). *Adverse effects* include rapid heart beat, fall in blood pressure on standing up after lying down, dizziness, weariness, nasal congestion, visual disturbances, and, rarely, stomach and bowel upsets, and failure to ejaculate. Leakage from injection can irritate surrounding tissues. Rarely it can produce a severe fall in blood pressure on intravenous infusion (an idiosyncratic reaction). *Precautions:* Do not use in patients who have had a stroke or recent heart attack. Use with caution in the elderly and in patients with congestive heart failure, heart disease, disorders of the circulation to the brain or kidney disease. Use with caution in pregnancy and do not use in patients with porphyria (a hereditary disorder of metabolism).

phenoxymethylpenicillin (penicillin V, Apsin, Tenkicin) is a penicillinase-sensitive penicillin ➤ penicillins.

Phensic is a pain-reliever containing aspirin and caffeine ➤ aspirin, caffeine.

phentolamine (phentolamine mesylate, Rogitine) is an alpha-blocker (see Chapter 25). It is used to treat episodes of raised blood pressure in patients suffering from a phaeochromocytoma (tumour of the sympathetic nervous system). *Adverse effects* include rapid beating of the heart, anginal pain, flushing, and a fall in blood pressure, dizziness, weakness, stomach and bowel upsets, nasal congestion, disorders of heart rhythm and chest pain. *Precautions:* Do not use in patients with a marked drop in blood pressure, an allergy to sulphites or in patients with coronary heart disease. It should be used with caution in pregnancy and in breastfeeding mothers, in patients with impaired kidney function, asthma, gastritis, peptic ulcers, or in the elderly. Blood pressure must be measured at regular intervals. *Interactions:* Other anti-blood pressure drugs, antipsychotic drugs.

phenylbutazone (Butacote) is a nonsteroidal anti-inflammatory drug (NSAID) used in hospital to treat rheumatic diseases such as ankylosing spondilitis. See Chapter 32. It also has pain-relieving properties and reduces a high temperature. It is metabolized and excreted slowly and therefore its effects are prolonged. *Adverse effects:* Phenylbutazone causes salt retention, blocks iodine uptake by the thyroid gland and interferes with several enzyme processes in the body. Adverse effects are common and occur even when the dose does not exceed 400 mg daily. They include rashes, nausea, stomach upset, fluid retention which may trigger heart failure, blurred vision, insomnia and diarrhoea. Ulcers in the mouth, oesophagus (gullet), stomach or duodenum may occur, leading to bleeding from these sites. Phenylbutazone may damage the pancreas, liver and bone marrow (causing serious blood disorders). Enlarged glands (including salivary glands) may occur and a generalized allergic reaction and kidney failure have been reported. It may cause serious skin disorders and damage the lungs. Adverse effects may occur within a few days of starting phenylbutazone and some patients may become sensitized so that a subsequent course of the drug may trigger adverse effects. *Precautions:* Phenylbutazone should not be given to patients with a history of peptic ulcers, heart disease, raised blood pressure, impaired kidney or liver function, bleeding disorders of the stomach

or intestine, blood disorders, porphyria (a hereditary disorder of metabolism), thyroid disease, children under fourteen or in pregnancy. It should be used with great caution in the elderly and breastfeeding mothers. Blood counts should be carried out before and at regular intervals during treatment. It should be used with caution by patients with impaired heart, liver or kidney function. It should not be used in patients allergic to aspirin or an NSAID; this warning includes patients who have developed asthma, angioedema (allergic swelling of the mouth and throat), nettle-rash or rhinitis (inflammation of the lining of the nose) to aspirin or an NSAID. *Interactions* ➤ NSAIDs.

phenylephrine (phenylephrine hydrochloride) is a sympathomimetic drug. See Chapter 9. It is used as a decongestant in cold remedies, nasal drops and sprays, to dilate the pupils, and to treat an acute fall in blood pressure. It is used in conjunction with local anaesthetics in order to prolong their effects. *Adverse effects* include raised blood pressure, headache, changes in heart rate and coldness of the hands and feet. It may cause pain and irritation at the site of injection. Overdose may cause headache, palpitation and vomiting. Nose drops may cause local irritation and eye drops may trigger glaucoma. *Precautions:* Phenylephrine injections should not be given to patients with severe heart disease or blood pressure. Injections should be used with caution in patients with over-active thyroid glands. *Interactions:* It should not be given during, or within two weeks of stopping treatment with an MAOI antidepressant drug.

phenylethyl alcohol (in Ceanel) is an antibacterial agent used as a preservative in eye drops.

phenylpropanolamine is an oral preparation used for nasal decongestion.

phenytoin (phenytoin sodium, Epanutin) is used to treat epilepsy. See Chapter 15. It is also used to treat disorders of heart rhythm, see Chapter 24. *Adverse effects* include dizziness, nausea, vomiting, headache, tremor and insomnia. High doses may cause loss of control over voluntary movements (ataxia), blurred vision and slurred speech. Occasionally it may cause tenderness and thickening of the gums, excessive hair growth, over-activity in young people, swollen glands, nystagmus (flicking movements of the eyeballs), skin rashes (stop if this occurs), sleepiness, allergic reactions, hallucinations and mental confusion. It may cause megaloblastic anaemia by interfering with folic acid metabolism. Phenytoin may irritate the lining of the stomach and should be taken with plenty of water preferably after meals (although it is more effective if given before meals). *Precautions:* It should not be used in patients with porphyria (a hereditary disorder of metabolism). It should be used with caution in patients with impaired liver function, in pregnancy and in breastfeeding mothers. The drug should be withdrawn gradually. *Interactions:* Coumarin anticoagulants, doxycycline, isoniazid, chloramphenicol, sulthiame and oral contraceptives. When used to treat disorders of heart rhythm it should not be used if the patient has AV heart block and it should be used with caution in pregnancy and breastfeeding mothers. ECG should be monitored and resuscitation equipment should be immediately to hand.

phenytoin sodium ➤ phenytoin.

Phillip's Milk of Magnesia is an antacid preparation ➤ magnesium.

Phimetin ➤ cimetidine.

pHiso-Med solution ➤ chlorhexidine

pholcodine (in Galenphol, Pavacol-D) is used as a cough suppressant. See Chapter 11. It is not as effective as codeine but it does not cause dependence and it produces less constipation ➤ codeine.

PhorPain ➤ ibuprofen.

Phosec tablets ➤ calcium.

phosphate-binding drugs Aluminium-containing and calcium-containing antacids are used to bind phosphates in the gut in the treatment of patients with kidney failure who have a high blood phosphate level. Calcium-containing phosphate-binders should not be used in patients with high levels of calcium in their blood or urine. Phosphate-binders that contain aluminium may cause a rise in blood aluminium levels in patients receiving kidney dialysis.

Phosphate-Sandoz effervescent tablets contain sodium acid phosphate, sodium bicarbonate and potassium bicarbonate. They are used to lower raised blood calcium levels due to over-active parathyroid glands, malignant tumours of plasma cells and certain cancers. They are also used to increase low levels of blood phosphates in rickets.

phosphate suppositories and enemas are used to clear the bowel before X-ray, endoscopy and surgery. They include Carbalax suppositories, Fleet Ready-to-use Enema and Fletchers Phosphate Enema. See Chapter 21.

phosphodiesterase inhibitors, see p. 123.

Phospholine Iodide ➤ ecothiopate iodide.

photofrin (Porfimer) is used for the treatment of lung cancer and cancer of the throat. See Chapter 51.

Phyllocontin Continus preparations ➤ aminophylline.

Physeptone ➤ methadone.

Physiotens ➤ moxonidine.

Phytex contains tannic acid, boric acid, salicyclic acid, methyl salicylate and acetic acid. It is used to treat fungal infections of the nails and skin. Do not use in pregnancy.

phytomenadione (Konakion, Konakion MM) is a vitamin K derivative. It is involved in blood clotting (see Chapter 28). It is used to treat bleeding diseases of the newborn caused by vitamin K deficiency, and bleeding due to low prothrombin in the blood (e.g. due to overdose of oral anticoagulants). *Adverse effects:* Overdose may cause jaundice in newborn babies. If given into a vein it should be given very slowly because it may produce sweating, flushing, a sense of suffocation, collapse and allergic reactions. *Precautions:* Use with caution in the elderly.

Picolax oral powder contains sodium picosulfate with magnesium citrate. It is used to evacuate the bowel before surgery, X-ray and endoscopy. See Chapter 21. *Precautions:* Do not use if the bowel is obstructed. Use with caution in patients with inflammatory bowel disease (e.g. ulcerative colitis). Take low residue diet before use and drink plenty of fluids during treatment.

pilocarpine (pilocarpine hydrochloride, pilocarpine nitrate, in Isopto Carpine, Minims Pilocarpine, Pilogel, Salagen, Sno Pilo) has effects and uses similar to those described under neostigmine. It is used in eye drops to constrict the pupil and decrease the pressure inside the eyeball in patients with glaucoma. See p. 63. *Adverse reactions* include temporary loss of visual acuity. *Precautions:* Do not use in patients with acute inflammation of the iris. Do not wear soft contact lenses.

Pilogel is a slow-release gel containing pilocarpine which is used to treat glaucoma ➤ pilocarpine.

pimozide (Orap) is an antipsychotic drug ➤ antipsychotic drugs.

pindolol (in Viskaldix, Visken) is a non-selective beta-blocker ➤ beta-blockers.

pioglitazone (Actos) is an anti-diabetic drug used in combination with metformin in obese patients, or with a sulphonylurea in patients for whom metformin is unsuitable, in Type II diabetes inadequately controlled by maximum tolerated doses of either. See Chapter 42. *Adverse effects* include anaemia, weight gain, headache, visual disturbance, pain in joints, blood in the urine, impotence, fluid retention, flatulence. *Precautions:* Do not use in patients undergoing dialysis, with liver damage, cardiac failure, in pregnancy or while breastfeeding.

piperacillin (piperacillin sodium, Pipril, in Tazocin) is a penicillin ➤ penicillins.

piperazine (Expilix, in Pripsen). Piperazine is used to treat threadworms and roundworm infection. *Adverse effects:* These are very rare unless high and prolonged dosage is used or kidney function is impaired. They include nausea, vomiting, diarrhoea, colic, vertigo, headache, blurred vision, nerve damage and allergic skin rashes. *Precautions:* Do not use in patients who suffer from epilepsy, kidney failure or liver failure. Use with caution if breastfeeding.

piperazine estrone sulphate (Harmogen) is a natural oestrogen used to treat symptoms of the menopause ➤ oestrogens ➤ HRT.

Piportil Depot oily injection ➤ pipotiazine.

pipothiazine ➤ pipotiazine.

pipotiazine (pipothiazine palmitate, Piportil Depot) is a phenothiazine antipsychotic drug ➤ antipsychotic drugs.

Pipril ➤ piperacillin.

piracetam (Nootropil) is used to treat myoclonus (involuntary spasms and jerkings of the muscles of the body) caused by a brain disorder. *Adverse effects* include nervousness, depression, insomnia, sleepiness, diarrhoea, rash, weight gain and over-activity. *Precautions:* Do not use in pregnancy, in breastfeeding mothers or in patients with severe impairment of kidney or liver function. Use with caution in patients with mild or moderate impairment of kidney function and in the elderly. Withdraw the drug slowly when stopping treatment. *Interactions:* Thyroid hormone.

Piriton ➤ chlorphenamine(chlorpheniramine).

piroxicam (Brexidol, Feldene, in Feldene gel, Fenbid Forte Gel, Kentene, Pirozip) is a non-steroidal anti-inflammatory drug (NSAID) ➤ non-steroidal anti-inflammatory drugs.

Pirozip ➤ piroxicam.

Pitressin ➤ argipressin.

pivmecillinam (Selexid) is an antibiotic used to treat urinary tract infections. See Chapter 49. *Adverse effects* include stomach and bowel upset, rash and allergic reactions. *Precautions:* Do not use in patients with carnitine deficiency, obstruction of the oesophagus or any obstruction in the digestive system. Use with caution in patients with kidney damage or in pregnancy.

pizotifen (pizotifen malate, Sanomigran) is a 5HT (serotonin) blocker (see p. 41). It is used to prevent migraine attacks (see Chapter 34). *Adverse effects* include drowsiness (children may be stimulated rather than made drowsy), increase of appetite and gain in weight, nausea, dizziness, flushing of the face, muscle pains and mood changes. *Precautions:* It should be used with caution in patients who are liable to retention of urine (e.g. men with enlarged prostate glands), in patients with glaucoma or impaired kidney function, in pregnancy and in breastfeeding mothers. It may cause drowsiness and affect the ability to drive and operate moving machinery. *Interactions.* Increases the effects of alcohol.

Placidex ➤ paracetamol.

Plaquenil ➤ hydroxychloroquine.

Plavix ➤ clopidogrel.

Plantago ovata (in Manevac) is used in the treatment of constipation. See Chapter 21. *Adverse effects* include flatulence, distension and diarrhoea. *Precautions:* Do not use in patients with an obstruction in the stomach or bowel.

Platinex ➤ cisplatin.

Plendil ➤ felodipine.

Plesmet syrup ➤ ferrous glycine sulphate.

Pneumovax II is a pneumoccal vaccine given by subcutaneous or intramuscular injection.

Pnu-Imune is a pneumoccal vaccine given by subcutaneous or intramuscular injection.

podophyllotoxin (Condyline, Warticon) is a cytotoxic (cell-destroying) drug used to treat external genital warts. It is obtained from the dried rhizomes and roots of *Podophyllum peltatum* (Berberidaceae). *Adverse effects:* It is irritant to the skin and very toxic if swallowed, producing nausea, vomiting, diarrhoea, blood disorders, hallucinations, confusion, stupor, convulsions and coma. The risk of toxic effects due to absorption from the skin is increased if large areas are treated and excessive amounts are used regularly over a prolonged period of time, or if the penile warts are bleeding or have been damaged (e.g. by biopsy). It may cause irritation where it is applied. *Precautions:* Avoid contact with healthy skin, open wounds, face and eyes. Do not use in pregnancy or in breastfeeding mothers.

podophyllum (podophyllin paint compound, podophyllum resin) is used to treat warts (see p. 262). *Adverse effects:* It is very irritant to the skin. If absorbed into the bloodstream it can cause serious brain and nerve damage, liver damage and blood disorders. *Precautions:* Do not take by mouth. Avoid contact with mucous membranes (e.g. the mouth, lining of the vagina), eyes and the face. The risk of absorption into the bloodstream from topical applications is increased if it is applied to large areas in extensive amounts for prolonged periods of time or if it is applied to warts that are bleeding, have been biopsied or are fragile. Avoid contact with normal skin. Do not use in pregnancy.

podophyllum resin (in Posalfilin) ➤ podophyllum.

poloxamer 188 (in Ailax, in Codalax) is a surface-active agent used as a faecal softener to treat constipation. See Chapter 21.

polyacrylic acid ➤ carbomer.

polyene (antifungal drugs) see Chapter 47.

polyethylene glycol (in Klean-prep, in Movical) ➤ macroyols.

Polyfax ointment contains the antibiotics polymyxin B and bacitracin zinc. It is used as an eye ointment to treat styes, infections of the conjunctiva and eyelids and to prevent eye infection after eye surgery. It is also used in skin ointments to treat skin infections, e.g. impetigo. *Adverse effects and Precautions:* Do not use on large, open wounds because of the risk of absorption producing kidney damage. Allergic reactions may occur ➤ polymyxin B.

polymyxin B (polymyxin B sulphate) is an antibiotic. See p. 271. It is used in the following topical preparations: Gregoderm, Maxitrol, Neosporin, Otosporin, Polyfax, Polytrim. *Adverse effects:* Because of the adverse effects it may produce by injection or by mouth (particularly nerve damage and kidney damage) its use is restricted to applications to the skin, ears and eyes. On the skin it should not be applied to large areas or to open wounds because of the risk of absorption into the bloodstream producing kidney damage.

polysaccharide-iron-complex drops (Niferex Elixier, Niferex Paediatric) are used to prevent and treat iron deficiency anaemia in infants born prematurely ➤ iron and see Chapter 35.

polystyrene sulphonate resins include calcium polystyrene sulphonate (Calcium Resonium) and sodium polystyrene sulphonate (Resonium A). They are ion exchange resins ➤ calcium polystyrene sulphonate, sodium polystyrene sulphonate.

Polytar preparations are used to treat dandruff, psoriasis, seborrhoea and eczema of the scalp. The main active ingredient is coal tar ➤ coal tar.

polythiazide (Nephril) is a thiazide diuretic ➤ thiazide diuretics.

Polytrim eye drops and ointment contain the antibacterial drugs trimethoprim and polymyxin B. They are used to treat bacterial infections of the eyes ➤ trimethoprim and polymyxin B. *Adverse effects:* Allergic reactions may occur very rarely. *Precautions:* Do not use in patients who are allergic to trimethoprim or polymyxin B.

Polyvinyl alcohol is used as a lubricant in Hypotears, Liquifilm Tears and Sno Tears.

Ponstan preparations ➤ mefenamic acid.

POP (progestogen-only pills), see Chapter 41.

poractant alfa (Curosurf) is a surface-active drug used to treat respiratory distress syndrome (hyaline membrane disease) in pre-term babies who are on a mechanical respirator. *Adverse effects* include bleeding in the lungs. *Precautions:* Continuously monitor heart rate and blood oxygen level (to prevent it going too high).

Porfimer ➤ photofrin.

Posalfilin ointment contains salicylic acid and podophyllum resin. It is used to treat warts ➤ salicylic acid and podophyllum. It is not suitable for warts around the anus or genitals, or for use in pregnancy.

Posiject ➤ dobutamine.

PostMI ➤ aspirin.

Potaba preparations contain potassium aminobenzoate. They are used to treat scleroderma and Peyronie's disease (conditions that involve excessive hardening of the tissues). *Adverse effects* include nausea and loss of appetite (stop if these occur). *Precautions:* Use with caution in patients with impaired kidney function. *Interactions:* Sulphonamides.

potassium supplements may be used in patients taking digoxin or anti-arrhythmic drugs, where potassium depletion may induce disorders of heart rhythm; in patients being treated with diuretics for fluid retention due to narrowing of a main artery to a kidney; cirrhosis of the liver; severe kidney damage (nephrotic syndrome) or severe heart failure. Potassium supplements may also be used in patients with excessive loss of potassium in the stools caused by chronic diarrhoea, laxative abuse or disorders of the intestine that affect absorption. Elderly patients may need potassium supplements and so may patients on drugs that cause a loss of potassium, e.g. corticosteroids. Rarely are they needed in patients taking loop or thiazide diuretics in small doses for a raised blood pressure. Patients on higher maintenance doses of a loop or thiazide diuretic for fluid retention should have a potassium-sparing diuretic added to their treatment rather than taking a potassium supplement. *Adverse effects:* Potassium salts are irritant and may cause nausea, vomiting and diarrhoea. They may occasionally cause ulcers in the oesophagus, stomach or intestine, with bleeding, perforation and scarring. When given with a thiazide diuretic they may cause similar effects. *Precautions:* Potassium salts should be used with caution in patients with impaired kidney function, underworking of the adrenal glands, heart disease or acute dehydration. *Note:* Potassium depletion is frequently associated with a loss of chloride causing alkalosis, therefore potassium chloride should be taken preferably in liquid or effervescent form.

potassium aminobenzoate (Potaba) is considered to belong to the B-group of vitamins. It is used in the treatment of various fibrotic disorders, such as sclerodema and Peyronie's disease that involve excessive hardening of tissues. *Adverse effects* include loss of appetite and nausea (stop the drug immediately if these symptoms occur). It should be used with caution in patients with impaired kidney function. *Interactions:* sulphonamides.

potassium bicarbonate is used in the prevention and treatment of potassium deficiency ➤ potassium.

potassium channel activators, see p. 116.

potassium chloride is used in the prevention and treatment of potassium deficiency. It is also used as a table salt substitute ➤ potassium supplements.

potassium citrate makes the urine less acid and is used to treat inflammation of the bladder and urethra. It may also be used as a potassium supplement ➤ potassium supplements.

potassium clorazepate ➤ clorazepate.

potassium hydroxyquinoline (potassium hydroxyquinoline sulphate) is used in skin applications as an antibacterial, antifungal deodorant and for removing dead skin. It is a constituent of Quinocort, Quinoderm preparations and Quinoped.

potassium permanganate has disinfectant, deodorizing and astringent properties. It is used as a cleansing agent and as a gargle or mouthwash when diluted with water. *Adverse effects:* It may cause corrosive burns.

Potter's Cleansing Herb is a laxative containing aloes, cascara and senna ➤ senna.

povidone (polyvinylpyrrolidone) is used in the preparation of tablets and as a carrier of drugs such as penicillin, insulin and iodine to prolong their action. It is also used in lubricant eye drops (Oculotect) and in solutions to make the wearing of contact lenses more comfortable.

povidone-iodine (Betadine preparations, Inadine, Savlon Dry Powder, Videne) is used in skin and mouth applications as an antiseptic ➤ iodine.

povidone (Oculotect) ➤ povidone.

Powergel ➤ ketoprofen.

PR Heat Spray is a heat rub containing ethyl nicotinate, methyl salicylate, camphor ➤ individual entry for each drug.

Pragmatar cream contains tar distillate, sulphur and salicylic acid. It is used to treat oily scalp conditions and scaly skin disorders. *Adverse effects* include irritation of the skin. *Precautions:* Avoid contact with eyes, genitals or inflamed or broken areas of skin ➤ coal tar, sulphur, salicylic acid.

Pralenal ➤ enalapril.

pralidoxime mesilate is used with atropine to treat poisoning by organophosphates. *Adverse effects* include dizziness, drowsiness, nausea, disturbances of vision, headache, rapid beating of the heart, hyperventilation and muscle weakness. *Precautions:* Do not use to treat poisonings due to carbamates or to organophosphate compounds that do not have anticholinesterase activity. Use with caution in patients with myasthenia gravis (muscle weakness due to neuromuscular abnormality) or impaired liver function.

pramipexole (Mirapexin) is used in combination with levodopa for the treatment of advanced idiopathic Parkinson's disease. See Chapter 16. *Adverse effects* include nausea, constipation, unpredictable sleep attacks (do not drive or operate machinery), drowsiness, hallucinations, abnormal or disordered movements. *Precautions:* Do not use while breastfeeding. Use with caution in patients with kidney damage, psychotic disorders, severe cardiovascular disease or in pregnancy. Any visual changes should be reported. Withdraw gradually.

pramocaine (pramoxine) is a local anaesthetic included in Anugesic-HC and Proctofoam HC.

pramoxine ➤ pramocaine.

pravastatin (Lipostat) is used to treat people with raised blood cholesterol levels (see Chapter 26) who have not responded to other treatments. It blocks the effects of an enzyme involved in the production of cholesterol. This reduces the blood level of cholesterol which stimulates an increase in low density lipoprotein (LDL) receptors, which in turn helps to reduce the level of LDL in the blood. It differs from similar drugs in so far as it is hydrophilic (attracted to water), which impedes its uptake by cells. This reduces its effects on cholesterol production by the cells and may reduce the risk of harmful effects (e.g. on the brain). However, it is actively taken up by the cells in the liver. *Adverse effects* include nausea, constipation, wind, insomnia, muscle damage, liver damage, angioedema (allergic swelling of the mouth and throat), vomiting, diarrhoea, fatigue, headache, chest pains and skin rashes. *Precautions:* It should not be used in pregnancy (confirm that patient is *not* pregnant before starting treatment and patients should avoid risk of getting pregnant during and for one month after stopping treatment). Do not use in breastfeeding mothers, or in individuals with active liver disease, or porphyria (a hereditary disorder of metabolism). It should be used with caution in people with a history of liver disease or heavy alcohol drinking. Tests of liver function should be carried out before and at regular intervals during treatment. Patients should report any muscle pains and avoid high alcohol intake. *Interactions:* Immunosuppressive drugs, nicotinic acid, erythromycin, rifampicin, gemfibrozil, other fibrates. Take one hour before or four hours after cholestyramine or colestipol. For risks of muscle damage ➤ simvastatin.

Praxilene ➤ naftidrofuryl.

prazosin (prazosin hydrochloride, Hypovase) is a selective alpha$_1$ blocker used to treat heart failure (see Chapter 23). It may also be used to treat raised blood pressure (see Chapter 25) and Raynaud's syndrome (See Chapter 27). It is also used to improve the flow of urine in men with enlarged prostate glands, see p. 284. *Adverse effects* include dizziness, headache, drowsiness, weakness, lack of energy, nausea, and palpitations. These are usually related to dose and may disappear on continuation of treatment or on reducing the dose. Blurred vision, frequency of passing urine, congestion of the nose, nervousness, depressed mood, constipation, skin rashes, diarrhoea, fainting, itching, sweating and impotence may occur very rarely. First dose may occasionally cause collapse due to a sudden drop in blood pressure. *Precautions:* Initial dose should be reduced in patients with kidney failure. Patients should lie down if they feel dizzy, sweaty or fatigued until these symptoms clear up. Take first dose on going to bed. Fainting while standing up to pass urine (micturition syncopy) may occur. Do not use to treat patients suffering from heart failure due to some obstruction (e.g. obstruction in the main artery (aorta) from the heart). Use with caution in the elderly, patients with impaired kidney function, in pregnancy and in breastfeeding mothers. *Interactions:* Anti-blood pressure drugs.

Preconceive ➤ folic acid.

Precortisyl and **Precortisyl Forte** ➤ prednisolone.

Predenema retention enema ➤ prednisolone.

Predfoam rectal foam ➤ prednisolone. *Precautions:* Protect the can from sunlight and do not expose to temperatures above 50°C. Do not pierce or burn the can.

Pred Forte eye drops ➤ prednisolone. They are used to treat inflammatory eye disorders. *Adverse effects* include rise in pressure inside the eyeball, thinning of the cornea, cataracts and secondary viral and fungal infections. *Precautions:* Do not use to treat viral, fungal or tuberculous eye infections. Do not use in patients with dendritic ulcers of the cornea or glaucoma. Do not use soft contact lenses.

prednisolone (prednisolone acetate, prednisolone sodium phosphate, Deltacortril, Deltastab, Minims prednisolone, Precortisyl, Precortisyl Forte, Predenema, Predfoam, Pred Forte, in Predsol, in Scheriproct) is a corticosteroid, see Chapter 37 on corticosteroids.

Predsol preparations ➤ prednisolone.

Predsol-N eye and ear drops contain neomycin (an aminoglycoside antibiotic) and prednisolone (a corticosteroid). Predsol N Ear Drops are used to treat inflammation of the outer ear. *Adverse effects:* Superinfection. *Precautions:* Do not use in patients with a perforated ear drum or untreated viral, fungal or tuberculous infection. Avoid long-term use in infants. Predsol N Eye Drops are used to treat infected inflammatory conditions of the eye. *Adverse effects* include a rise in pressure inside the eye, thinning of the cornea, cataract and allergic reactions. *Precautions:* Do not use in patients with dendritic ulcers, viral, fungal or tubercular infections or glaucoma. Use with caution in infants and if using for prolonged periods in pregnancy. Do not wear soft contact lenses.

Pregaday tablets contain ferrous fumarate and folic acid ➤ iron, folic acid.

Pregnyl ➤ chorionic gonadotrophin.

Premarin HRT preparations contain conjugated oestrogens ➤ HRT.

Premique and **Premique Cycle** are two HRT preparations that contain conjugated oestrogens and the progestogen medroxyprogesterone ➤ HRT.

Premiums is an antacid containing salts of aluminium, calcium and magnesium and light kaolin ➤ antacids.

Prempak-C contains conjugated oestrogens and the progestogen norgestrel. It is used as hormone replacement therapy (HRT). *Adverse effects and Precautions* ➤ HRT.

Prepadine ➤ dothiepin.

Preparation H gel is a haemorrhoidal preparation containing hamamelis water.

Preparation H ointment and **suppositories** are haemorrhoidal preparations containing shark liver oil and yeast cell extract.

Prescal ➤ isradipine.

Preservex ➤ aceclofenac.

Prestim preparations contain timolol (a non-selective beta-blocker) and bendrofluazide (a thiazide diuretic). They are used to treat raised blood pressure. See Chapter 25. *Adverse effects and Precautions* ➤ beta-blockers, thiazide diuretics.

Prevenar is a pneumococcal vaccine given by intramuscular injection.

Priadel ➤ lithium.

prilocaine (prilocaine hydrochloride, Citanest, in EMLA) is a local anaesthetic (see

Chapter 44) with similar effects and uses to lidocaine(lignocaine) but it produces fewer adverse effects. *Adverse effects:* Overdose may cause chemical change inside the red blood cells (methaemoglobinaemia) and it should therefore not be used in patients with anaemia. It may rarely produce allergic reactions. *Precautions:* It should be used with caution in patients with epilepsy, impaired liver, kidney or lung function or conductive defects of the heart. It should not be used in patients with anaemia or methaemaglobinaemia.

Primacor ➤ milrinone.

primaquine (primaquine phosphate) is an antimalarial drug. *Adverse effects* include loss of appetite, abdominal pains, nausea and vomiting. Rarely, it may cause blood disorders and jaundice. *Precautions:* Adverse effects on the blood occur more frequently in patients who are deeply pigmented or who have G6PD deficiency. Use chloroquine in pregnancy and delay use of primaquine until after delivery. Use with caution in patients suffering from disorders that may be associated with a low white cell count, e.g. rheumatoid arthritis, systemic lupus erythematosus (SLE – a disease of unknown cause with symptoms of fever, muscle and joint pain, blood disorders and skin eruptions). Use with caution in breastfeeding mothers.

Primaxin IV and IM contains imipenem with cilastatin. Imipenem (a beta-lactam antibiotic, see p. 266) is partially inactivated in the kidneys by certain enzymes which are blocked by cilastatin. *Adverse effects* include nausea, vomiting, diarrhoea, disturbances of taste, allergic reactions, blood disorders, colitis (inflammation of the bowel), convulsions, confusion, mental disturbances, changes in liver and kidney function tests, red coloration of urine in children, and pain, redness and swelling at site of injection. *Precautions:* Do not use in patients allergic to imipenem or cilastatin or in breastfeeding mothers. Use with caution in patients allergic to penicillins, cephalosporins or other beta-lactam antibiotics, in patients who suffer from epilepsy, colitis, impaired kidney function, in pregnancy, while breastfeeding or in patients with a low white blood cell count. Do not use IM preparations in patients allergic to lidocaine. *Interactions:* Probenecid, ganciclovir.

primidone (Mysoline) is used to treat epilepsy. See Chapter 15. It is metabolized to phenobarbitone in the liver ➤ phenobarbital. *Adverse effects* such as drowsiness, loss of control over voluntary movements (ataxia), nausea and visual disturbances usually clear up if treatment is continued.

Primolut N ➤ norethisterone.

Primoteston Depot ➤ testosterone.

Primperan ➤ metoclopramide.

Prioderm preparations ➤ malathion.

Priorix is a measles, mumps, rubella (MMR) vaccine which is given by deep subcutaneous or by intramuscular injection.

Pripsen preparations contain piperazine and sennosides A and B. They are used to treat threadworms and roundworms. *Adverse effects and Precautions* ➤ piperazine, sennosides.

Pripsen mebendazole ➤ mebendazole.

Pro-Banthine ➤ propantheline.

probenecid is used to treat gout. See Chapter 33. It increases the excretion of urates by the kidneys. This results in a reduction of the raised blood uric acid level (which occurs in gout) and slowly causes removal of urate deposits from the tissues. It is of no use in treating an acute attack of gout and is only used to prevent attacks. Treatment must usually be continued for life. Probenecid also reduces the excretion of penicillins and of the antibiotics cephalexin and cephalothin. It therefore increases the plasma level of these drugs, which is directly related to their effectiveness. *Adverse effects* include nausea, vomiting, increased frequency of passing urine, flushing, dizziness, sore gums, kidney stones and pain. Very rarely, allergic reactions, kidney damage, liver damage, blood disorders, skin rashes and fever may occur. Adverse effects are more likely with high doses or in patients with impaired kidney function. *Precautions:* Acute attacks of gout may be triggered in the first few weeks or months of treatment with probenecid, particularly with high doses. Daily dosage should not be interrupted because this allows the blood uric acid level to rise. Aspirin, citrates and salicylates should not be given with probenecid because they block its effects. Treatment should not be started during an acute attack. Do not use in patients with blood disorders or uric acid kidney stones. Use with caution in the elderly, in patients with peptic ulcers, impaired kidney function and in pregnancy. Drink plenty of fluids during treatment. *Interactions:* Aspirin and other salicylates, pyrazinamide, sulphonylurea antidiabetic drugs, beta-lactam antibiotics, indomethacin, methotrexate.

Probeta LA ➤ propranolol.

procainamide (procainamide hydrochloride, Pronestyl) is used to treat disorders of heart rhythm. See Chapter 24. *Adverse effects:* In high dosage by mouth it may cause loss of appetite, nausea, vomiting and diarrhoea. It may rarely cause depression, dizziness, mental symptoms, hallucinations and allergic reactions. Rapid injections into a vein may cause a sudden fall in blood pressure and disorders of heart rhythm. Prolonged use may cause systemic lupus erythematosis (SLE – a disease of unknown cause with symptoms of fever, muscle and joint pain, blood disorders and skin eruptions) and a reduced white blood cell count. *Precautions:* Procainamide should not be given to patients who are allergic to the drug, who have heart block, heart failure, SLE or to breastfeeding mothers. It should be used with caution in patients with impaired function of their liver or kidneys, with asthma, myasthenia gravis (muscle weakness due to neuromuscular abnormality) or in pregnancy. Regular tests for early SLE should be carried out.

procaine (procaine hydrochloride) is a short-acting local anaesthetic. See Chapter 44. It is seldom used.

procarbazine is an anti-cancer drug. See Chapter 51. *Adverse effects* include loss of appetite, nausea, vomiting, sore mouth and gums, diarrhoea, pain, fever and damage to the bone marrow causing blood disorders. *Precautions:* See Chapter 51 on anti-cancer drugs.

prochlorperazine (prochlorperazine maleate, Buccastem, Proziere, Stemetil) is a phenothiazine antipsychotic drug. See Chapter 3. It is also used to treat nausea and vomiting, vertigo and Ménière's disease (see p. 93). *Adverse effects and Precautions* ➤ antipsychotic drugs.

Proctofoam HC foam aerosol contains hydrocortisone (a corticosteroid) and pramocaine (a local anaesthetic). It is used to treat haemorrhoids and itching of the anus. *Adverse effects and Precautions:* see Chapter 37 on corticosteroids and ➤ pramocaine. Avoid prolonged use. Use with caution in pregnancy. Do not use if there is a viral, tubercular, fungal or bacterial infection.

Proctosedyl preparations contain hydrocortisone (a corticosteroid) and cinchocaine (a local anaesthetic). They are used to treat haemorrhoids and itching of the anus. *Adverse effects and Precautions:* see Chapter 37 on corticosteroids and ➤ cinchocaine. Avoid prolonged use. Use with caution in pregnancy. Do not use if there is a viral, tubercular, fungal or bacterial infection.

procyclidine (procyclidine hydrochloride, Arpicolin, Kemadrin) is an antimuscarinic drug used to treat parkinsonism. See Chapter 16. *Adverse effects and Precautions* are similar to those listed under benzhexol ➤ benzhexol.

Pro-Epanutin ➤ fosphenytoin.

Profasi ➤ chorionic gonadotrophin.

proflavine (proflavine hemisulphate) is an antiseptic used in skin applications and eye drops.

Proflex pain relief cream ➤ ibuprofen, topical anti-rheumatic applications.

progesterone (Crinone, Cyclogest, Gestone) is used to treat premenstrual syndrome and post-natal depression. See Chapter 40. *Adverse effects* include acne, urticaria (nettle-rash), weight gain, breast discomfort, stomach upsets, depression, chloasma (patchy brown pigmentation on the face), raised temperature, insomnia, sleepiness, hair loss, excessive hair growth, changes in libido, changes in menstrual cycle and occasionally jaundice. *Precautions:* Use suppositories vaginally if patient has inflammation of the anus or rectum. Use rectally if the patient has vaginal infection. Do not use in patients with a history of blood clots or blocked blood vessels, porphyria (a hereditary disorder of metabolism), undiagnosed vaginal bleeding, breast cancer or threatened miscarriage. It should be used with caution in breastfeeding mothers and in patients suffering from diabetes, raised blood pressure or kidney, liver or heart disease.

progestogen-only oral contraceptives, see Chapter 41.

progestogens are discussed in Chapter 40. *Adverse effects:* Progestogens may occasionally cause breast tenderness and milk production, itching and skin rashes, depression, acne, breakthrough bleeding, spotting, changes in menstrual flow, loss of periods, fluid retention, changes in weight, changes in libido, mental depression, rise in temperature, insomnia, nausea and sleepiness. Very rarely, they may cause changes in the neck of the womb, changes in liver function tests, jaundice, allergic reactions, excessive hair growth, hair loss, allergic skin rashes, eye damage, ectopic pregnancy and cysts of the ovaries. For potential harmful effects of using combined oestrogen/progestogen oral contraceptives, see Chapter 41. *Precautions:* Progestogens should not be used in anyone with inflammation in a vein or any type of blood clot or stroke, or who has a history of these disorders; they should

not be used in pregnancy, in breastfeeding mothers, in women with active liver disease or impaired liver function, with cancer of the breast or genitals, undiagnosed vaginal bleeding, threatened or incomplete miscarriage, severe arterial disease or as a diagnosis for pregnancy. Use with caution in women with diabetes, raised blood pressure, heart, liver or kidney disease, epilepsy, migraine, asthma or porphyria (a hereditary disorder of metabolism). *Interactions:* Cyclosporin, rifampicin.

Prograf preparations ➤ tacrolimus.

proguanil (proguanil hydrochloride, in Malarone, Paludrine) is used to prevent malaria. *Adverse effects* include nausea, vomiting, abdominal pain, skin rashes, hair loss, mouth ulcers and sore gums. Occasionally it may damage red blood cells (methaemaglobinaemia and haemolytic anaemia) especially in patients with G6PD deficiency. *Precautions:* Use with caution in patients with G6PD deficiency and disorders associated with a low white cell count, e.g. rheumatoid arthritis and systemic lupus erythematosus (SLE – a disease of unknown cause with symptoms of fever, muscle and joint pain, blood disorders and skin eruptions). Use with caution in pregnancy and in breastfeeding mothers and in patients with severe kidney failure.

Progynova ➤ estradiol.

Progynova TS skin patches contain oestradiol (an oestrogen). They are used as HRT. Patches need replacing only every seven days instead of the usual three to four days. *Adverse effects and Precautions* ➤ HRT.

Proleukin injection ➤ aldesleukin.

Proluton Depot ➤ hydroxyprogesterone.

promazine (promazine hydrochloride) is a phenothiazine antipsychotic drug ➤ antipsychotic drugs. It is principally used to relieve agitation and restlessness in the elderly.

promethazine is an antihistamine drug. See Chapter 17. It is structurally related to the phenothiazines. Promethazine hydrochloride is used as an antihistamine and to produce sleep (in Medised, in Pamergan P100, Phenergan, Sominex). Promethazine theoclate is used as an anti-vomiting drug (Avomine). *Adverse effects and Precautions* ➤ antihistamines. The commonest adverse effect is drowsiness, which can interfere with the ability to drive a motor vehicle or operate machinery. Stimulation may occur, particularly in children and infants, causing excitability and nightmares after even one dose.

Promictuline ➤ oxybutynin.

Prominal ➤ methylphenobarbital.

Pronestyl ➤ procainamide.

Propaderm skin preparations ➤ beclometasone.

propafenone (Arythmol) is used to treat disorders of heart rhythm. See Chapter 24. *Adverse effects* include nausea, vomiting, diarrhoea, constipation, bitter taste, headache, dizziness and fatigue. Rarely, allergic skin reactions, slowing of the heart rate and heart block may occur. *Precautions:* Do not use in patients with uncontrolled congestive heart failure, severe slowing of the heart, severe obstructive airways disease, marked low blood pressure, certain heart blocks, electrolyte disturbances, myasthenia gravis (muscle weakness due to neuromuscular abnormality), in breastfeeding mothers or in pregnancy. Use with caution in patients with heart failure and in patients with impaired kidney or liver function. It should be used with caution in the elderly and in patients with pacemakers. *Interactions:* Other class I anti-arrhythmic drugs, digoxin, warfarin, cimetidine, propranolol, metoprolol, rifampicin, tricyclic and related antidepressants, antipsychotic drugs, cyclosporin, theophylline.

Propain pain-relieving tablets contain codeine, paracetamol, diphenhydramine and caffeine ➤ codeine, paracetamol, diphenhydramine. The main adverse effect is drowsiness. It may increase the effects of alcohol and should be used with caution in patients with impaired liver and kidney function.

propamidine isethionate ➤ dibromopropamidine isethionate.

Propanix and **Propanix SR** ➤ propranolol.

propantheline (propantheline bromide, Pro-Banthine) is an antimuscarinic drug. See Chapter 9. It is used to treat peptic ulcers (see Chapter 19), irritable bowel syndrome and bedwetting (see Chapter 49). *Adverse effects and Precautions* ➤ antimuscarinic drugs. Do not use in patients with obstructive diseases of the stomach, bowel or bladder. Do not use in patients with glaucoma. Use with caution in patients with severe heart disease, active bowel ulceration (ulcerative colitis), in the elderly, in patients with impaired kidney or liver function or overactive thyroid gland. *Interactions:* Digoxin.

Propess ➤ dinoprostone.

Propine eye drops ➤ dipivefrin.

propiverine (Detrunorm) is used to treat instability in the bladder or damage to the nerves of the bladder from spinal cord injury, which cause a need to urinate frequently. See Chapter 49. *Adverse effects* include dry mouth, blurred vision, drowsiness, stomach and bowel upset, increased urine retention and tiredness. *Precautions:* Do not use in patients with significant bladder outflow obstruction, myasthenia gravis (muscle weakness due to neuromuscular abnormality), bowel obstruction, slowness of movement in the intestine, severe active bowel ulceration (ulcerative colitis), megacolon (distention of the bowel), glaucoma, liver or severe kidney damage, in pregnancy or while breastfeeding. Use with caution in patients with hyperthyroidism, heart disorders, enlarged prostate or hiatus hernia with heartburn.

propofol (Diprivan) is a general anaesthetic given by intravenous infusion. It is also used to sedate patients on a mechanical respirator for up to three days. Patients recover rapidly from its effects without hangover. There are rare reports of it causing allergic reactions and convulsions. It may occasionally cause severe slowing of the heart rate.

propranolol (propranolol hydrochloride, Angilol, Apsolol, Berkolol, Beta-Progane, Cardinol, Inderal preparations, in Inderetic, in Inderex, Probeta LA, Propanix, Syprol) is a non-selective beta-blocker ➤ beta-blockers.

propyl salicylate (in Monphytol) is a salicylate used for removing dead skin (a keratolytic). See p. 247.

propylthiouracil is a drug used to treat overworking of the thyroid gland. See Chapter 43. It has effects, uses and adverse effects similar to those described under carbimazole. It may, rarely, cause a tendency to bleed or serious skin disorders. The dose should be reduced in patients with impaired kidney function.

propyl undecenoate (in Monphytol) is an antifungal drug ➤ undecenoates.

Prosaid ➤ naproxen.

Proscar ➤ finasteride.

prostacyclin ➤ epoprostenol.

prostaglandins, see Chapter 52.

Prostap SR ➤ leuprorelin.

Prostin E2 ➤ dinoprostone.

Prostin F2 ➤ dinoprost.

Prostin VR ➤ alprostadil.

Prosulf ➤ protamine.

protamine (protamine sulphate, protamine sulfate, Prosulf) is prepared from sperm obtained from the testes of mature fish (*Clupeidi* or *Salmonidae*). It combines with heparin to form an inactive complex and is used as an antidote to heparin overdose. Rarely, intravenous injections of protamine, if given rapidly, may cause flushing, nausea, vomiting, fall in blood pressure, slow heart rate and breathlessness. Very rarely, allergic reactions may occur.

protective skin applications, see p. 237.

Prothiaden ➤ dosulupin.

protirelin (thyrotrophin-releasing hormone, TRH, TRH-Cambridge) is a natural hormone produced by the hypothalamus which acts on the pituitary gland to produce and secrete thyrotrophin. It is used to test thyroid function. *Adverse effects:* Rapid intravenous administration may cause nausea, dizziness, faintness, flushing, strange taste in the mouth, a strong desire to pass urine, increase in pulse rate and blood pressure and, rarely, wheezing. *Precautions:* Use with utmost caution in patients with asthma, chronic obstructive airways disease, coronary artery disease, severe underworking of the thyroid gland or in pregnancy.

Protium ➤ pantoprazole.

proton-pump blockers, see p. 97.

proton-pump inhibitors ➤ proton-pump blockers.

Provera ➤ medroxyprogesterone.

Provigil ➤ modafinil.

Pro-Viron ➤ mesterolone.

proxymetacaine (Minims Proxymetacaine) is a local anaesthetic used in eye drops. Because it causes less initial stinging than other local anaesthetics, it is useful for children.

Prozac ➤ fluoxetine.

Proziere ➤ prochlorperazine.

pseudoephedrine (pseudoephedrine hydrochloride, in Actifed, in Dimotane Plus, Galpseud, Galpseud Plus and Sudafed preparations) produces similar effects to those described under ephedrine. It is used in cold and cough medicines to relieve nasal and bronchial congestion. *Adverse effects and Precautions* ➤ ephedrine.

psoralen (methoxsalen, methoxypsoralen) is used to treat psoriasis. See p. 260. *Adverse effects* include nausea, mental depression and insomnia. It may cause itching, mild temporary redness, dizziness, headache and various types of skin rashes including blisters and acne-type rashes. The long-lasting risks include premature ageing of the skin, pigmentation and a risk of skin cancer. It may also affect the immune system, and cause cataracts. *Precautions:* Do not use with any other drug that sensitizes the skin to the sun's rays or in any disease triggered by the sun's rays (e.g. porphyria (a hereditary disorder of metabolism)). Do not use in patients with skin cancer and use with caution in patients with impaired liver function. The skin should be protected from the sun's rays for twenty-four hours before and eight hours after taking a psoralen by mouth. Use UVA wraparound glasses for twenty-four hours after taking by mouth. Eye examinations, blood counts, tests of liver and kidney function and tests for antibodies should be carried out before treatment and at regular intervals during treatment.

Psoriderm ➤ coal tar.

Psorin ointment contains dithranol, crude coal tar and salicylic acid. It is used to treat stable subacute and chronic psoriasis. See p. 258. *Adverse effects* ➤ dithranol, coal tar and salicylic acid. *Precautions:* Avoid direct sunlight. Do not use to treat unstable psoriasis. Do not use with topical corticosteroids.

Pulmicort preparations ➤ budesonide.

pulmonary surfactants act by wetting the surfaces of the lungs. They are used in the treatment of respiratory distress syndrome (hyaline membrane syndrome) in premature babies who are receiving mechanical respiration through a tube into the windpipe. Preparations include beractant (Survanta), poractant alpha (Curosurf) and pumactant (Alec).

Pulmo Bailly is a cough mixture containing codeine and guaicol ➤ codeine, guaicol.

Pulmozyme nebulizer solution ➤ dornase alfa.

Pulvinal Beclometasone ➤ beclometasone.

Pulvinal Salbutamol ➤ salbutamol.

Pump-Hep infusion ➤ heparin.

Puregon ➤ follitropin beta.

Puri-Nethol ➤ mercaptopurine.

PUVA therapy for psoriasis, see p. 260.

Pylorid contains ranitidine combined with bismuth citrate ➤ ranitidine and bismuth citrate. See Chapter 19.

Pyralvex oral paint contains anthraquinone glycosides and salicylic acid. It is used to treat mouth ulcers and denture irritation. *Adverse effects and Precautions* ➤ salicylic acid and anthraquilone glycosides.

pyrazinamide (in Rifater, Zinamide) is a drug used to treat tuberculosis. See Chapter 50. *Adverse effects:* Liver damage with fever, loss of appetite, nausea, vomiting, enlargement of the liver, jaundice, severe liver failure, painful joints, nettle-rash and sideroblastic anaemia. *Precautions:* It should not be given to patients with impaired liver function or porphyria (a hereditary disorder of metabolism). It should be used with caution in patients with impaired kidney function, gout and diabetes. Liver function tests and blood uric acid measurements must be carried out before treatment starts and at regular intervals during treatment. Stop treatment if liver damage or gout develop.

pyridostigmine (pyridostigmine bromide, Mestinon) is an anticholinesterase drug (see Chapter 9). It is used to treat myasthenia gravis (muscle weakness due to neuromuscular abnormality) and paralysis of the small intestine. *Adverse effects* include salivation, colic, nausea and diarrhoea. Increased muscular weakness is a symptom of overdosage. *Precautions:* It should not be used in patients with an intestinal or urinary obstruction and should be used with caution in patients with asthma, slow heart rate, recent heart attack, low blood pressure, peptic ulcers, kidney disease, epilepsy or parkinsonism. *Interactions:* Depolarizing muscle relaxants, cyclopropane, halothane.

pyridoxine (pyridoxine hydrochloride, Orovite Compliment B6) is vitamin B6, see p. 179.

pyrimethamine is combined with dapsone (in Maloprim) to prevent *Pliasmodium falciparum* malaria, and combined with sulfadoxone (Fansidar) to treat *Pliasmodium falciparum* malaria. A combination of pyrimethamine and sulphadiazine is used to treat toxoplasmosis. This combination should be avoided in pregnancy. *Pyrimethamine is unsuitable for travellers and should not be used on its own. Adverse effects:* Prolonged use may damage the production of red blood cells by interfering with folic acid uptake. Skin rashes and insomnia may occur occasionally. *Precautions:* It should be used with caution in patients with impaired liver or kidney function, in patients taking folic acid supplements or in breastfeeding mothers. Pregnant women should take folic acid supplements. Blood counts should be carried out before treatment starts and at regular intervals during treatment. *Interactions:* Co-trimoxazole, lorazepam.

pyrithione zinc has antibacterial and antifungal properties. It is used to treat excessive oily secretions on the scalp and dandruff, see p. 254. It is an ingredient of some proprietary shampoos. It may rarely cause contact dermatitis.

Pyrogastrone tablets contain carbenoxolone and the antacids magnesium trisilicate, aluminium hydroxide and a base containing sodium bicarbonate and alginic acid. They are used to treat inflammation of the oesophagus (oesophagitis) and acid reflux. See p. 101. *Adverse effects and Precautions* ➤ carbenoxolone and antacids.

Quellada M Preparations ➤ malathion.

Questran and **Questran Light** preparations ➤ cholestyramine.

quetiapine (Seroquel) is used to treat schizophrenia. See Chapter 3. *Adverse effects* include drowsiness, dizziness, constipation, light-headedness when standing up after sitting or lying down (postural hypotension), dry mouth, liver enzyme abnormalities, neuroleptic malignant syndrome (for symptoms see p. 331), tardive dyskinesia (➤ antimuscarinic drugs). *Precautions:* Do not use while breastfeeding. Use with caution in patients with kidney or liver damage, history of disorders of blood supply to the brain or heart, low blood pressure, epilepsy or in pregnancy.

quinagolide (Norprolac) is a dopamine blocker (see p. 40) used to reduce high blood levels of prolactin. Prolactin stimulates milk production in women and men. The commonest cause of an increased blood level of prolactin is over-production by a tumour of the pituitary gland. Raised blood levels of prolactin may also be caused by antipsychotic drugs (e.g. phenothiazines) and some anti-blood pressure drugs (e.g. methyldopa). Raised blood prolactin levels (hyperprolactinaemia) are associated with enlargement of the breasts and milk production in both men and women and loss of periods in women. *Adverse effects* include headache, dizziness, nausea, fatigue, loss of appetite, stomach and bowel upsets, congestion of the nose, flushing, insomnia, ankle-swelling, fall in blood pressure and severe mental reactions (psychotic reactions). *Precautions:* Do not use in patients with impaired kidney or liver function. Use with caution in patients with severe mental illness. Stop the drug if pregnancy occurs. Use non-hormonal contraception (e.g. a condom) if pregnancy is to be avoided. *Interactions:* Antipsychotic drugs, alcohol.

quinalbarbital sodium (secobarbital, secobarbitone, Seconal Sodium, in Tuinal) is a barbiturate sleeping drug. *Adverse effects, Precautions and Drug dependence* ➤ phenobarbital sodium.

quinabaritone ➤ quinabarbital.

quinapril (Accupro, in Accuretic) is an ACE inhibitor used to treat congestive heart failure (see Chapter 23) and raised blood pressure (see Chapter 25). *Adverse effects* include nausea, indigestion, abdominal pains, headache, dizziness, runny nose, cough, chest pain, fatigue, muscle pains, fall in blood pressure, and rarely, allergic reactions (angioedema). Stop the drug immediately if this occurs. *Precautions:* Do not use in pregnancy or in breastfeeding mothers. Do not use in patients with obstruction to the outflow of blood from the heart (e.g. aortic stenosis). Use with caution in patients with high blood pressure caused by kidney disease, severe congestive heart failure and patients with impaired kidney function. Tests of kidney function, measures of protein in the urine and white blood cell counts should be carried out before and at regular intervals during treatment. Use with caution during general anaesthesia. *Interactions:* Potassium-sparing diuretics, potassium supplements, NSAIDs, tetracyclines, lithium.

quinidine (quinidine bisulphate, Kinidin Durules) prolongs the resting period of the heart and reduces its rate. It is used to treat disorders of heart rhythm. See Chapter 24. *Adverse effects* include noises in the ears, vertigo, visual disturbances, headache, confusion, skin rash, loss of appetite, nausea, vomiting, diarrhoea, pain in the chest, abdominal cramps and fever. This group of symptoms is referred to as cinchonism. Quinidine may cause allergic reactions, disorders of heart rhythm, blood disorders and liver damage (hepatitis). *Precautions:* A test-dose for allergy should be given first. It should not be used in patients suffering from severe heart disorders, AV heart block, digoxin toxicity, myasthenia gravis (muscle weakness due to neuromuscular abnormality) or in pregnancy. Use with caution in patients with congestive heart failure, low blood potassium levels, slow heart rate, low blood pressure or blockage to the oesophagus. *Interactions:* Digoxin, digitoxin, oral anticoagulants, cimetidine, rifampicin, barbiturates, phenytoin, verapamil, amiodarone, nifedipine, desipramine, imipramine, procainamide, metoprolol.

quinine is used to treat falciparum malaria and night cramps. *Adverse effects:* Long-term use may cause cinchonism: noises in the ear (tinnitus), headache, nausea, hot and flushed skin and disturbed vision in the mild form; when severe, symptoms also include vomiting, abdominal pain, diarrhoea, vertigo, confusion, fever, itching and skin rashes. It may cause a fall in blood sugar level and some patients may be allergic to quinine. Rarely it may produce blood disorders and kidney damage. *Precautions:* Do not use in patients with inflammation of the optic nerve or haemoglobin in the urine. Use with caution in patients with heart disorders, G6PD deficiency and in pregnancy. Monitor blood glucose levels during injection of quinine. *Interactions:* Halofantrine, mefloquine and other antimalarial drugs, cimetidine, digoxin and related drugs, flecainide.

Quinocort cream contains potassium hydroxyquinoline sulphate (an antibacterial/antifungal drug) and hydrocortisone (a corticosteroid). It is used to treat eczema and dermatitis when infection is present. *Adverse effects and Precautions* see corticosteroid skin applications p. 241 and ➤ hydroxyquinolone.

Quinoderm cream and lotio-gel contains benzoyl peroxide (for removing dead skin) and potassium hydroxyquinoline sulphate (an antibacterial/antifungal drug) in an astringent base. They are used to treat acne, see p. 250. *Adverse effects and Precautions:* They may cause temporary irritation and peeling. Avoid contact with eyes, mouth and nose ➤ benzoyl peroxide, hydroxyquinoline.

quinolones, see p. 277.

Quinoped cream contains benzoyl peroxide (for removing dead skin) and potassium hydroxyquinoline sulphate (an anti-bacterial/antifungal drug). It is used to treat athlete's foot. *Adverse effects and Precautions:* May cause transient irritation and peeling. Avoid contact with eyes, mouth and nose ➤ benzoyl peroxide and hydroxyquinoline.

quinupristin is used in combination with dalfopristin in Synercid ➤ dalfopristin.

Qvar ➤ beclometasone.

rabeprazole (Pariet) is a proton-pump blocker used to treat duodenal and gastric ulcers. It is used with antibiotics to eradicate *H. Pylori* in peptic ulcer disease. See Chapter 19. *Adverse effects* include headache, stomach and bowel upset, rash, weakness, dry mouth. *Precautions:* Do not use in pregnancy or while breastfeeding. Use with caution in patients with severe liver damage.

rabipur is a freeze-dried rabies vaccine which is given by intramuscular injection.

Radian B muscle lotion, Radian B heat spray are heat rubs containing ammonium salicylate, camphor, menthol and salicylic acid ➤ rubefacients.

Radian B muscle rub is a heat rub containing camphor, capsicin, menthol and methyl salicylate ➤ rubefacients.

radioactive iodine ➤ iodine, radioactive.

Ralgex preparations are heat rubs: **Ralgex cream** contains capsicin, glycol monosalicylate and methyl nicotinate; **Ralgex low odour spray** contains glycol monosalicylate and methyl nicotinate; **Ralgex spray** contains glycol monosalicylate, methyl nicotinate, ethyl salicylate and methyl salicylate; **Ralgex stick** contains capsicin, ethyl salicylate, methyl salicylate and menthol ➤ rubefacients.

raloxifene (Evista) affects oestrogen receptors and is used to treat and prevent post-menopausal osteoporosis. See Chapter 40. *Adverse effects* include hot flushes, leg cramps, swelling of the fingers and ankles, decreased platelet counts. *Precautions:* Do not use in patients with a history of thrombosis (obstruction in the veins due to blood clots), liver or severe kidney damage, undiagnosed vaginal bleeding, endometrial or breast cancer, prolonged immobilization. Ensure adequate calcium and vitamin D intake.

raltitrexed (Tomudex) is a folate blocker used as an anti-cancer drug (see Chapter 51) to treat cancer of the bowel. Its effectiveness compares well with other treatments for this disorder. It causes a lower incidence of neutropenia (fall in white cell count) and mucositis (inflammation of the lining of the mouth, intestine, etc.) but produces a higher incidence of anaemia and impaired liver function tests – but the latter usually do not produce symptoms and are reversible. It is given by fifteen-minute intravenous infusions once every three weeks. *Adverse effects* include blood disorders, stomach and bowel upsets, weight loss, dehydration, rash, weakness, fever, headache, hair loss, sweating, muscle and joint pains, disturbances of taste, inflammation in the eye and changes in liver function tests. *Precautions:* Do not use in patients with severe impairment of kidney or liver function, in pregnancy or breastfeeding mothers. Use with caution in patients with stomach or bowel disorders, blood disorders, moderate impairment of liver function or bone-marrow damage or in the elderly. Carry out full blood counts, liver function tests and kidney function tests before each dose. *Interactions:* Folinic acid, folic acid, vitamin preparations.

ramipril (Tritace capsules, Triapin) is an ACE inhibitor used to treat mild to moderately high blood pressure (see Chapter 25) and heart failure (see Chapter 23). It is a prodrug, which means that it is inactive until it is activated in the liver to form ramiprilat, which is a long-acting ACE inhibitor. *Adverse effects* include nausea, vomiting, abdominal pains, diarrhoea, headache, dizziness, fatigue and cough. Rarely, it may cause a marked fall in blood pressure, faintness, allergic reactions and impaired kidney function. *Precautions:* It should not be used in individuals with a history of angioedema (allergic swelling in the mouth and throat), in pregnancy or in breastfeeding mothers. It should not be used in people with obstruction to the outflow of blood from the heart. It should be used with the utmost caution in individuals with congestive heart failure, blood disorders, impaired liver function and impaired kidney function. Kidney function should be checked before and at regular intervals during treatment and the dose reduced according to the degree of impaired function. Diuretic drugs should be stopped two–three days before starting treatment with ramipril, otherwise there is an increased risk of a marked fall in blood pressure. *Interactions:* Other anti-blood pressure drugs, potassium-sparing diuretics, potassium supplements, lithium, anti-diabetic drugs, NSAIDs, adrenergic blockers.

ranitidine (in Pylorid, Rantec, Ranitic, Zaedoc, Zantac) is an H$_2$ antihistamine (H$_2$ blocker) which blocks acid production in the stomach and is used to treat peptic ulcers and other disorders associated with an increased acid production. See Chapter 19. *Adverse effects* include headache, changes in bowel habits, tiredness, skin rashes and dizziness. Very rarely it may cause allergic reactions, blood disorders, liver damage, hallucinations and confusion. Painful enlargement of the breasts, in men, may occur occasionally. *Precautions:* It should be used with caution (lower doses) in patients suffering from impaired kidney function, during pregnancy and in breastfeeding mothers. Exclude stomach cancer before starting treatment because the drug may mask the symptoms.

ranitidine bismuth citrate (Pylorid) is an H$_2$ blocker (ranitidine) combined with a protective (bismuth citrate). It is used to treat duodenal and stomach ulcers. It is used with antibiotics to eradicate *H. Pylori* and to prevent relapse of peptic ulcers. See Chapter 19. *Adverse effects* include blackening of tongue and stools, stomach and bowel upset, headache, altered liver enzymes, mild anaemia, slow heart beat. Rarely, inflammation of the pancreas or liver, disorders of the blood, confusion, musculoskeletal disorders, allergic reactions, slow heart beat, heart block. *Precautions:* Do not use in patients with moderate to severe kidney damage, long-term maintenance therapy, history of acute porphyria (a hereditary disorder of metabolism), the elderly, in pregnancy or while breastfeeding.

Rantec ➤ ranitidine.

Rapamune ➤ sirolimus.

Rap-eze ➤ calcium carbonate.

Rapifen injection ➤ alfentanil.

Rapilysin ➤ reteplase.

Rapitil eye drops ➤ nedocromil sodium.

rasburicase (Fasturtec) is used to treat and prevent acute hyperuricaemia (high level of uric acid in the blood). *Adverse effects* include stomach and bowel upset, fever and rash. *Precautions:* Do not use in patients with G6PD deficiency, metabolic disorders causing anaemia, in pregnancy or while breastfeeding. Use with caution in patients with a hereditary predisposition to allergies.

rauwolfia are the plants from which reserpine is obtained.

razoxane is an anti-cancer drug. See Chapter 51. *Adverse effects:* Nausea, vomiting, diarrhoea, skin rashes, hair loss, blood disorders, inflammation of the oesophagus or lungs may occur in patients receiving radiotherapy to the chest. *Precautions:* It should not be used in pregnancy or in breastfeeding mothers. The white blood cell count should be monitored regularly (see Chapter 51 on anti-cancer drugs).

RBC is a topical antihistimine used in the treatment of insect bites. It contains antazoline, calamine, camphor, cetrimide and menthol.

Rebetol ➤ ribavirin.

Rebif ➤ interferon beta.

reboxetine (Edronax) is used to treat depression. See Chapter 4. *Adverse effects* include dry mouth, constipation, insomnia, sweating, rapid heart beat, dizziness, urinary retention, pain or burning on urination, impotence. *Precautions:* Do not use in pregnancy or while breastfeeding. Use with caution in patients with kidney or liver damage, history of epilepsy, patients with marked mood swings, urinary retention or glaucoma.

Recombinate (recombinant factor VIII) ➤ antihaemophilic factor VIII. *Adverse effects* include nausea, dizziness, fall in blood pressure, tightness in the chest, allergic reactions and the development of inhibitors which block its effects. *Precautions:* Do not use in patients who are allergic to beef, mouse or hamster proteins. Use with caution in pregnancy and in breastfeeding mothers. Monitor for factor VIII inhibitors at regular intervals.

rectified spirits (dilute alcohols) ➤ alcohol.

Redoxon ➤ vitamin C.

Reductil ➤ sibutramine.

Refacto ➤ factor VIII fraction, freeze-dried, Recombinate.

Refludan ➤ lepirudin.

Refolinon ➤ folinic acid.

Regaine liquid contains minoxidil (➤ minoxidil). It is used to treat male-type baldness in men and thinning of the hair in women (see baldness p. 253). *Adverse effects* include irritant dermatitis and allergic contact dermatitis. *Precautions:* Avoid contact with eyes, mouth and nose, do not apply to broken, infected or inflamed skin. Avoid inhalation of spray mist. See general adverse effects of minoxidil but only about 1.4% of the drug is absorbed from scalp applications. None the less, watch out for a fall in blood pressure and monitor patients being treated for raised blood pressure.

Regranex ➤ becaplermin.

Regulan ➤ ispaghula.

Regulose ➤ lactulose.

Regurin ➤ trospium.

Rehidrat oral rehydration salts contain sodium chloride, potassium chloride, sodium bicarbonate, citric acid, glucose, sucrose and fructose.

Relaxit micro-enema contains sodium citrate, sodium lauryl sulphate and sorbic acid in a viscous solution. It is used as a faecal softener to treat constipation. See Chapter 21.

Relaxyl preparations ➤ alverine.

Relcofen preparations ➤ ibuprofen.

Relenza ➤ zanamivir.

Relifex ➤ nabumetone.

Remedeine pain-relieving preparations contain paracetamol and dihydrocodeine ➤ paracetamol, dihydrocodeine.

Remegel preparations ➤ calcium carbonate.

Remicade ➤ infliximab.

remifentamil (Ultiva) is a pain reliever for use during induction or maintenance of general anaesthesia.

Reminyl ➤ galantamine.

Remnos ➤ nitrazepam.

Renagel ➤ sevelamer.

Rennies is an antacid ➤ calcium, magnesium.

ReoPro ➤ abciximab.

repaglinide (Novonorm) is an antidiabetic drug used to treat non-insulin dependent (Type II) diabetes not controlled by diet and exercise, in combination with metformin where control of high blood glucose levels is not satisfactory. See Chapter 42. *Adverse effects* include low blood glucose level (hypoglycaemia), visual disturbances, stomach and bowel upset, rash, temporary elevation in liver enzymes. *Precautions:* Do not use in patients with Type I diabetes, diabetic acidosis, severe kidney or liver damage, in pregnancy or while breastfeeding.

Replenate (human freeze-dried coagulation factor VIII) is used to treat haemophilia A. It has nominal antihaemophilic factor activity ➤ factor VIII fractions, dried.

Replenine-VF (human freeze-dried coagulation factor IX), is used to treat haemophilia B. It has nominal antihaemophilic factor activity ➤ factor IX fraction, dried.

Replens is a non-hormonal vaginal moisturizer used to treat menopausal dryness of the vagina. It has a high moisture content and its effects last for about twenty-four hours.

reproterol (reproterol hydrochloride, Bronchodil), is a selective beta₂ stimulant used to treat asthma. *Adverse effects and Precautions* ➤ salbutamol.

Requip ➤ ropinirole.

reserpine is obtained from the roots of rauwolfia. It depresses the brain, produces sedation, lowers the blood pressure and slows the heart rate. It was used to treat patients with high blood pressure.

Resolve is an analgesic preparation ➤ paracetamol.

Resonium A ➤ sodium polystyrene sulphonate.

resorcinol (resorcinol monoacetate, in Eskamel) is used to stop itching and is used in skin ointments because it causes skin peeling. Prolonged use of large amounts on the skin can cause underworking of the thyroid gland because it may be absorbed and interfere with the production of thyroid hormones.

Respacal ➤ tulobuterol.

respiratory stimulants (analeptic drugs) are occasionally used to treat depressed breathing when mechanical respiration is not suitable for the patient. They are only effective when given by intravenous injection or infusion and they have a short duration of action. They may arouse the drowsy or comatose patient sufficiently to enable them to cooperate in clearing out their breathing tubes. They may be harmful in respiratory failure because they stimulate all muscles in the body and not just those involved with breathing. Preparations include doxapram (Dopram). The previously used drug, nikethamide, is no longer used because of risks of convulsions.

Respontin ➤ ipratropium.

Restandol ➤ testosterone undecanoate.

reteplase (Rapilysin) is a fibrinolytic (clotbuster, see p. 117). It is used in the early treatment of a heart attack due to a blood clot in the coronary artery of the heart. *Adverse effects* include bleeding, fall in blood pressure, disorders of heart rhythm and, rarely, allergic reactions. *Precautions:* Do not use in patients with bleeding disorders, tumours in the brain, stroke, active peptic ulcers, severe impairment of liver or kidney function, inflammation of the pancreas, lining or muscles of the heart, bleeding disorders of the eye, within ten days of external cardiac massage, or within three months of severe bleeding, surgery or major injury. Use with caution in patients suffering from disorders of the circulation to the brain, raised blood pressure, recent bleeding from the stomach, intestines or bladder or in the elderly.

Retin-A ➤ tretinoin.

retinoids are vitamin A derivatives used to treat acne, see p. 250. They include tretinoin (Retin-A topical application) and the related isotreinoin (Isotrex topical application and Roaccutane capsules for use by mouth).

Retinova cream ➤ tretinoin.

Retrovir ➤ zidovudine.

Revasc ➤ desirudin.

reviparin (Clivarine) is a low molecular weight heparin (LMVH) used to prevent and treat thrombosis. See Chapter 28. *Adverse effects* include bleeding at high doses, decrease in number of platelets in the blood (thrombocytopenia), temporary raised liver enzymes, allergic reactions, osteoporosis with long-term use. *Precautions:* Do not use in patients with an allergy to heparin, a high risk of bleeding, blood disorders (thrombocytopenia), damaged blood vessels, imminent miscarriage, kidney stones, chronic alcoholism, spinal or peridural anaesthesia, surgery on the central nervous system, lumbar puncture or in pregnancy.

Rexocaine ➤ lidocaine.

Rheumacin LA ➤ indometacin.

Rheumacrodex intravenous infusion contains dextran in glucose solution or sodium chloride solution ➤ dextran infusion.

Rheumox ➤ azapropazone.

Rheumatac ➤ diclofenac.

Rhinocort Aqua preparations ➤ budesonide.

Rhinolast ➤ azelastine.

Rhuaka ➤ cascara.

Rhumalgan ➤ diclofenac sodium.

ribavirin (Virazid powder for nebulization, Virazole) is an antiviral drug (see Chapter 48) used to treat severe virus infections of the lungs caused by the syncytial virus (RSV). *Adverse effects:* It may make the lung condition worse and bacterial pneumonia may develop. *Precautions:* Both the patient and the breathing equipment should be monitored carefully because the drug may precipitate out from the nebulization solution and block the tubing, making it difficult for the patient to breathe. Do not use in pregnancy or in women of childbearing potential. Monitor blood electrolytes closely.

riboflavin (vitamin B_2) is a member of the vitamin B group. See Chapter 36.

Ridaura tablets ➤ auranofin.

Rideril ➤ thioridazine.

rifabutin (Mycobutin) is an antibacterial drug used to treat tuberculosis and non-tuberculous mycobacterial infections, and to prevent tuberculosis in patients with immune deficiency (e.g. AIDS). See Chapter 50. *Adverse effects* include stomach and bowel upsets, muscle and joint pains, orange-red discoloration of the skin, urine, saliva and other body secretions, blood disorders, changes in liver function, jaundice

and eye disorders (uveitis). Allergic reactions may occur producing fever, rash and wheezing. *Precautions:* Do not use in pregnancy or breastfeeding mothers. Use with caution in patients with severe impairment of liver or kidney function. Blood counts and liver function tests should be carried out at regular intervals. Do not wear soft contact lenses. *Interactions:* Oral contraceptives, anticoagulants, pain-relievers, corticosteroids, cyclosporin, digitalis, dapsone, oral anti-diabetic drugs, phenytoin, quinidine, zidovudine, macrolide antibiotics and triazole antifungal drugs.

Rifadin ➤ rifampicin.

rifampicin (Rifadin, in Rifater, in Rifinah, Rimactane, in Rimactazid) is used to treat tuberculosis (see Chapter 50), brucellosis, Legionnaire's disease and serious staphylococcal infections in combination with other drugs. It is also used to prevent meningitis (meningococcal and H. influenzae, Type B) in contacts. *Adverse effects* include loss of appetite, nausea, vomiting, diarrhoea (can be severe and produce severe inflammation of the bowel). Other adverse effects include flu-like symptoms (chills, fever, bone pains, dizziness), breathing difficulties, collapse, blood, liver and kidney disorders, jaundice, flushing, rashes, muscle weakness, menstrual disorders and yellow-red coloured urine, saliva and other body fluids. Inflammation in the vein may occur at the site of infusion. *Precautions:* It should not be used in patients with jaundice or porphyria (a hereditary disorder of metabolism). It should be given with caution in pregnancy, to breastfeeding mothers and to patients with impaired liver function, the elderly, the very young, malnutritioned, alcoholics and to patients who have had previous drug allergies. It may discolour soft contact lenses. *Interactions:* Anticoagulants, corticosteroids, digitalis, anti-diabetic drugs, cyclosporin, dapsone, phenytoin, quinidine, opiate pain-relievers.

Rifater tablets contain isoniazid, pyrazinamide and rifampicin, used to treat tuberculosis. See Chapter 50 and ➤ isoniazid, pyrazinamide, rifampicin.

Rifinah preparations contain rifampicin and isoniazid. It is used to treat tuberculosis. See Chapter 50 and ➤ rifampicin, isoniazid.

Rilutek ➤ riluzole.

riluzole (Rilutek) is used to extend life or the time before mechanical ventilation is used in patients suffering from amyotrophic lateral sclerosis (ALS), a form of motor neurone disease. Glutamate toxicity is a possible causative factor in this disease and riluzole helps to reduce the level of glutamate in the central nervous system. *Adverse effects* include weakness, headache, nausea, vomiting, abdominal pains, dizziness, sleepiness, fast heart rate, pins and needles around the mouth, reduced white blood cell count and changes in liver function tests. *Precautions:* Do not use in pregnancy or breastfeeding mothers, or in patients with severely impaired liver function. Use with caution in patients with mild or moderate impairment of liver function and monitor liver function tests at regular intervals. Stop the drug if there is an indication of liver damage (e.g. serum transaminase up five times normal). Use with caution in patients with impaired kidney function. Because of risk of reduced white blood cell count (neutropenia) patients should report any sore throat or fever immediately.

Rimacid ➤ indometacin.

Rimacillin ➤ ampicillin.

Rimactane ➤ rifampicin.

Rimactazid preparations contain rifampicin and isoniazid. They are used to treat tuberculosis. See Chapter 50 and ➤ rifampicin, isoniazid.

Rimafen ➤ ibuprofen.

Rimapam ➤ diazepam.

Rimapurinol ➤ allopurinol.

rimexolone ➤ Vexol.

Rimoxallin ➤ amoxicillin.

Rimso-50 ➤ dimethyl sulfoxide.

Rinatec nasal spray ➤ ipratropium.

Ringer-Lactate Solution (Hartman's solution) is a sterile solution of calcium chloride, potassium chloride, sodium chloride and sodium lactate in water.

Ringer's Solution contains chloride salts of calcium, potassium and sodium in water. The injection is used to correct fluid and electrolyte disturbances.

Rinstead gel contains benzocaine (a local anaesthetic) and chloroxylenol (an antiseptic). It is used to treat teething in infants ➤ benzocaine, chloroxylenol.

Rinstead pastilles ➤ chloroxylenol, menthol.

risedronate (Actonel) is biphosphorate used to prevent and treat osteoporosis in post-menopausal women and in those undergoing long-term corticosteroid therapy and to treat systemic Paget's disease. *Adverse effects* include abdominal pain, stomach and bowel upset, bone and muscle pain, headache, rash, temporary decrease in serum calcium and phosphate levels. Rarely, flu-like symptoms, chest pain, dizziness, tumour, peripheral oedema (swelling of the fingers and ankles due to fluid retention), weight loss, shortness of breath, bronchitis, sinusitis, inflammation of the iris or dimness of vision may occur. *Precautions:* Do not use in patients with calcium deficiency in the blood, severe kidney damage, in pregnancy or while breastfeeding. Use with caution in patients with a history of oesophageal disorders that cause difficulty swallowing, or disturbance of bone and mineral metabolism. Maintain adequate dietary intake of calcium and vitamin D.

Risperdal ➤ risperidone.

risperidone (Risperdal) is an antipsychotic drug. See Chapter 3. *Adverse effects* include dizziness, headache, anxiety, fatigue, stomach and bowel upsets, impaired concentration, agitation, rash, running nose, blurred vision, weight gain, rapid beating of the heart, fall in blood pressure on standing after sitting or lying down, menstrual disturbances, milk from the breasts (male and female), insomnia, sexual dysfunction, parkinsonism, tardive dyskinesia (➤ antipsychotic drugs). Very rarely it may cause neuroleptic malignant syndrome (for symptoms ➤ antipsychotic drugs), low blood sodium levels with water intoxication and fits. *Precautions:* Use with caution in patients who are elderly, with impaired kidney, liver or heart function, epilepsy or parkinsonism, in pregnancy and breastfeeding mothers. May affect ability to drive and operate machinery. Monitor carefully for tardive dyskinesia. *Interactions:* Levodopa and drugs that act on the brain ➤ antipsychotic drugs.

Ritalin ➤ methylphenidate.

ritodrine (ritodrine hydrochloride, Yutopar) is a beta-stimulant sympathomimetic drug which is used to relax the womb in premature labour (twenty-three–thirty-five weeks). This delays delivery until other measures can be used. *Adverse effects* include tremor, anxiety, vomiting, flushing, sweating, low blood pressure, rise in blood sugar, drop in blood potassium, blood disorders, rapid heart beat, chest pain, fall in white blood cells, enlarged salivary glands, disorders of heart rhythm and impaired liver function. If mother develops fluid on the lungs (pulmonary oedema) stop the drug immediately and give diuretics. *Precautions:* It should not be used in any condition where prolongation of labour may be dangerous or in mothers with heart disorders. Use with caution in mothers with diabetes, multiple pregnancy, over-active thyroid gland, raised blood pressure or infection. Avoid giving too much fluid. Monitor mother's and baby's heart rate. *Interactions:* MAOIs, tricyclic antidepressants, corticosteroids, sympathomimetic drugs, anaesthetics, potassium-loosing diuretics, beta-blockers.

ritonavir (in Kaletra, Norvir) is an antiviral drug used to treat patients suffering from HIV infection, see p. 280. *Adverse effects* include stomach and bowel upsets, taste disturbances, pins and needles around the mouth and in the hands and feet, flushing, weakness and headache. It may cause blood disturbances and changes in blood chemistry. *Precautions:* Do not use in children or in patients with severe impairment of liver function. Use with caution in patients with mild to moderate impairment of liver function, diarrhoea, haemophilia and in pregnancy. *Interactions:* rifabutin, sedatives, sleeping drugs, anti-anxiety drugs, saquinavir, clarithromycin, oral contraceptives, theophylline, desipramine. Avoid metronidazole or diltiazem with oral suspension of Norvir.

rituximab (Mabthera) is used to treat stage III–IV cancer of the lymph glands that has relapsed or has not responded to treatment with other drugs. See Chapter 51. *Adverse effects* include fever, chills, nausea, vomiting, allergic reactions, flushing, pain. *Precautions:* It should be used with caution in patients receiving chemotherapy which could be damaging to the heart, or with a history of coronary heart disease, because worsening of angina, abnormal heart rhythm and heart failure have been reported.

rivastigmine (Exelon) is an acetycholinesterase inhibitor used to treat the symptoms of mild to moderately severe Alzheimer's dementia. See Chapter 9. *Adverse effects* include weakness, anorexia, dizziness, drowsiness, abdominal pain, agitation, confusion, depression, sweating, trauma, generally feeling unwell, weight loss, tremor, headache, insomnia, respiratory or urinary tract infections. *Precautions:* Do not use in patients with severe liver damage or while breastfeeding. Use with caution in patients with disorders of heart rhythm, heart defects, predisposition to seizures, history or risk of ulcers in the stomach or bowel, asthma, obstructive pulmonary disease (lung disease causing severe difficulty breathing), bladder outflow obstruction, liver or kidney damage or in pregnancy.

Rivotril ➤ clonazepam.

rizatriptan (Maxalt) is used to treat the headache phase of migraine with or without associated aura. See Chapter 34. *Adverse effects* include dizziness, drowsiness, weakness, abdominal or chest pain, palpitations, rapid heart beat, stomach and bowel upset, musculoskeletal symptoms, sore throat, difficulty breathing, itching, sweating, blurred vision, hot flushes, tongue swelling, rash, bad taste in the mouth. *Precautions:* Do not use in patients with severe kidney or liver damage, a history of stroke or heart disease, coronary artery disease, certain types of angina, disorders of the circulation in the arms and legs, high blood pressure, basilar or hemiplegic migraine, unusual headache. Use with caution in patients with liver or kidney damage.

Roaccutane ➤ isotretinoin.

Robaxin ➤ methocarbamol.

Robitussin Chesty Cough contains guaifenesin; **Robitussin Chesty Cough with Congestion** contains guaifenesin and pseudoephedrine; **Robitussin Dry Cough** contains dextromethorphan; **Robitussin Junior Persistant Cough** contains dextromethorphan; **Robitussin Night Time** contains brompheniramine, codeine and pseudoephedrine. See Chapter 11.

Robinul preparations ➤ glycopyrronium.

Robinul-Neostigmine injection contains neostigmine and glycopyrronium. Neostigmine reverses the effects of non-depolarizing muscle-relaxants (see p. 37) and is used at the end of surgical operations. The glycopyrronium prevents adverse effects of neostigmine such as slowing of the heart rate and excessive salivation ➤ neostigmine and glycopyrronium.

Rocaltrol ➤ calcitrol.

Rocephin ➤ ceftriaxone.

rocuronium (rocuronium bromide, Esmeron) is a non-depolarizing muscle relaxant (see p. 42) used to produce paralysis under light anaesthesia in surgical operations ➤ muscle relaxants.

rofecoxib (Vioxx) is a non-steroidal anti-inflammatory drug used to relieve the symptoms of osteoarthritis. See Chapter 32. *Adverse effects* include abdominal pain, stomach and bowel upset, dizziness, fluid retention, high blood pressure, pain in the upper part of the stomach, headache, itching, increased liver enzymes. *Precautions:* Do not use in patients with active peptic ulcer or bleeding from the stomach and bowel, inflammatory bowel disease, severe congestive heart failure, severe liver or kidney damage, aspirin or anti-inflammatory-induced asthma or allergies, in the third trimester of pregnancy or while breastfeeding. Use with caution in patients with liver or kidney damage, heart failure which is not being treated, cirrhosis of the liver, heart disorders, fluid retention, a history of ulcers or bleeding in the stomach and bowel or in pregnancy.

Roferon-A ➤ interferon alfa.

Rogitine ➤ phentolamine.

Rohypnol ➤ flunitrazepam.

Rommix ➤ erythromycin.

ropinirole (Requip) is a dopamine stimulant used to treat Parkinson's disease (see Chapter 16). *Adverse effects* include nausea, abdominal pains, vomiting, fainting, fall in blood pressure, slowing of the heart rate, sleepiness and swollen ankles. *Precautions:* Do not use in patients with severely impaired kidney or liver function, in pregnancy or in breastfeeding mothers. Use with caution in patients with severe heart disease or psychotic disorders. Withdraw the drug gradually. *Interactions:* Anti-blood pressure drugs, anti-arrhythmic drugs, antipsychotic drugs, high doses of oestrogens, HRT, alcohol, other dopamine stimulants.

ropivacaine (Naropin) is used for surgical anaesthesia, including epidural blocks for surgery and Caesarean section, field blocks and major nerve blocks. See Chapter 44.

Adverse effects include confusion, respiratory depression, convulsion, low blood pressure, slow heart beat, allergic reactions. *Precautions:* Do not use in patients with epilepsy, liver or respiratory damage, heart defects, slow heart beat or porphyria (a hereditary disorder of metabolism).

rose bengal (Minims Rose Bengal) eye drops are deep red in colour and are used to stain the eyes as an aid to the detection of scars or ulcers of the cornea and to look for foreign bodies in the eye. May occasionally cause severe stinging.

rosiglitazone (Avandia) is an anti-diabetic drug used in combination with metformin in obese patients, or with a sulphonylurea in patients for whom metformin is unsuitable, in Type II diabetes inadequately controlled by maximum tolerated doses of either. See Chapter 42. *Adverse effects* include anaemia, low blood glucose level, weight gain, headache, stomach and bowel upset, fatigue, fluid retention, high cholesterol levels. *Precautions:* Do not use in patients with liver or kidney damage, raised liver enzymes, a history of heart failure, in pregnancy or while breastfeeding.

Roter is an antacid containing salts of bismuth and magnesium, sodium bicarbonate and frangula ➤ antacids.

Rowachol capsules contain the essential oils menthol, menthone, pinenes, camphene, cineole and borneol. They are used as additional treatment to chenodeoxycholic acid to dissolve stones in the common bile duct. See p. 102. *Interactions:* Oral anticoagulants, oral contraceptives.

Rowatinex capsules contain the essential oils camphene, pinenes, borneol, fenchone, anethol and cineole. They are used to treat kidney stones and mild urinary tract infections. *Interactions:* Oral anticoagulants, oral contraceptives.

Rozex gel ➤ metronidazole. It is used to treat acne rosacea.

rt-PA ➤ alteplase.

rubefacients are chemicals that cause redness, dilatation of the blood vessels and warmth when applied to an area of skin. This stimulation of sensory nerves in the skin diverts the feelings of pain from, for example, a painful underlying muscle providing relief. This process is referred to as *counter-irritation.* This counter-irritation produced by rubefacients provides some relief of pain from sprains, strains, stiffness and rheumatism. The ingredients of rubefacients include essential oils, pain-relievers such as salicylates, vasodilators such as nicotinates, histamine and capsicum. Menthol and camphor are also used as counter-irritants but they cool the skin rather than warm it. *Adverse effects:* Rubefacients may irritate the skin. *Precautions:* Avoid contact with eyes, lips, mouth or broken or inflamed skin. Do not use under non-permeable dressings. Wash hands immediately after use. Do not use large amounts and do not apply to large areas of skin. *Note:* Rubefacients work in a different way from topical NSAIDs ➤ topical anti-rheumatics.

Rusyde ➤ furosemide.

Rynacrom contains ➤ sodium cromoglicate; **Rynacrom Compound** contains sodium cromoglicate and xylometazoline ➤ individual entry for each drug.

Rythmodan and **Rythmodan Retard** ➤ disopyramide.

Sabril ➤ vigabatrin.

Saizen ➤ somatropin.

Salactol paint is used to treat warts (see p. 262), corns and calluses. It contains salicylic acid, lactic acid and inflexible collodion ➤ salicylic acid and lactic acid.

Salagen tablets are used to increase saliva in dry mouth and tear production in dry eyes ➤ pilocarpine.

Salamol ➤ salbutamol.

Salatac gel contains salicylic acid and lactic acid. It is used to treat warts, corns and calluses. See p. 262 ➤ salicylic acid and lactic acid. Do not use to treat warts on the genitals or anus. Avoid contact with healthy skin.

Salazopyrin preparations ➤ sulfasalazine.

Salbulin ➤ salbutamol.

salbutamol (salbutamol sulphate, in Aerocrom, Aerolin, Aerolin Autohaler, Airomir, Asmasal, Asmaven, in Combivent, Maxivent, Pulvinal Salbutamol, Salamol, Steri-Neb Salamol, Salbulin, Ventamax SR, in Ventide, Ventodisks, Ventolin, Volmax) is a selective beta$_2$ stimulant used to treat wheezing in asthma, chronic bronchitis and emphysema. See Chapter 14. Salbutamol is also used to relax the womb in premature labour. *Adverse effects* ➤ sympathomimetic drugs. Salbutamol may cause a fine tremor of the muscles (particularly of the hands), palpitations, muscle cramps, tenseness, headache, increased heart rate and flushing. Allergic reactions may occur (wheezing, nettle-rash, swelling in the mouth and throat) and intramuscular injections may cause pain. High doses of salbutamol and related drugs may cause a fall in blood potassium levels which can cause serious problems when given with other anti-asthma drugs, e.g. theophylline, corticosteroids or diuretics. This is because these drugs may also cause a fall in blood potassium levels. In addition, the fall in blood oxygen levels that occurs in severe asthma can also cause a fall in blood potassium. Therefore, blood potassium levels must be regularly monitored in patients being treated for severe asthma and any fall in potassium must be corrected. *Precautions:* It should be used with caution by patients with high blood pressure, coronary heart disease, disorders of heart rhythm, or overworking of the thyroid gland, in elderly people, in pregnancy and in breastfeeding mothers. Blood sugar levels should be carefully monitored in diabetics. *Interactions:* Sympathomimetic drugs.

salcatonin ➤ calcitonin (salmon).

salicylamide (in Intralgin) has effects and uses similar to those described under aspirin, but it is less effective.

salicylates are salts or esters of salicylic acid. Some relieve pain and bring down the temperature (e.g. sodium salicylate) and others are applied to the skin to remove dead skin or as a heat rub to relieve rheumatic pain (➤ rubefacients). Applied to the skin they can be mildly irritant. Aspirin is acetylsalicylic acid.

salicylic acid ➤ salicylates.

saline purgatives ➤ osmotic laxatives, see p. 109.

Salivace (artificial saliva) oral spray contains carmellose sodium, xylitol, calcium, potassium and sodium salts and methyl hydroxybenzoate. It is used to treat dry mouth caused by radiotherapy or sicca (dry) syndrome.

Saliveze (artificial saliva) contains electrolytes. It is used to treat dry mouth caused by radiotherapy or sicca (dry) syndrome.

Salivix sugar-free pastilles contain acacia, malic acid and other ingredients. They are used as artificial saliva to treat dry mouth caused by radiotherapy or sicca (dry) syndrome.

salmeterol (in Seretide, Serevent) is a selective beta$_2$-adrenoreceptor stimulant used in the long-term regular treatment of asthma, including asthma at night, exercise-induced asthma, and wheezing associated with bronchitis. It is formulated to remain at the site of action in order to produce long-lasting effects (twelve hours) so that it need only be taken twice daily. In addition to its bronchodilator effects, salmeterol helps to control the release of chemicals (e.g. histamine, prostaglandins) that produce inflammation. See Chapter 14. *Adverse effects* include tremor, headaches, palpitations, muscle cramps, chest pain, skin reactions, irritation where it is applied, painful joints, low blood potassium levels and paradoxical bronchospasm (wheezing). For other potential harmful effects ➤ salbutamol. *Precautions:* It should not be used in the emergency treatment of asthma attacks because it is not fast-acting. It should be added to corticosteroid or sodium cromoglycate treatment and *not* replace it. Do not reduce or stop the corticosteroid. Do not use if asthma is getting worse. It should be used with caution in pregnancy and in breast-feeding mothers, and in patients with over-active thyroid glands. For other precautions ➤ salbutamol.

Salofalk ➤ mesalazine.

Salonair spray contains methyl salicylate, glycol salicylate, menthol, camphor, squalane and benzyl nicotinate. It is used as a heat rub ➤ rubefacients.

Salonpas is a rheumatic rub containing methyl salicylate, glycol salicylate, menthol and camphor ➤ rubefacients.

salt substitutes contain significant amounts of *potassium chloride* (e.g. Lo-salt, Ruthmol). They should not be used by patients with impaired kidney function and may cause a general rise in blood potassium levels.

Sandimmun ➤ ciclosporin.

Sando-K effervescent tablets contain potassium bicarbonate and potassium chloride. They are used as a potassium supplement ➤ potassium supplements.

Sandocal preparations contain calcium lactate gluconate, calcium carbonate and citric acid. They are used as a calcium supplement ➤ calcium supplements.

Sandoglobulin injection, see human normal immunoglobulin p. 302.

Sandostatin ➤ octreotide.

Sandrena is an estradiol gel used for hormone replacement therapy ➤ HRT.

SangCya ➤ ciclosporin.

Sanomigran ➤ pizotifen.

saquinavir (Fortovase, Invirase) is an antiviral drug used to treat patients suffering from HIV infection, see p. 280. *Adverse effects* include headache, skin rashes, nerve damage, stomach and bowel upsets and weakness. *Precautions:* Do not use in breast-feeding mothers. Use with caution in pregnancy, in elderly patients and in patients suffering from severe impairment of liver or kidney function, haemophilia, chronic diarrhoea or disorders of the intestine that interfere with the absorption of nutrients. *Interactions:* Dexamethasone, carbamazepine, cisapride, calcium-channel blockers, rifampicin, rifabutin, phenobarbital, phenytoin, azole antifungal drugs, astemizole, clindamycin, dapsone, quinidine, triazolam, midazolam, ritonavir, terfenadine.

Saventrine IV ➤ isoprenaline.

Savlon Antiseptic Wound Wash ➤ chlorhexidine.

Savlon Dry Powder spray ➤ povidone iodine.

Scandonest is a local anaesthetic used in dentistry ➤ mepivacaine.

Schering PC4 is a post-coital (morning-after) oral contraceptive. Each tablet contains norgestrel (a progestogen) and ethinyloestradiol (an oestrogen). See p. 207.

Scheriproct preparations contain prednisolone (a corticosteroid) and cinchocaine (a local anaesthetic). They are used to treat haemorrhoids, itching of the anus and vaginal lips. *Adverse effects* see Chapter 37, Corticosteroids. *Precautions:* Avoid prolonged use. Use with utmost caution in pregnancy. Do not use if there is a viral, tubercular or fungal infection.

Scopoderm TTS ➤ hyoscine.

scopolamine ➤ hyoscine.

Sea-legs tablets ➤ meclozine.

Secadrex tablets contain acebutolol (a selective beta-blocker) and hydrochlorothiazide (a thiazide diuretic). They are used to treat raised blood pressure. *Adverse effects* *and Precautions* ➤ beta-blockers, thiazide diuretics.

secobarbital sodium ➤ quinalbarbitone sodium.

secobarbitone ➤ quinalbarbitone sodium.

Seconal Sodium ➤ quinalbarbitone sodium.

Sectral ➤ acebutolol.

Securon preparations ➤ verapamil.

sedatives, see Chapter 2.

Select-A-Jet Dopamine ➤ dopamine.

Selective serotonin re-uptake inhibitors (SSRIs) are antidepressants. See Chapter 4. These are also referred to as 5IIT re-uptake inhibitors (or blockers) or selective serotonin re-uptake blockers.

selegiline (selegiline hydrochloride, Centrapryl, Eldepryl, Zelapar) is a monoamine oxidase-B inhibitor. Unlike other monoamine oxidase inhibitors it does not cause episodes of raised blood pressure. It is used in the treatment of parkinsonism either alone or in conjunction with levodopa. See Chapter 16. *Adverse effects* include a fall in blood pressure, involuntary movements (if patient is also taking levodopa, reduce dose of levodopa), confusion, psychosis, agitation, nausea and vomiting. *Precautions:* The adverse effects of levodopa may be increased, and the dosage may need to be reduced. *Interactions:* Fluoxetine, pethidine, non-selective MAOIs.

selenium sulphide (selenium sulphide, Selsun) is used as a shampoo to treat dandruff and dermatitis of the scalp. See p. 254. *Adverse effects:* If taken by mouth it is very dangerous. Repeated use as a shampoo may result in irritation of the scalp, oiliness, discoloration and loss of hair. *Precautions:* It should not be used on inflamed or broken skin, or on extensive areas of the skin, and it should not enter the eyes. Do not use within forty-eight hours of waving or tinting the hair.

Selexid ➤ pivmecillinam.

Selsun preparations ➤ selenium sulphide.

Semi-Daonil tablets ➤ glibenclamide.

semisodium valporate ➤ valporic acid.

Semprex ➤ acrivastine.

senna ➤ sennosides.

sennosides A and **B** (in Boots Compound Laxative Syrup of Figs, Boots Senna tablets, in Califig, Ex-Lax Senna, in Fam-Lax Senna, in Manevac, in Nylax with Senna, in Potter's Cleansing Herb, in Pripsen, in Rhuaka, Senokot) are the principal active ingredients of senna fruit; used as a stimulant laxative. See Chapter 21.

Senokot ➤ sennosides.

Senselle is a non-hormonal vaginal moisturizer used to treat menopausal dryness of the vagina. It has a high moisture content and its effects last for about twenty-four hours.

Septanest ➤ articaine.

Septrin ➤ co-trimoxazole.

Serc ➤ betahistine.

Serenace ➤ haloperidol.

Seretide ➤ fluticasone, salmeterol.

Serevent ➤ salmeterol.

sermorelin (Geref) is chemically similar to the growth hormone-releasing hormone somatorelin (GHRH). It is used to test the production of growth hormone by the pituitary gland. *Adverse effects* include pain at injection site and flushing of the face. *Precautions:* Do not use in pregnancy or breastfeeding mothers. Discontinue growth hormone treatment one to two weeks before the test. Use with caution in patients with epilepsy, untreated underworking of the thyroid gland, obesity, high blood sugar, high blood cholesterol and fat levels and in patients on anti-thyroid drugs. *Interactions:* Avoid aspirin, indomethacin and NSAIDs.

Scroquel ➤ quetiapine.

serotonin re-uptake blockers ➤ serotonin re-uptake inhibitors.

Seroxat ➤ paroxetine.

sertraline (Lustral) is a 5HT re-uptake blocker used to treat depression. See Chapter 4. It increases the amount of the stimulant nerve transmitter 5-hydroxytryptamine (5HT, serotonin) in the brain by blocking its re-uptake by nerve cells. *Adverse effects* include dry mouth, nausea, diarrhoea, tremor, sweating, indigestion, delayed ejaculation, dizziness, insomnia, sleepiness, rash and generally feeling unwell. It may rarely cause convulsions (stop the drug if this happens), movement disorders, a fall in blood sodium levels and mania or hypomania. *Precautions:* It should not be used in individuals with impaired liver function. It should be used with caution in patients with impaired kidney function, in pregnancy, in breastfeeding mothers, in people with unstable epilepsy, or who are undergoing ECT.

Settlers is an antacid ➤ calcium.

Settlers Heartburn and Indigestion liquid contain calcium, sodium alginate and sodium bicarbonate ➤ antacids.

Settlers Wind-eze ➤ activated dimethicane.

sevelamer (Renagel) binds to phosphates in the gut contents. It is used to reduce high phosphate levels in the blood in blood dialysis. *Precautions:* Do not use in patients with bowel obstruction. Use with caution in patients with swallowing disorders, poor emptying of the stomach, active inflammatory bowel disease, gastric motility disorders, history of major surgery on the stomach or bowel, in pregnancy or while breastfeeding.

Sevoflurane is a rapid acting liquid anaesthetic.

Sevredol ➤ morphine.

sex hormones (female), see Chapter 40.

sex hormones (male), see Chapter 38.

sibutamine (Reductil) is used as a supplement to diet in obese patients with body mass index of at least $30kg/m^2$. See Chapter 8. Sibutamine is a slimming agent that acts on the brain to inhibit the re-uptake of serotonin and noradrenaline (norepinephrine) which helps patients feel satisfied with less food. *Adverse effects* include rapid heart beat, palpitations, raised blood pressure, flushing, constipation, nausea, haemorrhoids, dry mouth, insomnia, weakness, headache, anxiety, sweating, abnormal taste sensation. *Precautions:* Do not use in patients with an organic cause to their obesity, a history of eating disorders, psychiatric illness, Gilles de la Tourette's syndrome, heart disorders, hyperthyroidism, severe kidney or liver damage, enlarged prostate, phaeochromocytoma (tumour of the sympathetic nervous system), glaucoma, a history of drug or alcohol abuse, in pregnancy or while breastfeeding. Use with caution in patients with sleep apnoea syndrome (who stop breathing for a moment in their sleep), epilepsy, liver or kidney damage or a family history of tics.

sildenafil (Viagra) is used to treat erectile dysfunction. See Chapter 38. *Adverse effects* include headache, flushing, dizziness, indigestion, nasal congestion, visual disturbances, allergic reactions, bloodshot eyes, eye pain. Rarely, priapism (prolonged erection) or heart disorders. *Precautions:* Do not use in patients with pre-existing heart conditions where sexual activity is inadvisable, severe liver damage, low blood pressure, recent stroke or heart attack, hereditary degenerative disorders of the retina. Use with caution in patients with severe kidney damage, liver damage, abnormal penile anatomy, sickle cell anaemia, tumours of plasma cells, leukaemia, active peptic ulcer or bleeding disorders.

silicic acid (in Unguentum Merck) is a silicon compound used as a suspending agent.

silver nitrate is used as a caustic, astringent and antiseptic in skin applications. Continued application to surfaces leads to a blue-black discoloration (argyria) due to deposition of silver granules in the tissues.

silver sulfadiazine is a compound of silver and sulfadiazine (a sulphonamide). It has antibacterial and astringent properties. It is used in skin applications (Flamazine cream) to treat infected leg ulcers and pressure sores. *Adverse effects:* Allergic reactions may occur. *Precautions:* It should not be applied to large areas of damaged skin, especially in patients suffering from impaired kidney or liver function. Do not use in pregnancy, or in newborn babies. Do not use in patients allergic to sulphonamides. Use with caution in patients with impaired liver or kidney function. *Interactions:* Oral anti-diabetic drugs, phenytoin, sulphonamides.

Simeco antacid tablets contain aluminium hydroxide, magnesium carbonate co-dried gel, magnesium hydroxide and activated dimethicone ➤ antacids and activated dimethicone.

simethicone (activated dimethicone) is a mixture of liquid dimethicones containing finely divided silicone dioxide to increase the defoaming properties of the silicone. It reduces the surface tension of gas bubbles, causing them to come together into larger bubbles. It is used to treat wind and indigestion. See Chapter 19. It is also used in some skin preparations, e.g. Vaseline Dermacare and Vasogen cream.

simple eye ointment contains liquid paraffin, wool fat and yellow soft paraffin.

simple linctus cough preparations contain citric acid and monohydrate with anise flavouring. See Chapter 11.

Simplene eye drops contain adrenaline (epinephrine). They are used to treat open-angle glaucoma. See p. 63. *Adverse effects* include eye discomfort, headache, redness of the eye, skin reactions and pigmentation (melanosis) of the cornea and conjunctiva. General effects are rare. *Precautions:* Do not use to treat patients with closed-angle glaucoma or diabetes. *Interactions:* Beta-blockers, MAOIs, tricyclic antidepressants.

SimpleXx ➤ somatropin.

Simulect ➤ basiliximab.

simvastatin (Zocor) blocks an enzyme involved in the production of cholesterol and is used to treat patients with a high blood cholesterol who have not responded to a cholesterol-reducing diet. See Chapter 26. *Adverse effects* include headache, fatigue, nausea, indigestion, wind, constipation, stomach cramps, diarrhoea, skin rash, sensitivity of the skin to the sun's rays, hair loss, dizziness, muscle cramps and pains, nerve damage and liver or pancreatic damage. Rarely, muscle weakness (myopathy) may occur due to damage to muscle fibres – diagnosed from blood tests for an enzyme involved in the breakdown of muscle (creatinine phosphokinase). If this is raised, the drug should be stopped immediately. *Precautions:* Do not use in patients with active liver disease or porphyria (a hereditary disorder of metabolism). Do not use in pregnancy. To avoid pregnancy during treatment, women should abstain or use a mechanical form of contraceptive. An oral contraceptive should not be used. Avoid pregnancy for one month after treatment has stopped. Do not use in breast-feeding mothers. Use with caution in patients with a history of liver disease – liver function tests should be carried out before and every four–six weeks during treatment. An eye examination should be carried out every twelve months. Patients should report any muscle pains. *Interactions:* Digoxin, coumarin anticoagulants, cyclosporin, gemfibrozil and other fibrates, nicotinic acid, erythromycin, azole antifungal drugs, immunosuppressants. Use with caution in patients who have a high intake of alcohol. *Warning:* Statin drugs (fluvastatin, pravastatin, simvastatin) may damage muscles causing pain and a rise in the blood level of creatine phosphokinase (CPK) – an enzyme that is released when muscles are damaged. This damage is particularly likely to occur in patients with impaired kidney function or underworking of the thyroid gland and also if a fibrate or cyclosporin is taken at the same time. Patients must report any muscle pain and have their CPK blood level measured. This should also be measured at intervals during therapy.

Sinemet preparations ➤ co-careldopa.

Sinequan ➤ doxepin.

Singulair ➤ montelukast.

Sinthrome ➤ nicoumalone.

Sinutab contains paracetamol and phenylpropanolamine ➤ individual entry for both drugs.

Sinutab Nightime contains paracetamol, phenylpropanolamine and phenyltoloxamine ➤ individual entry for each drug.

Siopel barrier cream contains silicone and cetrimide ➤ individual entry for both drugs.

sirolimus (Rapamune) is used to prevent organ rejection in adults receiving kidney transplant, who are at low to moderate risk of organ rejection. It is initially used in combination with cyclosporin and corticosteroids. See Chapter 17. *Adverse effects* include lymphocele, abnormal healing, fluid retention, infections, rapid heart beat, stomach and bowel upset, disorders of the blood, metabolic or nutritional disorders, pain in joints, death of tissues in the bone, nosebleed, pneumonia, skin reactions, urinary tract infection, increased susceptibility to tumours of the lymph glands, inflammation of the lung. *Precautions:* Do not use in patients with a high risk of organ rejection, in pregnancy (ensure adequate contraception during and for twelve weeks after therapy) or while breastfeeding. Use with caution in patients with liver damage, at risk of skin cancer, with a high cholesterol level, in black patients or in the elderly.

Skelid ➤ tiludronic acid.

Skinoren ➤ azelaic acid.

Slow-Fe ➤ ferrous sulphate.

Slow-Fe Folic tablets contain ferrous sulphate and folic acid in a slow-release form ➤ iron and folic acid.

Slofedipine and **Slofedipine XL** ➤ nifedipine.

Slofenac ➤ diclofenac.

Slo-Indo ➤ indometacin.

Slow-K ➤ potassium chloride.

Slo-Phyllin ➤ theophylline.

Slow-Sodium ➤ sodium chloride.

Slow-Trasicor ➤ oxprenol.

Slozem ➤ diltiazem.

Sno Phenicol eye drops contain chloramphenicol. They may cause allergic reactions where they are applied and, very rarely, aplastic anaemia ➤ chloramphenicol.

Sno Tears eye drops contain polyvinyl alcohol. They are used to lubricate the eyes. *Adverse effects* include transient stinging and blurred vision. *Precautions:* Do not wear soft contact lenses.

Sodiofolin ➤ disodium folinate.

sodium acid phosphate is given by mouth to make the urine more acid. It is also given with sodium phosphate in the treatment of high blood calcium levels. It is poorly absorbed from the intestine and retains water in it. It is administered rectally as an enema to clear the bowel before operations and it is used as a saline laxative by mouth. It is a constituent of Carbalax, Fleet Phosphosoda, Fletchers' Phosphate Enema and Phosphate-Sandoz (a phosphate supplement).

sodium alendronate ➤ alendronic acid.

sodium alginate (in Algitec, in Gastrocote, in Gaviscon liquid, in Peptac, in Pyrogastrone) is a salt of alginic acid ➤ alginic acid.

sodium alkylsulphoacetate is an ingredient in Micralax disposable enema.

Sodium Amytal ➤ amylobarbitone sodium.

sodium aurothiomalate (Myocrisin) ➤ gold.

sodium bicarbonate is used as an antacid ➤ antacids.

sodium calcium edetate (Ledclair) is used to treat poisoning by heavy metals, especially lead. *Adverse effects* include nausea and cramps. In overdose it may cause kidney damage. *Precautions:* Use with caution in patients with impaired kidney function.

sodium carboxymethylcellulose ➤ carboxymethylcellulose.

sodium chloride is used in water for hydration. **Sodium chloride solution** 0.9% is isotonic (in harmony with the body) and is used for sterile irrigation of the eye or bladder and for general skin and wound cleaning. It is also used in nasal drops and mouthwashes.

sodium citrate (Micolette, Micralax, Mictral, Relaxit) is used to make the urine less acid to relieve the symptoms of cystitis (see Chapter 49), it is in some osmotic laxatives and enemas (see Chapter 21), used to stop blood from clotting in laboratory instruments and to wash out the bladder after surgery on the bladder.

sodium clodronate (Bonefos, Loron) is used to keep blood calcium levels within normal ranges in individuals suffering from a high blood calcium caused by certain cancers (e.g. cancer of the breast, kidney, bronchus) in which the calcium is dissolved from bone into the bloodstream and also reabsorbed by the kidneys out of the urine and back into the blood. Sodium clodronate decreases blood calcium levels by suppressing the dissolving of bone and increasing the excretion of calcium in the urine without affecting the laying down of calcium in the bone. *Adverse effects:* Oral treatment may cause nausea or mild diarrhoea which may improve by dividing the daily dose and taking it twice daily instead of once daily. Rarely, allergic reactions may occur, infusions may cause protein in the urine, and the blood calcium may fall below normal levels. It may cause a rise in the blood levels of parathyroid hormone, creatinine,

lactate dehydrogenase and transaminase. *Precaution:* It should not be used in individuals with moderate to severe impairment of kidney function, or by mouth in people with inflammatory intestinal disorders, in pregnancy or in breastfeeding mothers. Use with caution in patients with moderate impairment of kidney function. Drink plenty of fluids. Blood calcium and phosphates should be measured during infusions. Kidney function tests should be carried out before and during treatment by mouth or infusion. *Interactions:* Other bisphosphonates, antacids, mineral supplements, NSAIDs.

sodium cromoglicate (in Aerocrom, Cromogen, Hay-Crom, Intal Compound, Intal Syncroner, Nalcrom, Opticrom, Rynacrom, Rynacrom Compound, Vividrin) is an anti-inflammatory drug used to prevent attacks of asthma (see Chapter 14), hayfever (see Chapter 17), food allergies and to treat allergic conjunctivitis (Viz-on). See p. 88. *Adverse effects:* By inhalation it may cause transient cough, irritation of the throat and, rarely, wheezing. By nasal spray it may cause transient irritation of the nose and, rarely, wheezing. Applied to the eyes it may cause transient stinging and by mouth it may cause nausea, skin rashes and joint pains.

sodium cromoglycate ➤ sodium cromoglicate.

sodium feredetate (Sytron) is used to treat and prevent iron deficiency anaemia. See Chapter 35 ➤ iron.

sodium fluoride (EndeKay, Fluorigard) ➤ fluoride.

sodium fusidate (in Fucibet, Fucidin, in Fucidin H, Fucithalmic) is a salt of fusidic acid (➤ fusidic acid). It is used as an antibacterial drug. See Chapter 46. It is effective against bacteria which have developed a resistance to penicillin. *Adverse effects:* By mouth or injection it may cause mild stomach and bowel upsets and rarely skin rashes and jaundice. *Precautions:* Stomach and bowel upsets are reduced if the drug is given with food. Regular tests of liver function should be carried out while on treatment by mouth or injection. Eye drops may cause transient irritation and allergic reactions.

sodium heparin (Pump-Hep) ➤ heparin.

sodium hyaluronate (Cystistat, Fermathron, Healonid, Hyalgan, Ophthalin, Orthovisc, Supartz, Suplasyn) is a viscoelastic polymer normally present in the fluid in the eyes (aqueous and vitreous humour). It is used during surgical operations on the eye and in arthritis of the knee and shoulder. *Adverse effects:* Because it is obtained from the eyes of birds it can occasionally cause allergic reactions and a temporary rise in pressure in the eyes.

sodium iron edetate ➤ sodium feredetate.

sodium lactate is metabolized to sodium bicarbonate after it is absorbed into the bloodstream. It is used as an alternative to sodium bicarbonate in the treatment of acidosis and to make the urine more alkaline. See Chapter 49.

sodium lauryl sulphate is used as a detergent skin cleanser, in shampoos and as a wetting agent. It is included in Relaxit micro-enemas. See Chapter 21.

sodium lauryl sulphoacetate is used in Micolette and Fleet micro-enemas. See Chapter 21.

sodium nitrate is used in conjunction with sodium thiosulphate to treat poisoning with cyanides.

sodium nitroprusside dilates blood vessels to treat heart failure (see Chapter 23), episodes of severe raised blood pressure (see Chapter 25), and to maintain a low blood pressure during surgery. *Adverse effects:* Rapid reduction in blood pressure may cause nausea, vomiting, retching, sweating, apprehension, headache, abdominal pain, dizziness, palpitations and chest pain (reduce the infusion rate). Occasionally it may cause a fall in the platelet count and temporary inflammation of the vein at the site of injection. *Precautions:* It should be used with caution in patients suffering from an under-active thyroid, severe impairment of kidney function, impaired circulation to the brain, or in the elderly. It should not be used in patients with liver failure or vitamin B_{12} deficiency (e.g. pernicious anaemia). As it is converted into cyanide in the body it is important that blood-level monitoring should be carried out. Blood pressure should be carefully monitored and it should be used with caution in pregnancy, in breastfeeding mothers and in patients with coronary artery disease.

sodium perborate (Bocasan) dissolves in water, releasing oxygen and hydrogen peroxide. It has mild antiseptic and deodorant properties and is made up into a mouthwash for treating mouth and gum conditions. Do not use in patients with impaired kidney function.

sodium phenylbutyrate (Ammonaps) is used as additional therapy in urea cycle disorders in patients with complete enzyme deficiencies presenting within first twenty-eight days of life or partial enzyme deficiencies presenting after first twenty-eight days of life. *Adverse effects* include irregular or no menstruation, pH imbalance in the blood, increase in chloride content of the blood, abnormally low concentrations of phosphates in the blood, decreased appetite, body odour, bad taste in the mouth or taste aversion. *Precautions:* Do not use in pregnancy or while breastfeeding. Use with caution in patients with congestive heart failure, sodium retention with oedema, liver or kidney damage.

sodium phosphate (in Fleet enemas, in Fleet Phospho-soda, in Fletchers' phosphate enemas) when taken by mouth acts as a saline laxative and produces a watery evacuation of the bowels. It can be used as an enema. See Chapter 21. It may be given by mouth or intravenously as a phosphate supplement.

sodium picosulfate (Laxoberal, in Picolax) is broken down in the intestinal tract to form an irritant compound that acts as a laxative. See Chapter 21.

sodium polystyrene sulphonate (Resonium-A) is an ion-exchange resin that is taken by mouth; in the intestine it exchanges sodium ions for potassium ions. The exchange resin is excreted in the faeces. It is used to treat high blood potassium levels associated with reduced kidney function and kidney dialysis. *Adverse effects:* Occasionally, loss of appetite, nausea, vomiting and diarrhoea may occur. Constipation may occur in elderly people; and the resin may block the bowel (impaction). It may cause severe potassium deficiency, resulting in muscle weakness, irritability, confusion and disorders of heart rhythm. It may also cause a loss of other ions (e.g. calcium), and cause high blood levels of sodium, especially in patients with impaired kidney function; this may cause congestive heart failure. *Precautions:* Blood potassium, sodium, calcium and other electrolytes should be measured before and at regular intervals during treatment. It should be used with caution in patients who suffer from any disorder which could be made worse by a high blood sodium – for example, heart failure, raised blood pressure. Do not use in patients with an obstructed bowel or in newborn babies with reduced movements of the intestine.

sodium stibogluconate (Pentostam) is used to treat Leishmaniasis. *Adverse effects* include loss of appetite, nausea, vomiting, abdominal pains, cough, pain in the chest (ECG changes may occur), severe allergic reactions, fever, sweating, flushing, vertigo, rash, bleeding nose and gums and changes in liver function. Intramuscular injections are painful. Intravenous injections are also painful and may cause thrombosis at the site of injection. *Precautions:* Do not use in breastfeeding mothers or in patients with severe impairment of kidney function. Use with caution in patients with impaired liver function, heart disease or Leishmaniasis affecting the skin, mouth and nose (it may cause severe swelling around the infected

area which could be life-threatening if the throat or trachea are involved – corticosteroids may be required). Use with caution in pregnancy. Intravenous injections must be given slowly over five minutes and stopped if coughing or chest pains develop. Any other infection (e.g. pneumonia) should be treated with appropriate antibiotics.

sodium sulphate (Glauber's salts, in Klean-prep) is used as a saline laxative. See Chapter 21.

sodium tetraborate ➤ borax.

sodium tetradecyl sulphate injection (STD, Fibro-Vein) is injected into varicose veins to shrink them. *Adverse effects:* It may cause allergic reactions including anaphylactic shock (allergic crisis), see p. 87. *Precautions:* Do not use if patient is unable to walk, has acute inflammation of a vein, is taking an oral contraceptive or has obese legs.

sodium thiosulphate is used with sodium nitrite to treat patients suffering from cyanide poisoning.

sodium valproate (Convulex, Epilim) is an anti-epileptic drug. See Chapter 15. *Adverse effects:* Liver damage, sometimes causing death, may rarely occur, particularly in children under the age of three, or children with brain damage, seizures and mental retardation, or certain metabolic disorders. This serious risk occurs mainly in the first six months of treatment (maximum risk two– twelve months) and usually involves the use of more than one anti-epileptic drug. Laboratory tests are not very useful in predicting which patients will be at risk or in spotting the early signs of trouble. It is best to rely on early signs and symptoms of liver damage. The onset of an acute illness, especially within the first six months, which may include vomiting, lethargy, weakness, drowsiness, loss of appetite, jaundice or loss of seizure control, is an indication for stopping the drug *immediately*. A temporary rise in blood ammonia without liver damage may occur, causing vomiting, lack of coordination of movement and clouding of consciousness. If this occurs, the drug should be stopped *immediately*. Rarely, damage to the pancreas (pancreatitis) may occur in the first six months of treatment; this may produce severe stomach pains. Very rarely, damage to the bone marrow affecting red cell and white cell production may occur; the stickiness of platelets may be affected and cause the bleeding time to be prolonged, resulting in easy bruising and bleeding. It may cause an increase in appetite and weight, and some patients may develop stomach upsets at the start of treatment. Loss of periods, rashes, drowsiness, irregular periods and swelling of the breasts (in males) may occur. Temporary loss of hair may occur, which does not appear to be related to the dose. Regrowth of hair starts in about six months and the hair may be more curly than before. Occasionally it may cause lack of coordination of movement, tremor, lethargy, confusion, stupor, hallucinations, aggression, increased alertness, hyperactivity and disorders of behaviour. *Precautions:* Do not use in patients with active liver disease or a family history of liver dysfunction. Tests of liver function should be carried out before treatment and at regular intervals (every two weeks) during the first six months of treatment, particularly in patients with a history of liver disease, or in children with severe epilepsy associated with brain damage. Use with caution in patients with severe impairment of kidney function, in pregnancy, in breastfeeding mothers and in patients with systemic lupus erythematosis (SLE – a disease of unknown cause with symptoms of fever, muscular and joint pain, blood disorders and skin eruptions) or porphyria (a hereditary disorder of metabolism). The drug may cause a false positive urine test for diabetes. Blood tests including platelet counts should be carried out before treatment and at regular intervals during treatment. If the prothrombin time (which gives an indication of the risk of bleeding) is prolonged the patient must be carefully monitored and if it becomes abnormally prolonged the drug should be stopped. Platelet counts should be carried out before major surgery to assess the risk of bleeding. *Interactions:* Antidepressants, other antiepileptic drugs, anticoagulants, cimetidine, cholestyramine.

Sofradex eye and ear drops contain the aminoglycoside antibiotics framycetin and gramicidin and the corticosteroid dexamethasone. They are used in ear drops to treat otitis externa (inflammation of the outer ear) and in eye drops to treat inflammatory conditions of the eye when preventive antibiotic treatment is required. *Adverse effects:* Ear drops may cause superinfection and eye drops may cause a rise in pressure inside the eye, thinning of the cornea, cataract and fungal infections. *Precautions:* Do not use ear drops if patient has a perforated ear drum. Do not use eye drops if patient has glaucoma or a fungal, tubercular, viral or pus-filled bacterial infection. Use both preparations with caution in pregnancy and in infants – avoid prolonged use. See Chapter 37, Corticosteroids and ➤ aminoglycosides.

Soframycin ➤ framycetin.

Sofra-Tulle gauze dressing is impregnated with framycetin ➤ framycetin.

Solareze ➤ diclofenac sodium.

Solarcaine is a local anaesthetic cream containing benzocaine and tricloson ➤ benzocaine, tricloson.

Solian ➤ amisulpride.

Solpadeine contains paracetamol, codeine and caffeine ➤ individual entry for each drug.

Solpadeine Max contains paracetamol and codeine ➤ paracetamol, codeine.

Solpadol effervescent pain-relieving tablets contain paracetamol and codeine ➤ paracetamol, codeine.

Solpaflex contains ibuprofen and codeine ➤ ibuprofen, codeine.

Soltamox ➤ tamoxifen.

Solu-Cortef ➤ hydrocortisone for injection.

Solu-Medrone ➤ methylprednisolone for injection.

Solvazinc effervescent tablets ➤ zinc sulphate.

Somatostatin analogues are similar to somatostatin which blocks the release of hormones from the hypothalamus. They are used for the relief of symptoms associated with neuroendocrine tumours and acromegaly (disease in which excessive growth hormone is secreted).

somatotrophin (growth hormone of human origin, HGH) has been replaced by *somatropin* produced by DNA biotechnology.

somatropin (Genotropin, Humatrope, Kabivial, Norditropin, Saizen, Simplex, Zomacton) is a bio-synthetic human growth hormone which has replaced growth hormone of human origin (HGH, somatotrophin). It is used to treat short stature in children due to growth hormone deficiency. It is also used to treat growth hormone deficiency in adults and Turner's syndrome (a chromosome disorder producing short stature and various deformities) in children. Must only be used in adults if there is evidence of one other pituitary hormone deficiency (excluding prolactin) and this deficiency must be treated before starting somatropin therapy. *Adverse effects* include fluid retention (may show as swollen ankles and fingers), painful joints and muscles and underworking of the thyroid gland. Occasionally the formation of antibodies to somatropin may occur and reduce its effectiveness. Leukaemia in children with growth hormone deficiency has been reported. Rarely the blood pressure in the brain may increase producing severe or recurrent headaches, visual disturbances, nausea and vomiting. This is called benign intracranial hypertension. Wasting of fat under the skin at sites of injection may pro-duce denting of the skin. *Precautions:* Rotate sites of injection to avoid fat wasting. Do not use in pregnancy. Use with caution in patients with other pituitary hormone deficiencies or diabetes. Use in children *before* the bone ends have closed. Do not use in patients wih an active pituitary tumour. Check thyroid function at regular intervals. Do not use after kidney transplant.

Somatuline LA ➤ lanreotide.

Sominex ➤ promethazine.

Somnite ➤ nitrazepam.

Sonata ➤ zaleplon.

Soneryl ➤ butobarbital.

Soothelip ➤ aciclovir.

soothing skin applications, see p. 236.

sorbic acid (in Micralax, in Relaxit) has antibacterial and antifungal properties and is used as a preservative in cosmetics, medicines and foods.

Sorbid SA ➤ isosorbide dinitrate.

sorbitol is used as a sugar substitute in diabetic food. It is used as a sweetening agent in drug preparations and is present in some creams and toothpastes. Excessive amounts in the diet may cause wind, abdominal distension and diarrhoea.

Sotacor ➤ sotalol.

sotalol (sotalol hydrochloride, Beta-cardone, Sotacor) is a non-selective beta-blocker ➤ beta-blockers.

Sovol is an antacid which contains aluminium, magnesium and activated dimeticone ➤ individual entry for each drug.

soya oil (Balneum, in Balneum with tar) is prepared from soya beans; it has a high content of unsaturated fatty acids. It is given intravenously to patients who are unable to take any nutrients orally. It is also used as a base in bath oils.

Spasmonal ➤ alverine.

SPF sun protection factor, see p. 238.

Spiro-Co ➤ co-flumactone.

spironolactone (in Aldactide, Aldactone, in co-flumactone, in Lasilactone, in Spiro-Co, Spirospare) is a potassium-sparing diuretic (see Chapter 29). It inhibits the effects of aldosterone, which is produced by the adrenal glands. Since aldosterone produces retention of sodium and loss of potassium from the urine, spironolactone does the reverse, and thus increases sodium loss and potassium retention. It is therefore used as a diuretic to treat patients with fluid retention caused by increased production of aldosterone by the adrenal glands in disorders such as cirrhosis of the liver, kidney disease (nephrotic syndrome), congestive heart failure and a primary disorder of the adrenal glands leading to an increased production of aldosterone. *Adverse effects* include headache, stomach and bowel upsets, loss of control over voluntary movements (ataxia), mental confusion, deepening of voice, irregular periods, swelling of the breasts (in males), impotence, rashes, blood disorders, liver damage, osteomalacia (adult rickets), raised blood potassium levels and a fall in blood sodium levels. *Precautions:* Do not use in patients with severe kidney failure, a raised blood potassium or low blood sodium level, or Addison's disease (underworking of the adrenal glands), or in patients not producing urine (anurea). Do not use in breastfeeding mothers or in pregnancy and use with caution in patients with impaired kidney or liver function, and for long-term use in young people. Blood chemistry and kidney function tests should be carried out at regular intervals in young patients on long-term treatment. *Interactions:* Potassium supplements, potassium-sparing diuretics, ACE inhibitors, digoxin and related drugs, carbenoxolone, NSAIDs.

Spirospare ➤ spironolactone.

Sporanox preparations ➤ itraconazole.

Sprilon spray contains dimethicone and zinc oxide in a propellant. It is used as a barrier application to protect the skin from urine and faeces and to treat pressure sores, leg ulcers and eczema ➤ dimethicone and zinc oxide.

squill is used as a cough expectorant, it is derived from the bulb of a lily that grows at the sea-shore, Urginea maritima. It is used in a wide variety of cough medicines, but it may cause nausea and vomiting in high doses, see Chapter 11.

SSRIs ➤ serotonin re-uptake inhibitors.

SST tablets are used for the treatment of dry mouth. They contain citric acid, malic acid in a sorbital base.

Stafoxil ➤ flucloxacillin.

stanozolol (Stromba) is an anabolic (body-building) steroid (see Chapter 39) used in the treatment of Behcet's disease and to prevent hereditary allergic swelling on the face, hands and feet. *Adverse effects* include headache, hair loss, depression, euphoria, cramps, indigestion, rashes and, rarely, jaundice. May cause virilization in women and pre-pubertal children (see Chapter 38). *Precautions:* Do not use in patients with cancer of the prostate, severe liver disease, male breast cancer, porphyria (a hereditary disorder of metabolism), diabetes, during pregnancy or in patients with raised blood pressure, epilepsy or migraine. Use with caution in children and pre-menopausal women, and in patients with impaired liver, heart or kidney function. Tests of liver function should be carried out before treatment and at regular intervals during treatment. Bone growth should be monitored in young people. *Interactions:* Oral anticoagulants, oral anti-diabetic drugs.

Staril ➤ fosinopril.

Starlix ➤ nateglinide.

statins, see Chapter 26. For risk of muscle damage ➤ simvastatin.

stavudine (Zerit) is an antiviral drug used to treat patients suffering from HIV infection, see p. 280. *Adverse effects* include headache, fever, generally feeling unwell, stomach and bowel upsets, skin irritation, swollen glands, damage to nerves, inflammation of the pancreas and risk of cancer. *Precautions:* Do not use in pregnancy or in breastfeeding mothers. Use with caution in patients with impaired kidney function, history of nerve damage or inflammation of the pancreas, in the elderly or in patients with lactose intolerance. Stop treatment at the earliest signs of nerve damage (e.g. pins and needles) or damage to the pancreas. If symptoms clear up restart drug at a lower dose.

STD ➤ sodium tetradecyl sulphate.

Stelazine ➤ trifluoperazine.

Stemetil ➤ prochlorperazine.

Sterac (sterile water) and **Sterac Sodium Chloride** are used to irrigate wounds.

sterculia (in Alvercol, Normacol, in Normacol Plus, Prefil, Spasmonal Fibre) is a vegetable gum. It absorbs large amounts of water and swells and can be used as a bulk laxative. See Chapter 21. It is also used to treat diarrhoea. See Chapter 20. Because it swells it is claimed that it can make people feel full so that they can reduce their calorie intake when trying to lose weight; there is little evidence to support this claim. See Chapter 8. *Adverse effects:* It may cause wind, abdominal distension and obstruction of the bowel. *Precautions:* Sterculia should be swallowed with a large drink of water and not taken just before going to bed. Do not use in patients with difficulty in swallowing or an obstruction of the intestine.

Sterexidine solution ➤ chlorhexidine.

Steri-Neb Cromogen nebulizer solution ➤ sodium cromoglicate.

Steri-Neb Ipratropium nebulizer solution ➤ ipratropium.

Steri-Neb Salamol nebulizer solution ➤ salbutamol.

Steri-Neb Sodium Chloride is used to dilute nebulizer solutions.

Steripod Blue ampoules contain sterile sodium chloride solution for washing out the eyes and for flushing wounds and burns. **Steripod Yellow** ampoules contain the antiseptics chlorhexidine and cetrimide. **Steripod Pink** ampoules contain chlorhexidine. Yellow and pink are used to wash wounds and burns. They must not be used in the eyes. *Adverse effects and Precautions* ➤ chlorhexidine and cetrimide.

Steripoule saline ➤ sodium chloride.

Ster-Zac Bath Conc ➤ triclosan.

Ster-Zac DC skin cleanser cream ➤ hexachlorophene.

Ster-Zac Powder ➤ hexachlorophene.

Stesolid injection ➤ diazepam.

Stiedex preparations ➤ desoxymetasone.

Stiemycin contains erythromycin in alcohol solution, for treating acne ➤ erythromycin.

Stimlor ➤ naftidrofuryl.

stilboestrol ➤ diethylstilboestrol.

Stilnoct ➤ zolpidem.

stimulants, respiratory ➤ respiratory stimulants.

St John's Wort ➤ hypericum peroratum.

Strefen lozenges ➤ flurbiprofen.

Strepsils contains amylmetacresol and diochlorobenzyl alcohol; **Strepsils Extra** contains hexylresorcinol and menthol; **Strepsils Pain Relief Plus** contains amylmetacresol, diochlorobenzyl alcohol and lidocaine(lignocaine); **Strepsils Pain Relief Spray** contains lidocaine(lignocaine) ➤ individual entry on each drug.

Streptase ➤ streptokinase.

streptodornase (in Varidase) is an enzyme that dissolves the protein of dead cells. It is used in combination with streptokinase to clean wounds.

streptokinase (Kabikinase, Streptase, in

Varidase) is an enzyme that dissolves the protein fibrin in thrombi (clots in blood vessels). It is used as a clot-buster to treat deep-vein thrombosis, thrombosis in the arteries, clotted blood dialysis shunts, and in the early treatment of heart attack due to a coronary thrombosis (blood clot in the coronary arteries of the heart) (see Chapter 22). *Adverse effects* include nausea, vomiting, bleeding, rashes, fever, allergic reactions, fall in blood pressure, nerve damage and disorders of heart rhythm. *Precautions:* Bleeding is usually limited to the site of injection but bleeding into the brain or other sites may occasionally occur. If the bleeding is severe the drug should be stopped and an antifibrinolytic drug given. See p. 144. Allergic reactions can occasionally be very severe causing shock, and treatment for an allergic emergency should be to hand. See p. 87. Streptokinase should not be used in patients within ten days of a haemorrhage, injury or surgery (including dental extraction). Do not use in patients with a bleeding disorder (e.g. haemophilia), aortic dissection, coma, stroke, severe raised blood pressure, active peptic ulcer, acute inflammation of the pancreas, bacterial inflammation of the lining of the heart, severe liver disease, heavy vaginal bleeding, serious lung disease with lung cavities, or distended veins (varices) in the oesophagus. Do not use in patients allergic to the drug or who have had the drug from five days to twelve months previously. Do not continue the drug beyond four days. Do not use in patients with severe diabetes, severe kidney failure, brain tumour or in pregnancy. *Interactions:* Anticoagulants and drugs that affect platelet function.

streptomycin (streptomycin sulphate) is an aminoglycoside antibiotic. See p. 270. It is used to treat tuberculosis in combination with other drugs. See Chapter 50. *Adverse effects:* After intramuscular injections the patient may develop pain at the site of injection, peculiar sensations around the mouth, vertigo, headache and weariness. Allergic reactions are common and patients may develop skin rashes, swollen glands and fever. More severe adverse effects may result from streptomycin's effects upon the nerves supplying the ear and organ of balance. These may come on suddenly and disappear when the drug is withdrawn, but permanent deafness and damage to the organ of balance may develop slowly and even come on after the drug has been stopped. In high doses kidney damage, blood disorders and liver damage may develop. *Precautions:* Great caution is needed when giving streptomycin to patients with impaired kidney or liver function, to the elderly, and to premature infants. It should not be used in pregnancy because the baby could be born deaf. It should not be used in patients who are blind, or with ear disorders, or disorders of their organ of balance, or in patients who are allergic to it. See also aminoglycoside antibiotics.

Stromba ➤ stanozolol.

Stugeron and **Stugeron Forte** ➤ cinnarizine.

Sublimaze injection ➤ fentanyl.

Subutex ➤ buprenorphine.

sucralfate (Antepsin) protects the surface of the stomach (cytoprotective) and is used to treat peptic ulcers. See Chapter 19. *Adverse effects* include diarrhoea, constipation, nausea, indigestion, back pain, itching, dry mouth, dizziness, vertigo, insomnia, drowsiness, and skin rash. *Precautions:* It should be used with caution in patients with impaired kidney function, in pregnancy and in breastfeeding mothers. It should not be used in patients with severe impairment of kidney function. *Interactions:* Leave two hours between taking sucralfate and the following drugs – tetracyclines, phenytoin, cimetidine, digoxin, tube feeds.

Sudafed-Co contains paracetamol and pseudoephedrine ➤ paracetamol, pseudoephedrine.

Sudafed Nasal Spray ➤ oxymetazoline.

Sudafed Plus preparations are used to treat

hayfever symptoms. See p. 87. They contain pseudoephedrine (a sympathomimetic drug used as a decongestant) and triprolidine (an antihistamine). *Adverse effects* ➤ antihistamines and sympathomimetic drugs. It may cause drowsiness, skin rash, disturbed sleep and rarely hallucinations. *Precautions:* Do not use in patients with coronary artery disease or severe raised blood pressure. Use with caution in patients with glaucoma, over-active thyroid, diabetes or enlarged prostate gland. *Interactions:* MAOIs, sympathomimetic drugs, alcohol, sleeping drugs, sedatives, anti-anxiety drugs or any drug that depresses brain function.

Sudocrem cream contains benzyl alcohol, benzyl benzoate, benzyl cinnamate, wool fat and zinc oxide. It is an antiseptic skin softener used to treat nappy rash, pressure sores, varicose ulcers, eczema, minor wounds and abrasions.

Sulazine ➤ sulfasalazine.

sulconazole nitrate (Exelderm cream) is an antifungal drug used in skin applications to treat fungal infections of the skin. See p. 243. It may irritate the skin (stop immediately). Avoid contact with eyes.

Suleo-M lotion ➤ malathion.

sulfa- see also sulpha-.

sulfa drugs ➤ sulphonamides.

sulfacetamide (sulphacetamide sodium) is a sulphonamide drug ➤ sulphonamides.

sulfadiazine is a sulphonamide drug ➤ sulphonamides.

sulfadiazine, silver ➤ silver sulfadiazine.

sulfadoxine is a sulphonamide drug. It has a long duration of action and is used to treat leprosy. It is given with pirimethamine (in Fansidar) to treat and prevent falciparum malaria. *Adverse effects and Precautions* ➤ sulphonamides.

sulfamethoxazole is a sulphonamide. It is frequently combined with trimethoprim as

co-trimoxazole ➤ co-trimoxazole, sulphonamides.

sulfametopyrazine (Kelfizine W) is a long-acting sulphonamide drug. It is used to treat chronic bronchitis and urinary tract infections. *Adverse effects and Precautions* ➤ sulphonamides.

sulfasalazine (sulphasalazine, Salazopyrin, Sulazine, Ucine) is used to treat ulcerative colitis and Crohn's disease (severe diarrhoeal disorders), and occasionally rheumatoid arthritis. See Chapter 32. It is a salicylate/sulphonamide compound. *Adverse effects* include nausea, vomiting, loss of appetite, stomach pains, headache, vertigo, noises in the ears (tinnitus), rashes and fever. Very rarely, it may cause blood disorders, nerve damage, liver damage, flare-up of colitis, inflammation of the pancreas, serious skin disorders, lung damage, kidney damage, sensitivity of the skin to sunlight, damage to arteries and a reduced sperm count. Urine may be coloured orange, so may contact lenses. *Precautions:* It should not be given to patients with a known allergy to salicylates and/or sulphonamides or to children under two years of age. It should be used with caution in pregnancy and in breastfeeding mothers, in patients with impaired kidney or liver function, with porphyria (a hereditary disorder of metabolism) or G6PD deficiency. Adequate fluid intake must be maintained to prevent crystals developing in the kidneys. Patients should report immediately if they develop unexplained bleeding or bruising, sore throat, generally feeling unwell or fever. If blood disorders are suspected a full blood test should be carried out. Full blood tests and liver function tests should be carried out at start of treatment and at monthly intervals for the first three months of treatment and then at less frequent intervals. *Interactions:* Digoxin, folate (folic acid).

sulfathiazole (in Sultrin) is a sulphonamide ➤ sulphonamides.

sulfinpyrazone (Anturan) reduces the blood uric acid level and is used as long-term treatment for gout. See Chapter 33. It increases uric acid excretion by the kidneys. It is no use for treating acute attacks of gout. *Adverse effects:* It may cause nausea, vomiting and abdominal pain, and aggravate peptic ulcers. At the beginning of treatment it may trigger acute attacks of gout. Rarely, it may cause kidney stones, bleeding from the stomach or intestine, kidney damage, liver damage, jaundice, fluid and salt retention, skin rashes and blood disorders. *Precautions:* It should not be used in patients with active peptic ulcers, with a history of peptic ulcers, during acute attacks of gout or in patients with a severe impairment of kidney or liver function, blood disorders, porphyria (a hereditary disorder of metabolism), bleeding disorders, or who are allergic to it or related drugs. It should be given with caution to patients with mild to moderate impaired kidney function, who are allergic to aspirin or other NSAIDs, or who have heart failure. It should be used with caution in pregnancy and breastfeeding mothers. Patients should drink plenty of fluids while on treatment, and have regular blood counts and tests of kidney function. *Interactions:* Salicylates (e.g. aspirin), anticoagulants, anti-diabetic drugs, sulphonamides, penicillins, theophylline, phenytoin.

sulindac (Clinoril) is a non-steroidal anti-inflammatory drug (NSAID) ➤ non-steroidal anti-inflammatory drugs.

Sulparex ➤ sulpiride.

sulpha drugs ➤ sulphonamides.

sulphabenzamide (in Sultrin) is a sulphonamide drug ➤ sulphonamides.

sulphacetamide ➤ sulfacetamide.

sulphadiazine ➤ sulfadiazine.

sulphadiazine, silver ➤ silver sulfadiazine.

sulphamethoxazole ➤ sulfamethoxazole.

sulphasalazine ➤ sulfasalazine.

sulphathiazole ➤ sulfathiazole.

sulphinpyrazone ➤ sulfinpyrazone.

sulphonamides are antibacterial drugs used principally to treat infections of the urinary tract (see Chapter 46). *Adverse effects* include nausea, vomiting and diarrhoea, allergic skin rashes, sensitivity of the skin to sunlight, and, very rarely, Stevens-Johnson syndrome (a disease causing severe inflammation of the skin and mucous membranes), contact dermatitis, systemic lupus erythematosis (SLE – a disease of unknown cause with symptoms of fever, muscle and joint pain, blood disorders and skin eruptions), kidney damage, blood disorders, and severe allergic reactions affecting blood vessels, the heart, liver and other tissues and organs, nerve damage and eye disorders. *Precautions:* Do not use in pregnancy, in infants under six months of age, in patients with impaired kidney or liver function, jaundice, blood disorders or patients sensitive to the sun's rays. They should be used with caution in the elderly and in breastfeeding mothers. Also ➤ co-trimoxazole.

sulphonylureas are oral anti-diabetic drugs. They are discussed in Chapter 42. *Adverse effects* are generally mild and infrequent. They include headache, hunger, and stomach and bowel upsets – nausea, vomiting, loss of appetite and diarrhoea. Allergic reactions may occur (usually in the first six–eight weeks of treatment) and include itching, nettle-rash and other rashes; rarely, dermatitis, fever and jaundice may occur. Sensitivity of the skin to sunlight (photosensitivity) has been reported with chlorpropamide. Very rarely, there may be damage to the bone marrow, producing blood disorders. Any of the sulphonylureas may cause a fall in blood glucose level (hypoglycaemia) four hours or more after eating. Most hypoglycaemic reactions to the sulphonylureas occur in people over fifty years of age, and are more likely to occur in anyone who has liver or kidney disease. Overdose or inadequate and irregular meals may trigger an attack. Elderly patients are particularly prone to develop hypoglycaemia with long-acting sulphonylureas such as chlorpropamide and glibenclamide and these should be replaced with gliclazide or tolbutamide which are shorter-acting. There is no evidence that any one sulphonylurea is better than all the others. Selection should therefore depend on age, the patient's kidney function and personal preference. *Precautions:* Sulphonylureas should be used with the utmost caution in elderly people. They should not be used in pregnancy, in breastfeeding mothers, in patients with severely impaired kidney or liver function or to treat insulin-dependent diabetes. Chlorpropamide causes nausea, flushing and palpitations if it is taken with alcohol. The attack comes on within twenty minutes of taking alcohol and lasts up to an hour. The individual may also feel light-headed and breathless. It is rare in insulin-dependent diabetics and in people without diabetes. It seems to be associated with non-insulin-dependent diabetes and may be an inherited characteristic. Some individuals may become allergic to sulphonylurea drugs; if this happens, a sulphonylurea drug should not be used in future. A sulphonylurea drug should not be used in patients suffering from diabetic ketoacidosis, whether they are in coma or not. This condition should be treated with insulin. The short-acting tolbutamide may be used in patients with impaired kidney function, as may gliclazide and gliquidone which are principally broken down in the liver. Insulin should be used temporarily in patients who develop an infection, suffer an injury, undergo surgery, have a heart attack or in pregnancy. Patients on sulphonylureas tend to gain weight and they should only be prescribed if poor sugar control and symptoms persist despite a strict antidiabetic diet. They should not be used in patients with porphyria (a hereditary disorder of metabolism). *Interactions:* Beta-blockers, corticotrophin, corticosteroids, MAOIs, diuretics, oral contraceptives, alcohol (only chlorpropamide), bezafibrate, clofibrate, oral anticoagulants, aspirin, phenylbutazone, cyclophosphamide, rifampicin, sulphonamides, chloramphenicol, glucagon.

sulphur is used as a mild antiseptic in skin applications.

sulpiride (Dolmatil, Sulparex, Sulpitil) is an antipsychotic drug ➤ antipsychotic drugs.

Sulpitil ➤ sulpiride.

Sultrin cream and vaginal tablets contain the sulphonamide drugs sulphathiazole, sulphacetamide and sulphabenzamide. They are used to treat bacterial infections of the vagina. *Adverse effects:* They may produce allergic reactions. The cream may damage latex condoms and diaphragms. *Precautions:* Do not use in pregnancy or in patients with kidney disease ➤ sulphonamides.

sumatriptan (Imigran) is used to treat acute migraine with or without an aura (see Chapter 34) and also to treat cluster headaches. It is a 5HT-like receptor stimulant which selectively constricts blood vessels inside the head including those that supply the covering of the brain (the dura mater). It is given by mouth or injection under the skin using a special device (auto-injector). *Adverse effects* include transient pain at the injection site, sensations of heat, heaviness, tingling, tightness in various parts of the body, flushing, dizziness, weakness, pins and needles and fatigue. A temporary rise in blood pressure or fall in blood pressure may occur and slowing of the heart rate, nausea, vomiting, convulsions and severe allergic reactions have been reported. Chest pain and tightness may be intense and involve the throat mimicking angina. The spasm of arteries that it produces may cause disorders of heart rhythm or a heart attack (myocardial infarction). If these symptoms occur the drug should be stopped and the patient should be checked to assess whether he/she has had a heart attack or a severe allergic reaction (anaphylaxis). *Precautions:* It should not be used in patients with coronary artery disease (e.g. angina) or who have (or have had) a heart attack (myocardial infarction), uncontrolled hypertension, or in patients with hemiplegic migraine (migraine producing weakness in an arm or leg). It should be used with caution in pregnancy, in breastfeeding mothers and in patients with impaired kidney or liver function. The dosage directions should be carefully followed. It should be used with caution in patients with epilepsy or brain lesions, allergy to sulphonamides and in patients with a history of misuse of other anti-migraine drugs. It should *not* be taken with any other anti-migraine drug, especially ergotamine. It should not be used within twenty-four hours of stopping an ergotamine-containing drug and such a drug should not be taken within six hours of stopping sumatriptan. Drowsiness may affect ability to drive. *Interactions:* MAOIs, 5HT re-uptake blockers, lithium, ergotamine.

sunblocks, see p. 237.

sun protection factor (SPF), see p. 237.

sunscreen and anti-sunburn skin preparations, see p. 237.

Supartz is used in the treatment of osteoarthritis of the knee and periarthritis of the shoulder ➤ sodium hyaluronate.

Suplasyn is used in the treatment of osteoarthritis of the knee ➤ sodium hyaluronate.

Supralip ➤ fenofibrate.

Suprane ➤ desflurane.

Suprax ➤ cefixime.

Suprecur nasal spray ➤ buserelin.

Suprefact ➤ buserelin.

suramin is used to treat the early stages of African trypanosomiasis (sleeping sickness) which is transmitted by tsetse flies. It is also used to treat onchocerciasis caused by infestation with onchocerca (filarial worms). It is given by slow intravenous infusion. *Adverse effects* include nausea, vomiting, abdominal pains, skin rash, itching and allergic reactions. Later adverse effects include severe skin rashes, nerve damage producing numbness and pins and needles of the palms and soles, watery eyes, discomfort on looking in the light (photo-

phobia) and very rarely blood disorders and damage to the adrenal glands. *Precautions:* A small test dose should be given before treatment starts because in some patients it can cause collapse. Use only under skilled medical supervision. Do not use in patients with impaired kidney function. The urine should be tested before each dose and treatment stopped if there are signs of kidney damage (e.g. protein and casts).

Surgam ➤ tiaprofenic acid.

surgical spirit contains methyl salicylate, diethyl phthalate and castor oil in industrial methylated spirits.

Surmontil ➤ trimipramine.

Survanta suspension ➤ beractant.

Suscard ➤ glyceryl trinitrate.

Sustac ➤ glyceryl trinitrate.

Sustanon injections contain three testosterone compounds formulated so that blood levels are maintained for a long period after injection ➤ testosterone.

Sustiva ➤ efavirenz.

suxamethonium (succinylcholine chloride, suxamenthonium bromide, suxamethonium chloride, Anectine, Scoline) is a depolarizing voluntary muscle relaxant used in anaesthesia. It mimics the action of acetylcholine (see Chapter 9). It has a five-minute duration of action and is used to allow the insertion of a breathing tube into the lungs ready for a general anaesthetic. *Adverse effects and Precautions:* It may cause muscle pain (particularly in patients who are up and about), slowing of the heart rate, irregularities of heart rhythm, fever and allergic reactions, a rise in temperature and a rise in blood potassium may very rarely cause arrest of the heart. Prolonged paralysis may occur in some patients due to a low level of the enzyme which breaks it down (see Chapter 9). This low level may occur in patients with impaired liver function and severe anaemia. The drug should not be used in such patients and it should not be used for eye surgery. It causes a rise in pressure in the eyes and should not be used in patients with glaucoma. Do not use in patients with high blood potassium, e.g. after major injury or major burns. It is important to read the manufacturer's guidelines on its use.

Symbicort is an inhaler combining a beta$_2$-stimulant (formoterol) and a corticosteroid (budesonide) for the treatment of asthma ➤ formoterol, budesonide.

Symmetrel ➤ amantadine.

sympathomimetic drugs are discussed in Chapter 9. *Adverse effects* include anxiety, restlessness, palpitations, rapid beating of the heart, tremors, weakness, dizziness, headache, coldness of the hands and feet and breathlessness. These harmful effects may occur in people particularly sensitive to adrenaline (e.g. anxious and tense, or with an over-active thyroid gland). Overdosing may produce disorders of heart rhythm, fluid on the lungs (pulmonary oedema) and brain haemorrhage. Local constriction of arteries may be so severe following an injection as to cause damage and death to the surrounding tissue. In people with arteriosclerosis (hardening of the arteries) or raised blood pressure, these drugs may occasionally trigger a brain haemorrhage. In anyone with coronary artery disease (e.g. angina), they may trigger an attack of angina or a heart attack. *Precautions:* Sympathomimetic drugs should not be used in anyone with closed-angle glaucoma, raised blood pressure, coronary artery disease or prostatic enlargement. *Interactions:* Adrenaline(epinephrine) and isoprenaline may cause disorders of heart rhythm if given with volatile liquid anaesthetics, and if given with tricyclic antidepressants they may cause a rise in blood pressure and disorders of heart rhythm (adrenaline(epinephrine) used in local anaesthetic injections appears safe); dangers of severe rise in blood pressure (see p. 19) if given with MAOIs or beta-blockers; increased risk of toxicity when isomethep-

tene or phenylpropanolamine is given with dopexamine. *Note:* Increased risk of a fall in blood potassium levels when salbutamol and related drugs are given with corticosteroids or potassium-loosing diuretics.

Synacthen and **Synacthen Depot** ➤ tetracosactrin.

Synagis ➤ palivizumab.

Synalar preparations ➤ fluocinolone.

Synalar C preparations contain fluocinolone (a corticosteroid) and clioquinol (an antibacterial/antifungal). They are used to treat infected eczema and dermatitis. *Adverse effects and Precautions:* See corticosteroid skin applications p. 241 and ➤ clioquinol.

Synalar N preparations contain fluocinolone (a corticosteroid) and neomycin (an aminoglycoside antibiotic). They are used to treat infected eczema and dermatitis. *Adverse effects and Precautions:* See corticosteroid skin applications p. 241 and ➤ aminoglycoside antibiotics.

Synarel ➤ nafarelin.

Syndol tablets contain the pain-relievers paracetamol and codeine, the antihistamine doxylamine and caffeine ➤ paracetamol, codeine, doxylamine.

Synercid is a combination of quinupristin and dalfopristin ➤ dalfopristin.

Synflex ➤ naproxen.

Synphase is a triphasic oral contraceptive. See p. 217.

Syntaris nasal spray ➤ flunisolide.

Syntocinon ➤ oxytocin.

Syntometrine contains ergometrine and oxytocin. It is used in the routine management of the third stage of labour ➤ ergometrine, oxytocin.

Syprol ➤ propanolol.

Syscor MR ➤ nisoldipine.

Sytron Elixir ➤ iron.

tacalcitol (Curatoderm) is related to calcitrol (vitamin D₃). It binds to vitamin D₃ receptors in the keratin-making cells of the skin and slows down their division. It is used as an ointment to treat psoriasis which is characterized by an overgrowth of keratin-making cells which form thickened, scaling plaques. *Adverse effects:* It may cause transient localized skin irritation, itching, redness, tingling and a burning sensation. *Precautions:* Do not use in patients with disorders of calcium metabolism. Use with caution in patients with impaired kidney function, who are at risk of developing a rise in their blood calcium levels or who have extensive, pustular or exfoliative (skin peeling) psoriasis, in pregnancy or in breastfeeding mothers. Use with caution when applying to face – avoid contact with eyes. Apply only to the lesions and wash hands thoroughly after application. Monitor blood calcium levels in patients with impaired kidney function. *Interactions:* Ultraviolet light.

tacalcitrol (Curatoderm) is used as an ointment to treat psoriasis. It is similar to vitamin D which inhibits cell proliferation and stimulates differentiation of keratinocytes correcting the abnormal cell turnover that characterises psoriasis. *Precautions:* Should not be used in patients with high calcium levels in the blood.

tacrolimus (Prograf) is an immunosuppressant drug. See Chapter 17. Unlike cyclosporin it is not dependent upon the presence of bile for its absorption from the intestine. It is used to prevent rejection in liver and kidney transplants and when other immunosuppressive drugs lose their effectiveness. *Adverse effects* include tremor, headache, raised blood pressure and blood sugar, impaired kidney function, risk of infection, disorders of the heart and circulation, blood disorders, nervous disorders (mood changes, agitation, dream and thinking abnormalities), eye disorders, chest disorders, diabetes and changes in blood potassium levels. *Precautions:* Do not use in pregnancy. Use non-hormonal contracep-

tion. Exclude pregnancy before starting treatment. Do not use in breastfeeding mothers. Do not use with cyclosporin. Do not use if patient has had an allergic reaction to a macrolide antibiotic e.g. azithromycin, erythromycin, clarithromycin, spiramycin.

Tagamet preparations ➤ cimetidine.

talc is used in dusting powders and skin applications. Prolonged and intense use may cause scarring of the lungs through inhalation. Contamination of wounds and body cavities may cause scar tissues to develop.

Tambocor ➤ flecainide.

Tamofen ➤ tamoxifen.

tamoxifen (Emblon, Fentamox, Nolvadex, Soltamox, Tamofen) is an anti-oestrogen (see Chapter 40). It is used to treat cancer of the breast with secondaries, and also to treat infertility due to failure to ovulate. *Adverse effects* include hot flushes, vaginal bleeding and discharge, itching vagina, loss of periods, stomach and bowel upsets, visual disturbances (stop the drug if this occurs), light-headedness and fluid retention. It may rarely cause hair loss, rashes, uterine fibroids, blood disorders and liver damage. *Precautions:* It should not be given in pregnancy or to breastfeeding mothers. High blood calcium levels and bone pain may occur in patients with secondary bone tumours treated with tamoxifen. Use with caution in pre-menopausal women with cystic ovarian swellings and in women with porphyria (a hereditary disorder of metabolism). There is an increased risk of blood clots when used with anti-cancer drugs. Women who develop vaginal bleeding or discharge and irregular periods should be examined to exclude a cancer of the lining of the womb, even though this risk is only slight. (Tamoxifen in a dose of 20 mg daily substantially increases survival in early breast cancer and these benefits far outweigh the small risk of cancer of the womb.) *Interactions:* Warfarin.

Tampovagan pessaries contain diethylstilboestrol (an oestrogen) and lactic acid. They are used to treat menopausal vaginitis ➤ diethylstilboestrol ➤ HRT.

tamsulosin (Flomax MR) is used to relieve symptoms caused by an enlarged prostate gland (benign prostatic hypertrophy, BPH). See p. 284. Tamsulosin specifically blocks certain adrenoreceptors in the prostate gland. This stops sympathetic stimulation and relaxes the muscles in the prostate and outlet from the bladder with the result that resistance to the outflow of urine is reduced and there is an improvement in passing urine. *Adverse effects* include dizziness, headache, weakness, palpitations and a fall in blood pressure on standing or sitting up after lying down (postural hypotension). It may affect ejaculation. *Precautions:* Do not use in patients with a severe impairment of liver function or who suffer from fainting when they stand to pass urine (micturition syncope). Use with caution in patients with a low blood pressure. *Interactions:* alpha adrenoreceptor blockers, diclofenac, warfarin.

Tanatril ➤ imidapril.

tar (in Gelcosal, in Gelcotar, in Polytar) is used as an anti-itching drug in skin applications. It is used to treat eczema and psoriasis ➤ coal tar.

Targocid ➤ teicoplanin.

Tarivid ➤ ofloxacin.

Tarka is used in the treatment of hypertension in patients stabilized on trandolapril and verapamil ➤ trandolapril, verapamil.

Tavanic ➤ levofloxacin.

Tavegil ➤ clemastine.

Taxol ➤ paclitaxel.

Taxotere ➤ docetaxel.

tazarotene (Zorac) is a retinoid used to treat mild to moderate plaque psoriasis. See Chapter 45. *Adverse effects* include skin irritation, skin peeling, rash, dermatitis. Stop using if irritation occurs. *Precautions:* Do not use in pregnancy (adequate contracep-

tion must be used during therapy) or while breastfeeding. Avoid skin folds, face, scalp, normal or inflamed skin, eyes and excess UV light.

tazobactam is a betalactamase blocker that inactivates the penicillinase produced by penicillin-resistant bacteria. It therefore enhances the effects of the penicillin (piperacillin) with which it is combined in Tazocin. *Adverse effects and Precautions* ➤ penicillins. Allergic reactions, stomach and bowel upsets, rashes, and superinfection may occur. Use with caution in pregnancy, in breastfeeding mothers or in patients with kidney failure or a low blood potassium level. *Interactions:* Anticoagulants, probenecid.

Tazocin preparations contain piperacillin and tazobactam ➤ tazobactam, penicillins. *Adverse effects* include stomach and bowel upsets, skin rashes, allergic reactions and rarely, a fall in the white blood cell count, kidney damage and a severe form of colitis (pseudomembranous colitis). *Precautions:* Use with caution in patients with kidney failure, with low blood potassium levels, in pregnancy and in breastfeeding mothers. *Interactions:* Probenecid, drugs affecting blood clotting, methotrexate, nondepolarizing muscle relaxants.

TCP pastilles ➤ phenols.

tears artificial ➤ artificial tears.

Tears Naturale contain dextran and hypromellose. It is used to treat tear deficiency. Do not wear soft contact lenses ➤ dextran, hypromellose.

Teejel applications contain choline salicylate (pain-reliever) and cetalkonium (antiseptic). Use to treat mouth ulcers and other painful lesions in the mouth. Do not use in children under four months of age ➤ choline salicylate, cetalkonium.

tegafur/uracil (Uftoral) is used to treat secondary cancer of the bowel in combination with calcium folinate. See Chapter 51. *Adverse effects* include stomach and bowel disorders, weakness, fever, headache, generally feeling unwell, chills, pain, fungal infections, dehydration, severe weakness and emaciation, bad taste in the mouth, watery eyes, conjunctivitis, swelling of the fingers and ankles, inflammation of veins or throat, difficulty breathing, hair loss, skin reactions. *Precautions:* Do not use in patients with severe liver damage, bone marrow suppression, liver CYP2A6 deficiency, in pregnancy or while breastfeeding. Use with caution in the elderly, in patients with kidney or liver damage, signs of bowel obstruction, inflammation of the liver or heart disease.

Tegretol ➤ carbamazepine.

teicoplanin (Targocid) is a glycopeptide antibiotic. See Chapter 46. *Adverse effects* include nausea, vomiting, diarrhoea, dizziness, headache, fever, skin rashes and wheezing. It may cause redness and swelling at the site of injection, serious allergic reactions (anaphylaxis), noises in the ears (tinnitus), mild hearing loss, vertigo, blood disorders and affect kidney and liver function. *Precautions:* Do not use in patients who are allergic to it or to vancomycin. Use with caution in the elderly (reduce the dose). Do not use in pregnancy or in breastfeeding mothers. Blood tests, hearing tests and tests of liver and kidney function should be carried out before and at regular intervals during treatment.

Telfast ➤ fexofenadine.

telmisartan (Micardis) is an angiotensin II receptor antagonist used to treat high blood pressure. See Chapter 25. *Adverse effects* include headache, upper respiratory tract infection, dizziness, pain, fatigue, stomach and bowel upset, fever, urinary tract infection. *Precautions:* Do not use in patients with biliary obstruction, severe liver or kidney damage, intolerence to fructose, in pregnancy or while breastfeeding. Use with caution in patients with kidney disorders, intravascular volume depletion, primary aldosteronism, narrowing of the aorta (main artery from the heart) or mitral valve,

hypertropic cardiomyopathy (enlargement of the muscles of the heart), high level of potassium in the blood, liver disease or ulcerated bowel.

temazepam (Normison) is a benzodiazepine drug ➤ benzodiazepines.

Temgesic preparations ➤ buprenorphine.

Temodal ➤ temozolomide.

temozolomide (Temodal) is used to treat malignant or benign tumours, showing recurrence or progression after standard therapy. See Chapter 51.

Tenben is a combination of the beta-blocker atenolol and the thiazide diuretic bendrofluazide used in the treatment of high blood pressure. See Chapter 25 and ➤ beta-blockers, thiazide diuretics.

Tenchlor ➤ co-tenidone.

tenecteplase (Metalyse) is an enzyme activator that helps dissolve the protein fibrin in thrombi (blood clots). It is used as a clot-buster in the early treatment of heart attack due to a coronary thrombosis. See Chapter 22. *Adverse effects* include severe bleeding, nausea, vomiting, allergic reactions. *Precautions:* Do not use in patients with bleeding disorders, severe high blood pressure which is not being treated, significant physical trauma within the last two months, severe inflammation of heart tissue, pancreas or liver damage, peptic ulcer, a history of stroke, heart attacks, dementia.

Tenif is used to treat angina (see Chapter 22) and raised blood pressure (see Chapter 25). It contains atenolol (a selective beta-blocker) and nifedipine (a calcium-channel blocker). *Adverse effects and Precautions* ➤ beta-blockers and nifedipine.

Tenkicin ➤ phenoxymethylpenicillin.

Tenkorex ➤ cefalexin.

Tenoret-50 tablets contain atenolol (a selective beta-blocker) and clortalidone (a thiazide diuretic). They are used to treat raised blood pressure. See Chapter 25.

Adverse effects and Precautions ➤ beta-blockers, thiazide diuretics.

Tenoretic tablets contain atenolol (a selective beta-blocker) and clortalidone (a thiazide diuretic). They are used to treat raised blood pressure. See Chapter 25. *Adverse effects and Precautions* ➤ beta-blockers, thiazide diuretics.

Tenormin ➤ atenolol.

tenoxicam (Mobiflex) is a non-steroidal anti-inflammatory drug (NSAID) ➤ non-steroidal anti-inflammotry drugs.

Tensipine MR ➤ nifedipine.

Tensium ➤ diazepam.

Tensopril ➤ captopril.

Teoptic eye drops contain carteolol, a beta-blocker used to treat glaucoma. See p. 62. *Adverse effects and Precautions:* ➤ beta-blockers. The eye drops may cause irritation, burning, pain and redness of the eyes. They may cause blurred vision and occasionally damage the surface of the cornea. Do not wear soft contact lenses.

terazosin (Hytrin) is used to treat raised blood pressure. It is a selective alpha-receptor blocker. See Chapter 25. *Adverse effects* include dizziness, headache, frequency of passing urine, lack of energy, ankle-swelling and a fall in blood pressure upon standing from a sitting or lying position (postural hypotension). *Precautions:* It should be used with caution in patients with impaired liver function and in patients with a history of fainting. The first dose may cause collapse due to a fall in blood pressure; therefore, take the first dose on retiring to bed. Lie flat if symptoms of low blood pressure occur e.g. faintness, dizziness, light-headedness, fatigue, sweating. Remain lying down until all symptoms have gone. Terazosin is also used to improve passing urine in patients with an enlarged prostate gland ➤ Hytrin BPH.

terbinafine (Lamisil) is an antifungal drug (see Chapter 47) taken by mouth or applied as a cream to treat fungal infections of the skin (e.g. ringworm). *Adverse effects* by mouth include nausea, loss of appetite, diarrhoea, headache, disturbances of taste and nettle-rash, occasionally painful muscles and joints and rarely, liver damage and jaundice. It may rarely cause very serious disorders affecting the skin (e.g. Stevens-Johnson syndrome). The drug should be stopped if a skin rash gets worse. It may sensitize the skin to the sun's rays. *Precautions:* It should be used with caution in patients with impaired kidney or liver function, in pregnancy and in breastfeeding mothers. *Interactions:* Cimetidine, rifampicin. *Skin applications* may cause redness, stinging, itching and rarely, allergic reactions.

terbutaline (terbutaline sulphate, Bricanyl, Bricanyl SA, Monovent) is a selective beta-stimulant sympathomimetic drug used to treat asthma. See Chapter 14. It is also used to treat uncomplicated premature labour. *Adverse effects and Precautions* are similar to those listed under salbutamol ➤ salbutamol.

terfenadine is a non-sedative antihistamine drug (see Chapter 17). *Adverse effects* ➤ antihistamines. They include headache, stomach and bowel upsets, hair loss, allergic reactions, palpitations, dizziness, rashes, visual disturbances, fatigue, wheezing and pins and needles. High doses may cause a serious disorder of heart rhythm (ventricular tachycardia). *Precautions* and *interactions:* Because of the risk of serious disorders of heart rhythm, do not exceed the recommended dose and do not use in patients with impaired liver function. Avoid using drugs that may cause the blood level of terfenadine to increase by affecting liver function (e.g. ketoconazole, itraconazole, other imidazole antifungal drugs, erythromycin and related drugs), at the same time as using terfenadine. Do not use if blood potassium is low and if the ECG shows a prolonged QT interval. Also avoid use of any drug that may help to trigger a disorder of heart rhythm e.g. anti-arrhythmic drugs, antipsychotic drugs, tricyclic antidepressant drugs and drugs likely to cause a fall in blood potassium levels or changes in other electrolytes, e.g. diuretics. If the person taking it faints, stop the drug and check for a disorder of heart rhythm. Do not give with astemizole or with grapefruit juice. Use with caution in pregnancy and in breastfeeding mothers ➤ antihistamines.

Teril CR ➤ carbamazepine.

terlipressin (in Glypressin) is a derivative of vasopressin which is used to treat distended veins (varices) in the oesophagus that are bleeding ➤ vasopressin.

Terra-Cortril ointment contains hydrocortisone (a corticosteroid) and oxytetracycline (a tetracycline antibiotic). It is used to treat infected eczema, insect bites and infected rash on skin folds (for no more than seven days). *Adverse effects and Precautions:* See corticosteroid skin applications p. 241 and ➤ tetracycline antibiotics.

Terra-Cortril Nystatin contains Terracortril with the anti-fungal drug nystatin ➤ Terra-cortril, nystatin.

Terramycin ➤ oxytetracycline.

Tertroxin ➤ liothyronine.

Testoderm ➤ testosterone.

testosterone (testosterone phenylpropionate, testosterone propionate, testosterone undecenoate, Andropatch, Primoteston Depot, Restandol, Sustanon, Testoderm, Virormone) is a male sex hormone (see Chapter 38). It is used to treat underdevelopment of the testes in males and to treat cancer of the breast in females. *Adverse effects* include increase in skeletal weight, salt and water retention, increased number of small blood vessels in the skin, raised blood calcium, increased bone growth, prolonged erections of the penis (priapism), stunting of growth, precocious sexual development in boys before puberty, prostate trouble in elderly men, and reduced sperm production. Prolonged use of high doses in women produces masculinization – excessive hairiness, deep voice, decrease in breast size, enlargement of the clitoris, increased libido and acne. *Precautions:* It should not be used in men with cancer of the breast, liver or prostate, in pregnancy, in breastfeeding mothers, in patients with a high blood calcium level or severe kidney disease. It should be used with caution in patients with impaired kidney, heart, liver function, raised blood pressure, epilepsy, migraine, in the elderly, in pre-pubertal boys, in patients with secondary cancer in bone (risk of a rise in blood calcium), and in patients with coronary artery disease. Intramuscular depot injections are preferred for replacement treatment in under-developed testicles.

Tetabulin is a tetanus immunoglobulin given by intramuscular injection.

tetrabenazine (Xenazine) reduces the concentration of dopamine in the brain and is used to treat movement disorders due to Huntington's chorea, senile chorea and related disorders. *Adverse effects* include drowsiness, stomach and bowel upsets, depression, fall in blood pressure and parkinsonism-like effects. *Precautions:* Do not use if breastfeeding and use with caution in pregnancy. May affect ability to drive.

tetracaine(amethocaine) (Ametop aqueous gel, in Eludril Spray, Minims amethocaine) is a local anaesthetic used in eye and skin preparations. It is more toxic than procaine by injection and cocaine by local application, but it is relatively safer because its local anaesthetic action is greater and it can, therefore, be used in smaller concentrations. It is rapidly absorbed and should not be applied to inflamed or injured surfaces.

tetracosactide (Synacthen, Synacthen Depot, tetracosactide) is a synthetic adrenal-stimulating hormone ➤ corticotrophin. It is structurally similar to natural corticotrophin, which is usually obtained from pigs and may produce allergic reactions. There are fewer allergic reactions with tetracosactide and it may be used in patients allergic to pig corticotrophin. It is occasionally used to treat rheumatoid arthritis, ulcerative colitis and Crohn's disease. *Adverse effects* see Chapter 37, Corticosteroids.

tetracosactrin ➤ tetracosactide.

tetracycline (tetracycline hydrochloride, Achromycin, in Deteclo, Economycin, Topicycline) is a tetracycline antibiotic ➤ tetracyclines.

tetracyclines are discussed in Chapter 46. *Adverse effects:* Nausea, vomiting and diarrhoea commonly occur, particularly if high doses are given by mouth. Very rarely, capsules and tablets of a tetracycline may irritate the oesophagus and produce ulceration, especially if they are swallowed with only a small sip of water. Thrush infections of the mouth, vagina and anus may occur and, rarely, a severe inflammation of the bowel (pseudomembranous colitis). Tetracyclines increase protein breakdown and may produce signs of kidney failure in patients with impaired kidney function (e.g. the elderly). Very rarely, severe liver and pancreatic damage may occur in pregnant women given a tetracycline intravenously to treat a kidney infection, and in patients with kidney failure who have been given high doses. Tetracyclines may damage the teeth of children (see Chapter 46), occasionally cause allergic reactions, sensitivity of the nails and skin to sunlight (especially demeclocycline) and blood disorders. Visual disturbances may occur and may be a sign that the blood pressure in the brain has increased (intracranial hypertension). Damage to the pancreas may occur occasionally. *Precautions:* Do not use in patients with impaired function of their kidneys. Tetracyclines are deposited in growing bones and teeth, causing staining of the teeth and occasionally underdevelopment of teeth and therefore they should not be given to children under twelve years of age, in pregnancy or to breastfeeding mothers. They should not be used in patients suffering from systemic lupus erythematosus (SLE – a disease of unknown cause with symptoms of fever, muscle and joint pain, blood disorders and skin eruptions). Do not use intravenously if liver function is impaired. Doxycycline and minocycline may be used in patients with impaired kidney function. Minocycline may cause dizziness and vertigo (especially in women), pigmentation of the skin, liver damage and very severe peeling skin rashes. Avoid doxycycline and oxytetracycline in patients with porphyria (a hereditary disorder of metabolism). *Interactions:* Milk, antacids, mineral supplements, oral contraceptives, penicillins, anticoagulants.

Tetralysal ➤ lymecycline.

Teveten ➤ eprosartan.

T/Gel shampoo ➤ coal tar.

Theo-Dur tablets ➤ theophylline.

theophylline (in Do-Do Chesteze, in Franol, in Franol Plus, Nuelin, Nuelin SA, Slo-Phyllin, Theo-Dur, Uniphyllin Continus) is a xanthine used to treat bronchial asthma (see Chapter 14). *Adverse effects* depend on the blood levels and include palpitations, nausea, vomiting, loss of appetite, rapid heart beat, insomnia, headache and stomach upsets. With very high blood levels severe adverse effects may occur – cramps, convulsions, and disorders of heart rhythm. *Precautions:* Use with caution in patients with fever, impaired liver function, raised blood pressure, epilepsy, heart disease, peptic ulcers, in pregnancy, in breastfeeding mothers, and in elderly patients. *Interactions:* When theophylline is given with beta$_2$-stimulant bronchodilators (see p. 68) the combination may cause an increased risk of adverse effects including a fall in blood potassium levels. Theophylline is broken down in the liver and this process can be slowed down (causing high blood levels) in patients with heart failure, cirrhosis of the liver, viral infections, and by cimetidine, ciprofloxacin, erythromycin and oral contraceptives. Breakdown of theophylline is speeded up in smokers, heavy drinkers and by phenytoin, carbamazepine, rifampicin and barbiturates. These differences in the rate of breakdown and therefore concentration of theophylline in the blood are important because there is a narrow margin of safety between an effective blood level and a toxic blood level.

thiamine (aneurine hydrochloride, thiamine hydrochloride, thiamine mononitrate, vitamin B, Benerva) is vitamin B$_1$. See Chapter 36.

thiazide diuretics are discussed in Chapter 29. *Adverse effects* include loss of appetite, stomach upsets, nausea, vomiting, diarrhoea, a fall in blood sodium, potassium and magnesium, dehydration, changes in the acidity of the blood, raised blood uric acid levels, raised blood sugar, and an increase in blood cholesterol levels. They may, rarely, cause a rise in blood calcium levels. Occasionally, thiazide diuretics may cause skin rashes, impotence, liver damage with jaundice, sensitivity of the skin to sunlight, muscle spasm, weakness, restlessness, blurred vision, allergic reactions, damage to blood vessels, damage to the pancreas and blood disorders. *Precautions:* Thiazide diuretics should not be used in people who suffer from severe liver or kidney impairment, Addison's disease (underworking of the adrenal glands), porphyria (a hereditary disorder of metabolism), from high blood calcium levels, persistently low blood sodium or potassium levels or raised blood uric acid levels causing symptoms, or in patients allergic to sulphonamides. They may cause a low blood potassium level and, because of their effects on increasing the blood sugar level, they may trigger diabetes in a susceptible person and may cause problems in the treatment of diabetes. Because of their effects on increasing blood uric acid levels, they may trigger an acute attack of gout in a susceptible individual. They may worsen an impairment of kidney or liver function and trigger liver coma in someone suffering from advanced cirrhosis of the liver. Potassium supplements should be given to anyone who is taking high and regular doses of thiazides and/or when the diet is low in potassium. (See p. 149.) Harmful effects of thiazide diuretics may be more frequent and severe in elderly people, especially if used in high doses and/or regularly every day for prolonged periods of time. Elderly people are particularly sensitive to changes in the body's water and salts; therefore regular tests of the chemistry of their blood should be carried out, with particular emphasis on blood sodium and potassium levels and glucose levels. These tests of blood chemistry should be carried out before treatment starts, after one month of treatment and then preferably every three–six months during treatment. Use with caution in patients with systemic lupus erythematosus (SLE – a disease of unknown cause with symptoms of fever, muscle and joint pain, blood disorders and skin eruptions). *Interactions:* Lithium, digoxin and related drugs, corticosteroids, carbenoxolone, tubocurarine, NSAIDs, anti-diabetic drugs, alcohol, barbiturates, opiates.

thioguanine ➤ tioguanine.

thiopental sodium is a fast-acting barbiturate which is used by intravenous injection as a general anaesthetic.

thiopentone ➤ thiopental sodium.

thioridazine (thioridazine hydrochloride, Melleril) is a phenothiazine antipsychotic drug ➤ antipsychotic drugs.

thiotepa is an anti-cancer drug. See Chapter 51. *Adverse effects* include nausea, vomiting, headache, fever, allergic reactions, loss of hair (alopecia), loss of periods (amenorrhoea) and reduced sperm production. It is very damaging to bone marrow, producing severe blood disorders. *Precautions:* See anti-cancer drugs, Chapter 51.

Throaties Family Cough Linctus is a cough expectorant containing ipecacuanha ➤ ipecacuanha.

thrombolytics, see p. 144.

thurfyl salicylate (in Transvasin) is a heat rub ➤ rubefacients.

thymol is obtained from the essential oil of the plant thyme. It is used as an antiseptic in mouthwashes, gargles and skin applications. It may irritate the skin and lining of the mouth and throat. It is included in Karvol capsules for vapour inhalation.

thymoxamine ➤ moxisylyte.

thyroid antagonists ➤ anti-thyroid drugs.

thyroid extract (dry thyroid) is powdered thyroid gland from domesticated animals used as food by man. Its use to treat under-working of the thyroid gland has been re-placed by thyroxine and liothyronine. See Chapter 43.

thyroid hormones, see Chapter 43.

thyroid-stimulating hormone ➤ thyro-trophin.

thyrotrophin (thyroid-stimulating hor-mone, TSH) is produced by the pituitary gland. It controls the release of thyroid hormones by the thyroid gland. See Chap-ter 43. It is controlled by thyrotrophin-releasing hormone from the hypothalamus which responds to the level of thyroid hor-mone in the bloodstream.

thyrotrophin-releasing hormone ➤ pro-tirelin.

thyroxine is one of the two thyroid hor-mones produced by the thyroid gland. The other thyroid hormone is tri-iodothyronine. Their production and secretion by the thy-roid is under the control of thyrotrophin produced by the pituitary gland. Thyroxine is used to treat underworking of the thyroid gland in the form of *levothyroxine sodium*.

thyroxine sodium ➤ levothyroxine sod-ium.

tiagabine (Gabitril) is used as additional therapy for partial seizures with or with-out secondary generalization which have not been controlled by optimal doses of at least one other anti-epileptic drug. See Chapyter 15. *Adverse effects* include dizzi-ness, tiredness, nervousness, tremor, diar-rhoea, difficulty in concentrating, depressed mood, fluctuations in emotions, slowness in speech. *Precautions:* Do not use in patients

with severe liver damage. Use with caution in patients with moderate kidney damage, a history of serious behavioural problems, in pregnancy or while breastfeeding.

tiaprofenic acid (Surgam) is a non-steroidal anti-inflammatory drug (NSAID) ➤ non-steroidal anti-inflammatory drugs.

tibolone (Livial) is used to treat hot flushes which may occur during the menopause. These hot flushes are caused by a reduction in female sex hormones (oestrogens and progesterone). They are usually treated with hormone replacement therapy (HRT). Tibolone is a gonadomimetic; it mimics the effects of sex hormones to produce weak oestrogenic, progestogenic and androgenic effects. Unlike HRT it appears not to affect significantly the lining of the womb or increase the risk of thrombosis. It is given continuously without having to take a pro-gestogen. See HRT. *Adverse effects* include headache, dizziness, stomach and bowel upsets, changes in bodyweight, vaginal bleeding, seborrhoeic dermatitis (excessive oily conditions on the skin), increased growth of hair on the face, migraine, visual disturbances, skin rashes, itching, swelling of the skin on the front of the legs (pretibial oedema) and changes in the results of liver function tests. *Precautions:* It should not be used in women with hormone-dependent cancers, undiagnosed vaginal bleeding, a history of coronary heart disease, stroke, thrombophlebitis or thrombotic disorders (blood clots and swelling in the veins), jaun-dice, severely impaired liver function, in pregnancy or in breastfeeding mothers. It should be used with caution in patients with impaired kidney function, epilepsy, mig-raine, diabetes, or raised blood cholesterol. The drug should be stopped immediately if signs of blood clots develop, if liver func-tion tests become abnormal, or if jaundice develops. A progestogen should be used to produce withdrawal bleeding before trans-ferring a woman from HRT on to tibolone. Irregular periods may occur if tibolone is started within twelve months of the last natural period. *Interactions:* Anticoagulants, phenytoin, carbamazepine, rifampicin.

ticarcillin (ticarcillin disodium, in Timentin) is an anti-pseudomonal penicillin antibiotic ➤ penicillins.

Ticlid ➤ ticlopidine.

ticlopidine (Ticlid) is an antiplatelet drug used to reduce the stickiness of platelets. It is used to prevent thrombosis in patients at risk of thromboembolism, especially following stroke. *Adverse effects* include a decrease in the number of white blood cells in the blood (neutropenia and agranulcytosis), bleeding disorders, diarrhoea, nausea, skin rashes. *Precautions:* Do not use in patients with a tendency to bleed, active peptic ulcer, stroke, prolonged bleeding or blood disorders. Use with caution in patients with liver or kidney disorders, in pregnancy or while breastfeeding.

Tiger Balm is a heat rub containing cajuput oil, camphor, clove oil, menthol, peppermint oil.

Tiger Balm Red Extra Strength is a heat rub containing cajuput oil, camphor, clove oil, menthol, peppermint oil and cinnamon oil ➤ rubefacients.

Tilade preparations ➤ nedocromil.

Tiloryth ➤ erythromycin.

Tildiem, Tildiem LA and **Tildiem Retard** preparations ➤ diltiazem.

tiludronic acid (Skelid) is used to treat Paget's disease of bone in which there is an increased dissolving of bone by special bone cells called osteoclasts. Tiludronic acid is a biophosphonate that blocks osteoclasts and stops the bones from dissolving. It produces fewer adverse effects on bone than other biophosphonates (e.g. bone softening, osteomalacia (adult rickets)). *Adverse effects* include stomach and bowel upsets and rarely headache, dizziness, weakness and skin rashes. *Precautions:* Do not use in patients with severe impairment of kidney function, juvenile Paget's disease, or in pregnancy. Use with caution in patients with mild or moderate impairment of kidney function or disorders of calcium metabolism. Ensure adequate intake of calcium in the diet and vitamin D. *Interactions:* Calcium-rich foods, calcium salts, antacids, indomethacin.

Timentin injections contain clavulanic acid (a betalactamase inhibitor) and ticarcillin (an anti-pseudomonal penicillin). It is used to treat severe infections in hospital patients who are immunodeficient. *Adverse effects and Precautions* ➤ penicillins. May cause stomach and bowel upsets, allergic reactions, liver damage and jaundice (which is possibly associated with the clavulanic acid). See also entry on co-amoxyclav. Use with utmost caution in patients with severely impaired liver function.

Timodine cream contains hydrocortisone (a corticosteroid), nystatin (an antifungal drug), benzalkonium (an antiseptic) and dimethicone (a water repellent). It is used to treat skin disorders (e.g. eczema) and nappy rash infected by thrush. *Adverse effects and Precautions:* See corticosteroid skin applications p. 241 and ➤ benzalkonium, nystatin.

timolol (Betim, in Cosopt, Moducren, in Prestim, Timoptol and Glaucol eye drops, Glau-opt) is a non-selective beta-receptor blocker ➤ beta-blockers.

Timoptol eye drops contain the beta blocker timolol (➤ timolol). They are used to treat glaucoma. See p. 62. *Adverse effects* include irritation of the eyes, flare-up of myasthenia gravis (muscle weakness due to neuromuscular abnormality) and general beta-blocker effects ➤ beta-blockers. *Precautions* ➤ beta-blockers. Do not wear soft contact lenses when using metered-dose preparations of timolol. Withdraw treatment gradually. Use with caution in pregnancy and in breastfeeding mothers.

Timonil Retard ➤ carbamazepine.

Timpron ➤ naproxen.

Tinaderm and **Tinaderm-M** cream contain the antifungal drugs tolnaftate and nystatin ➤ tolnaftate and nystatin. It is used to treat fungal infections of the skin and nails. See p. 243.

tinidazole (Fasigyn) is a nitroimidazole antibacterial drug similar to metronidazole. See p. 272. It is used to treat anaerobic bacterial infections. *Adverse effects and Precautions* ➤ metronidazole.

tinzaparin (Innohep) is a low molecular weight heparin (see Chapter 28) used to prevent blood clots in veins during surgery, especially orthopaedic surgery. It has a long duration of action and is given once daily under the skin (subcutaneous injection) for seven to ten days. *Adverse effects* include skin rashes, bruising and increased risk of bleeding, fall in blood platelets and changes in liver function tests. *Precautions:* Do not use in patients with bleeding tendencies, severe blood pressure, active peptic ulcer or septic endocarditis (infection of the lining membrane of the heart). Use with caution in patients with severely impaired kidney or liver function, asthma, in pregnancy and in breastfeeding mothers. *Interactions:* Anticoagulants, anti-platelet drugs.

tioconazole (Trosyl) is an imidazole antifungal drug (see Chapter 47) used to treat fungal infections of the nails. *Adverse effects* include mild irritation and allergic reactions where it is applied. *Precautions:* Do not use in patients allergic to the drug or to other related drugs (imidazoles). Do not use in pregnancy.

tioguanine (Lanvis) is an anti-cancer drug used in the treatment of acute leukaemia. See Chapter 51. *Adverse effects and precautions* are similar to those described under mercaptopurine.

tirofiban (Aggrastat) is used to prevent early heart attack in patients with unstable angina or non-Q-wave heart attack It should be used with aspirin and unfractionated heparin. See Chapter 28. *Adverse effects* include excessive internal and external bleeding, decrease in platelet counts, nausea, fever, headache, rash. *Precautions:* Do not use in patients with a history of stroke or bleeding within the last thirty days, a history of brain disease, severe high blood pressure, trauma or surgery within last six weeks, blood disorders, severe liver failure, in pregnancy or while breastfeeding. Use with caution in patients with severe kidney failure, mild liver damage, a recent organ biopsy, severe trauma or major surgery, active peptic ulcer, untreated high blood pressure, blood or heart disorders, female, elderly or underweight patients.

Tisept antiseptic solution contains chlorhexidine and cetrimide ➤ chlorhexidine, cetrimide.

titanium (titanium dioxide) is a white pigment used as a skin protective and also as a sunscreen agent. It is included in some face powders and cosmetics.

Titralac tablets contain calcium carbonate and glycine. They are used as a calcium supplement ➤ calcium supplements.

Tixycolds is a cough medicine ➤ diphenhydramine, pseudoephedrine.

Tixylix preparations are cough medicines. **Tixylix Catarrh** contains diphenhydramine and menthol; **Tixylix Chesty Cough** contains guaifenesin; **Tixylix Cough and Cold** contains chlorphenamine, pholcodeine and pseudoephedrine; **Tixylix Daytime** contains pholcodeine; **Tixylix Night-time** contains pholcodeine and promethazine ➤ individual entry for each drug.

Tixymol ➤ paracetamol.

tizanidine (Zanaflex) is a central alpha$_2$ stimulant (see p. 130) used to treat extreme muscle tension associated with multiple sclerosis, spinal cord injury or disease. *Adverse effects* include drowsiness, fatigue, dizziness, dry mouth, stomach and bowel upset, low blood pressure, insomnia, slow heart beat, hallucinations, raised liver enzymes, liver damage. *Precautions:* Do not use in patients with liver damage. Use with caution in patients with kidney damage, in pregnancy or while breastfeeding.

Tobi ➤ tobramycin.

Tobradex eye drops are used to prevent infection and reduce inflammation following cataract surgery. They contain tobramycin (an antibiotic) and dexamethasone (a corticosteroid) ➤ tobramycin, dexamethasone.

tobramycin (Nebcin, Tobi, Tobradex) is an aminoglycoside antibiotic ➤ aminoglycoside antibiotics. Tobradex eye drops may cause stinging in the eyes.

tocopherols ➤ vitamin E, Chapter 36.

Tocopheryl ➤ vitamin E, Chapter 36.

Tofranil ➤ imipramine.

tolbutamide is a sulphonylurea oral antidiabetic drug ➤ sulphonylureas.

tolfenamic acid (Clotam Rapid) is a non-steroidal anti-inflammatory drug (NSAID) used to treat migraine. See Chapter 34. *Adverse effects* include stomach and bowel upset, skin reactions and a burning sensation on passing water. *Precautions:* Do not use in patients with active peptic ulcer, allergy to aspirin or other NSAIDs, liver or kidney impairment or in the third trimester of pregnancy.

tolnaftate (Tinaderm-M preparations) is an antifungal drug. See p. 243. It is used in applications to treat athlete's foot and other fungal infections of the skin. It may, very rarely, cause an allergic reaction.

tolterodine (Detrusitol) is an antimuscarinic drug used to treat unstable bladder conditions with symptoms of urgency, frequency or urge incontinence. See Chapter 49. *Adverse effects* include dry mouth, stomach and bowel upset, headache, xerophthalmia (a dry and thickened condition of the conjunctiva), dry skin, drowsiness, nervousness, abnormal sensations such as tingling, burning or tightness. *Precautions:* Do not use in patients with urinary retention, uncontrolled narrow angle glau-

coma, myasthenia gravis (muscle weakness due to neuromuscular abnormality), severe ulcerative colitis (active bowel ulcer), distension of the bowel, in pregnancy or while breastfeeding. Use with caution in patients with an obstruction of the bladder outlet, stomach or bowel obstruction, kidney or liver damage, autonomic neuropathy (damage to the nerves of the autonomic nervous system) or hiatus hernia.

Tomudex ➤ raltitrexed.

tonics, see Chapter 7.

Topal tablets contain dried aluminium hydroxide, light magnesium carbonate and alginic acid ➤ antacids, alginic acid.

Topamax ➤ topiramate.

topical antirheumatic (non-steroidal anti-inflammatory drug (NSAID)) applications are used to treat sprains, strains, rheumatic aches and pains, muscle aches and neuralgia. See p. 164. Preparations are applied as creams, gels or sprays and the active NSAID penetrates through the skin to relieve pain and inflammation in the affected tissue. *Adverse effects:* They may cause irritation where they are applied and occasionally itching, dermatitis and sensitivity of the treated skin to the sun's rays (photosensitivity). Rarely, sufficient of the drug may be absorbed into the bloodstream to cause general adverse effects such as asthma, allergy and kidney damage (➤ non-steroidal anti-inflammatory drugs). *Precautions:* Avoid contact with eyes, lips, mouth or broken or inflamed skin. Do not use under non-permeable dressings. Do not use large amounts and do not apply to large areas of skin because of the risk of absorption producing adverse effects. Do not use in pregnancy or in breastfeeding mothers. Avoid extensive exposure of the area of skin that has been treated to the sun because of the risk of photosensitivity. Do not use in children. Wash hands immediately after application. Do not use in individuals allergic to aspirin or an NSAID. Do not take an

NSAID by mouth at the same time as using an NSAID topical anti-rheumatic.

Topicycline solution ➤ tetracycline. It is used to treat acne. See p. 250. *Adverse effects* include stinging and burning. *Precautions:* Avoid contact with eyes and mouth. Use with caution in pregnancy, breastfeeding mothers and patients with impaired kidney function.

topiramate (Topamax) is an anti-epileptic drug. See Chapter 15. *Adverse effects* include confusion, dizziness, fatigue, impaired concentration, ataxia (loss of control over voluntary movements), pins and needles, sleepiness, emotional upsets, depression and rarely, kidney stones and loss of weight. *Precautions:* Do not use in breastfeeding mothers. Use with caution in patients with impaired kidney function, those at risk of developing kidney stones (drink plenty of fluids) and pregnancy. Stop drug gradually, not suddenly. *Interactions:* Phenytoin, carbamazepine, digoxin, oral contraceptives, drugs that may cause kidney stones.

topotecan (Hycamtin) is an anti-cancer drug used to treat secondary cancer of the ovaries where other therapies have failed. See Chapter 51. *Adverse effects* include damage to the bone marrow producing blood disorders, hair loss, nausea, vomiting, diarrhoea, constipation, sore mouth and gums, abdominal pains, fatigue and weakness. *Precautions:* Do not use in patients with severe myelosuppression (suppression of blood cell production), in pregnancy or in breastfeeding mothers. Use with caution in patients with kidney or liver damage. Monitor red blood cell, white blood cell and platelet counts. Do not give if white cell count or platelet count are low.

Toradol injections ➤ ketorolac.

torasemide (Torem) is a loop diuretic (see Chapter 29) used to treat congestive heart failure (see Chapter 23) and fluid retention caused by liver or kidney disease, fluid on the lungs and raised blood pressure. *Adverse effects and Precautions* are similar to those listed under furosemide(frusemide) ➤ furosemide.

Torem ➤ torasemide.

toremifene (Fareston) is an anti-oestrogen drug (see p. 198) used to treat oestrogen-dependent secondaries from cancers of the breast in post-menopausal women. *Adverse effects* include hot flushes, nausea, sweating, dizziness, fluid retention, vomiting and white vaginal discharge. *Precautions:* Do not use in pregnancy, in breastfeeding mothers, in women with severe liver failure or with overgrowth of the lining of the womb (pre-existing endometrial hyperplasia). Use with caution in women with impaired liver function, untreated heart failure, severe angina, secondary bone deposits, severe thrombotic disease, diabetes. *Interactions:* Thiazide diuretics, phenobarbitone, phenytoin, carbamazepine, anticoagulants, ketoconazole, erythromycin, troleandomycin.

Totaretic ➤ co-tenidone.

TPA ➤ alteplase.

Tracrium ➤ atracurium.

Tractocile ➤ atosiban.

tramadol (Dromadol SR, Tramake, Zamadol, Zamadol SR, Zydol, Zydol SR, Zydol XL) is an opiate-related drug used to relieve moderate to severe pain. See Chapter 30. *Adverse effects* include nausea, vomiting, dry mouth, dizziness, drowsiness, fatigue, rash, confusion, headache, mood changes, and hallucinations. Rarely it may cause heart and breathing problems, blood disorders, drug dependence and convulsions. *Precautions:* Do not use in pregnancy or breastfeeding mothers. Use with caution in the elderly, in patients with impaired liver or kidney function, head injury, raised pressure in the skull, depressed breathing or previous history of convulsions. *Interactions:* Alcohol, sleeping drugs, sedatives or other drugs that depress brain function, MAOIs and carbamazepine.

Tramake ➤ tramadol.

tramazoline (in Dexa-Rhinaspray) is a sympathomimetic drug (see Chapter 9) used as a nasal decongestant. It is similar to naphazoline.

Trandate ➤ labetalol.

trandolapril (Gopten, Odrik, in Tarka) is an ACE inhibitor used to treat raised blood pressure. See Chapter 25. It is also used to treat dysfunction of the left ventricle of the heart after a heart attack. See Chapter 22. To avoid the risk of the blood pressure falling, diuretic drugs should be stopped before starting trandolapril. *Adverse effects* include dizziness, headache, weakness, fall in blood pressure, rash, cough, palpitations and rarely allergic reactions (e.g. angioedema) and blood disorders. *Precautions:* Do not use if patient has had an allergic reaction (e.g. angioedema) to another ACE inhibitor. Do not use in pregnancy, breastfeeding mothers or in patients with outflow obstruction from the heart (e.g. aortic stenosis). Use with caution in patients with impaired kidney or liver function, on kidney dialysis or with congestive heart failure. Kidney function should be checked before and at regular intervals during treatment. Use with caution in patients whose blood volume or blood salt is decreased. *Interactions:* Potassium-sparing diuretics, NSAIDs, potassium supplements, lithium, anti-diabetic drugs, antidepressants, antipsychotics and andrenergic blockers.

tranexamic acid (Cykolkapron) is an anti-fibrinolytic drug (see Chapter 28) used to treat bleeding as a result of overdose with fibrinolytic drugs (drugs that dissolve blood clots). It is also used to treat heavy menstrual periods (menorrhagia), nosebleeds and bleeding from dental extractions in haemophiliacs. *Adverse effects:* It may cause nausea, vomiting and diarrhoea. The blood pressure may fall (causing giddiness) if intravenous injections are given too rapidly. It may cause disturbance of colour vision (stop the drug if this occurs). *Precautions:* Do not use in patients with thromboembolic disease (see Chapter 28). Use with caution if kidney function is impaired or the patient has blood in the urine particularly from haemophilia. Patients on long-term treatment (patients with hereditary angioedema) should have regular eye check-ups and tests of liver function.

tranquillizers ➤ anti-anxiety drugs.

tranquillizers, major ➤ antipsychotic drugs.

tranquillizers, minor ➤ anti-anxiety drugs.

Transiderm-Nitro patches ➤ glyceryl trinitrate.

Transvasin Cream contains ethyl nicotinate, hexyl nicotinate, thurfyl salicylate and benzocaine ➤ rubefacients.

Tranxene ➤ clorazepate potassium.

tranylcypromine (tranylcypromine sulphate, Parnate) is an MAOI antidepressant drug. See Chapter 4. Unlike other drugs of this group, its effects persist for only about two–three days after withdrawal. *Adverse effects and Precautions* are similar to those listed under phenelzine ➤ phenelzine and see entry on MAOIs in Chapter 4. It may cause insomnia if given in the evening. Episodes of a rise in blood pressure with throbbing headaches occur more frequently than with phenelzine. Liver damage occurs less frequently than with phenelzine.

Trasicor ➤ oxprenolol.

Trasidrex tablets contain oxprenolol (a non-selective beta-blocker) and cyclopenthiazide (a thiazide diuretic). They are used to treat raised blood pressure. See Chapter 25. *Adverse effects and Precautions* ➤ beta-blockers and thiazide diuretics.

trastuzumab (Herceptin) is used to treat secondary breast cancer either on its own following two or more chemotherapy regimens or as first line treatment in combination with paclitaxel in patients for whom anthracyclines are unsuitable. See Chapter 51. *Adverse effects* include abdominal, chest, back, musculoskeletal and neck pain, flu-like syndrome, headache, stomach and bowel upset, skin reactions, infection, generally feeling unwell, mastitis, allergic reactions, weight loss, heart or lung problems, liver tenderness or damage, dry mouth, disorders of the blood. *Precautions:* Do not use in patients with an allergy to murine proteins, with laboured breathing or who are breastfeeding. Use with caution in patients with heart disorders, coronary artery disease, a history of high blood pressure or in pregnancy.

Trasylol ➤ aprotinin.

Travasept 100 antiseptic solution contains chlorhexidine and cetrimide ➤ chlorhexidine and cetrimide.

Traxam clear gel contains the non-steroidal anti-inflammatory drug felbinac, used to treat sprains and strains ➤ topical antirheumatic applications.

trazodone (trazodone hydrochloride, Molipaxin) is an antidepressant drug. See Chapter 4. *Adverse effects* include nausea, vomiting, constipation, diarrhoea, loss of weight, dry mouth, tremor, weakness, changes in the heart rate, fall in blood pressure on standing up after sitting or lying (postural hypotension), headaches, drowsiness, blurred vision, restlessness, dizziness, insomnia, confusion and skin rash. It may produce a persistent erection of the penis (priapism), blood disorders and liver damage. *Precautions:* It should be used with utmost caution in patients who drive motor vehicles or operate moving machinery. It should be used with caution in patients with impaired function of kidneys or liver, or with epilepsy. *Interactions:* Muscle relaxants, anaesthetic gases, alcohol, sleeping drugs, sedatives, anti-anxiety drugs and other drugs that depress brain function, MAOIs, clonidine, digoxin, phenytoin.

Trental ➤ pentoxifylline.

treosulfan (Treosulfan) is an anti-cancer drug. See Chapter 51. *Adverse effects* include depression of bone-marrow function producing blood disorders, abdominal pain, nausea and vomiting, skin rashes and loss of hair (alopecia). Stomatitis may occur if patients chew the capsules. *Precautions:* See anti-cancer drugs, Chapter 51.

tretinoin (Acticin, in Aknemycin Plus, Retin-A, Retinova, in Vesanoid) is a derivative of vitamin A which causes the top layer of skin to peel off more quickly. It is used to treat acne (see p. 250) and to remove creases from the skin. *Adverse effects* include stinging, a feeling of warmth on the skin, increased sensitivity of the skin to sunlight and increased or decreased pigmentation of the skin. Excessive use may cause redness (erythema) at the site of application. *Precautions:* Avoid contact with eyes and lining of the nose and mouth. Do not use in patients with eczema or on damaged skin. Avoid excessive exposure to sunlight; patients who have got sunburned should not apply tretinoin until the sunburn has healed. Do not use in pregnancy or in patients with a personal or family history of skin cancer. *Interactions:* Avoid use of any other skin application that may cause peeling or irritation of the skin, e.g. benzoyl peroxide, and do not use a UVL lamp.

TRH thyrotrophin-releasing hormone ➤ protirelin.

Tri-Adcortyl preparations contain triamcinolone (a corticosteroid), nystatin (an antifungal drug) and gramicidin (an antibiotic). They are used to treat infected eczema and other infected, inflamed skin disorders. *Adverse effects and Precautions:* See corticosteroid skin applications p. 241 and ➤ nystatin, gramicidin.

triadcortyl-otic ➤ triamcinolone.

Triadene is a triphasic oral contraceptive. See p. 217.

TriamaxCo ➤ co-triamterzide.

triamcinolone is a corticosteroid (see Chapter 37, Corticosteroids). It is used as **triamcinolone acetonide** in injections (Kenalog). Injections are also used locally to treat inflamed joints or tendons (Adcortyl). Triamcinolone acetonide is included in Adcortyl cream and ointment to treat eczema and psoriasis (*Adverse effects and Precautions*, see corticosteroid skin applications p. 241). It is also included with antibiotics in Audicort, Aureocort and Tri-Adcortyl and with antifungal drugs in Nystadermal. Adcortyl in Orabase is used to treat mouth ulcers. See entry on each product. It is used as a nasal spray (Nasocort) for the treatment of hayfever and allergic rhinitis. See Chapter 17. *Adverse effects* include nose bleed, nasal irritation, swelling of the throat and headache. *Precautions:* Use with caution when transferring patients from systemic steroids, in patients with untreated nasal infection, in pregnancy or while breastfeeding.

Triam-Co tablets ➤ co-triamterzide.

triamterene (in co-triamterzide in Dyazide, Dytac, in Dytide, in Frusene, in Kalspare, in Triamax Co, in Triam-Co) is a potassium-sparing diuretic (see Chapter 29). *Adverse effects:* It may cause nausea, vomiting, diarrhoea, headache, fall in blood pressure, dry mouth, skin rashes, dizziness, cramps, blood disorders. Loss of calcium in the urine, raised blood potassium levels and reversible kidney failure (very rare) may occur. *Precautions:* Do not use in patients with raised blood potassium, progressive kidney or liver failure or Addison's disease (underworking of the adrenal glands). Use with caution in patients with impaired kidney or liver function, gout or acidosis. Use with the utmost caution in pregnancy, in breastfeeding mothers, in the elderly and in patients with diabetic kidney disease. It may cause fluorescent blue coloration of the urine. Blood potassium levels and kidney function should be measured before treatment starts and at regular intervals during treatment. *Interactions:* Potassium supplements, potassium-sparing diuretics, anti-blood pressure drugs, indometacin, ACE inhibitors.

Triapin ➤ ramipril.

tribavirin ➤ ribavirin.

triclofos is used as a sleeping drug. See Chapter 1. It has effects similar to those described under dichloralphenazone. *Adverse effects, Precautions and Drug dependence:* These are similar to those described under dichloralphenazone. Headache and skin rashes may occur and triclofos may increase the effects of alcohol.

triclosan (Aquasept, Manusept, in Oilatum Plus, Ster-Zac Bath Concentrate) has antiseptic properties and is used in surgical scrubs, soaps, deodorants and skin applications. Very rarely, it may cause contact dermatitis. Avoid contact with the eyes.

tricyclic antidepressants are discussed in Chapter 4. *Adverse effects* of tricyclic antidepressant drugs vary between different patients. They also vary in frequency and in type. Some harmful effects are directly related to the dose and some are related to how a particular individual reacts. Some harmful effects may be more likely to occur, or to occur with greater intensity, according to what other disorders the patient is suffering from. It is important, therefore, that treatment is tailored to each individual's particular needs and responses. Not all of the following harmful effects have been reported with every tricyclic antidepressant drug, but they have been reported with one or more of them and should always be borne in mind whenever these drugs are used. They include dry mouth, blurred vision, constipation, difficulty in passing urine, weariness, weakness, fatigue, lack of energy, confusion, inability to concentrate, disorientation, dizziness, restlessness, drowsiness, nervousness, insomnia, nightmares, numbness, and pins and needles in the hands and feet, tremors, noises in the ears, parkinsonism-like effects, changes in weight, sweating, allergic skin reactions, fall in blood pressure on standing up after lying or sitting down (may produce dizziness and faintness), rapid beating of the heart, palpitations, disorders of heart rhythm, heart attacks, convulsions, strokes, allergic skin rashes (e.g. nettle-rash), sensitivity of the skin to sunlight, angioedema (allergic reactions), nausea, stomach upsets, vomiting, loss of appetite, a peculiar taste in the mouth, diarrhoea and black tongue. Very rarely, tricyclic antidepressant drugs may damage the bone marrow, producing blood disorders; they may damage the liver, producing jaundice. Other reported effects include swelling of the testicles and breasts in men; breast enlargement and leakage of milk in women; increased or decreased sexual drive (libido), impotence, changes in blood sugar levels, loss of hair (alopecia) and changes in weight. Some patients may become manic, and symptoms of schizophrenia may be triggered, especially in elderly people. Tricyclic antidepressants that produce *sedation* include amitriptyline, dothiepin, doxepin and trimipramine; those that produce *little sedation* include amoxapine, butriptyline, clomipramine, desipramine, imipramine, lofepramine and nortriptyline. Those that produce *stimulation* include protriptyline. All tricyclic antidepressants cause some anticholinergic effects (e.g. dry mouth, difficulty in passing urine, blurred vision, constipation) and harmful effects on the heart; however, lofepramine appears to produce fewer of these effects than others. Some tricyclic antidepressants are particularly associated with certain harmful effects. For example, *amitriptyline* is associated with serious disorders of heart rhythm and may be a factor in the sudden death of patients with heart disease. *Amoxapine* may cause tardive dyskinesia (➤ antipsychotic drugs), irregular periods, breast enlargement and milk production in women. *Doxepin* should not be used in breastfeeding mothers. *Lofepramine* may cause liver damage and should not be used in patients with impaired liver function or severe impairment of kidney function. *Protriptyline* causes more anxiety, agitation, rapid beating of the heart and fall in blood pressure than the others. It also causes sensitivity of the skin to the sun's rays causing a rash. Do not go in the direct sunlight. Also there is an increased risk of adverse effects on the heart in elderly patients. *Trimipramine* causes marked antimuscarinic effects (dry mouth, blurred

vision, constipation) and numbness and pins and needles in the hands and feet. Neuroleptic malignant syndrome (for symptoms see p. 331) may occur very rarely in patients on tricyclic antidepressants. *Precautions:* Do not use in patients allergic to tricyclics, who have had a recent heart attack (myocardial infarction), who suffer from a disorder of heart rhythm, coronary artery disease or severe liver disease. Do not use in the manic phase of mental illness and and do not use in pregnancy. They should be used with caution in people with mild or moderate impairment of liver function, diabetes, heart disease, history of epilepsy, in breastfeeding mothers, in patients with thyroid disease, a history of mania, schizophrenia, closed-angle glaucoma, difficulty passing urine (e.g. due to an enlarged prostate gland), porphyria (a hereditary disorder of metabolism), raised blood pressure, tumours of the adrenal medulla, epilepsy, constipation, kidney disease, or in anyone at risk of committing suicide. Adverse effects of tricyclic antidepressants may be more frequent and severe in elderly people; in particular they can affect the heart and circulation, and cause difficulty in passing urine, they may trigger glaucoma and affect the brain, producing confusion, restlessness and drowsiness. Their effects on lowering the blood pressure may be harmful in elderly people, causing faintness and light-headedness on standing up after sitting or lying down. They should therefore be used with caution and in lower doses than normal. Tricyclic antidepressants affect the function of the brain; therefore do not drive or operate machinery until you know how the particular drug affects you. Liver function tests and heart tests should be carried out at regular intervals in patients on long-term treatment. *Interactions:* Alcohol, sleeping drugs, sedatives, carbamazepine, phenytoin, antipsychotic drugs, barbiturates, other antidepressants, antimuscarinic drugs, local anaesthetics containing adrenaline(epinephrine) or noradrenaline (norepinephrine), cimetidine, quinidine, oestrogens, anti-blood pressure drugs. They should not be used with, or within fourteen days of taking, a MAOI (a high temperature, convulsions and deaths have occurred from some such combinations); with clomipramine, imipramine, or desipramine there should be a delay of twenty-one days.

Tridestra preparations contain oestradiol (an oestrogen) and medroxyprogesterone (a progesterone). They are used as HRT ➤ HRT.

trientine (trientine hydrochloride) is a copper chelating agent used to treat Wilson's disease which is a progressive disease that runs in families. It is a disorder of metabolism that causes copper to accumulate in the body with damaging effects on the brain and liver. It may cause iron deficiency and therefore iron treatment should be given at the same time. *Adverse effects* include nausea. *Precautions:* It should be used only to treat patients with Wilson's disease who are intolerant to penicillamine. It should not be used to treat rheumatoid arthritis or cystinurea (➤ penicillamine). Use with caution in pregnancy. Penicillamine-induced systemic lupus erythematosus (SLE – a disease of unknown cause with symptoms of fever, muscle and joint pain, blood disorders and skin eruptions) may not clear up on treatment with trientine.

trifluoperazine (trifluoperazine hydrochloride, in Parstelin, Stelazine) is a phenothiazine antipsychotic drug ➤ antipsychotic drugs. It is also used to treat nausea and vomiting. See Chapter 18.

Trifyba is a bulk laxative containing concentrated extract of wheat husk. See Chapter 21.

triglycerides, omega 3 ➤ Maxepa.

trihexyphenidyl(benzhexol) (benzhexol hydrochloride, Broflex) is an antimuscarinic drug. It is used to treat parkinsonism and drug-induced parkinsonism. See Chapter 16. *Adverse effects* include dizziness, dryness of the mouth, nausea, vomiting, blurred vision, retention of urine, rapid heartbeat, skin rashes and nervousness. High doses may cause mental confusion, excitement and psychiatric disturbances. These symptoms are dose-related and disappear when the dose is reduced. *Precautions:* Benzhexol should not be used in patients suffering from closed-angle glaucoma, obstruction of the bowel or untreated retention of urine. It should be used with caution in patients with an enlarged prostate, heart disease or impaired kidney or liver function. It should be withdrawn slowly. It may affect driving skills and patients may abuse its use. *Interactions:* Phenothiazines, antihistamines, tricyclic antidepressants. Also ➤ antimuscarinic drugs.

tri-iodothyronine (L tri-iodothyronine, T_3) is the natural form of one of the two main thyroid hormones. See Chapter 43. The other one is thyroxine. It is also known as *liothyronine sodium*. It has a higher potency and more rapid onset of action than thyroxine and is used when a rapid response is required.

Trileptal ➤ oxcarbazepine.

Trilostane (Modrenal) stops the synthesis of both mineralocorticoids and glucocorticoids by the adrenal glands. See Chapter 37. It is used to treat over-active adrenal glands (Cushing's disease) and primary hyperaldosteronism. It may be used to treat breast cancer in post-menopausal women who have relapsed following the use of anti-oestrogens. Corticosteroids will also be needed in these patients. *Adverse effects* include flushing, nausea, diarrhoea, runny nose, tingling and swelling in the mouth, vomiting, rashes and a fall in white blood cell count. *Precautions:* Do not use in pregnancy (use a mechanical form of contraception but not the pill), in breastfeeding mothers, in patients with severe impairment of liver or kidney function or with a tumour of the pituitary gland producing ACTH (see p. 186). Use with caution in patients with mild to moderate impairment of kidney or liver function. The blood levels of corticosteroids and electrolytes should be carefully monitored. *Interactions:* Aldosterone antagonists, amiloride, triampterine, potassium supplements.

trimeprazine ➤ alimemazine.

trimetaphan is a ganglion blocking drug which causes a fall in blood pressure (see Chapter 25). It is used to keep the blood pressure low during surgical procedures. *Adverse effects* include rapid beating of the heart, dilatation of the pupils, depression of breathing, rise in pressure in the eyes and constipation. *Precautions:* Do not use in patients with severe hardening of the arteries (arteriosclerosis), severe heart disease, pyloric stenosis (obstruction to the outlet from the stomach) or in pregnancy. Use with caution in patients with impaired kidney or liver function, diabetes, Addison's disease (underworking of the adrenal glands), cerebral or coronary artery disease or degenerative disorders of the brain.

trimethoprim (in Chemotrim, in cotrimoxazole, in Fectrim, Ipral, Monotrim, in Polytrim, in Septrin, Trimopan) is an antibacterial drug. It is often given combined with the sulphonamide sulphamethoxazole. This combination is known as cotrimoxazole. See p. 273. *Adverse effects:* Nausea, vomiting and diarrhoea, itching and rashes. When used over a prolonged period it may produce anaemia because it interferes with the body's use of folic acid, which is essential for the manufacture of red blood cells. *Precautions:* It should not be given to patients with a severe impairment of kidney function. Do not use in pregnancy or in breastfeeding mothers, in newborn babies or in patients with blood disorders. It should be given with caution to patients with impaired kidney function, folic acid deficiency, patients suffering from porphyria (a hereditary disorder of metabolism) and elderly patients. When it is used over a prolonged period, blood tests for anaemia should be carried out at regular intervals. *Interactions:* Cyclosporin, rifampicin, phenytoin, digoxin, immunosuppressants.

trimetrexate (Neutrexin) is used with folinic acid to treat moderate to severe *Pneumocystis carinii* pneumonia in patients suffering from AIDS which has not responded to standard treatment. Trimetrexate kills cells by blocking the production of an enzyme that requires folic acid for its production – it is an anti-folate drug. Folinic acid enters the cells of the body to provide a source of folic acid and protects the cells from being killed by trimetrexate. However, it cannot enter the *Pneumocystis carnii* organisms and so does not protect them from being killed by the anti-folate effects of trimetrexate. *Adverse effects* include vomiting, diarrhoea, skin rashes, confusion, itching at the site of injection and fever. It may cause blood disorders and liver and kidney damage. *Precautions:* Do not use in patients allergic to the drug. Do not use without folinic acid (given as its calcium salt: calcium folinate), therefore do not use in patients allergic to folinic acid. Do not use in pregnancy or in breastfeeding mothers. Females of childbearing potential and males should take contraceptive precautions during and for six months after stopping treatment. Use with utmost caution in patients with blood disorders, impaired liver or kidney function or with any drug that may also damage the liver or kidneys or cause blood disorders. Blood counts and tests of liver and kidney function should be carried out before treatment and twice weekly during treatment. *Warning:* Trimetrexate must be used with folinic acid (as calcium folinate) to avoid potentially serious and life-threatening damage to bone marrow, liver and kidneys, ulceration of the mouth, stomach and intestine. Folinic acid (as calcium folinate) must be given during treatment with trimetrexate and continued for seventy-two hours after the last dose. *Interactions:* Any drug that may cause blood disorders, kidney or liver damage ➤ folinic acid.

Tri-Minulet is a triphasic oral contraceptive. See p. 217.

trimipramine (trimipramine maleate, Surmontil) is a tricyclic antidepressant drug ➤ tricyclic antidepressants.

Trimopan ➤ trimethoprim.

Trimovate cream contains clobetasone (a corticosteroid), nystan (an antifungal drug) and oxytetracycline (a tetracycline antibiotic). It is used to treat infected eczema and other infected, inflamed skin disorders. *Adverse effects and Precautions:* See corticosteroid skin applications p. 241 and ➤ nystatin, tetracyclines.

Trinordiol is a triphasic oral contraceptive. See p. 217.

TriNovum is a triphasic oral contraceptive. See p. 217.

tripotassium dicitratobismuthate (bismuth citrate) ➤ DeNoltab.

triprolidine (triprolidine hydrochloride, in Actifed, in Sudafed Plus) is an antihistamine drug ➤ antihistamines.

Triptafen and **Triptafen-M** contain amitriptyline (a tricyclic antidepressant) and perphenazine (a phenothiazine antipsychotic drug). They are used to treat depression with anxiety. *Adverse effects and Precautions* ➤ tricyclic antidepressants, antipsychotic drugs.

triptorelin (Decapeptyl SR) is a gonadotrophin releasing hormone analogue (➤ gonadorelin). It is used to treat advanced cancer of the prostate gland that is dependent on male sex hormones for growth ➤ leuprorelin. *Adverse effects* include swelling in the vein, dry mouth, stomach pain, a temporary rise in blood pressure, recurrence of asthma, fever, itching, sweating, pins and needles, insomnia, excessive salivation, difficulty passing urine, vertigo, slight hair loss, and pain, redness and swelling at the site of injection. *Precautions:* Do not use in patients with compression of their spinal cord or with secondary cancer of the spine. Symptoms caused by secondaries from advanced cancer of the prostate may flare up at the start of treatment due to the rise in male sex hormone levels, therefore use an anti-androgen for three days before treatment starts and for two to three weeks into treatment with triptorelin. Monitor patients at risk of kidney stones and spinal compression carefully for first month of treatment.

Trisequens are different coloured tablets containing different doses of oestriol and oestradiol (natural oestrogens) and norethisterone (a progestogen). They are used as HRT ➤ HRT.

trisodium edetate (Limclair) is used by injection to treat high blood calcium levels and also to remove calcium deposits in the cornea. It is also used to treat disorders of heart rhythm caused by digoxin. *Adverse effects* include nausea, diarrhoea and cramps; overdose may produce kidney damage. *Precautions:* It should be used with caution in patients suffering from tuberculosis. Repeated measurements of blood calcium level should be carried out during treatment. It should not be used in patients with impaired kidney function.

Tritace ➤ ramipril.

Trizivir contains three antiviral agents, abacavir, lamivudine and zidovudine ➤ abacavir, lamivudine, zidovudine.

Tropergen ➤ co-phenotrope.

tropicamide eye drops (Minims tropicamide, Mydriacyl) are used to dilate the pupils. See p. 61. Tropicamide is an antimuscarinic drug (➤ antimuscarinic drugs). The drops may cause stinging as they are applied. They should not be used in closed-angle glaucoma. In infants, pressure should be applied on the tear-producing sac for one minute after applying the drops.

tropisetron (Navoban) is a 5HT3 blocker used to treat nausea and vomiting caused by anti-cancer drugs. See Chapter 18. *Adverse effects* include dizziness, headache, fatigue, allergic reactions, nettle-rash, tightness of the chest, wheezing, flushing of the face, constipation and stomach and bowel upsets. *Precautions:* Do not use in pregnancy or in breastfeeding mothers or in children. Use with caution in patients with raised blood pressure that has not been controlled by drugs. Dizziness and drowsiness may affect ability to drive.

Tropium ➤ chlordiazepoxide.

trospium chloride (Regurin) is used to treat urinary frequency, urgency and urge incontinence. See Chapter 49. *Adverse effects* include dry mouth and constipation. *Precautions:* Do not use in patients with urinary retention, glaucoma, rapid heart beat not being controlled by drugs, myasthenia gravis (muscle weakness due to neuromuscular abnormality), severe ulcerative colitis, megacolon (distension of the bowel), liver or kidney damage or in patients undergoing dialysis. Use with caution in patients with obstruction of the stomach or bowel, obstructed urinary outflow, disorders of the autonomic nervous system, hiatus hernia or hyperthyroidism.

Trosyl nail solution ➤ tioconazole.

Trusopt eyedrops ➤ dorzolamide.

tryptophan (Optimax) is an amino acid that is an essential constituent of the diet. It is used by the body to manufacture a neurotransmitter in the brain called *serotonin* or *5hydroxytryptamine* (5HT). This transmitter is involved in our mood and in giving pleasant feelings of satisfaction after eating a meal. A fall in the serotonin level in the brain is associated with depression and tryptophan was a popular antidepressant, especially when taken with pyridoxine (vitamin B_6) and ascorbic acid (vitamin C) which are involved in the metabolism of tryptophan. Unfortunately the use of tryptophan to treat depression was associated with dangerous side-effects (eosinophilia-myalgia syndrome (EMS – fever, skin rashes, painful muscles, fluid retention and damage to the lungs and nervous system)) and it was withdrawn from the market. It has recently been reintroduced under strict hospital supervision. See Chapter 4. *Adverse effects* include drowsiness, nausea, headache, light-headedness and EMS. *Precautions:* Do not use in patients who suffered oesinophilia-myalgia due to taking tryptophan in the past. Monitor blood counts for an increase in oesinophils and check for any muscle symptoms. Stop immediately if symptoms of EMS develop. Use with caution in pregnancy and in breastfeeding mothers, in patients with impaired kidney or liver function, and in the elderly. Patients and prescribing doctors must register with the Optimax Information and Clinical Support (OPTICS) Unit. *Interactions:* 5HT re-uptake blockers, MAOIs, phenothiazine antipsychotic drugs, benzodiazepines.

Tuinal capsules contain equal quantities of the barbiturates quinalbarbital and amylobarbital. *Adverse effects and Precautions* ➤ phenobarbital sodium.

tulobuterol (Respacal) is a selective beta$_2$ adrenoreceptor stimulant used to treat asthma and other reversible airways disease. See Chapter 14. It is taken by mouth and each dose produces effects for up to six hours. *Adverse effects* include tremor, palpitations, rapid beating of the heart and mild tension. It may cause a potentially serious fall in the blood potassium level. *Precautions:* It should not be used in patients with moderate to severe impairment of kidney function, acute liver failure, or chronic liver diseases. It should be used with caution in patients with diabetes, raised blood pressure, over-active thyroid gland, heart disease or epilepsy. For other adverse effects and precautions ➤ salbutamol.

Tums is an antacid ➤ calcium.

Turbohaler dry powder inhaler ➤ terbutaline.

Twinrix is a vaccine against hepatitis A and hepatitis B which is given by intramuscular injection.

Tylex pain-relieving preparations contain paracetamol and codeine ➤ paracetamol, codeine.

Typherix is a vaccine against typhoid which is given by intramuscular injection.

Typhim VI is a vaccine against typhoid which is given by intramuscular injection.

tyrothricin is an antibiotic used in skin applications and throat lozenges (e.g. in Tyrozets).

Tyrozets throat lozenges contain tyrothricin (an antibiotic) and benzocaine (a local anaesthetic). They are used to treat mild mouth and throat infections. *Adverse effects* include superinfection and blackening or soreness of the tongue.

Ubretid ➤ distigmine.

Ucerax ➤ hydroxyzine.

Ucine ➤ sulfasalazine.

Uftoral ➤ tegafur.

ulcer-healing drugs, see Chapter 19.

Ultec ➤ cimetidine.

Ultiva ➤ remipentanil.

Ultrabase skin softening cream contains white soft paraffin, liquid paraffin and stearyl alcohol ➤ liquid paraffin and white soft paraffin.

Ultralanum preparations ➤ fluocortolone.

Ultramol is a pain reliever containing paracetamol, codeine and caffeine ➤ paracetamol, codeine.

Ultraproct preparations contain cinchocaine (a local anaesthetic) and fluocortolone (a corticosteroid). They are used for the short-term relief of symptoms of haemorrhoids, itching of the anus and vagina. *Adverse effects and Precautions:* See Chapter 37 on Corticosteroids. Do not use in patients with a fungal, viral or tuberculous infection. Use with caution in pregnancy and avoid prolonged use.

undecenoic acid (undecylenic acid, in Ceanel) is an antifungal drug used in skin applications. See p. 243.

undecenoic acid esters are antifungal and are included in Monphytol paint, which is used to treat athlete's foot. See p. 243.

Unguentum cream contains silicic acid, liquid and white soft paraffin, cetostearyl alcohol, polysorbate-40, glyceryl monostearate, saturated neutral oils, sorbic acid, propylene glycol, sodium hydroxide and purified water. It is used to soften the skin (see p. 236) to treat dermatitis, nappy rash and dry, scaly skin.

Uniflu with Gregovite C comprises a composite pack of pairs of tablets: Uniflu lilac tablets contain caffeine, codeine, diphenhydramine, paracetamol and phenylephrine; Gregovite C yellow tablets contain ascorbic acid (vitamin C). They are used to relieve symptoms in colds and coughs. *Adverse effects and Precautions* ➤ each constituent drug and see Chapter 10.

Uniphyllin Continus tablets ➤ theophylline.

Uniroid-HC ointment and suppositories contain cinchocaine (local anaesthetic) and hydrocortisone (a corticosteroid). They are used for the short-term relief of symptoms caused by haemorrhoids and itching of the anus. *Adverse effects and Precautions* ➤ cinchocaine and see Chapter 37 on Corticosteroids. Do not use in patients with a fungal, viral or tuberculous infection. Avoid prolonged use and use with caution in pregnancy.

Unisept antiseptic solution ➤ chlorhexidine.

Univer ➤ verapamil.

Uprima ➤ apomorphine.

Urdox ➤ ursodexycholic acid.

urea (carbamide, in Alphaderm, Aquadrate, Balneum Plus cream, in Calmurid, in Calmurid HC, Euceris, Nutraplus) is used in skin creams as a skin softener and to improve the penetration of a drug (e.g. hydrocortisone) into the skin. It is also included in ear drops used for dissolving wax (e.g. in Exterol, in Otex).

urea hydrogen peroxide is a compound chemical of urea combined with hydrogen peroxide. It is present in Exterol and Otex ear drops used to remove ear wax. See p. 57. *Adverse effects:* It may effervesce in the ear canal. Stop if it causes irritation of the lining. *Precautions:* Do not use in patients with a perforated ear drum.

Uriben ➤ nalidixic acid.

uricosuric drugs, see Chapter 33.

Uriflex C catheter solution ➤ chlorhexidine.

Urispas ➤ flavoxate.

urofollitrophin ➤ urofollitropin.

urofollitropin (Metrodin High Purity) is an extract of urine from post-menopausal women containing follicle stimulating hormone (FSH). It is given by injection to treat infertile women whose pituitary gland is not functioning effectively or who have not responded to clomiphene. It is also used in IVF treatment to stimulate the ovaries to produce eggs for fertilization and used in males to stimulate sperm production. *Adverse effects:* Ovarian hyperstimulation (➤ Humegon), multiple pregnancies and allergic reactions (may also occur in males). *Precautions:* Do not use in men who suffer from a testicular or pituitary tumour or in women who suffer from an ovarian tumour or pituitary tumour ➤ gonadotrophins.

Uromitexan ➤ mesna.

Uro-Tainer Saline catheter solution contains sodium chloride. **Uro-Tainer Chlorhexidine** solution contains chlorhexidine. **Uro-Tainer Mandelic acid** contains mandelic acid. **Uro-Tainer Suby G** contains citric acid, light magnesium oxide, sodium bicarbonate and disodium edetate. **Uro-Tainer Solution R** contains citric acid, gluconolactone, light magnesium carbonate, and disodium edetate. **Uro-Tainer M** contains sodium chloride. These sterile preparations are used to prevent and reduce infection caused by catheters inserted in the bladder.

ursodeoxycholic acid (Destolit, Urdox, Ursofalk, Ursogal) is used to dissolve cholesterol gallstones. See p. 102. *Adverse effects and Precautions* ➤ chenodeoxycholic acid. Diarrhoea occurs less frequently than with chenodeoxycholic acid and liver damage has not been reported. It may be used (as Ursofalk) to treat primary biliary cirrhosis (a slowly developing liver disease that causes swelling and blockage of the internal bile ducts in the liver). It slows the progression of the disease and reduces fatigue and itching.

Ursofalk ➤ ursodeoxycholic acid.

Ursogal ➤ ursodeoxycholic acid.

uterine relaxants (myometrial relaxants) ➤ beta$_2$-adrenoreceptor stimulants.

uterine stimulants are used to induce abortion or help labour and to minimize the loss of blood from the site of placenta (afterbirth). They include oxytocin, ergometrine and prostaglandins (Chapter 52).

Utinor ➤ norfloxacin.

Utovlan ➤ norethisterone.

vaccines ➤ Chapter 53.

Vagifem pessaries contain oestradiol. They are used to treat shrinkage of the vagina due to oestrogen deficiency in post-menopausal women. They may rarely cause slight vaginal bleeding, vaginal discharge and skin rash ➤ oestrogens ➤ HRT.

Vaginyl ➤ metronidazole.

Vagisil cream contains a local anaesthetic ➤ lidocaine(lignocaine).

valaciclovir (Valtrex) is an antiviral drug. See Chapter 48. It is a pro-drug of acyclovir. It is taken as tablets to treat initial and recurrent genital herpes, shingles (herpes zoster) and herpes simplex of the skin and lining of the mouth and nose. *Adverse effects and Precautions* ➤ aciclovir. It may cause nausea and headache. Use with caution in pregnancy, in breastfeeding mothers and in patients with impaired kidney function.

Valclair suppositories ➤ diazepam.

Valda ➤ menthol, thymol.

Valium ➤ diazepam.

Vallergan ➤ alimemazine.

Valoid ➤ cyclizine.

valproate ➤ sodium valproate.

valproic acid (Convulex, Depakote) is an anti-epileptic drug. See Chapter 15. *Adverse effects* include blood clotting, stomach and bowel upsets and liver damage. *Precautions:* Do not use in patients with impaired liver function. Use with caution in pregnancy. Carry out liver function tests and blood coagulation tests before starting treatment and at two-monthly intervals. Also repeat tests before increasing the dose. *Interactions:* Barbiturates, antidepressant drugs, antipsychotic drugs, alcohol, anticoagulants, other anti-epileptic drugs.

valsartan (Diovan) is a specific angiotensin II receptor blocker used to treat raised blood pressure. See Chapter 25. *Adverse effects* include fatigue, decrease in certain kinds of white blood cells, high levels of creatinine and bilirubin. *Precautions:* Do not use in pregnancy, in patients with severe impairment of liver function, cirrhosis of the liver or obstruction to the bile ducts. Use with caution in patients with mild to moderate impairment of liver function, moderate to severe impairment of kidney function, narrowing of a main artery to a kidney (renal stenosis), low blood sodium level, low blood volume or while breastfeeding. Monitor potassium levels in elderly patients and in patients with impaired kidney function if they are taking potassium supplements.

Valtrex ➤ valaciclovir.

Vancocin preparations ➤ vancomycin.

vancomycin (vancomycin hydrochloride, Vancocin) is an antibiotic (see p. 272). It is given by injection to treat serious infections caused by bacteria resistant to other antibiotics and given orally to treat inflammation of the bowel caused by antibiotics. *Adverse effects:* Infusions may cause flushing and severe allergic reactions. Leakage into the surrounding tissues at the site of injection can cause pain and tissue damage. The drug may cause nausea, chills, fever and skin rashes and large doses or prolonged treatment may cause irreversible deafness, particularly in patients with impaired kidney function. *Precautions:* It should be used with caution in patients with impaired kidney function, previous hearing loss, in the elderly and in pregnancy. Regular tests of the level of the drug in the blood, hearing tests and tests of kidney function should be carried out. *Interactions:* There is an increased risk of damage to hearing and to the kidneys if given with aminoglycoside antibiotics or capreomycin and increased risk of damage to hearing if given with loop diuretics.

Vaqta injection is a hepatitis A vaccine which is given by intramuscular injection.

Varidase powder contains streptokinase and streptodornase. It is used to clean dead skin and debris off wounds ➤ streptokinase, streptodornase. Do not use if the wound is bleeding. It may also be used to dissolve clots in the bladder and in urinary catheters. It may cause burning sensations.

Vascace ➤ cilazapril.

Vaseline Dermacare cream contains dimethicone and white soft paraffin. The **lotion** contains dimethicone, liquid paraffin and white soft paraffin. It is used to moisturize the skin (see p. 236) to treat dry skin and eczema ➤ liquid paraffin, dimethicone.

vasoconstrictors are used to constrict blood vessels in order to decrease the blood flow and increase the blood pressure. They are mainly sympathomimetic drugs (see p. 38). They are used as nasal decongestants (see p. 47), to prolong the duration of action of local anaesthetics (see p. 231) and to treat heart failure (see p. 123).

vasodilators are drugs that dilate blood vessels and increase the flow of blood. They are used to treat angina (see Chapter 22), to lower raised blood pressure (see Chapter

25) and to improve the circulation (see Chapter 27).

Vasogen is a barrier cream used to treat nappy rash, pressure sores and is also used in ileostomy and colostomy care. It contains dimeticone, calamine, zinc oxide ➤ individual entry for each drug.

vasopressin (anti-diuretic hormone, ADH) is a hormone produced by the posterior lobe of the pituitary gland that works on the kidneys to increase the reabsorption of water from the urine back into the bloodstream. It helps to control the water content of the body. Vasopressin (Pitressin injections) is used to treat diabetes insipidus, which is a disease characterized by excessive drinking of water and the passing of a large volume of urine. It is caused by any disorder of the nerve tracks supplying the posterior lobe of the pituitary gland. Other vasopressin-related drugs used to treat diabetes insipidus include lypressin (Syntopressin nasal spray) and desmopressin (DDAVP nasal drops and injections, Desmospray nasal spray). Terlipressin (Glypressin injections) is a vasopressin derivative that is used for its constricting effects on blood vessels to treat bleeding from distended veins (varices) in the oesophagus. *Adverse effects* produced by vasopressin include pallor, nausea, abdominal cramps, bleeding, a desire to have the bowels opened, allergic reactions, and constriction of arteries which may cause anginal attacks in patients with coronary artery disease. *Precautions:* Do not use in patients with diseases of the arteries, especially coronary artery disease or in patients with chronic kidney disease (chronic nephritis) until kidney tests have been carried out and show reasonable kidney function. Use with caution in patients with asthma, heart failure or epilepsy, or migraine or any other disorder that could be made worse by water retention. Use with caution in pregnancy and avoid overloading the body with fluid. Nasal applications may cause congestion of the nose and injections may cause itching, lumps and redness at the site of injection. *Interactions:* Indomethacin, tri-cyclic antidepressants, chlorpromazine, carbamazepine. *Adverse effects and Precautions* of desmopressin, lypressin and terlipressin ➤ entry under each drug. *Warning:* Vasopressin may cause convulsions due to a fall in blood sodium levels. Children and adults taking vasopressin (Desmospray, Desmotabs or DDAVP) for bedwetting (see p. 283) should not drink excessive amounts of fluids. If patient develops diarrhoea or vomiting the drug should be stopped temporarily. Do not give tricyclic antidepressants with vasopressin. These drugs promote secretion of vasopressin and therefore increase the risk of developing a fall in blood sodium levels.

Vasoxine ➤ methoxamine.

Vectavir ➤ penciclovir.

vecuronium bromide (Norcuron) is a non-depolarizing muscle-relaxant (see p. 42) used during surgical operations. It has a short to medium duration of action.

Veganin pain-relieving tablets contain aspirin, paracetamol and codeine ➤ individual entry for each drug.

Velbe ➤ vinblastine.

Velosef ➤ cephradine.

venlafaxine (Efexor) is a 5HT/noradrenaline(norepinephrine) re-uptake blocker used to treat depression. See Chapter 4. *Adverse effects* include nausea, flushing, headache, dizziness, weakness, sweating, sleepiness, agitation, nervousness, pins and needles, insomnia, loss of appetite, nausea, constipation, indigestion, abdominal pains, anxiety, tremor, impotence, visual disturbances, dry mouth, chills, changes in blood pressure and changes in liver function tests, skin rashes, and convulsions (stop drug if these occur). *Precautions:* Do not use in pregnancy, breastfeeding mothers or in patients with severe impairment of liver or kidney function. Use with caution in patients with mild or moderate impaired kidney or liver function, a history of epilepsy, drug abuse or heart attacks. Blood pressure should be checked at regular intervals when high doses are used. If the drug has been taken for one month or more it should be stopped slowly by reducing the dose daily over a period of at least one week. *Interactions:* MAOIs, stimulant drugs.

Venofer is an iron injection ➤ iron.

Venos for Dry Coughs, **Venos Expectorant** and **Venos Honey and Lemon** all contain guaifensin ➤ guaifensin.

Ventmax SR ➤ salbutamol.

Ventide inhalations contain salbutamol (a selective beta₂ stimulant) and beclometasone (a corticosteroid). They are used to treat asthma. See Chapter 14. *Adverse effects and Precautions* ➤ salbutamol and see Chapter 37 on corticosteroids. Inhalation of corticosteroids may cause a hoarse voice and thrush of the mouth and throat.

Ventodisks ➤ salbutamol.

Ventolin preparations ➤ salbutamol.

Vepesid ➤ etoposide.

Veracur gel ➤ formaldehyde.

verapamil (verapamil hydrochloride, Cordilox, Ethimil SR, Securon, in Tarka, Univer, Verapress MR, Vertab SR, Zolvera) is a calcium-channel blocker. It is used to treat angina (see Chapter 22), raised blood pressure (see Chapter 25), migraine (see Chapter 34) and disorders of heart rhythm (see Chapter 24). *Adverse effects* include nausea, vomiting, constipation, headache, impairment of liver function, flushing, dizziness, fatigue, ankle-swelling and allergic reactions. After intravenous injection it may cause a drop in blood pressure, slowing of the heart rate and transient heart block if injected rapidly. *Precautions:* It should not be used in acute heart disorders, severe heart block, severe slowing of the heart rate, in certain types of disordered heart rhythm or in patients with porphyria (a hereditary disorder of metabolism). It should be used with caution in patients with low blood pressure, slow heart rate, partial heart block,

impaired liver or kidney function, in the early stages of an acute heart attack (especially if the patient has a slow heart rate), in pregnancy or in breastfeeding mothers. Verapamil should not be injected into patients recently treated with a beta-blocker because of the risk of a severe fall in blood pressure and the heart stopping (asystole). Avoid giving verapamil and a beta-blocker together by mouth unless there is no evidence of heart disease. *Interactions:* Beta-blockers (see above), quinidine, digoxin.

Verapress MR ➤ verapamil.

Vermox ➤ mebendazole.

Verrugon preparations contain salicylic acid and glycerol. They are used to treat plantar warts. See p. 262. *Adverse effects and Precautions* ➤ salicylic acid. Do not use on facial or anogenital warts. Avoid contact with healthy skin.

Vertab SR ➤ verapamil.

vertoporfin (Visudyne) is used to treat subfoveal choroidal neovascularization (a condition where blood vessels form abnormally on the retina) due to age-related loss of clear central vision (macular degeneration) or following on from short-sightedness caused by disease (pathological myopia). *Adverse effects* include visual disturbances (including blurred vision, flashing lights, visual-field defects), nausea, back pain, weakness, itching, excess cholesterol in the blood. *Precautions:* Do not use in patients with porphyria (a hereditary disorder of metabolism), sensitivity to the sun, liver damage, biliary obstruction, in pregnancy or while breastfeeding.

Vesanoid ➤ tretinoin.

Vexol ➤ rimexolone.

Viagra ➤ sildenafil.

Viatim is a combined vaccine against typhoid fever and hepatitis A.

Viazem XL ➤ diltiazem.

Vibramycin preparations ➤ doxycycline.

Vicks Medinight contains paracetamol, dextromethorphan, doxylamine and ephedrine; **Vicks Sinex** contains xylometazoline; **Vicks Ultra Chloraseptic** contains benzocaine ➤ each constituent drug.

Videne preparations ➤ povidone-iodine.

Videx ➤ didanosine.

vigabatrin (Sabril) is an anti-epileptic drug. See Chapter 15. *Adverse effects* include fatigue, dizziness, drowsiness, nervousness, irritability, depression and headache. Children may become excited and agitated. Patients with myoclonic seizures may develop an increased frequency of attacks. *Precautions:* Do not use in pregnancy or in breastfeeding mothers. Use with caution in patients with impaired kidney function and in elderly people. Patients should be carefully monitored. The drug should be withdrawn slowly over a period of two–four weeks. Use with caution in patients with a history of psychosis, behaviour disorders or brain or nerve disorders. *Interactions:* Phenytoin.

Vigam S ➤ human normal immunoglobulin. See p. 302.

Vigranon B is a complex of vitamin B in liquid form. It contains the B vitamins thiamine, riboflavin, nicotinamide, pyridoxine and panthenol.

vinblastine (vinblastine sulphate, Velbe) is used as an anti-cancer drug. See Chapter 51. *Adverse effects* include nausea, vomiting, diarrhoea, mood changes, loss of hair (alopecia) and nerve damage. It damages bone marrow, producing blood disorders. Injections may be painful and can produce itching, swelling and redness at the site. *Precautions:* See Chapter 51 on anti-cancer drugs.

vinca alkaloids are obtained from the periwinkle plant (Vinca rosea). They are used as anti-cancer drugs. See Chapter 51.

vincristine (vincristine sulphate, Oncovin) is used as an anti-cancer drug. See Chapter 51. *Adverse effects* include nausea, vomiting, constipation, mood changes, loss of hair (alopecia) and nerve damage. It damages bone marrow, producing blood disorders. Injections may be painful and can produce itching, swelling and redness at the site. *Precautions:* See Chapter 51 on anti-cancer drugs.

vindesine (Eldisine) is an anti-cancer drug. See Chapter 51. *Adverse effects* include difficulty in swallowing, loss of appetite, nausea, vomiting, constipation, skin rashes, loss of hair (alopecia), blood disorders, generally feeling unwell, fever, chills, and nerve damage. *Precautions:* See anti-cancer drugs, Chapter 51.

vinorelbine (Navelbine) is used on its own or in combination with other drugs for first line treatment of stage 3 or 4 non-small cell lung cancer. It is also used to treat stage 3 or 4 advanced breast cancer which has relapsed or does not respond to treatment with anthracycline. See Chapter 51. *Adverse effects* include decrease in certain kinds of white blood cells (neutropenia), anaemia, decrease in the number of platelets in the blood, intestinal weakness, stomach and bowel upset, allergic reactions, swelling at injection site, hair loss, jaw pain. *Precautions:* Do not use in patients with severe liver damage, in pregnancy or while breastfeeding. Use with caution in patients with moderate liver impairment. Symptoms of fever, sore throat or infection should be reported.

Vioform-Hydrocortisone preparations contain clioquinol (an antibacterial and antifungal drug) and hydrocortisone (a corticosteroid). They are used to treat infected eczema and dermatitis. *Adverse effects and Precautions* ➤ clioquinol and see corticosteroid skin applications p. 241. Do not use in patients with a viral, fungal or tubercular infection. Use with caution in pregnancy and avoid prolonged use.

Vioxx ➤ rofecoxib.

Viracept ➤ nelfinavir.

Viraferon injection ➤ interferon alfa-2b.

Viralief ➤ aciclovir.

Viramune ➤ nevirapine.

Virasorb ➤ aciclovir.

Virazid powder ➤ ribavirin(tribavirin).

Virazole ➤ ribavirin(tribavirin).

Virgan ➤ ganciclovir.

Viridal Duo ➤ alprostadil.

Virormone ➤ testosterone.

Visclair ➤ mecysteine.

Viscotears ➤ carbomer 940.

Viskaldix tablets contain pindolol (a non-selective beta-blocker) and clopamide (a thiazide diuretic). They are used to treat raised blood pressure. See Chapter 25. *Adverse effects and Precautions* ➤ beta-blockers, thiazide diuretics.

Visken ➤ pindolol.

Vista-Methasone ear drops contain betamethasone (a corticosteroid). They are used to treat non-infected inflammatory conditions of the ear. Avoid long-term use in infants and pregnancy. See Chapter 37 on corticosteroids.

Vista-Methasone N ear drops contain betamethasone (a corticosteroid) and neomycin (an aminoglycoside antibiotic). They are used to treat infected inflammatory conditions of the ear. *Adverse effects:* Super-infection. *Precautions:* Do not use in patients with a perforated ear drum. Avoid long-term use in infants and during pregnancy. See Chapter 37 on corticosteroids and ➤ aminoglycosides.

Vista-Methasone eye drops contain betamethasone (a corticosteroid). They are used to treat non-infected inflammatory conditions of the eye.

Vista Methasone N eye drops are used to treat infected inflammatory conditions of the eye. They contain neomycin (an aminoglycoside antibiotic) as well as betamethasone. *Adverse effects* of both preparations include rise in pressure inside the eye, thinning of the cornea, cataract and fungal infections. *Precautions:* Do not use to treat viral, fungal, tuberculous or bacterial infections. Do not use in patients with glaucoma. Do not wear soft contact lenses. Avoid prolonged use in pregnancy and in infants.

Vistide ➤ cidofovir.

Visudyne ➤ venteporfin.

vitamins, see Chapter 36.

Vitravene ➤ fomivirsen.

Vividrin preparations ➤ sodium cromoglycate.

Vivioptal capsules are a multivitamin preparation containing a range of vitamins, minerals and trace elements.

Vivotif is a live oral vaccine of typhoid. It is given in capsule form on days one, three and five.

Viz-on ➤ sodium cromoglycate.

Volmax ➤ salbutamol.

Volraman ➤ diclofenac sodium.

Volsaid Retard sustained-released tablets ➤ diclofenac.

Voltarol preparations ➤ diclofenac. *Note:* Voltarol intramuscular injections and intravenous infusions are available to treat post-operative pain.

Voltarol Emulgel (diclofenac) ➤ topical anti-rheumatic applications.

Voltarol Ophtha eye drops contain the NSAID diclofenac sodium. The preparation is used to stop the pupil constricting during eye surgery and to treat post-operative inflammation ➤ non-steroidal anti-inflammatory drugs.

warfarin (warfarin sodium, Marevan) is a coumarin anticoagulant drug (see Chapter 28). *Adverse effects* include small patches of dead skin (skin necrosis), purple toes, loss of hair, nausea, vomiting, diarrhoea, skin rashes, jaundice, allergic reactions and damage to the pancreas. Early signs of overdosage are bleeding from the gums or elsewhere and red blood cells in the urine. *Precautions:* It should not be given to patients with impaired liver or kidney function, severe raised blood pressure, bacterial endocarditis (inflammation of the lining membrane of the heart), peptic ulcers, bleeding disorders, in pregnancy, within twenty-four hours of surgery or childbirth or if patient is allergic to it. It should be used with caution in patients with raised blood pressure, in the elderly, in acute illness or in patients with vitamin K deficiency. Prothrombin times should be determined at least twice weekly for the first two weeks of treatment and then every two to three weeks. *Interactions:* NSAIDs, oral anti-diabetic drugs, sulphonamides, quinidine, antibiotics, cimetidine, corticosteroids, imidazole antifungal drugs, tamoxifen.

Warticon preparations ➤ podophyllotoxin.

Wasp-Eze ointment ➤ antazoline.

Wasp-Eze spray contains mepyramine and benzocaine ➤ individual entries for each drug.

Waxsol ear drops ➤ docusate sodium.

Welldorm elixir ➤ chloral hydrate.

Welldorm tablets ➤ chloral betaine.

Wellvone ➤ atovaquone.

Whitfield's ointment ➤ benzoic acid.

Woodward's colic drops ➤ activated dimeticone.

Woodward's teething gel contains cetylpyridinium and lidocaine(lignocaine) ➤ cetylpyridinium, lidocaine(lignocaine).

Xalatan ➤ lantanoprost.

Xanax ➤ alprazolam.

xanthine bronchodilators, see Chapter 14.

xanthine-oxidase inhibitors, see Chapter 33.

Xanthomax ➤ allopurinol.

Xatral ➤ alfuzosin.

Xefo ➤ lornoxicam.

Xeloda ➤ capecitabine.

Xenazine ➤ tetrabenazine.

Xenical ➤ orlistat, see Chapter 8.

Xepin is a cream containing the tricyclic antidepressant doxepin hydrochloride and is used to treat itching associated with eczema ➤ doxepin hydrochloride.

xipamide (Diurexan) is a thiazide-like diuretic. See Chapter 29. *Adverse effects and Precautions* are similar to those listed under thiazide diuretics ➤ thiazide diuretics.

Xylocaine Antiseptic Gel contains lidocaine(lignocaine) (a local anaesthetic) and chlorhexidine (an antibacterial drug). It is used for local anaesthesia ➤ lidocaine(lignocaine), chlorhexidine.

xylometazoline is a sympathomimetic drug (➤ sympathomimetic drugs). It is used as a nasal decongestant (Afrazine, Dristan, Otradrops, Otraspray, Otrivine preparations, Vicks Sinex). It may rarely cause stinging, dry nose, headache, palpitations and insomnia. Prolonged use may cause rebound congestion of the lining of the nose. See Chapter 10. It is combined with the antihistamine antazoline in Otrivine-Antistin eye drops to treat allergic conjunctivitis ➤ Otrivine Antistin. In Rynacrom Compound spray it is combined with sodium cromoglycate to treat hayfever ➤ Rynacrom Compound.

Xyloproct preparations contain aluminium acetate, hydrocortisone (a corticosteroid), lidocaine(lignocaine) (a local anaesthetic) and zinc oxide. They are used for the short-term relief of symptoms of haemorrhoids, itching of the anus, anal fissure and fistula. *Adverse effects and Precautions* ➤ lidocaine (lignocaine) and see Chapter 37 on corticosteriods. It may cause dermatitis. Avoid prolonged use. Use with caution in pregnancy and in patients with a viral, fungal or tubercular infection.

Xylotox ➤ lidocaine(lignocaine).

Xyzal ➤ levocetirizine.

8Y ➤ factor VIII fraction, dried.

Yutopar ➤ ritodrine.

Zacin is a heat rub containing the counter-irritant capsaicin. It is used to relieve the symptoms of osteoarthritis ➤ rubefacients.

Zaditen ➤ ketotifen.

zaedoc ➤ ranitidine.

zafirlukast (Accolate) is used to treat asthma. See Chapter 14. *Adverse effects* include headache, stomach and bowel upset, rash, increased serum transaminases and increased respiratory infections in elderly patients. *Precautions:* Do not use in patients with liver damage, allergies or while breast-feeding. Do not substitute for steroid therapy or use for acute attacks. Use with caution in patients with severe kidney damage, in the elderly or in pregnancy.

zalcitabine (Hivid) is an antiviral drug (see Chapter 48) used to treat HIV infection in adults who cannot take zidovudine because it has damaged the bone marrow, producing anaemia and a reduced number of white blood cells or in patients in whom zidovudine is not working. *Adverse effects* include nerve damage, mouth ulcers, nausea, vomiting, difficulty in swallowing, loss of appetite, diarrhoea, constipation, abdominal pains, muscle and joint pains, sweating, fatigue, weight loss, skin rash, itching, blood disorders and rarely oesophageal ulcers, damage to the pancreas (pancreatitis), liver damage and jaundice. *Precautions:* Do not use in patients with peripheral nerve damage (peripheral neuropathy), or in breast-feeding mothers. Use with caution in patients who are at risk of developing nerve damage or pancreatitis, with a low CD4 cell count, in patients with impaired liver or kidney function, heart failure or a history of alcohol abuse. Monitor blood count, blood chemistry and pancreatic and liver function at regular intervals. Women of childbearing potential should not be pregnant and should avoid getting pregnant while on treatment. *Interactions:* Drugs likely to cause nerve damage, didanosine, amphotericin, foscarnet, IV aminoglycosides, pentamidine.

zaleplon (Sonata) is used to treat insomnia in patients who have difficulty falling asleep, when the disorder is severe, disabling, or extremely distressing. See Chapter 1. *Adverse effects* include tolerance, dependence, rebound insomnia and anxiety, amnesia, headache, weakness, drowsiness, dizziness, unusual psychiatric reactions. *Precautions:* Do not use in patients with severe liver damage, sleep apnoea syndrome (failure to breathe for a moment while sleeping), myasthenia gravis (muscle weakness due to neuromuscular abnormality), severe breathing problems, psychoses, suicidal tendency, in pregnancy or while breastfeeding. Use with caution in patients with moderate liver damage, breathing problems, depression, a history of alcohol or drug abuse or in the elderly.

Zamadol and **Zamadol SR** ➤ tramadol.

Zanaflex ➤ tizanidine.

zanamivir (Relenza) is used to treat influenza A and B. See Chapter 48. *Adverse effects* include rarely, acute bronchospasm, breathing difficulties (stop immediately) and swelling at the back of the throat. *Precautions:* Do not use while breastfeeding. Use with caution in pregnancy. Patients with asthma or COPD (chronic obstructive pulmonary disease) should have a fast-acting bronchodilator to hand.

Zanidip ➤ levcanidine.

Zantac ➤ ranitidine.

Zarontin ➤ ethosuximide.

Zavedos ➤ idarubicin.

ZeaSORB dusting powder contains dihydroxyallantoinate, chloroxylenol and cellulose. It is used to treat sweaty feet ➤ chloroxylenol, dihydroxyallantoinate.

Zeffix ➤ lamivudine.

Zelapar ➤ selegiline.

Zemtard XL ➤ diltiazem.

Zenalb is a concentrated solution of human albumin.

Zenapax ➤ daclizumab.

Zerit ➤ stavudine.

Zestoretic contains the ACE inhibitor lisinopril and the thiazide diuretic hydrochlorothiazide. It is used to treat raised blood pressure. See Chapter 25. *Adverse effects and Precautions* ➤ lisinopril, thiazide diuretics.

Zestril ➤ lisinopril.

Ziagen ➤ abacavir.

Zida-Co ➤ co-amilozide.

Zidoval is a vaginal gel ➤ metronidazole.

zidovudine (in Combivir, Retrovir, in Trizivir) is an antiviral drug. See Chapter 48. It is used to treat AIDS, AIDS-related complex and HIV positive women over fourteen weeks pregnant. The use of zidovudine on its own to treat HIV positive patients in the hope of preventing or delaying the onset of AIDS has not been successful. A study of its use (in HIV patients) combined with other antiviral drugs is under way. *Adverse effects* include damage to the blood-forming tissues in the bone marrow affecting red blood cell production causing anaemia and affecting the production of white blood cells. It also causes nausea, vomiting and loss of appetite, headache, abdominal pain, skin rash, fever, painful muscles, pins and needles, insomnia, generally feeling unwell, weakness, damage to muscles (myopathy), pigmentation of the nails, skin and lining of the mouth, liver damage and lactic acidosis. *Precautions:* Blood tests should be carried out before and every two weeks during the first three months of treatment, and then every month after that. It should not be used in patients who are allergic to it, or in patients with very low numbers of white blood cells or with severe anaemia. It should not be used in breastfeeding mothers. Use with caution in pregnancy, in elderly patients and in patients with impaired kidney or liver function. *Interactions:* Regular, long-term use of pain-relievers, especially paracetamol. Any drug that affects liver function or damages the kidneys, immunosuppressive drugs, probenecid, phenytoin, tribavirin.

Zileze ➤ zopiclone.

Zimbacol ➤ bezafibrate.

Zimovane ➤ zopiclone.

Zinacef ➤ cefuroxime.

zinamide ➤ pyrazinamide.

zinc acetate is used as a source of zinc in patients being tube-fed.

zinc oxide is applied to the skin as a mild astringent and a soothing protective. It is included in numerous preparations to treat eczema, nappy rash and urinary rashes.

zinc paste preparations contain zinc oxide, white soft paraffin combined with ichthamol, coal tar, gelatin, salicylic acid or calamine.

zinc sulphate (in Efalith, in Fefol Z, in Fesovit Z, Solvazinc) is used as a source of zinc and as an astringent in skin applications, mouth-washes and eye lotions. It has been given by mouth in the treatment of pressure sores. It irritates mucous membranes (lining of mouth and nose) and may produce inflammation, ulceration and perforation of the stomach.

Zineryt acne solution contains erythromycin (an antibiotic) and zinc acetate (an astringent). It is used to treat acne (see p. 250) ➤ erythromycin. *Adverse effects:* It may cause itching where it is applied. *Precautions:* Avoid contact with eyes and mucous membranes (e.g. lining of mouth and nose).

Zinga ➤ nizatidine.

Zinnat ➤ cefuroxime.

Zirtek ➤ cetirizine.

Zispin ➤ mirtazapine.

Zita ➤ cimetidine.

Zithromax ➤ azithromycin.

Zocor ➤ simvastatin.

Zofran ➤ ondansetron.

Zoladex depot injection ➤ goserelin.

zolendronic acid (Zometa) is used to treat high calcium levels caused by cancer. *Adverse effects* include reduction in blood cells, confusion, nausea, fatigue, pain in the joints, slowing of heart beat, fever, unusual taste sensations, thirst, low blood calcium and phosphate levels. *Precautions:* Do not use in pregnancy or while breastfeeding. Use with caution in patients with severe liver or kidney damage or heart failure. It is important to monitor serum calcium, phosphate and magnesium levels.

Zoleptil ➤ zotepine.

zolmitriptan (Zomig) is a 5HT blocker used to treat migraine with or without aura. See Chapter 34. *Adverse effects* include nausea, dizziness, warm sensation, weakness, dry mouth, drowsiness, heaviness or pressure in throat, neck, limbs and chest, pain in muscles, muscle weakness, abnormal sensations such as tingling, burning or tightness. *Precautions:* Do not use in patients with uncontrolled high blood pressure or heart disorders. Use with caution in patients with liver damage, in pregnancy or while breastfeeding.

zolpidem (zolpidem hemitartrate, Stilnoct) is a sleeping drug. See Chapter 1. *Adverse effects* include stomach and bowel upsets, headache, dizziness, drowsiness, restlessness in the night, confusion, depression, tremors, memory loss, nightmares, double vision and ataxia (loss of control over voluntary movements). *Precautions:* Do not use in patients with sleep apnoea (failure to breathe for a moment while sleeping), myasthenia gravis (muscle weakness due to neuromuscular abnormality), severe liver or lung disorders. Use with caution in patients with mild or moderate impairment of liver function, impaired kidney function, depression, a history of drug or alcohol abuse, in pregnancy or in breastfeeding mothers. Daytime drowsiness may affect driving ability. Rebound insomnia and other withdrawal symptoms may occur when the drug is stopped suddenly. Reduce dose slowly and monitor patient because of the risk of dependence.

Zolvera ➤ verapamil.

Zomacton ➤ somatropin.

Zomig ➤ zolmitriptan.

Zomorph ➤ morphine.

Zometa ➤ zolendronic acid.

zopiclone (Zileze, Zimovane) is a sleeping drug. See Chapter 1. It is a cyclopyrrolone. *Adverse effects* include nausea and vomiting, a mild bitter and metallic taste in the mouth, dry mouth, dizziness, light-headedness, incoordination, headache, hallucinations, nightmares, loss of memory (amnesia), aggression, drowsiness, irritability, confusion, depressed mood and allergic reactions. *Precautions:* It should not be used in pregnancy or in breastfeeding mothers, or in patients suffering from myasthenia gravis (muscle weakness due to neuromuscular abnormality), respiratory failure, severe sleep apnoea syndrome (failure to breathe for a moment while sleeping), severe impairment of liver function. Use with caution in patients with impaired kidney function, mild to moderate impairment of liver function, a history of drug abuse or psychiatric illness. It should not be used regularly for more than four weeks, and when stopped patients should be monitored for withdrawal symptoms. It may impair the ability to drive motor vehicles and to operate moving machinery. *Interactions:* Alcohol, sedatives and other drugs that depress brain function, trimipramine.

Zorac ➤ tazarotene.

zotepine (Zoleptil) is used to treat schizophrenia. See Chapter 3. *Adverse effects* include weakness, fever, headache, generally feeling unwell, infections, pain, disorders of the heart, stomach, bowel, nerves or skin; breathing or musculoskeletal disorders, altered appetite, weight changes, prolactin increase, blood or biochemical changes, fluid retention, thirst. *Precautions:* Do not use in patients who are drunk, have gout, a history of nephrolithiasis (build-up of calcium in the kidney) or who are breast-feeding. Use with caution in patients with a history or family history of epilepsy, with heart disease, hypokalaemia (potassium deficiency in the blood), changes on the electrocardiograph, low blood pressure, liver or kidney damage, enlarged prostate, urinary retention, narrow-angle glaucoma, paralysis of the small intestine, adrenal tumours, Parkinson's disease or in pregnancy.

Zoton ➤ lansoprazole.

Zovirax preparations ➤ aciclovir.

Zoxin ➤ flucloxacillin.

zuclophenthixol (Clopixol) is a thioxanthene antipsychotic drug ➤ antipsychotic drugs. Do not use in patients with porphyria (a hereditary disorder of metabolism).

Zumenon ➤ oestradiol.

Zyban ➤ amfebutamone.

Zydol, Zydol SR and **Zydol XL** ➤ tramdol.

Zyloric ➤ allopurinol.

Zyomet gel ➤ metronidazole.

Zyprexa ➤ olanzapine.

Zyvox ➤ linezolid.

Update

New Medicines on the Market since Preparation of Main Text

anakinara (Kineret) injection is an immunosuppressant which is used in combination with methotrexate to treat the symptoms of rheumatoid arthritis in patients for whom methotrexate alone is not sufficient. *Adverse effects* include injection site reactions, headache, serious infections and blood disorders (neutropenia). *Precautions:* It should not be used in patients with severe kidney impairment, in pregnancy or while breastfeeding. Treatment should not be initiated in patients with a history of neutropenia or recurring infections. It should be used with caution in the elderly.

Arcoxia ➤ etoricoxib in this Update.

Arixtra ➤ fondaparinux sodium in this Update.

Asmanex Twisthaler ➤ mometasone furoate in this Update.

Avodart ➤ dutasteride in this Update.

benperidol (Benquil) belongs to the group of drugs known as the butyrophenones and it is used to control deviant antisocial sexual behaviour. *Adverse effects* include lack of muscle tone, loss of perception of movement, parkinsonism-like syndrome, slowness of movement, dry mouth, nasal stuffiness, difficulty in urination, rapid heart beat, constipation, blurring of vision, low blood pressure, weight gain, impotence, excessive or spontaneous flow of milk, low body temperature, development of breasts in males. *Precautions:* Do not use in patients with depression, Parkinson's disease, lesions of the basal ganglia. Use with caution in patients with liver or kidney failure, epilepsy, disturbed thyroid function, phaeochromocytoma (a tumour of the sympathetic nervous system), severe heart disease, potassium deficiency in the blood, abnormal ECG, in pregnancy or while breastfeeding.

Benquil ➤ benperidol in this Update.

bexarotene (Targretin) is used to treat certain types of skin tumours which are at an advanced stage. *Adverse effects* include blood disorders, thyroid disorders, high lipid and cholesterol levels. *Precautions:* It should not be used in patients with a history of inflammation of the pancreas, high cholesterol levels, liver damage, infection, during pregnancy (barrier contraception must be used by both sexes during and for one month after treatment) or while breastfeeding.

bimatoprost (Lumigan) is a prostaglandin used to treat open-angle glaucoma and high blood pressure in the eye where other treatments have failed or are not tolerated. See Chapters 13 and 52. *Adverse effects* include blurred vision, red eye, a feeling that something is in the eye and changes in the colour of the eyes. The iris becomes increasingly brown due to the deposit of the brown pigment melanin. This occurs predominantly in patients with mixed coloured eyes and rarely in patients with eyes of one colour. *Precautions:* Do not use while wearing contact lenses, in pregnancy or while breastfeeding. Use with caution in patients with congenital glaucoma, disorders of the lens and severe asthma. Do not use within five minutes of other eye-drop preparations.

Bondronat ➤ ibandronic acid in this Update.

bosentan (Tracleer) is used in the treatment of hypertension in the arteries supplying the lungs and this helps to improve the ability of patients to exercise. *Adverse effects* include chest infections, inflammation of the nasal passages, pneumonia, oedema, palpitations, upset stomach, dry mouth, headache, flushing, hypotension, itching (pruritus), fatigue, anaemia, heartburn and rectal haemorrhage. *Precautions:* Do not use in pregnancy or while breastfeeding or in liver disease.

Buccastem M tablets ➤ prochlorperazine in A–Z of Medicines.

calcitriol topical (Silkis) is synthetic vitamin D. It is used to treat mild to moderate psoriasis. It stops the over-growth of cells in the surface (epidermis) of the skin that occurs in psoriasis and helps to restore a normal turnover of the surface cells. It has more effect on the calcium metabolism in the body than other synthetic vitamin D preparations (e.g. calcipotriol) and therefore the risks of a raised blood calcium, calcium in the urine and bone softening are increased. *Adverse effects* include transient irritation and, rarely, dermatitis of the face or around the mouth. It may also cause itching, make the psoriasis worse, sensitize the skin to sunlight and cause a rise in blood

calcium levels. *Precautions:* It should not be used in patients with disorders of calcium metabolism. It should not be applied to the face, and the hands should be washed after application. It should not be used in pregnancy and by breastfeeding mothers. It is not recommended for children.

Ceprotin ➤ human protein C in this Update.

Cialis ➤ tadalafil in this Update.

Cipralex ➤ escitalopram in this Update.

citostanzal (Pletal) is a vasodilator used to improve the maximal and pain-free walking distances in patients who get a cramping pain in the calf and leg muscles which is induced by exercise and relieved by rest; this is caused by an inadequate supply of blood to the affected muscle (intermittent claudication). *Adverse effects* include headache, diarrhoea, abnormal stools, bruising, oedema, dizziness, palpitations, tachycardia, angina, arrhythmia, rhinitis. *Precautions:* Do not use in pregnancy or while breastfeeding. It should not be used where there is kidney or liver disease, congestive heart failure, history of ventricular arrhythmia or a predisposition to bleeding. Patients should report any incidence of bleeding, bruising or heart flutter.

Clearsore cream ➤ aciclovir in A–Z of Medicines.

clindamycin (topical) (Zindaclin) is an antibiotic used to treat acne. *Adverse effects* include dry skin and reddening of the skin. *Precautions:* Avoid applying to eyes, ears, nose or mouth ➤ clindamycin in A–Z of Medicines.

Concerta XL ➤ methylphenidate in A–Z of Medicines.

Coversyl Plus is a combination of perindopril and indapamide used in the treatment of blood pressure which is not adequately treated by perindopril alone ➤ perindopril, indapamide in A–Z of Medicines.

Dandrid shampoo ➤ ketoconazole in A–Z of Medicines.

Dovobet ointment contains a combination of calcipotriol and betamethasone and is used in the topical treatment of psoriasis ➤ calcipotriol, betamethasone in A–Z of Medicines.

drospirenone (Yasmin) is an oral contraceptive, see Chapter 41 for information on oral contraceptives.

dutasteride (Avodart) is used to treat an enlarged prostate gland. It blocks the enzyme that converts the male sex hormone, testosterone, into a more potent form (dihydrotestosterone). This reduces the amount in the body which helps to reduce the size of the prostate gland. This improves passing urine in men with benign enlargement of their prostate gland. *Adverse effects* include impotence, decreased libido, reduced amount of ejaculate, tenderness and enlargement of breasts and allergic reactions. *Precautions:* Do not use to treat cancer of the prostate. Women who are pregnant or of childbearing potential should *not* handle the capsules. Dutasteride is excreted in the semen, therefore a condom should be worn if sexual partner is pregnant or of childbearing potential.

Dynastat ➤ parecoxib in this Update.

Ebixa ➤ memantine in this Update.

eletriptan (Relpax) is used to treat acute migraine with or without an aura (see Chapter 34). It is a 5HT-like receptor stimulant which selectively constricts blood vessels inside the head including those that supply the covering of the brain (the dura mater). *Adverse effects* include heaviness, tingling, tightness in various parts of the body, flushing, dizziness, weakness, pins and needles and fatigue. A *temporary* rise or fall in blood pressure may occur. Slowing of the heart rate, nausea, vomiting, convulsions and severe allergic reactions have been reported. Chest pain and tightness may be intense and involve the throat, mimicking angina. The spasm of arteries that it produces may cause disorders of heart rhythm or a heart attack (myocardial infarction). If these symptoms occur the drug should be stopped and the patient should be checked to assess whether he/she has had a heart attack or a severe allergic reaction (anaphylaxis). *Precautions:* It should not be used in patients with coronary artery disease (e.g. angina) or who have (or have had) a heart attack, uncontrolled hypertension, or in patients with hemiplegic migraine (migraine producing weakness in an arm or leg). It should be used with caution in pregnancy, in breastfeeding mothers and in patients with impaired kidney or liver function. The dosage directions should be carefully followed. It should be used with caution in patients with epilepsy or brain lesions, allergy to sulphonamides and in patients with a history of misuse of other antimigraine drugs. It should not be taken with any other anti-migraine drug, especially ergotamine. It should not be used within twenty-four hours of stopping an ergotamine-containing drug and such a drug should not be taken within six hours of stopping eletriptan. Drowsiness may affect ability to drive.

Elidel ➤ pimecrolimus in this Update.

Epaxal is a vaccine for immunization against hepatitis A.

ertapenem (Invanz) is a beta-lactam antibiotic (see Chapter 46) used for intra-abdominal infection, pneumonia or acute gynaecological infection. *Adverse effects* include nausea, vomiting, diarrhoea, abdominal pain, headache, itching, rashes, pins and needles, convulsions, blood disorders and disturbances of liver function. Rarely it may cause thrush infections and colitis. It may cause pain and inflammation at the site of injection. *Precautions:* Do not use in pregnancy. Use with caution in patients allergic to penicillins, cephalosporins or other beta-lactam antibiotics, in patients with impaired liver or kidney function, history of colitis or in breastfeeding mothers.

escitalopram (Cipralex) is a 5HT re-uptake

blocker used to treat depression. See Chapter 4. *Adverse effects* include nausea, dry mouth, sleepiness, tremor, sweating, reduced appetite, sexual dysfunction, yawning. *Precautions:* Do not use in breastfeeding mothers. Use with caution in pregnancy and in patients with severe impairment of kidney or liver function. *Interactions:* MAOIs, 5HT stimulants, lithium, tryptophan and antipsychotic drugs. Also see adverse effects and precautions listed under fluoxetine (Prozac) in A–Z of Medicines.

etoricoxib (Arcoxia) is a non-steroidal anti-inflammatory drug used to relieve the symptoms of arthritis (see Chapter 32) and to treat pain. *Adverse effects* include abdominal pain, stomach and bowel upset, dizziness, oedema (fluid retention), high blood pressure, pain in the upper part of the stomach, headache, itching, increased liver enzymes. *Precautions:* Do not use in patients with active peptic ulcer or bleeding from the stomach and bowel, inflammatory bowel disease, severe congestive heart failure, severe liver or kidney damage, aspirin or anti-inflammatory-induced asthma or allergies, in pregnancy, while trying to become pregnant, or while breastfeeding. Use with caution in patients with liver or kidney damage, heart disorders, fluid retention, a history of ulcers, or of bleeding in the stomach or bowel, or in pregnancy.

finasteride (Propecia) is used to treat baldness in men. *Adverse effects* include impotence, decreased volume of semen, decreased libido, pain in the testicles, breast tenderness and enlargement, skin rashes. *Precautions:* It should not be used by women, and women should avoid handling the tablets ➤ finasteride in A–Z of Medicines.

fondaparinux sodium (Arixtra) is used to prevent blood from clotting during major surgery on the hips or knees. *Adverse effects* include bleeding, fluid retention (oedema) and anaemia. It may cause a drop in blood platelets (thrombocytopenia). *Precautions:* It should not be used in patients with bleeding disorders, severe kidney or liver disease or in women who are breastfeeding. It should be used with caution in the elderly, in pregnancy or in patients with a low body weight.

Glivec ➤ imatinib in this Update.

HBVaxPro ➤ hepatitis B surface antigen in this Update.

hepatitis B surface antigen (HBVaxPro) is a vaccine used to give active immunization against hepatitis B virus. *Adverse effects* include injection site reactions, fever, malaise (generally feeling unwell), flu-like symptoms, fatigue, muscle weakness (myalgia), pain in the bone (arthralgia, nausea and dizziness). *Precautions:* Do not use in patients with severe febrile infections. Use with caution in pregnancy.

Hiberix is a vaccine for immunization against Haemophilus influenzae Type b infection.

human protein C (Ceprotin) is used to treat severe and rapidly worsening bleeding in the skin and in the mucosa (purpura fulminans) which may occur in very severe bacterial and viral infections, especially in children. It is also used to treat skin that is dying (necrosis) in patients with severe congenital protein C deficiency.

ibandronic acid (Bondronat) is used to treat raised blood calcium levels caused by cancer or secondary cancer deposits in bone, bone loss and bone pain associated with secondary breast cancer. *Adverse effects* include flu-like symptoms, bone, joint and muscle pains, skin reactions at the site of injection, headache, blood disorders and low blood magnesium and calcium levels. *Precautions:* Do not use in pregnancy, in breastfeeding mothers, in patients with impaired kidney function, or heart disease. Changes in blood chemistry may possibly trigger convulsions. Blood chemistry and kidney function should be monitored during use.

Idrolax ➤ macrogol in this Update.

imatinib (Glivec) is used to treat certain types of leukaemias usually when treatment with interferons has not worked. *Adverse effects* include severe reactions to the medicine, blood disorders, stomach and bowel upset, anorexia, headache, dizziness, taste disturbance, abnormal sensations such as tingling, prickling, burning, tightness (paraesthesia), insomnia, conjunctivitis, excessive tears (lacrimation). *Precautions:* Do not breastfeed. It should be used with caution in patients with kidney or liver damage, heart disorders. Pregnancy should be avoided (contraception must be used).

Immucyst ➤ bacillus Calmette-Guérin (BCG) in A–Z of Medicines.

Insulatard InnoLet ➤ insulin in A–Z of Medicines.

Invanz ➤ ertapenem in this Update.

Ispagel ➤ ispaghula husk in A–Z of Medicines.

Ketek ➤ telithromycin in this Update.

ketotifen (Zaditen eye drops) is used for the treatment of allergic conjunctivitis. *Adverse effects* include transient stinging or burning in the eye.

Kineret injection ➤ anakinara in this Update.

Lantus ➤ insulin in A–Z of Medicines.

Levitra ➤ vardenafil in this Update.

Lumigan ➤ bimatroprost.

macrogol (Idrolax) is used in the treatment of constipation. *Adverse effects* include nausea and bloating. *Precautions:* It should not be used where there is obstruction of the bowel (paralytic ileus) or inflammation or dilation of the large intestine (toxic megacolon).

memantine (Ebixa) is used in the treatment of dementia associated with Alzheimer's disease. *Adverse effects* include hallucinations, confusion, dizziness, headache and tiredness. *Precautions:* It should not be used in kidney disease or by breastfeeding mothers. It should be used with caution in pregnancy, epilepsy, untreated heart failure or hypertension.

Menoring (estradiol) is used to relieve urogenital symptoms in post-menopausal women who have had their womb removed ➤ estradiol in A–Z of Medicines.

Mixtard InnoLet ➤ insulins in A–Z of Medicines.

mometasone furoate (Asmanex Twisthaler) is used in the prevention of asthma. *Adverse effects* include oral thrush, sore throat, headache. *Precautions:* Do no use in pregnancy or when breastfeeding. There is a risk of immunosuppression and if used in adolescents their growth should be monitored.

Monomax XL tablets ➤ isosorbide mononitrate in A–Z of Medicines.

Novofem ➤ estradiol in A-Z of Medicines.

NovoMix ➤ insulin in A–Z of Medicines.

Nyogel ➤ timolol in A–Z of Medicines.

octyl methoxycinnamate (Sunsense Ultra) is a sun block, see p. 238.

Omacor contains omega-3 acid ethyl esters and is used, in addition to other medicines, in the prevention of the recurrence of heart attacks. It is also used in the treatment of high levels of triglycerides in the body (hypertriglyceridaemia). *Adverse effects* include upset stomach. *Precautions:* It should not be used in bleeding disorders, pregnancy or when breastfeeding.

Orbifen ➤ ibuprofen in A–Z of Medicines.

oseltamivir (Tamiflu) is used to treat influenza when the virus is prevalent in the community. See Chapter 48. *Adverse effects* include upset stomach, respiratory infection, dizziness, fatigue, headache, insomnia. *Precautions:* Do not use while breastfeeding or in pregnancy.

parecoxib (Dynastat) is a non-steroidal anti-inflammatory drug used to relieve pain after an operation ➤ non-steroidal anti-inflammatory drugs in the A–Z of Medicines.

Pegasys is a peginterferon alfa ➤ interferon in A–Z of Medicines.

pimecrolimus (Elidel) is used to treat mild to moderate eczema and it can be used long-term, intermittently, for prevention of progression to flares. *Adverse effects* include burning sensation, itching (pruritus), reddening of the skin (erythema), increased skin sensitivity, tingling, alcohol intolerance, increased risk of inflammation of hair follicles (folliculitis), acne and herpes simplex. *Precautions:* It should not be used in pregnancy or while breastfeeding. It should be used with caution in patients with liver failure, or generalized skin reddening (erythroderma). Avoid contact with eyes and mucous membranes.

Piriteze allergy tablets ➤ cetirizine in A–Z of Medicines.

Pletal ➤ citostazol in this Update.

Propecia ➤ finasteride in this Update and also in A–Z of Medicines.

Protopic ➤ tacrolimus (topical) in this Update.

Relpax ➤ eletriptan in this Update.

Riamet tablets are a combination of artemether and lumefantrine, used in the treatment of malaria. *Adverse effects* include headache, dizziness, abdominal pain and anorexia. *Precautions:* It should not be used in patients with kidney or liver disorders, in pregnancy or while breastfeeding, or in patients with a family history of heart rhythm disorders.

salmonella typhi (Viatim) is a vaccine used to give active immunization against typhoid fever and hepatitis A. *Adverse effects* include injection site reactions, asthenia (general weakness), headache, malaise (generally feeling unwell), fever, stomach and bowel upset, muscle weakness (myalgia), joint weakness (arthralgia). *Precautions:* Do not

use in patients with acute flu-like illness or in pregnancy or breastfeeding.

Silkis ➤ calcitriol (Topical) in this Update.

Spiriva ➤ tiotropium in this Update.

Sulpor ➤ sulpiride in A–Z of Medicines.

Sunsense Ultra ➤ octyl methoxycinnamate in this Update.

tacrolimus (topical) (Protopic) is used to treat moderate to severe atopic dermatitis in patients who are not responding adequately to, or are intolerant of, conventional treatments. *Adverse effects* include burning sensation, itching (pruritus), reddening of the skin (erythema), increased skin sensitivity, tingling, alcohol intolerance, increased risk of inflammation of hair follicles (folliculitis), acne and herpes simplex. *Precautions:* It should not be used in patients who are hypersensitive to maclolides or who have genetic skin defects, in pregnancy or while breastfeeding. It should be used with caution in patients with liver failure, or generalized skin reddening (erythroderma). Avoid contact with eyes and mucous membranes.

tadalafil (Cialis) is used to treat erectile dysfunction. See Chapter 38. *Adverse effects* include headache, flushing, dizziness, indigestion, nasal congestion, visual disturbances, allergic reactions, bloodshot eyes, eye pain. Rarely, priapism (prolonged erection) or heart disorders. *Precautions:* Do not use in patients with pre-existing heart conditions where sexual activity is inadvisable, severe liver damage, low blood pressure, recent stroke or heart attack, hereditary degenerative disorders of the retina. Use with caution in patients with severe kidney damage, liver damage, abnormal penile anatomy, sickle cell anaemia, tumours of plasma cells, leukaemia, active peptic ulcer or bleeding disorders.

Tamiflu ➤ oseltamivir in this Update.

Targretin ➤ bexarotene in this Update.

telithromycin (Ketek) is an antibiotic used

in the treatment of mild or moderate pneumonia, acute bouts of chronic bronchitis, acute sinusitis, tonsillitis, or pharyngitis as an alternative when penicillin antibiotics are not appropriate. *Precautions:* It should be used with special caution in patients with a family history of long QT interval. It should not be used in pregnancy or by breastfeeding mothers.

tenofovir disoproxil (Viread) is an antiviral agent used in combination with other antiviral medicines to treat patients infected with HIV. *Adverse effects* include stomach and bowel upset and hypophosphatemia (low phosphate levels). *Precautions:* It should not be used in patients with severe kidney damage or while breastfeeding. It should be used with caution in patients with mild to moderate kidney damage, liver damage, in pregnancy or in the elderly.

tiotropium (Spiriva) is an antimuscarinic drug used to treat chronic obstructive pulmonary disease COPD (see Chapter 14). *Adverse effects and Precautions:* See antimuscarinic drugs in A–Z of Medicines. It is used by inhalation which may cause dry mouth. It may also cause difficulty in passing urine and constipation. It should not be used by women who are pregnant or are breastfeeding. It should be used with caution in patients with glaucoma or enlarged prostate glands.

Tracleer ➤ bosentan in this Update.

Transtec patches ➤ buprenorphine in A–Z of Medicines.

Travatan ➤ travoprost in this Update.

travoprost (Travatan) is a prostaglandin used to treat open-angle glaucoma and high blood pressure in the eye where other treatments have failed or are not tolerated. See Chapters 13 and 52. *Adverse effects* include blurred vision, red eye, a feeling that something is in the eye and changes in the colour of the eyes. The iris becomes increasingly brown due to the deposit of the brown pigment melanin. This occurs predominantly in patients with mixed coloured eyes and rarely in patients with eyes of one colour. *Precautions:* Do not use while wearing contact lenses, in pregnancy or while breastfeeding. Use with caution in patients with congenital glaucoma, disorders of the lens and severe asthma. Do not use within five minutes of other eye-drop preparations.

Valcyte ➤ valganciclovir in this Update.

valganciclovir (Valcyte) is an antiviral drug used to treat sight-threatening cytomegalovirus (CMV) infections in patients suffering from AIDS. *Adverse effects* include blood disorders, itching, fever, rash and abnormal liver function tests. It may also cause nausea, vomiting, diarrhoea, mouth ulcers, loss of appetite, bleeding in the gut, chest and abdominal pains, chills, generally feeling unwell, fluid retention, changes in blood pressure and heart rate, headache, breathlessness, nervousness, confusion, drowsiness, mental disorders, loss of control over voluntary movements (ataxia), nerve damage, tremor, urinary symptoms, fall in blood sugar level, blood in urine, changes to kidney function, eye pain, deafness, hair loss, acne, sweating, itching, pain and swelling at the injection site and detachment of retina in AIDS patients with inflammation of the retina. *Precautions:* Do not use in pregnancy and avoid getting pregnant while on treatment. Men should use a condom during and for ninety days after treatment has stopped. Do not breastfeed until seventy-two hours after the last dose. Do not use in patients allergic to ganciclovir or with a low white blood cell count. Blood counts should be carried out every two weeks and if counts for white cells and/or platelets are low the drug should not be given.

vardenafil (Levitra) is used to treat erectile dysfunction. See Chapter 38. *Adverse effects* include headache, flushing, dizziness, indigestion, nasal congestion, visual disturbances, allergic reactions, bloodshot eyes, eye pain. Rarely, priapism (prolonged erection) or heart disorders. *Precautions:* Do not use in patients with pre-existing heart conditions where sexual activity is inadvisable, severe liver damage, low blood pressure, recent stroke or heart attack, hereditary degenerative disorders of the retina. Use with caution in patients with severe kidney damage, liver damage, abnormal penile anatomy, sickle cell anaemia, tumours of plasma cells, leukaemia, active peptic ulcer or bleeding disorders.

Vfend ➤ voriconazole in this Update.

voriconazole (Vfend) is an antifungal drug. See Chapter 47. *Adverse effects* include flu-like symptoms, headache, dizziness and visual disturbance, indigestion, abdominal pains, peripheral and facial oedema, allergic reactions. *Precautions:* Do no use in pregnancy. Sexual intercourse should be avoided or contraceptives used during and for one month after treatment. Do not use when breastfeeding. Use with caution in patients

with impaired liver function. *Interactions:* Avoid astemizole, terfenadine and cisapride. Other interactions include carbamazepine, phenytoin, rifabutin, rifampicin, quinidine, ergot preparations and sirolimus.

Viatim ➤ salmonella typhi in this Update.

Viread ➤ tenofovir disoproxil in this Update.

Vivicrom ➤ eye drops ➤ sodium cromoglicate in A–Z of Medicines.

Xalacom contains latanoprost and timolol ➤ latanoprost, timolol in A–Z of Medicines.

Yasmin ➤ drospirenone in this Update.

Zaditen eye drops ➤ ketotifen in this Update.

Zindaclin ➤ clindamycin (topical) in this Update.

Medicines removed from the Market since Preparation of Main Text

Achromycin	Eppy
Acticin	Equagesic
Amoran	Forcaltonin
Anquil	Fybozest
Aureomycin	Ganda
Britaject	Gelcosal
Butacote	Gelcotar
Calcidrink	Guarem
Carbachol tablets and injection	HB-Vax II
Carbomix	Hep-Flush
Chemotrim	Heplok
Clarityn	Hespan
Cloburate	Hexalen
Cortisyl	HibTITER
Cytosar	Honvan
Decadron injection	HydroSaluric
Diarrest	Isocard
Dirythmin SA	Isordil
Disprol Paediatric	Jectofer
Diumide K continus	Kabikinase
Dutonin	Kelfizine W
Efallith	Konsyl
Efamast	Lactitol
Epogam	Lentaron

Lentizol
Lexotan
Lipobay
Liqui-Char
Lomexin
LoperaGen
Loxapac
Maalox
Maloprim
Masnoderm
Mexitil PL
Mictral
Monozide 10
Moraxen
Motipress
Mucaine
Nephril
Neutrastop
Neutrexin
Norditropin
Noritrate
Nova-T
Nuvelle TS
Okacyn
Optimine
Ostram
Ovran 30
Oxypertine
Papulex
Pavulon
Pentaspan
Percuvac

Pevaryl lotion
Pipril
Precortisyl Forte
Proluton Depot
Prominal
Pump-Hep
Quinocort
Quinoped
Respacal
Salivace
Saventrine IV
Schering PC4
Semprex
Simplene
Sorbid SA
Sno Phenicol
Stromba
Sulparex
Tamofen
Terramycin
Testoderm
Theo-Dur
Ticlid
Tropergen
Valium
Vaqta
Vasoxine
Ventide
Virormone patches
Vitravene
Volraman
Zita

Main Active Ingredients in Over-the-Counter Medicines

Acne The main active ingredient in OTC acne preparations is *benzoyl peroxide*. Other active ingredients include *salicylic acid, sulphur, resorcinol, triclosan* and *chlorhexidine*.

Antiseptics and Disinfectants The main active ingredients in OTC antiseptic and disinfectant preparations are *cetrimide, chlorhexidine, chlorxylonol, povidone-iodine, triclosan, phenol* and *hydrogenated phenols*.

Athlete's Foot The main active ingredients in OTC preparations to treat athlete's foot are the antifungal drugs *clotrimazole, miconazole, econazole, lotrimazole, undecenoic acid* and *tolnaftate*.

Colds and Flu These are mostly compound mixtures containing *paracetamol* or *ibuprofen*, with one or more of the following – an oral decongestant (*phenylephrine, phenylpropanolamine, pseudoephedrine*), an antihistamine (*brompheniramine, chlorpheniramine, diphenhydramine* or *tripolidine*), a cough suppressant (*dextromethorphan*), or a cough expectorant (*guaifenesin*). Most nasal decongestant sprays contain *oxymetazoline*.

Cold Sores OTC cold sore preparations contain various ingredients such as *aromatic ammonia solution, liquefied phenol, choline salicylate, cetalkonium chloride, povidone-iodine, phenol, menthol, cetrimide, chlorocresol,* or *lidocaine(lignocaine)*. These may produce some relief of symptoms, but the most effective drug is *aciclovir*.

Constipation Main active ingredients in OTC laxative preparations include *phenolphthalein, liquid paraffin, bisacodyl, aloin, senna, methyl cellulose, docusate sodium, lactulose, sodium picophosphate, ispaghula, sodium sulphate, sodium phosphate, sodium citrate,* or *magnesium hydroxide*.

Corns and Calluses The main active ingredient in OTC applications to treat corns and calluses is *salicylic acid*.

Coughs OTC cough preparations contain one or more ingredients from the following groups of drugs – cough suppressants (*codeine, dextromethorphan, pholcodeine*), cough expectorants (*guaifenesin, squill, ammonium chloride, ipecacuanha*), decongestants (*ephedrine, pseudoephedrine, phenylpropanolamine*) or antihistamines (*chlorpheniramine, brompheniramine, diphenhydramine, tripolidine*).

Cystitis The main active ingredients in OTC preparations used to treat cystitis are *sodium citrate* and *potassium citrate*. These salts reduce the acidity of the urine (make it alkaline) which relieves some of the symptoms but does nothing to treat the underlying infection or the cause of the infection.

Do not self-treat cystitis, especially in men and children.

Diarrhoea The main active ingredient in OTC anti-diarrhoeal preparations is *loperamide*. Some preparations contain *morphine* and some contain a bulking agent (*activated attapulgite* or *light kaolin*). *Rehydration fluids* contain *glucose* and *salts of sodium and potassium*.

Ears The main ingredients in OTC ear preparations for removing ear wax are *urea hydrogen peroxide, docusate sodium, dioctyl sodium sulphosuccinate* and oils such as *arachis, almond* and *turpentine*.

Eyes The main active ingredients in OTC eye preparations are anti-infectives (*dibromopropamidine, propamidine*), anti-allergics (*sodium cromoglycate, antazoline*), vasoconstrictors (*phenylephrine, naphazoline, xylometazoline*) and lubricants (*polyvinyl alcohol, hypromellose, mineral oil, liquid paraffin, hydroxyethyl cellulose* and *carbomer*).

Haemorrhoids OTC haemorrhoidal preparations contain a combination of ingredients such as local anaesthetics (*benzocaine, lidocaine(lignocaine), cinchocaine*), various astringent antiseptic and soothing agents such as *allantoin, lauromacrogol, heparinoid, balsam of Peru, zinc oxide, benzyl benzoate* and *compound tincture of benzoin*. Some contain a corticosteroid (*hydrocortisone*).

Hayfever The active ingredients in OTC hayfever preparations include: non-sedative antihistamines (*astemizole, cetrizine, loratadine*), sedative antihistamines (*azatadine, antazoline, brompheniramine, chlorpheniramine, clemastine, phenindamine, pheniramine, promethazine, triprolidine*), decongestants (*phenylpropanolamine, pseudoephedrine, phenylephrine* and *oxymetazoline*), the anti-allergic drug *sodium cromoglycate* and the corticosteroids *beclomethasone* and *flunisolide*.

Indigestion The main active ingredients in OTC indigestion mixtures are *antacids*. Some preparations also contain an anti-foaming agent (e.g. *dimethicone*) and/or a demulcent (*alginic acid* or one of its salts), a carminative (e.g. *peppermint oil*). Preparations of H_2 blockers include *cimetidine, famotidine* and *ranitidine*.

Insect Bites The main active ingredients in local OTC applications to treat insect bites and stings include local anaesthetics (*benzocaine*), antihistamines (*diphenhydramine, antazoline, mepyramine*), corticosteroids (*hydrocortisone*) and anti-infectives (*dibromopropamidine, triclosan, phenol*).

Iron The main iron salts used in OTC iron preparations include *ferrous sulphate, ferrous fumarate* and *sodium iron edetate*.

Mouth Ulcers and Oral Hygiene OTC preparations used to treat mouth ulcers and painful disorders of the gums and mouth include a variety of ingredients such as local anaesthetics (*benzocaine, lidocaine (lignocaine)*), antiseptics (*povidone-iodine, chlorhexidine, cetalkonium, chloroxylenol, phenols, hydrogenated phenols, chlorocresol, cetyl pyridinium* and *thymol*), pain-relievers (*methyl salicylate, benzydamine, chlorbutol*), corticosteroids (*hydrocortisone* and *triamcinolone*) and ulcer healing drugs (e.g. *carbenoxolone*).

Nappy Rash The main active ingredients in OTC nappy rash preparations include soothing and protective ingredients (*cod-liver oil, liquid paraffin, wool fat, soft paraffin, calamine, zinc oxide, dimethicone, silicone*), antiseptics (*cetrimide* and *benzalkonium*) and the antifungal drug *clotrimazole*.

Pain-relievers (and anti-fever) The three main ingredients in OTC pain-relieving preparations are *aspirin, paracetamol* and *ibuprofen*. Some preparations contain added *codeine* or *dihydrocodeine*.

Period Pains and PMS OTC preparations used to relieve period pains and symptoms of PMS include diuretics (*ammonium chloride* and *caffeine*), antispasmodics (*alverine* and *hyoscine*), pain-relievers (*paracetamol* and *codeine*), NSAIDs (*ibuprofen*) and vitamin B_6 (*pyridoxine*).

Scabies The main active ingredients include *benzyl benzoate, malathion* and *permethrin*. See entry on each drug. *Crotamiton* is used to prevent itching.

Scalp The main active ingredients in OTC scalp applications include *coal tar, salicylic acid, sulphur, benzalkonium, selenium sulphide* and *pyrithione zinc*.

Skin The main groups of drugs in OTC skin applications are emollients and protectives (e.g. *liquid paraffin, lanolin, wool fat, urea, zinc oxide, glycine, arachis oil*). Depending on their use, some contain an antihistamine (e.g. *chlorpheniramine, dipheniramine, mepyramine*); a local anaesthetic (*amethocaine, benzocaine, lidocaine, tetracaine*); an antiseptic (e.g. *cetrimide, benzalkonium, triclosan, chlorhexidine*); a corticosteroid (*hydrocortisone*); a water repellent (*dimethicone*); an anti-itching drug (*crotamiton*) and/or an antiperspirant (e.g. *aluminium chloride hexahydrate*).

Sleep OTC preparations used to treat temporary sleep disturbances include the antihistamines *diphenhydramine* and *promethazine*.

Sore Throats The main active ingredients in OTC sore throat preparations include local anaesthetics (*benzocaine, lidocaine (lignocaine)*), anti-infective drugs (*povidone-iodine, benzalkonium, domiphen, dequalinium, thymol, amylometacresol, phenol,*

hydrogenated phenols, cetylpyridinium, and *tyrothrycin*), and other chemicals such as *menthol, eucalyptus, benzoin, glycerine, peppermint oil* and *camphor*.

Teething The main active ingredients in OTC teething preparations are local anaesthetics (*lidocaine(lignocaine)*), pain-relievers (*choline salicylate*), and anti-infective drugs (*cetalkonium, cetylpyridinium, chlorocresol*).

Tonics The main active ingredients in OTC tonics are *minerals, vitamins* and *glycerophosphates*.

Travel Sickness The main ingredients in OTC travel sickness preparations are *promethazine, dimenhydrinate, hyoscine, meclozine* and *cinnarizine*.

Vaginal Thrush The main ingredients in OTC preparations used to treat vaginal thrush are the antifungal drugs *clotrimazole, econazole, fluconazole* and *miconazole*.

Vitamins and Minerals The contents are listed on the container.

Warts The main active ingredient in OTC wart preparations is *salicylic acid*. Other caustic/keratolytic drugs include *lactic acid, formaldehyde, glutaraldehyde, silver nitrate* and *potassium nitrate*.

Worms The main active ingredients in OTC worm preparations are *mebendazole* and *piperazine*.

Index

Readers' Note
Page numbers in bold indicate chapters devoted to particular topics. Most drugs are not included in the index and will be found in the A–Z section.